BLUE PRINTS

Family Medicine

FOURTH EDITION

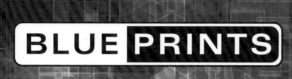

Family Medicine

FOURTH EDITION

Mitchell S. King, MD

Professor
Family and Community Medicine
University of Illinois
College of Medicine
Rockford, Illinois

Martin S. Lipsky, MD

Chancellor
South Jordan Campus
Roseman University of Health Sciences
South Jordan, Utah
Professor Emeritus
University of Illinois
College of Medicine
Rockford, Illinois

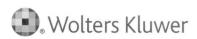. Wolters Kluwer

Philadelphia · Baltimore · New York · London
Buenos Aires · Hong Kong · Sydney · Tokyo

Acquisitions Editor: Matthew Hauber
Developmental Editor: Andrea Vosburgh
Editorial Coordinator: Lindsay Ries
Senior Production Project Manager: Alicia Jackson
Team Lead, Design: Stephen Druding
Manufacturing Coordinator: Margie Orzech-Zaranko
Prepress Vendor: S4Carlisle Publishing Services

Fourth Edition

9 8 7 6 5 4 3 2 1

Printed in China

Library of Congress Cataloging-in-Publication Data

Names: Lipsky, Martin S., author. | King, Mitchell S., author.
Title: Blueprints family medicine / Martin S. Lipsky, Mitchell S. King.
Other titles: Family medicine | Blueprints.
Description: Fourth edition. | Philadelphia: Wolters Kluwer Health, [2018] |
   Series: Blueprints | Includes bibliographical references and index.
Identifiers: LCCN 2017060977 | ISBN 9781496377883
Subjects: | MESH: Family Practice | Primary Health Care | Examination
   Questions
Classification: LCC RC59 | NLM WB 18.2 | DDC 616—dc23 LC record available at https://lccn.loc.gov/2017060977

LWW.com

Contents

PART I: PRINCIPLES OF FAMILY MEDICINE — 1

PART II: COMMON SIGNS AND SYMPTOMS — 35

PART III: COMMON MEDICAL CONDITIONS 148

Fourth Edition Contributors

Braden Adamson, PharmD
Assistant Professor of Pharmacy Practice
College of Pharmacy
Roseman University of Health Sciences
South Jordan, Utah

Zena Alyashae, MD
Resident
Family Medicine
University of Illinois
College of Medicine
Rockford, Illinois

Allison Beatty, PharmD, BCPP
Assistant Professor of Pharmacy Practice
College of Pharmacy
Roseman University of Health Sciences
South Jordan, Utah

Manika Bhateja, MD
Assistant Professor
Pediatrics
University of Illinois
College of Medicine
Rockford, Illinois

Medha Chunduru, MD
Resident
Family Medicine
University of Illinois
College of Medicine
Rockford, Illinois

Catherine Cone, PharmD, BCPS
Associate Professor
Assistant Dean for Assessment
College of Pharmacy
Roseman University of Health Sciences
South Jordan, Utah

Tim Drake, PharmD, BCPS
Assistant Professor of Pharmacy Practice
College of Pharmacy
Roseman University of Health Science
South Jordan, Utah

Aesha Drozdowski, PharmD, BCPS
Assistant Professor of Pharmacy Practice
College of Pharmacy
Roseman University of Health Sciences
South Jordan, Utah

Megan Fleischman, PharmD
Clinical Assistant Professor
University of Illinois
College of Medicine
Rockford, Illinois

Dustin Tate Grant, PharmD, BCPS
Assistant Professor of Pharmacy Practice
Director of Admissions and Student Affairs
College of Pharmacy
Roseman University of Health Sciences
South Jordan, Utah

Clarissa Gregory, PharmD, BCACP, BCGP, CACP
Assistant Professor of Pharmacy Practice
College of Pharmacy
Roseman University of Health Sciences
South Jordan, Utah

Andrew J. Gross, PhD, DMD
Postdoctoral Fellow
Roseman University of Health Sciences
College of Dental Medicine
South Jordan, Utah

Vasudha Gupta, PharmD, BCACP, CDE
Assistant Professor of Pharmacy Practice
College of Pharmacy
Roseman University of Health Sciences
Henderson, Nevada

Mark J. Harper, BS, PharmD, BCCCP
Assistant Professor
College of Pharmacy
Roseman University of Health Sciences
South Jordan, Utah

Arlene Holland, RN, MSN-EDU
Assistant Professor
Director of Clinical Resources
College of Nursing
Roseman University of Health Sciences
South Jordan, Utah

Thomas Hunt, MD
Professor and Chair
Department of Family Medicine
Roseman University College of Medicine
Las Vegas, Nevada

Joyce Johnson, MD
Assistant Professor
Family and Community Medicine
University of Illinois
College of Medicine
Rockford, Illinois

Khyati Kadia, MD
Resident
Family Medicine
University of Illinois
College of Medicine
Rockford, Illinois

Manu Khare, PhD
Research Assistant Professor
Family and Community Medicine
University of Illinois
College of Medicine
Rockford, Illinois

Mitchell S. King, MD
Professor
Family and Community Medicine
University of Illinois
College of Medicine
Rockford, Illinois

Bernadette Kiraly, MD
Associate Professor, Clinical
Division of Family Medicine
Department of Family and Preventive Medicine
University of Utah School of Medicine
Salt Lake City, Utah

Alhang Konyak, MD
Assistant Professor
Family and Community Medicine
University of Illinois
College of Medicine
Rockford, Illinois

Martin S. Lipsky, MD
Chancellor
South Jordan Campus
Roseman University of Health Sciences
South Jordan, Utah
Professor Emeritus
University of Illinois
College of Medicine
Rockford, Illinois

Jason Major, DNP, MSN, APRN
Assistant Professor
College of Nursing
Roseman University of Health Sciences
South Jordan, Utah

Jonathan Martins, MD
Resident
Family Medicine
University of Illinois
College of Medicine
Rockford, Illinois

Tania Mathews, MD
Resident
Family Medicine
University of Illinois
College of Medicine
Rockford, Illinois

Tressa McMorris, PharmD, BCPS
Assistant Professor of Pharmacy Practice
College of Pharmacy
Roseman University of Health Sciences
South Jordan, Utah

Chike Okolo, PharmD, BCPS
Assistant Professor of Pharmacy Practice
College of Pharmacy
Roseman University of Health Sciences
Henderson, Nevada

Toral Ramaiya, MD
Resident
Family Medicine
University of Illinois
College of Medicine
Rockford, Illinois

David Rebedew, MD
Assistant Professor
Family and Community Medicine
University of Illinois
College of Medicine
Rockford, Illinois

Joe Ross, MD
Assistant Professor
Residency Program Director
Family Medicine Residency
University of Illinois
College of Medicine
Rockford, Illinois

Guarav Sharma, MD
Physician
Mississauga, Ontario, Canada

Karan Verma, MD
Physician
Mississauga, Ontario, Canada

Natasha Verma, MD
Resident
Family Medicine
University of Illinois
College of Medicine
Rockford, Illinois

Velliyur Viswesh, PharmD, BCPS
Assistant Professor of Pharmacy Practice
College of Pharmacy
Roseman University of Health Sciences
Henderson, Nevada

Susan Watson, PhD, FNP-C, RN
Associate Professor
Campus Dean Associate Professor
College of Nursing
Roseman University of Health Sciences
South Jordan, Utah

Evan Williams, PharmD, MBA, BCPS, BCACP
Assistant Professor of Pharmacy Practice
College of Pharmacy
Roseman University of Health Sciences
Henderson, Nevada

Darice Zabak-Lipsky, MD, FAAFP
Adjunct Faculty
College of Nursing
Roseman University of Health Sciences
South Jordan, Utah

Third Edition

Daniel Cortez

Cassandra Lopez, MD

Second Edition

Adam W. Bennett, MD

Joanna Turner Bisgrove, MD

Sheila E. Bloomquist, MD

Sandra V. Doyle, DO

Priyah Gambhir, MD

Ati Hakimi, MD

Purvi Patel, MD

Leslie Mendoza Temple, MD

Darice Zabak-Lipsky, MD

First Edition

Adam W. Bennett, MD

Jasmine Chao, DO

Arden Fusman, MD

Daria Majzoubi, MD

Sanjaya P. Sooriarachchi, MD

Leslie Mendoza Temple, MD

Preface

In 1997, the first five books in the Blueprints series were published as board review for medical students, interns, and residents who wanted high-yield, accurate clinical content for USMLE Steps 2 and 3. More than a decade later, the Blueprints brand has expanded into high-quality trusted resources covering the broad range of clinical topics studied by medical students and residents during their primary, specialty, and subspecialty rotations.

The Blueprint series was conceived as a study aid created by students, for students. In keeping with this concept, the editors of the current edition of the Blueprints books recruited resident contributors and reviewers to ensure that the series continues to offer the information and approach that made the original Blueprints a success. We asked our contributors to boil their material down to the key concepts students on a family medicine clerkship should master. The goal we sought was to develop a book that enables a student to easily read and master the material during a 4 to 6 week family medicine clerkship. As such, it specifically focuses on key concepts rather than being a detailed resource. Students are encouraged to go to the medical literature to supplement Blueprints when reading about individual patients they encounter.

We are pleased that readers report that Blueprints are useful for every step of their medical career—from their clerkship rotations and subinternships to a board review for USMLE Steps 2 and 3. Residents studying for USMLE Step 3 often use the books for reviewing areas that were not their specialty. Students from a wide variety of health care specialties, including those in physician assistant, nurse practitioner, and osteopathic programs, use Blueprints either as a course companion or to review for their licensure examinations.

Now in its fourth edition, Blueprints Family Medicine has been revised and updated to bring you the most current treatment and management strategies. The feedback we have received from our readers has been tremendously helpful in guiding the editorial direction of the fourth edition. In addition to updating material, this edition also includes more case vignettes and a new section about the 25 most commonly prescribed drugs in the primary care setting.

We continue to be grateful to the many medical students and residents who have responded with in-depth comments and highly detailed observations to previous editions. We value this input and try to address these comments as we revise the book.

Martin S. Lipsky
Mitchell S. King

Acknowledgments

We would like to thank all of those who helped make the fourth edition of this book possible. If our readers feel this book contributes to their understanding of family medicine, it is largely due to the many people who played a role in making this new and updated version possible.

We would like to thank Matthew Hauber of Wolters Kluwer for supporting the development of a fourth edition and for his help in developing new ideas and material. Lindsey Ries, our editorial coordinator, was instrumental in converting our draft material into a completed and attractive book. We also appreciate Jeethu Abraham for her careful copy editing and thoughtful queries to eliminate errors and to make charts and table more easily understandable. We also want to thank Dr. Catherine Cone for her help in reviewing and editing the section we added to this edition on commonly use drugs in family medicine.

Finally and most importantly, both of us gratefully acknowledge the support of our family and friends, especially our wives, Darice Zabak-Lipsky and Jackie King. Darice's thoughtful comments, careful review, and skilled proofing were all invaluable. Without Jackie and Darice, this and other projects would not be possible.

Martin S. Lipsky
Mitchell S. King

Abbreviations

AAFP	American Academy of Family Physicians
AC	acromioclavicular
ACE	angiotensin-converting enzyme
ACEi	ACE inhibitors
Ach	acetylcholine
ACL	anterior cruciate ligament
ACOG	American College of Obstetricians and Gynecologists
ACP	American College of Physicians
ACS	American Cancer Society
ACS NSQIP	American College of Surgeons National Surgical Quality Improvement Program
ACTH	adrenocorticotropic hormone
AD	atopic dermatitis
ADHD	attention-deficit hyperactivity disorder
ADA	American Diabetes Association
ADLs	activities of daily living
AGCUS	atypical glandular cells of undetermined significance
AIDS	acquired immunodeficiency syndrome
AIS	adenocarcinoma in situ
ALT	alanine aminotransferase
AlzD	Alzheimer disease
ANA	antinuclear antibody
ANCA	antineutrophil cytoplasmic antibody
anti-CCP	anticyclic citrullinated peptide
AOM	acute otitis media
ARB	angiotensin receptor blocker
ARF	acute renal failure
AROM	active range of motion
ART	antiretroviral therapy
ASC-H	atypical squamous cells that cannot exclude HSIL
ASCUS	atypical squamous cells of undetermined significance
ASCVD	arteriosclerotic cardiovascular disease
ASO	antistreptolysin O
AST	aspartate aminotransferase

AT1	angiotensin 1
ATA	American Thyroid Association
AV	arteriovenous
AV	atrioventricular
BAER	brainstem auditory evoked response
BALs	blood alcohol levels
BBs	beta blockers
BCC	basal cell carcinoma
BMD	bone mineral density
BMI	body mass index
BNP	Brain natriuretic peptide
BP	blood pressure
BPH	benign prostatic hypertrophy
BPV	benign positional vertigo
BRAT	bananas, rice, applesauce, and toast
BUN	blood urea nitrogen
BV	bacterial vaginosis
BZD	benzodiazepine
CAD	coronary artery disease
CAGE	cut down, annoyed, guilty, and eye opener
CAP	community-acquired pneumonia
CBC	complete blood count
CCBs	calcium channel blockers
CDC	Centers for Disease Control and Prevention
CFS	chronic fatigue syndrome
CHD	congenital heart disease
CHF	congestive heart failure
CIWA	Clinical Institute Withdrawal Assessment for Alcohol
CKD	chronic kidney disease
CMV	cytomegalovirus
CNS	central nervous system
COMM	current opioid misuse measure
COPD	chronic obstructive pulmonary disease
COWS	clinical opioid withdrawal scoring
COX-2	cyclooxygenase-2
CPAP	continuous positive airway pressure
CPK	creatine phosphokinase
CPPS	chronic pelvic pain syndrome

CPR	cardiopulmonary resuscitation
CrCl	creatinine clearance
CRF	chronic renal failure
CRH	corticotropin-releasing hormone
CRL	crown–rump length
CRP	C-reactive protein
CSF	cerebrospinal fluid
CSOM	chronic suppurative otitis media
CT	computed tomography
CTPA	computed-tomographic pulmonary angiography
CU	chronic urticaria
CV	cardiovascular
CVA	cerebrovascular accident
CXR	chest x-ray
CYP	cytochrome P
D2	dopamine-2
DBP	diastolic blood pressure
DEXA	dual energy x-ray absorptiometry
DHE	dihydroergotamine
DHEA-S	dehydroepiandrosterone sulfate
DJD	degenerative joint disease
DMSA	dimercaptosuccinic acid
DNA	deoxyribonucleic acid
DPP-4	dipeptidyl peptidase-4 inhibitors
DRE	digital rectal examination
dsDNA	double-stranded DNA
DSM-V	*Diagnostic and Statistical Manual of Mental Disorders*, fourth edition
DTaP	diphtheria, tetanus, acellular pertussis
DTP	diphtheria, tetanus, pertussis
DTs	delirium tremens
DUB	dysfunctional uterine bleeding
DUI	driving under the influence
DVT	deep venous thrombosis
DWI	driving while intoxicated
EAA	exercise-associated amenorrhea
EBV	Epstein–Barr virus
ECC	endocervical curettage
ECG	electrocardiogram
EDD	estimated date of delivery
EEG	electroencephalogram
EGD	esophagogastroduodenoscopy
EMA	endomysial antibody
ENT	ear-nose-throat
EPS	extrapyramidal side effects
ERCP	endoscopic retrograde cholangiopancreatography
ESR	erythrocyte sedimentation rate
FDA	U.S. Food and Drug Administration
FEV1	forced expiratory volume in 1 second
FSH	follicle-stimulating hormone
FTA-Abs	fluorescent treponemal antibody absorption
FTT	failure to thrive
FVC	forced vital capacity
G6PD	glucose-6-phosphate dehydrogenase
GABA	gamma-aminobutyric acid
GAD7	Generalized Anxiety Disorder Assessment
GDM	gestational diabetes mellitus
GERD	gastroesophageal reflux disease
GFR	glomerular filtration rate
GGT	gamma glutamyl transferase
GI	gastrointestinal
GLP-1	glucagon-like peptide-1
GnRH	gonadotropin-releasing hormone
GTT	glucose tolerance test
GU	genitourinary
H1	histamine 1
HbA1C	hemoglobin A_{1C}
HBV	hepatitis B virus
HC	homocysteine
Hct	hematocrit
HCTZ	hydrochlorothiazide
HDL	high-density lipoprotein
HEPA	high-efficiency particulate air
HF	heart failure
HHS	hyperglycemic hyperosmolar state
HIV	human immunodeficiency virus
HPF	high-power field
HPV	human papillomavirus
HRSA	The Health Resources and Services Administration
HRT	hormone replacement therapy
HSV	herpes simplex virus
HTN	hypertension
IADLs	instrumental activities of daily living
IBD	inflammatory bowel disease
IBS	irritable bowel syndrome
ICHD-3	*International Classification of Headache Disorders*, third edition
ICs	inhaled corticosteroids
ICU	intensive care unit
IE	infective endocarditis
IF	intrinsic factor
IFE	immunofixation electrophoresis
IgA	immunoglobulin A
IgE	immunoglobulin E
IM	intramuscular
INR	international normalized ratio
IPV	inactivated polio vaccine
ISA	intrinsic sympathomimetic activity
IUD	intrauterine device

IV	intravenous
IVP	intravenous pyelogram
JNC	Joint National Committee
JVD	jugular venous distention
KOH	potassium hydroxide
LABA	long-acting beta 2 agonist
LAMAs	long-acting antimuscarinic agents
LARC	long-acting reversible contraception
LB	Lewy body
LDCT	low-dose CT
LDL-C	low-density lipoprotein cholesterol
LEEP	loop electroexcision procedure
LES	lower esophageal sphincter
LFT	liver function test
LH	luteinizing hormone
LH-RH	luteinizing hormone-releasing hormone
LMP	last menstrual period
LMWH	low-molecular-weight heparin
LN	lymph node
LRI	lower respiratory tract infection
LTC	long-term-care
LTRA	leukotriene receptor antagonist
LVEF	left ventricular ejection fraction
LVH	left ventricular hypertrophy
LVSD	left ventricular systolic dysfunction
MAOI	monoamine oxidase inhibitor
MASH	medications, allergies, surgeries, and hospitalizations
MCTD	mixed connective tissue disease
MCV	mean corpuscular volume
MET	metabolic equivalent of task
MI	myocardial infarction
MME	morphine milligram equivalents
MMR	measles, mumps, rubella (vaccine)
MMSE	Mini Mental Status Examination
MRA	magnetic resonance angiography
MRCP	magnetic resonance cholangiopancreatography
MRI	magnetic resonance imaging
MRSA	methicillin-resistant *Staphylococcus aureus*
MS	multiple sclerosis
MSAFP	maternal serum alpha fetoprotein
MVA	motor vehicle accident
NCAA	National Collegiate Athletic Association
NGU	nongonococcal urethritis
NH	nursing home
NICU	neonatal intensive care unit
NIH	National Institutes of Health
NMDA	*N*-methyl-D-aspartate
NMS	neuroleptic malignant syndrome
NNRTI	nonnucleoside reverse transcriptase inhibitor
NRTI	nucleoside reverse transcriptase inhibitor
NSAID	nonsteroidal anti-inflammatory drug
NTD	neural tube defect
OCD	obsessive-compulsive disorder
OCPs	oral contraceptive pills
OCs	oral contraceptives
OME	otitis media with effusion
ONJ	osteonecrosis of the jaw
ORT	opioid risk tool
OSA	obstructive sleep apnea
OTC	over-the-counter
OWI	operating while intoxicated
PAC	premature atrial contraction
PAD	peripheral artery disease
Pap	Papanicolaou
PCMH	patient-centered medical home
PCOS	polycystic ovarian syndrome
PCV	pneumococcal conjugate vaccine
PD	Parkinson disease
PE	pulmonary embolus
PEF	peak expiratory flow
PI	protease inhibitor
PID	pelvic inflammatory disease
PMDD	premenstrual dysphoric disorder
PMI	point of maximal impulse
PND	paroxysmal nocturnal dyspnea
PO	by mouth
PPD	purified protein derivative
PPE	preparticipation health examination
PPI	proton pump inhibitor
PPV	pneumococcal polysaccharide vaccine
PR	per rectum
PROM	passive range of motion
PSA	prostate-specific antigen
PT	prothrombin time
PTCA	percutaneous transluminal coronary angioplasty
PTH	parathyroid hormone
PTSDs	posttraumatic stress disorders
PTT	partial thromboplastin time
PTU	propylthiouracil
PVC	premature ventricular contraction
PVD	peripheral vascular disease
PVL	plasma viral load
PVR	postvoid residual
RA	rheumatoid arthritis
RADT	rapid antigen detection test
RAIU	radioactive iodine uptake

RAST	radioallergosorbent test	**Td**	tetanus-diphtheria vaccine
RBCs	red blood cells	**Tdap**	tetanus, diphtheria, and pertussis
REM	rapid-eye-movement (sleep)	**TIA**	transient ischemic attack
RNA	ribonucleic acid	**TIBC**	total iron-binding capacity
ROM	recurrent otitis media	**TIg**	tetanus immunoglobulin
RPR	rapid plasma regain (test)	**TJD**	temporomandibular joint dysfunction
RSV	respiratory syncytial virus	**TM**	tympanic membrane
SABAs	short-acting beta 2 agonists	**TMJ**	temporomandibular joint
SAH	subarachnoid hemorrhage	**TMP/SMX**	trimethoprim/sulfamethoxazole
SAMAs	short-acting antimuscarinic agents	**TNF**	tumor necrosis factor
SBE	subacute bacterial endocarditis	**TPO**	thyroid peroxidase
SD	standard deviation	**TPOAb**	thyroid peroxidase antibodies
SGL2	sodium glucose cotransporter 2	**TRH**	thyrotropin-releasing hormone
SHEP	Systolic HTN in the Elderly Program	**TSH**	thyroid-stimulating hormone
SIDS	sudden infant death syndrome	**TSI**	thyroid-stimulating immunoglobulin
SIL	squamous intraepithelial lesion	**tTG**	tissue transglutaminase
SLE	systemic lupus erythematosus	**TUG**	timed up and go
SLR	straight leg raising	**TURP**	transurethral resection of the prostate
SNRIs	serotonin norepinephrine reuptake inhibitors	**UA**	urinalysis
		UFH	unfractionated heparin
SOAPP-R	Revised Screening and Opioid Assessment for patients with pain	**UI**	urinary incontinence
		UPEP	urine protein electrophoresis
SPEP	serum protein electrophoresis	**URI**	upper respiratory tract infection
SQ	subcutaneous	**US**	ultrasound
SSRI	selective serotonin reuptake inhibitor	**USPSTF**	U.S. Preventive Services Task Force
STD	sexually transmitted disease	**UTI**	urinary tract infection
STIs	sexually transmitted infections	**UV**	ultraviolet
SUs	sulfonylureas	**V/Q**	ventilation/perfusion
T1DM	type 1 diabetes mellitus	**VCUG**	voiding cystourethrogram
T2DM	type 2 diabetes mellitus	**VDRL**	Venereal Disease Research Laboratory
T3	triiodothyronine	**VLDL**	very-low-density lipoprotein
T4	thyroxine	**VTE**	venous thromboembolic disease
TB	tuberculosis	**VZIG**	varicella zoster immune globulin
TBG	thyroxine-binding globulin	**WBC**	white blood cell
TCA	tricyclic antidepressant	**WIC**	women, infants, and children
TD	tardive dyskinesia	**WPW**	Wolff–Parkinson–White

1 | Elements of Family Medicine

DEFINITIONS

Family medicine is a medical specialty that provides continuing and comprehensive health care for individuals and families. It is a broad specialty that integrates the biologic, clinical, and behavioral sciences. The scope of family medicine encompasses all ages, sexes, organ systems, and disease entities. The specialty evolved as an enhanced expression of general medical practice and is uniquely defined in the family context.

A family physician is a practitioner in the field of family medicine. At present, family physicians complete a 3-year residency in family practice. This prepares them to manage the broad scope of problems involving patients, from newborns to the elderly. On average, about 15% of a family physician's practice is devoted to the care of infants and children. Some family physicians, about 15%, also deliver babies.

Family medicine is one of the primary care specialties. Currently, the most widely accepted definition of primary care is the one developed by the National Academy of Sciences Institute of Medicine in 1996. It defined primary care as the provision of integrated, successful health care services by clinicians who are accountable for addressing a large majority of personal health care needs, helping to sustain partnerships with patients, and practicing in the context of family and community. In addition to family medicine, general pediatrics and general internal medicine are considered primary care fields.

HISTORY OF FAMILY MEDICINE

After World War II, the United States saw a rapid movement toward specialization among physicians. In 1938, about 20% of U.S. physicians designated themselves as specialists and 80% considered themselves generalists. In contrast, by 1970, about 75% of physicians considered themselves specialists. By the late 1960s, this trend toward specialization was noted and the public perceived a need for generalist physicians who could coordinate care and serve as the entry point or "first contact" into the health care system.

The findings of three commissions—the Folsom Report, the Mills Report, and the Willard Report, referred to by the names of their chairmen—were published in 1966. These reports all affirmed the need for general practitioners who could ensure the integration and continuity of all medical services for patients.

In 1969, family practice was approved as the 20th medical specialty, and the American Board of Family Practice was established. From these early beginnings, family medicine has grown to become the second largest specialty in the United States, with over 500 residency programs and more than 120,000 physicians, students, and resident members of the American Academy of Family Physicians. Practitioners in family medicine care for more patients each day than do physicians in any other specialty. Family and general physicians manage about one-quarter of outpatient visits in the United States. In comparison, general internists accounted for 15% of patient visits and pediatricians 13%. Of patients making visits to family physicians, only 6.3% required referral to another discipline.

COMPONENTS OF FAMILY MEDICINE

A successful family physician incorporates several components of patient care, including accessibility, medical diagnosis and treatment, comprehensiveness, communication, coordination of care, continuity of care, and patient advocacy. The family physician is often the patient's first contact and is available if the patient has an urgent or chronic problem. Accessibility includes being financially affordable and geographically accessible.

As the patient's first contact, the family physician must be knowledgeable about a broad array of diseases and have the skill and judgment to determine the scope, site, and pace of medical evaluation. The family physician typically provides a broad range of services, including acute and chronic disease management in the office, hospital, or nursing home, or by telephone. Family medicine incorporates the biologic perspective as well as the social and psychological aspects of care. The large number of visits to family physicians for psychosocial and behavioral issues underscores the relationship between emotion and illness.

Communication and coordination of care are also essential elements. These topics are covered in greater detail in Chapter 2.

Continuity is an important component of family medicine. Family physicians typically develop long-term relationships with patients, maintain longitudinal records of patients' problems, and promote healthy lifestyles. These require that the physician see each patient for acute episodes of illness as well as periodically for health maintenance. Continuity nourishes a trusting long-term relationship between patient and physician. This relationship is a valuable tool for improving patient adherence to treatment recommendations. Assessing disease risk, screening for illness, and promoting health to prevent disease and disability are inherent parts of a successful continuous

relationship. Early intervention—through health education, behavioral change, and the promotion of a healthy lifestyle—can serve to prevent morbidity and mortality.

Finally, advocacy is a key responsibility for the family physician. Once a patient has been accepted into his or her practice, the family physician must serve as the patient's advocate. In addition, the physician is responsible for educating the patient about treatment outcomes and prognoses, incorporating the patient's preferences into treatment plans, and assuming responsibility for the patient's total care during times of health and illness. This includes helping the patient to make wise health care decisions and to find the needed health care resources.

MEDICAL HOME

A new model of medical care that embraces the components of family medicine is the concept known as the "Medical Home." Also known as the Patient-Centered Medical Home (PCMH), the PCMH is defined as comprehensive team-based primary care model that facilitates partnerships between patients and physicians by connecting each individual to a personal physician who is trained to provide continuous and comprehensive care. The personal physician serves as the patient's first contact and assumes responsibility for coordinating and integrating an individual's care across the entire spectrum of health care providers, agencies, and facilities with the goal to enhance access while maintaining a focus on quality and safety.

KEY POINTS

- Family medicine is a medical specialty that provides continuing and comprehensive health care for individuals and families, including all ages, sexes, organ systems, and disease entities.

- Practitioners in family medicine care for more patients each day than do physicians in any other medical specialty.

- A successful family physician incorporates several components into caring for his or her

patients, including accessibility, medical diagnosis and treatment, comprehensiveness, communication, coordination of care, continuity of care, and patient advocacy.

- Continuity nourishes a trusting long-term relationship between patient and physician. This relationship is a valuable tool for improving patient adherence to treatment recommendations.

2 | Patient Communication and Coordination of Care

Despite advances in technology, effective communication remains the family physician's most powerful diagnostic tool. An old adage is that up to 90% of the time, the diagnosis is made from a complete and accurate history. The key to obtaining a good history is the ability to communicate effectively and empathetically with patients. Good doctor–patient communication also fosters effective treatment. The rule of thirds applies to patient adherence: that is, approximately one-third of the patients will follow recommendations, another one-third will partially follow recommendations, and the remaining one-third will ignore most recommendations. The ability to explain clearly, in lay terms, the results of a test and the available treatment options increases the likelihood that a patient will accept the diagnosis, adhere to the treatment, and return for follow-up. Finally, good communication reduces the risk of malpractice.

In addition to patient–physician communication, the family physician plays a critical role in coordinating patient care. This requires effective communication, both oral and written, with peers, co-workers, and ancillary personnel.

THE PATIENT INTERVIEW

The goal of the patient interview is to obtain information, establish good rapport, and provide an opportunity to educate patients about their health. An important part of this process is projecting a nonjudgmental attitude and creating an environment that allows the patient to feel comfortable and secure about sharing personal information. Establishing good eye contact and maintaining a relaxed manner are important. Nodding occasionally and periodically summarizing what you have been told allow the patient to correct information that you may have misunderstood. Closing the doors of the examination room, minimizing discussion about patients in open areas, and providing written information in the waiting room that explains office procedures are steps that can help to create an atmosphere of confidentiality.

OPEN-ENDED QUESTIONS

The patient interview should begin with an open-ended question. This has two effects: first, it allows patients to express what they feel is important and, second, it helps provide a global view of their medical and psychological issues. It also allows patients to feel more in control and comfortable with providing personal information. Despite this time-honored principle, numerous studies show that physicians interrupt patients <10 seconds into their opening remarks.

TARGETED QUESTIONS

Once a patient expresses his or her chief complaint or the reason for the visit, it is important to start narrowing down the scope of the problem by asking more specific questions. The mnemonic PQRST in Box 2-1 can serve to guide targeted questions for pain symptoms.

New patients must be asked about their medical, surgical, family, and social history. Medications and allergies should be reviewed and a review of systems

BOX 2-1. The PQRST Mnemonic

What *p*rovokes and *p*alliates the pain?
What is the *q*uality of the pain?
Does the pain *r*adiate?
What is the *s*everity of the pain?
What is the *t*emporal course of the discomfort?

conducted. If time is limited, obtaining a MASH history (of *m*edications, *a*llergies, *s*urgeries, and *h*ospitalizations) is a way to acquire key information quickly.

PHYSICAL EXAMINATION

Communication can be further enhanced during the physical examination. Ensuring that the patient's physical needs are met (by having a comfortable room temperature and providing appropriate draping) is important for establishing rapport. Subtle clues can also be gleaned from the patient's reaction during an examination. For example, a woman or child with an unusual bruise or burn who gives an evasive answer may very well be the victim of abuse.

PATIENT COUNSELING

Many patients have aspects of their lives that they want to change. Counseling patients about healthy lifestyle behaviors requires a systematic approach that evaluates the patient's readiness for change and offers information appropriate to his or her frame of mind. A commonly used approach to behavioral counseling is the "stages of readiness" model presented in Table 2-1, which uses smoking cessation as an example. This model is also widely used to help patients start exercising and changing their diets.

ELDERLY PATIENTS

Communicating with elderly patients poses special challenges because of problems such as hearing loss and cognitive impairment. If you suspect a hearing loss, it is important to sit directly in front of the patient and to speak loudly (do not shout) and clearly. Many hearing-impaired patients unconsciously read lips. Women who work with elderly patients can help by making a special effort to wear lipstick, and men should be careful to ensure that their facial hair is neatly trimmed and does not obscure the mouth. Patients with hearing aids should be instructed to bring them to their office appointments. For cognitively impaired patients, having a family member or other responsible individual present is critical to obtaining an accurate history and planning treatment.

Another key issue to address with elderly patients is advanced directives. These directives are a set of instructions, usually written, intended to allow a patient's current preferences to shape medical decisions during a future period of incompetence. All patients admitted to a hospital or long-term-care facility should be asked about their treatment preferences in an open fashion should they become unable to speak for themselves. If patients designate a durable power of attorney for health care, it is important that they be encouraged to discuss their treatment preferences

TABLE 2-1. Patients' Stages of Readiness and Smoking Cessation

Stage	Example of Intervention
Precontemplation	
Not considering quitting smoking	Ask about smoking
May not believe they can quit	Ascertain knowledge about risks
Do not believe that they are susceptible to severe illness	
Contemplation	
Considering quitting	Encourage patients to quit
Recognize dangers of smoking	Provide materials about quitting
May be upset about failed attempt	
Preparation	
Ready to make change by setting goal	Encourage patients to set a quit date
	Offer nicotine replacement or other appropriate therapy
Action	
Are in the cessation process	Provide support and positive reinforcement
	Discuss relapse strategies
Maintenance	
Maintain former-smoker status	Continue support and reinforcement
	Be available for help if relapse occurs

with the person who will have this responsibility. The office setting provides the opportunity to initiate discussions about advanced directives when the patient is not acutely ill or otherwise distressed.

INTERPRETERS

Family physicians may encounter patients who do not speak English. Hospitals are required by federal law to offer patients competent interpreters. Patients may decline using an outside interpreter and prefer a family member or friend. However, it is often preferable to use a competent and unbiased interpreter to assure that information is being shared completely. Family members may add their own biases to the translation, which can negatively affect the ability to obtain an accurate history. For example, a husband interpreting for his wife may not be willing to tell the interviewer about her history of a mental disorder, or a family member who is not familiar with medical terminology may translate information incorrectly. Finally, an underage child should not interpret for a parent or older family member.

All physicians' offices should have contact numbers for interpreter agencies or qualified individual interpreters. In the case of deaf patients, a state-licensed sign language interpreter may have to be called in. A useful way to know whether an interpreter will be needed is if the patient enlists a proxy in calling for an appointment. Instruct the receptionist to be alert for such situations and to ask why the patient is not making the call.

INFORMED CONSENT

Patients undergoing surgery or other invasive medical treatments must grant informed consent. The elements of informed consent include describing the nature of the patient's condition and its consequences, such as whether it is life threatening or potentially disabling. Recommended treatment and alternatives should be reviewed, including benefits, risks, costs, discomfort, and side effects. Finally, possible outcomes of nontreatment—including benefits, risks, discomfort, costs, and side effects—should be discussed. Informed consent is one of the cornerstones of preserving patient autonomy and is an important aspect of patient communication and treatment.

COORDINATION OF CARE

"Coordination of care" refers to the organization of health care services to meet the needs of the patient. A key element of this is the referral of the patient to a specialist. Although approximately 95% of patient problems seen in the outpatient family practice setting can be handled by a family physician, 5% will need specialist attention.

RESPONSIBILITIES FOR A REFERRING PHYSICIAN

The family physician is responsible for handling several aspects of the referral process, including selection of the desired specialist. The patient may request a certain specialist or may rely on the advice of the family physician for this choice. The family physician must provide required referral information and specify whether he or she wants the specialist to evaluate and treat or to limit the input to a consultation and recommendations about the patient's condition. Referrals should also specify the number of visits and treatments. In this regard, the physician should work with the patient's insurance guidelines as to preauthorization and address in-network versus out-of-network referrals. In the referral, the family physician should provide the consultant with information regarding the nature of the complaint as well as important elements of the history, physical examination, and previously obtained test results. More importantly, the family physician should pose any specific questions he or she wants to have answered by the specialist.

In addition to written information, it is often helpful to call the specialist directly. This gives the family physician the opportunity to discuss the patient with the specialist and allows the specialist to ask specific questions or to request information (e.g., old records) that may be helpful in preparing for the consultation.

SPECIALIST RESPONSIBILITIES

It is the responsibility of the specialist to see any referred patient in a timely manner. Emergency consultations should be held that day, urgent consultations usually within 24 to 48 hours, and nonurgent consultations within 1 to 2 weeks.

Specialists should attempt to answer any specific questions and offer treatment options if this is requested by the family physician. Specialists should then send a follow-up letter and, when necessary, discuss on phone their findings and recommendations as well as any treatments that might have been initiated.

CASE MANAGEMENT

The family physician often has the difficult but critically important task of coordinating information from several different health care providers, all of whom are participating in the care of one patient. In this situation, it becomes critical that the family physician provides oversight, so that medications and treatments do not interact adversely with one another. In addition, the family physician should review with the patient the findings of other health care providers and specialists and make sure he or she understands and agrees with the treatment options. Often, patients with complex care issues need the support of a trusted personal physician to help guide them through the complexities of modern-day health care.

KEY POINTS

- The rule of thirds applies to patient adherence, that is approximately one-third of patients will follow recommendations, another one-third will partially follow the recommendations, and remaining one-third will ignore most recommendations.

- The goal of the patient interview is to obtain information and to establish good rapport; it should begin with an open-ended question.

- Communicating with elderly patients provides special challenges that must be addressed.

- About 95% of patient problems seen in an outpatient family practice setting can be handled by a family physician, 5% will need specialist attention.

3 | Screening

Preventive health care and screening for various diseases are parts of routine medical care at all ages. Disease prevention can be primary, secondary, or tertiary. Primary prevention seeks to prevent a disease or condition from developing. An example of primary prevention is vaccination, where an infectious disease is prevented through immunization. Secondary prevention involves early detection of a disease before symptoms develop and is synonymous with screening. Examples of screening tests are mammography and testing for occult fecal blood (for early detection of breast and colon cancers, respectively), in the hope that early intervention can improve outcomes. Another example of screening is cholesterol and blood pressure testing in order to lower risk for future cardiovascular disease. Included within the context of primary and secondary prevention are screening and counseling for behaviors such as smoking or substance abuse that affect an individual's health.

"Tertiary prevention" refers to rehabilitation as well as efforts to limit complications of a disease after it has developed, such as an exercise program in a patient who recently underwent coronary artery bypass surgery.

CRITERIA FOR USE OF SCREENING TESTS

In order for a screening test to be of value for routine use in patient care, several criteria should be met. First, the disease or condition screened for must be common and have a sufficient impact on an individual's health to justify the risks and costs associated with the testing. Second, effective prevention or treatment measures must be available for the condition, and earlier detection must improve clinical outcome. The screening and treatment benefits should outweigh any risks associated with testing and therapy. Finally, there must be a screening test that is readily available, safe, and accurate. The overall cost-effectiveness of a screening program will be a factor in terms of insurers' and individuals' willingness to pay for the test or procedure. The availability and acceptability of the test affects whether or not patients will actually undergo screening. For example, an individual may refuse colonoscopy because he or she finds the procedure distasteful.

TEST CHARACTERISTICS

Screening tests should be accurate at detecting the intended disease or condition. Accuracy is a term that considers several different testing measures—namely, sensitivity, specificity, positive predictive value, and negative predictive value (Table 3-1). Sensitivity is a measure of the percentage of cases that a test is able to detect. Specificity measures the percentage of patients testing negative who do not have the disease. These test characteristics are factors in determining the value of screening tests. Desirable characteristics of screening tests include high levels of both sensitivity and specificity.

By combining disease prevalence with these test characteristics, the clinician can determine the predictive

TABLE 3-1. Determining Sensitivity and Specificity

	Disease Present	Disease Absent
Positive test	a	b
Negative test	c	d
Sensitivity	a/a + c or [TP/(TP + FN)]	
Specificity	d/b + d or [TN/(FP + TN)]	

FN, false negative; FP, false positive; TN, true negative; TP, true positive.

TABLE 3-2. Calculating Predictive Values

	Disease Present	Disease Absent
Positive test	9500	4500
Negative test	500	85,500
Sensitivity 9500/9500 + 500 = 95%		Positive predictive value (PPV) 9500/9500 + 4500 = 68% or PPV = TP/(TP + FP)
Specificity 85,500/4500 + 85,500 = 95%		Negative predictive value (NPV) 85,500/500 + 85,500 = 99.4% or NPV = TN/(TN + FN)

Total number of patients = 100,000.
FN, false negative; FP, false positive; TN, true negative; TP, true positive.

values of a screening test. The positive predictive value is the percentage likelihood that a patient with a positive test actually has the disease; conversely, a negative predictive value indicates that a person with a negative test is disease-free. Disease prevalence critically affects the predictive value, as shown by the following example of screening for a disease with a prevalence of 10% in 100,000 patients, using a test that is 95% sensitive and 95% specific. In this instance, the positive and negative predictive values for the test would be 68% and 99.4%, respectively (Table 3-2).

Thus, for every 9500 cases detected, an additional 4500 patients would have to undergo additional testing to determine that they were disease-free. However, a negative test provides 99.4% assurance that the patient is truly disease-free. For diseases with a potentially fatal outcome and where effective treatments are available, this screening would be acceptable. However, if the prevalence of the disease was 1% instead of 10%, the positive predictive value would fall to 16% and the vast majority of patients with positive results would actually be disease-free. The associated health care costs, risks of additional procedures, and patient anxiety may not justify the use of this screening test in this instance, where the disease prevalence and positive predictive value of the test are low.

CLINICAL IMPLEMENTATION OF SCREENING

For preventive health care measures to be effective, health care providers, patients, and society must all agree that screening and prevention are priorities in providing good health care. Conflicting recommendations by government organizations and professional societies have led to uncertainty on the part of providers regarding both what guidelines to follow and the effectiveness of the various screening tools. The reasons for these different recommendations include different methods of assessing evidence, different criteria for defining benefit, and different patient populations. In addition, professional interests may play a role. Some authorities may represent groups that treat high-risk individuals, giving them a different perspective or a financial stake in screening. Time constraints and lack of reimbursement for preventive health care are additional barriers to providers offering screening tests to patients. It is important that providers keep abreast of the current preventive health care recommendations and prioritize incorporating screening into their everyday practice. Subsequent chapters will outline recommendations for health screening at different ages. These recommendations are largely based on those of the U.S. Preventive Services Task Force (USPSTF), representing input from the various medical specialties, and utilize an evidence-based approach with analysis of disease prevalence, screening, and treatment effectiveness, as well as overall cost-effectiveness. After evaluating the available information, the USPSTF updated the grading system in 2012. They assign one of five letter grades to each of its recommendations (A, B, C, D, or I). The task force also grades the strength of evidence behind the recommendation on a three-point scale, good, fair, or poor. Table 3-3 outlines the recommendation grades and evidence levels in greater detail.

To provide primary care to their patients effectively, providers must educate their patients regarding preventive health care and the benefits of different screening tests as well as healthy behaviors. This is often accomplished by scheduling a periodic health examination, which comprises a comprehensive prevention-focused history and physical examination. During this visit, the provider can provide counseling about unhealthy behaviors, give immunizations if required, and provide or order indicated screening tests. These issues can also be incorporated into visits triggered by other health concerns.

TABLE 3-3. Grade Definitions and Suggestions for Practice

Grade	Definition	Suggestions for Practice
A	The USPSTF recommends the service. There is high certainty that the net benefit is substantial.	Offer or provide this service.
B	The USPSTF recommends the service. There is high certainty that the net benefit is moderate or there is moderate certainty that the net benefit is moderate to substantial.	Offer or provide this service.
C	The USPSTF recommends selectively offering or providing this service to individual patients based on professional judgment and patient preferences. There is at least moderate certainty that the net benefit is small.	Offer or provide this service for selected patients depending on individual circumstances.
D	The USPSTF recommends against the service. There is moderate or high certainty that the service has no net benefit or that the harms outweigh the benefits.	Discourage the use of this service.
I statement	The USPSTF concludes that the current evidence is insufficient to assess the balance of benefits and harms of the service. Evidence is lacking, of poor quality, or conflicting, and the balance of benefits and harms cannot be determined.	Read the clinical considerations section of USPSTF Recommendation Statement. If the service is offered, patients should understand the uncertainty about the balance of benefits and harms.

The USPSTF updated its definitions of the grades it assigns to recommendations and now includes "suggestions for practice" associated with each grade. The USPSTF has also defined levels of certainty regarding net benefit. These definitions apply to USPSTF recommendations voted on after July 2012.

Quality of Evidence
The USPSTF grades the quality of the overall evidence for a service on a three-point scale based on the certainty of the recommendations having an effect on health care. The USPSTF defines certainty as "likelihood that the USPSTF assessment of the net benefit of a preventive service is correct." The net benefit is defined as benefit minus harm of the preventive service as implemented in a general, primary care population. The USPSTF assigns a certainty level based on the nature of the overall evidence available to assess the net benefit of a preventive service (high, moderate, and low).
High level of certainty indicates that available studies are well-designed and well-conducted and they are representative of primary care populations.
Moderate: Evidence is sufficient to determine effects on health outcomes, but the strength of the evidence is limited by the number, quality, or consistency of the individual studies, generalizability to routine practice, or lack of coherence among the findings of the evidence on health outcomes. These recommendations may change in the future.
Low: Evidence is insufficient to assess the effects on health outcomes because of limited number or power of studies, important flaws in their design or conduct, gaps in the chain of evidence, or lack of information on important health outcomes. More information is required to evaluate the effect on health outcomes.
USPSTF, U.S. Preventive Services Task Force.
Source: Grading and definitions of screening recommendations can be found at: Internet Citation: Grade Definitions. U.S. Preventive Services Task Force. June 2016. https://www.uspreventiveservicestaskforce.org/Page/Name/grade-definitions

KEY POINTS

- Primary, secondary, and tertiary preventive strategies can prevent and limit the effects of many diseases.

- Criteria for the use of screening tests include the following: (a) the disease is common and significantly affects individuals and society, (b) effective treatments for the disease are available,

and (c) the screening tests or procedures are accurate and reasonable in terms of cost, comfort, and complications.

- Characteristics that measure the accuracy of screening tests include sensitivity, specificity, and positive and negative predictive values.

4 | Immunizations

Childhood vaccinations are among the most successful preventive measures of modern medicine. Once-common infections, such as polio, are now rare because of vaccination; however, there has been resurgence in the United States of vaccine preventable disease such as chicken pox and whooping cough because of a decrease in vaccination. Important considerations in deciding whether a vaccine is recommended for routine use are disease prevalence, disease morbidity and mortality, economic costs to society, vaccine efficacy, and adverse reactions to the vaccine. New and improved vaccines along with changes in disease prevalence mean that immunization recommendations change. The Advisory Committee on Immunizations makes annual recommendations by age, and the Center for Disease Control (CDC) publishes updated immunization recommendations annually at: https://www.cdc.gov/vaccines/schedules. The American Academy of Family Physicians also provides updates to clinicians about appropriate vaccine schedules.

The schedule of recommended ages for routine administration of currently licensed childhood vaccines is shown in Figure 4-1.

SPECIFIC IMMUNIZATIONS

HEPATITIS B VACCINE

Hepatitis B is a blood-borne viral infection associated with an acute illness; it progresses to a carrier state or chronic liver disease in about 5% of infected individuals. Since the introduction of universal hepatitis B vaccination of infants, children, and high-risk adults in the United States, there has been a decline in the annual infection rate from 200,000 to 300,000 people per year before 1982 to 19,200 reported cases of acute hepatitis B in 2013. Hepatitis B vaccine is available in both a monovalent form or in combination with other vaccines.

For adults and children, three intramuscular injections are given, the second and third doses administered 1 and 6 months, respectively, after the first dose.

Hepatitis B vaccination prevents up to 90% of neonatal infections. Infants born to hepatitis B virus (HBV)–infected mothers require hepatitis B vaccine and hepatitis B immune globulin within 12 hours of birth to protect them from infection. Administering the first dose of hepatitis B vaccine soon after birth to all infants decreases the risk of perinatal infection when maternal HBsAg status is unknown. In addition to universal vaccination for children, adults at higher risk requiring vaccination include those who use intravenous drugs, patients with multiple sexual partners or a history of a sexually transmitted disease, men who have sex with men, those with sexual partners with chronic hepatitis B infection, household contact with hepatitis B carriers, hemodialysis patients, inmates of correctional facilities, people who receive clotting factor concentrates, and health care workers or other individuals who are at occupational risk for exposure to blood. The benefits of vaccination appear to confer long-term protection against acute and chronic HBV infection.

DIPHTHERIA AND TETANUS VACCINE

The number of tetanus cases has decreased >95% since the incorporation of the tetanus toxoid vaccine in wound treatment. Although only 233 cases were reported from 2001 to 2008, there was a mortality rate of 13.2%. Providers should ensure that tetanus immunization is up to date, especially in intravenous drug users and those >65 years of age with diabetes who are at increased risk for infection. Diphtheria cases have decreased from >200,000 annually in 1921 to <5 cases in the past decade.

Vaccine	Birth	1 mo	2 mos	4 mos	6 mos	9 mos	12 mos	15 mos	18 mos	19-23 mos	2-3 yrs	4-6 yrs	7-10 yrs	11-12 yrs	13-15 yrs	16 yrs	17-18 yrs
Hepatitis B[1] (HepB)	1st dose	←----2nd dose----→			←--------------------3rd dose--------------------→												
Rotavirus[2] (RV) RV1 (2-dose series); RV5 (3-dose series)			1st dose	2nd dose	See footnote 2												
Diphtheria, tetanus, & acellular pertussis[3] (DTaP: <7 yrs)			1st dose	2nd dose	3rd dose			←-----4th dose-----→				5th dose					
Haemophilus influenzae type b[4] (Hib)			1st dose	2nd dose	See footnote 4		←--3rd or 4th dose,--→ See footnote 4										
Pneumococcal conjugate[5] (PCV13)			1st dose	2nd dose	3rd dose		←-----4th dose-----→										
Inactivated poliovirus[6] (IPV: <18 yrs)			1st dose	2nd dose	←--------------------3rd dose--------------------→							4th dose					
Influenza[7] (IIV)					Annual vaccination (IIV) 1 or 2 doses									Annual vaccination (IIV) 1 dose only			
Measles, mumps, rubella[8] (MMR)					See footnote 8		←----- 1st dose-----→					2nd dose					
Varicella[9] (VAR)							←----- 1st dose-----→					2nd dose					
Hepatitis A[10] (HepA)							←----- 2-dose series, See footnote 10 -----→										
Meningococcal[11] (Hib-MenCY ≥6 weeks; MenACWY-D ≥9 mos; MenACWY-CRM ≥2 mos)				See footnote 11										1st dose		2nd dose	
Tetanus, diphtheria, & acellular pertussis[12] (Tdap: ≥7 yrs)														Tdap			
Human papillomavirus[13] (HPV)														See footnote 13			
Meningococcal B[11]															See footnote 11		
Pneumococcal polysaccharide[5] (PPSV23)												See footnote 5					

| | Range of recommended ages for all children | | Range of recommended ages for catch-up immunization | | Range of recommended ages for certain high-risk groups | | Range of recommended ages for non-high-risk groups that may receive vaccine, subject to individual clinical decision making | | No recommendation |

NOTE: The above recommendations must be read along with the footnotes of this schedule which can be viewed at https://www.cdc.gov/vaccines/schedules/hcp/imz/child-adolescent.html.

FIGURE 4-1. Pediatric immunizations. (From Robinson CL, Romero JR, Kempe A, et al. Advisory committee on immunization practices recommended immunization schedule for children and adolescents aged 18 years or younger—United States, 2017. *MMWR Morb Mortal Wkly Rep.* 2017;66:134–135.)

Although each vaccine can be administered alone, most individuals receive tetanus and diphtheria vaccines in combination. The vaccine for diphtheria given to children differs from that given to an adult. Before 2005, the only available combined adult booster formulation of tetanus–diphtheria was Td. Today, there are boosters that contain tetanus, diphtheria, and pertussis (Tdap), and after the primary series has been completed, a booster dose of Tdap is recommended at age 11 to 12 years. Adults who did not get Tdap in their teenage years should get one dose of Tdap instead of a Td when due for their next regularly scheduled tetanus booster. Getting vaccinated with Tdap is especially important for families with new infants. After this one-time dose of Tdap, adults resume getting Td boosters every 10 years.

Fully immunized individuals who have received a booster in the previous 10 years and who sustain a clean, minor wound do not require repeat vaccination. If an individual has a potentially contaminated wound and more than 5 years have lapsed since the last dose, a booster shot should be given. In unimmunized individuals with high-risk wounds, passive immunization with tetanus immunoglobulin in addition to starting the primary series is indicated at initial presentation for wound care.

PERTUSSIS VACCINE

Before the introduction of pertussis vaccine, more than 100,000 cases of pertussis per year were reported in the United States. The introduction of pertussis vaccines reduced the number of reported cases to fewer than 10,000 by 1965. During the 1980s, pertussis reports began increasing gradually, and by 2014 more than 32,000 cases were reported nationwide. Infants aged <1 year, who are at greatest risk for pneumonia (22%), seizures (3%), encephalopathy (1%), or death (0.3%), continue to have the highest reported rate of pertussis. Children aged 7 to 10 years continue to account for a significant proportion of reported pertussis cases. Adults who were not vaccinated with the newer acellular pertussis vaccine, provided in combination with diphtheria and tetanus, also contribute to the increase in disease prevalence.

The acellular version of the vaccine is recommended for U.S. children younger than 7 years who do not have a contraindication to vaccination. There are several vaccines available, but experts recommend using the same brand of pertussis vaccine whenever possible because there are few data on safety or efficacy when different formulations are interchanged. Formerly, pertussis vaccine was given in combination with diphtheria and tetanus toxoids as DTP (diphtheria, tetanus, pertussis); however, vaccines are available that include combinations with other vaccines. Although the pertussis vaccine is highly effective and saves many lives, its protection wanes after a few years. Although childhood is the time of greatest risk, waning immunity has resulted in the emergence of a large pool of susceptible adults and adolescents. In addition to creating a primary reservoir for pertussis, there are an increasing number of pertussis infections among adults. Coupled with the development of a safer vaccine, health authorities now recommend giving a pertussis booster in combination with tetanus and diphtheria to preteens and adults, except to those individuals with contraindications to pertussis vaccination.

Contraindications to pertussis vaccination include an immediate anaphylactic reaction to the vaccine or any of its components or the occurrence of encephalopathy within 7 days of vaccination. Relative contraindications include seizures with or without fever that occur within 3 days of vaccination, persistent inconsolable screaming, or any of the following within 48 hours of vaccination: crying for 3 or more days, a shock-like state, and an unexplained temperature of greater than or equal to 40.5°C (104.8°F). These relative contraindications and benefits should be discussed with parents before the vaccine is given.

POLIOVIRUS VACCINE

Polio has been eliminated from the United States because of widespread polio vaccination, and the last reported case of wild poliovirus infection in the United States was in 1979. However, the disease has been brought into the country by travelers with polio. In addition, there are approximately eight cases per year of vaccine-related infection caused by the live attenuated oral vaccine. As a result, since January 2000, the United States has recommended using inactivated poliovirus vaccine (IPV) for routine vaccinations. IPV is extremely safe and can be given in combination with other vaccines. IPV is administered as a shot in either the arm or the leg, and mild local reactions such as redness and swelling are the primary adverse effect. In rare instances, more serious reactions may occur in those allergic to the trace amounts of antibiotics (streptomycin, neomycin, polymyxin B) present in the vaccine. Because IPV is a killed vaccine, it can be given to immunodeficient persons and their household contacts.

MEASLES, MUMPS, AND RUBELLA VACCINE

Mumps is a childhood viral illness associated with orchitis, pancreatitis, myocarditis, and encephalitis. These complications are unusual, and death and long-term sequelae from mumps are rare. Measles is associated with significant morbidity and mortality. Some 1 to 3 patients per 1000 of those with measles infections die as a result of respiratory and neurologic complications. Rubella is associated with congenital anomalies in the children of infected women. These children are born with ophthalmologic, cardiac, and neurologic defects, including mental retardation. The vaccines for these three illnesses have led to a 99% reduction in the incidence of infection. They were once administered as a single vaccine dose; however, outbreaks of measles in the late 1990s led to a recommendation for a second booster shot administered before school entry at ages 4 to 6 years. Individuals born after 1956 or those previously receiving killed measles vaccine must be given two doses of live attenuated measles vaccine at least 1 month apart before being considered immune.

Because measles, mumps, and rubella (MMR) is a live attenuated virus vaccine, it should not be given to pregnant women, and conception should be avoided for 4 weeks postimmunization. Immunocompromised persons with cancer or other medical conditions, a transplant, or radiation or drug treatment (such as steroids or cancer chemotherapy) should not be immunized. Because measles can cause severe and even fatal disease in patients infected with human immunodeficiency virus (HIV), MMR is recommended for children with HIV who are not severely immunocompromised and for household contacts that lack immunity to measles. Other contraindications include allergic reactions to any vaccine component. Children who are severely allergic to eggs are considered at risk for anaphylactic reactions in measles-containing vaccines. MMR should be delayed for 3 months or longer following the administration of blood products or immunoglobulin. If indicated, a tuberculin skin test should be given either before or together with MMR because the vaccine may temporarily suppress tuberculin sensitivity.

VARICELLA VACCINE

Varicella, or chicken pox, is generally a self-limited childhood infection. However, despite its reputation as a benign childhood disease, before implementation of varicella vaccination chicken pox caused approximately 4 million cases of disease, 11,000 hospitalizations, and a number of deaths each year in the United States. The most common sequelae of varicella are skin infections among children and pneumonia among adults. Physicians should give live attenuated varicella vaccine (Varivax) to children age 12 months and older or adults who do not have a confirmed history of chicken pox and have no contraindication to vaccination. Varicella vaccine is 95% or more effective against severe disease. The absolute duration of immunity is unknown, although exposure to wild-type varicella zoster virus boosts antibody levels. The varicella vaccine should not be given to patients with a history of hypersensitivity. Pregnant and immunocompromised or immunosuppressed individuals should not receive the vaccine. Adverse reactions to the vaccine include fever, occurring in up to 15% of recipients; local reactions, seen in 20% of recipients; and a varicella-like rash containing virus that develops in 3% to 5% of recipients and can be spread to others by direct contact with lesions. In 2017, the ACIP voted to recommend a newly released herpes zoster vaccine (Shingrix) for the prevention of shingles in adults 50 and older based on evidence that it is more effective than the older one dose herpes vaccine recommended for adults age 60 or more. The newer vaccine is a non-live, recombinant subunit vaccine given IM in a two dose series, with the second dose given two to six months after the first. The CDC also recommends the vaccine for adults who previously received the older shingles vaccine (Zostavax).

PNEUMOCOCCAL VACCINE

Streptococcus pneumoniae is a bacterium that can cause respiratory infection, bacteremia, and meningitis in both adults and children. It is one of the most common bacterial causes of community-acquired pneumonia and meningitis in addition to being the predominant bacterium causing sinusitis and otitis media. Two kinds of pneumococcal vaccines are available in the United States: Pneumococcal conjugate vaccine (PCV13 or Prevnar13) and Pneumococcal polysaccharide vaccine (PPSV23 or Pneumovax23).

PCV13 is recommended as the primary series for all babies and children younger than 2 years and is given once to all adults 65 years or older. PPSV23 is recommended for all adults 65 years or older 1 year after receiving PCV13, for people between 2 and 64 years old who are at increased risk for disease because of certain medical conditions, and adults 19 through 64 years old who smoke cigarettes. PPSV23 is recommended for those with chronic illnesses such as cardiovascular disease, pulmonary disease, diabetes mellitus, alcoholism, liver disease, cerebrospinal fluid leaks, or cochlear implants. It is also indicated for patients with functional or anatomic asplenia and for those living in special environments or social settings, such as Alaskan natives, American Indians, and residents of long-term-care facilities. It should be given at least 2 weeks prior to elective splenectomy or the initiation of immunosuppressive therapy.

PCV13 consists of purified capsular polysaccharide of 13 serotypes of *S. pneumoniae*. PPSV23 is composed of purified preparations of pneumococcal capsular polysaccharide and contains polysaccharide antigen from 23 types of pneumococcal bacteria. PCV13 is safe and reduces invasive disease caused by the included vaccine serotypes by 97%. Overall, the PPSV23 is 60% to 70% effective in preventing invasive disease caused by serotypes included in the vaccine. Pneumococcal vaccines are well tolerated, with local reactions as the primary adverse effect.

INFLUENZA VACCINE

The influenza virus generally causes mild respiratory illness in young healthy adults; however, in high-risk groups of older patients (over age 65), children under 2 years of age, and those with cardiac disease, chronic respiratory illness, renal disease, diabetes mellitus, or cancer, it may lead to severe respiratory illness, pneumonia, and death. During influenza season, millions of people get the flu, hundreds of thousands of people are hospitalized, and thousands or tens of thousands of people die from flu-related causes. CDC estimates that annual flu-related hospitalizations since 2010 ranged from 140,000 to 710,000, whereas flu-related deaths are estimated to have ranged from 12,000 to 56,000. The vaccine must be administered annually because of the antigenic variation in the influenza viruses from year to year. The vaccine's efficacy will vary depending on the accuracy of the antigen match for the particular year, with an efficacy of approximately 70% to 80%. In February 2008, CDC and the Advisory Committee on Immunization Practice voted to recommend annual vaccination of all children aged 6 months to 18 years along with the current recommendation of immunization for all adults. Different formulations of influenza vaccines both live and inactivated are available that are directed toward the three or four different viral strains thought to be active in the community. Included in these are recombinant vaccines or vaccines grown in mammalian culture media allowing those with egg allergies to be vaccinated. One form of vaccination utilizes a live attenuated virus as an intranasal vaccine spray. It is approved for healthy individuals between 2 and 49 years of age without underlying medical conditions that predispose them to influenza complications. This vaccine should be avoided in health care workers and immunocompromised individuals as well as those in close contact with immunocompromised patients, because the virus can be shed for up to 7 days after administration. Although the flu vaccine is recommended for all adults without a contraindication, it is especially important for persons who are at high risk for influenza complications, including those 65 years or older; residents of chronic-care facilities; adults and children with chronic cardiovascular or pulmonary problems (including asthma); adults and children with chronic metabolic diseases such as diabetes mellitus, renal disease, hemoglobinopathies, or immunosuppression (e.g., HIV); women who will be in the second or third trimester of pregnancy during flu season; and those requiring chronic aspirin therapy. Health care workers and persons providing care to individuals in high-risk groups and household contacts with persons at risk should also be given the influenza vaccine. Although local reactions occur in up to 20% of patients, serious reactions are rare. Those with severe egg allergies should receive the egg-free vaccines.

HEPATITIS A VACCINE

Hepatitis A is a viral infection that usually causes a mild, self-limited illness with symptoms including nausea, anorexia, fever, malaise, or abdominal pain. There is no chronic form of this infection. Person-to-person transmission through the fecal–oral route is the primary means of hepatitis A virus transmission in the United States. Most infections result from close personal contact with an infected household member or sex partner. Common-source outbreaks and sporadic cases can also occur from exposure to fecally contaminated food or water. Hepatitis A rates have declined by 95% in the United States, since the vaccine became available. Hepatitis A is an inactivated viral vaccine. Vaccination is recommended for unvaccinated adults traveling to or living in areas with high endemic rates of disease, users of illicit drugs, and men who have sex with men. Universal administration is recommended for all children aged 1 year and is given as 2 doses at least 6 months apart. Catch-up vaccination is also recommended for older children who are at increased risk for infection. The vaccine has an efficacy of 94% to 100% and causes local reactions as the primary adverse effect.

MENINGOCOCCAL VACCINE

Neisseria meningitidis causes invasive bacterial disease and meningitis in 1 per 100,000 in the population. Although not a common disease, meningococcal disease is associated with very high morbidity and mortality and tends to occur in outbreaks. There are three types of meningococcal vaccines available in the United States: Meningococcal conjugate vaccines (Menactra, Menveo, and MenHibrix); Meningococcal polysaccharide vaccine (Menomune); and Serogroup B meningococcal vaccines (Bexsero and Trumenba).

All 11- to 12-year-olds should be vaccinated with a meningococcal conjugate vaccine (Menactra or Menveo). A booster dose is recommended at age of 16 years. High-risk teens and young adults (16 through 23 year olds) may also be vaccinated with a serogroup B meningococcal vaccine. High-risk groups include patients with anatomic or functional asplenia, military recruits, those with complement component deficiencies, and travelers to endemic regions. Vaccine administration does not substitute for antimicrobial chemoprophylaxis for close contacts of an infected individual.

ROTAVIRUS VACCINE

Rotavirus can cause severe watery diarrhea, vomiting, fever, and abdominal pain. Each year in the United States, rotavirus results in more than 200,000 emergency room visits, approximately 60,000 hospitalizations, and between 20 and 60 deaths. Children who get rotavirus disease can become dehydrated and may need to be hospitalized for intravenous fluids. About 70% of children vaccinated for rotavirus are protected from the illness, and 90% of children will be protected from severe illness. Two live attenuated rotavirus vaccines are currently licensed for use in infants in the United States: RotaTeq (RV5), which is given in 3 doses at ages 2, 4, and 6 months; and Rotarix (RV1),which is given in 2 doses at ages 2 and 4 months. Both vaccines are given orally. The first dose of either vaccine is most effective when given before a child is 15 weeks old. Children should receive all doses of rotavirus vaccine before they turn 8 months old. Vaccination is contraindicated for those children with severe allergy to the vaccine or any component of the vaccine or with a latex allergy. An infant who has had a severe (life-threatening) allergic reaction to a dose of rotavirus vaccine should not get another dose. Infants with "severe combined immunodeficiency" should not get rotavirus vaccine and infants who have had intussusception should not get rotavirus vaccine. Infants who are moderately or severely ill should wait to get the vaccine until they recover. This includes infants with moderate or severe diarrhea or vomiting. Babies who are mildly ill can get the vaccine.

HUMAN PAPILLOMAVIRUS

Human papillomavirus (HPV) is the most common sexually transmitted disease in the United States. It can cause anogenital warts and low-grade cervical cytologic changes. HPV infections are often subclinical, and although most resolve without significant sequelae, some HPV infections can lead to cancer. Nearly 80 million people—about one in four—are currently infected with HPV in the United States. About 14 million people, including teens, become infected with HPV each year. Over 30,000 people in the United States each year are affected by a cancer caused by HPV infection. Although screening is available for cervical cancer for women, there is no screening for the other cancers linked to HPV infection such as cancers of the mouth/throat, anus/rectum, penis, vagina, or vulva. HPV vaccination provides safe, effective, and lasting protection against the HPV infections that are most commonly associated with cancer. A quadrivalent vaccine is available that protects against HPV types 16 and 18, which account for 70% of the cases of cervical cancer, and types 6 and 11, which are responsible for 90% of cases of genital warts. HPV vaccine is administered as a three-shot series and is composed of surface proteins and is not infectious. The CDC recommends HPV vaccination for girls and boys at age 11 or 12 years to protect against cancers caused by HPV infections. The CDC encourages clinicians to recommend HPV vaccination the same way and same day they recommend other routinely recommended vaccines for adolescents.

KEY POINTS

- The implementation of routine childhood vaccinations is one of the most successful preventive measures in modern-day medicine.

- Considerations in deciding whether a vaccine is recommended for routine use are disease prevalence, disease morbidity and mortality, economic cost to society, vaccine efficacy, and adverse reactions to the vaccine.

5 | Preventive Care: 19 to 64 Years

The focus of preventive care is age and gender dependent, reflecting the changes in disease prevalence across the adult life span. Although many available guidelines can assist practitioners in making decisions about appropriate preventive care, they should not replace medical judgment. In addition to primary prevention, secondary prevention to prevent or limit future disease is important. A common dilemma for secondary prevention of an asymptomatic illness such as hypertension is that the consequences may not be seen for years after a person develops high blood pressure. For example, blood pressure evaluation and treatment is a preventive measure for future disease that may not manifest itself until the patient is 70 years of age or beyond.

LEADING CAUSES OF DEATH

The leading causes of death in young men (19 to 35 years) are unintentional injuries (includes unintentional fall deaths, motor vehicle accidents, and unintentional poisoning deaths), suicides, and homicides, whereas the leading causes of death in young women (19 to 35 years) are unintentional injuries, suicide, and cancer. In addition, diseases that increase in prevalence and contribute to morbidity and mortality in this age range include heart disease and some forms of cancer. Lifestyle assessment is important for young adults since this is the time they often acquire habits that can both affect their current health and place them at risk for future disease. For example, unsafe sexual behavior may result in sexually transmitted diseases, including HIV. Smoking may lead to a lifelong habit and increased risk for stroke, heart disease, and lung disease. Alcohol and drug abuse may place the individual at risk for hepatitis, liver disease, and accidents or injuries.

Leading causes of death in all adult men 35 to 44 years of age are unintentional injuries, heart disease, and suicide. For men 45 to 64 years of age, heart disease is the leading cause of death, followed by cancer and unintentional injuries. In comparison, leading causes of death in women 35 to 44 years of age are cancer, unintentional injuries, and heart disease. From 45 to 54 years of age, heart disease ranks second followed by unintentional injuries. From ages 55 to 64, chronic lower respiratory disease ranks third after cancer and heart disease.

IMMUNIZATIONS AND PREVENTIVE CARE

Recommended vaccinations for adults by age and medical condition are presented in Figure 5-1. Patients' medical history may indicate a need for vaccination (e.g., hepatitis B and MMR). Patients with medical problems such as diabetes or asthma should receive pneumococcal and influenza vaccines. Those who have never had chicken pox may wish to consider the varicella vaccine.

In addition to reviewing the medical history, reviewing family history and social history will provide information that may lead to counseling or screening measures. For example, individuals with a family history of premature coronary artery disease or hyperlipidemia should be screened for hyperlipidemia. Patients with a family history of skin cancer and those with fair skin should be counseled about limiting sun exposure. Individuals with a history of substance abuse or smoking should be counseled about the potential consequences associated with these behaviors.

Diagnostic care is when patients see their provider to evaluate a symptom or because of a known health problem. In contrast, a preventive care visit focuses

Vaccine	19–21 years	22–26 years	27–59 years	60–64 years	≥ 65 years
Influenza[1]	1 dose annually				
Td/Tdap[2]	Substitute Tdap for Td once, then Td booster every 10 yrs				
MMR[3]	1 or 2 doses depending on indication				
VAR[4]	2 doses				
HZV[5]					1 dose
HPV–Female[6]	3 doses				
HPV–Male[6]	3 doses				
PCV13[7]					1 dose
PPSV23[7]	1 or 2 doses depending on indication				1 dose
HepA[8]	2 or 3 doses depending on vaccine				
HepB[9]	3 doses				
MenACWY or MPSV4[10]	1 or more doses depending on indication				
MenB[10]	2 or 3 doses depending on vaccine				
Hib[11]	1 or 3 doses depending on indication				

Recommended for adults who meet the age requirement, lack documentation of vaccination, or lack evidence of past infection

Recommended for adults with additional medical conditions or other indications

No recommendation

NOTE: The above recommendations must be read along with the footnotes of this schedule which can be viewed at https://www.cdc.gov/vaccines/schedules/hcp/imz/adult-conditions.html.

FIGURE 5-1. Recommended adult immunization schedule by vaccine and age group, 2017. (From Kim DK, Riley LE, Harriman KH, et al. Advisory committee on immunization practices recommended immunization schedule for adults aged 19 years or older—United States, 2017. *MMWR Morb Mortal Wkly Rep*. 2017;66:136–138.)

on preventing health problems. There is no consensus about the optimal interval for routine preventive care visits. A common recommendation for adults ages 10 to 64 years is about every 1 to 3 years depending on risk and patient preferences.

Although patients may not schedule preventive care visits, preventive care should be incorporated into a visit when patients are in the office for other reasons. At each visit, height, weight, and blood pressure should be checked and deviations from normal ranges should be addressed. Measurements of height and weight can be used to calculate the body mass index and along with a dietary history help to screen for obesity as well as the risk for osteoporosis. Sexually active individuals may require counseling about contraception and preventing sexually transmitted diseases. High-risk individuals, for example, sexually active women under age 24, may merit screening. Those who own firearms should be counseled about their safe storage. Those presenting with an acute injury may be reminded about injury prevention measures, such as the use of bicycle helmets and seat belts. Patients should be reminded about good dental care practices and the importance of regular dental visits. Assessment and screening for depression, substance use, intimate partner violence, and trauma should be incorporated into the history taking, and any concerns should prompt referrals and counseling.

Identification and, when possible, treatment of risk factors for various diseases is a focus of routine health care visits. For some diseases, there are no recommendations to screen for the actual disease, but there are recommendations to screen for risk factors. For example, routine screening for heart disease is not recommended, but screening for cardiac risk factors is recommended. Risk factors for heart disease include modifiable factors such as smoking, hypertension, diabetes mellitus, obesity, and hyperlipidemia. For other diseases, such as osteoporosis, screening is recommended only for those with risk factors. Some nonmodifiable risk

PREVENTIVE VISIT ALGORITHM: PATIENTS AGES 18-64*

Patient check-in

- Verify that 1 year has passed since patient's last visit.
- Verify that visit is covered by insurance and that patient is willing to pay if visit is not covered.

Comprehensive history**

Comprehensive exam**

Age 18-34	Age 35-44	Age 45-49	Age 50-54	Age 55-64

Screening†

Blood pressure

Obesity

DM 2 screen for adults (age 40-70 who are overweight/obese)

Depression

Alcohol misuse

Syphilis, HIV (high risk)   Gonorrhea (F sexually active, high risk)

Hep B viral infection (non-pregnant, high risk)

Hep C screening (high risk and those born 1945-1965)

Age 18-34	Age 35-44	Age 45-49	Age 50-54 / Age 55-64
Cholesterol (M & F ≥ 20 y high risk)	Cholesterol (M)	Cholesterol (M)	Cholesterol (M)
Pap (F ≥ 21 y every 3 years)	Cholesterol (F high risk)	Cholesterol (F high risk)	Cholesterol (F high risk)
Chlamydia (F ≤ 24 y sexually active; F ≥ 25 y high risk)	Pap (F every 3 years)	Pap (F every 3 years)	Pap (F every 3 years)
	Breast cancer (F ≥ 40 y)	Breast cancer (F)	Colorectal cancer
	Chlamydia (F high risk)	Chlamydia (F high risk)	Breast cancer (F)
			Chlamydia (F high risk)

Immunizations††

Td or Tdap with booster every 10 years

Varicella if not immune

Yearly influenza

Pneumococcal (high risk)

Age 18-34				Age 55-64
HPV (F ≤ 26 y; M ≤ 21 y; M 22-26 y high risk)				Zoster (≥ 60 y)

Counseling†

Healthy diet (high risk)

Folic acid supplementation (F capable of pregnancy)

Obesity (BMI ≥ 30)

Sexually transmitted infections (high risk)

Tobacco use

Alcohol misuse

		Age 45-49	Age 50-54	Age 55-64
				Daily aspirin (F ≥ 55 y, when benefit exceeds risk)
		Daily aspirin (M, when benefit exceeds risk)	Daily aspirin (M, when benefit exceeds risk)	

*Pregnancy-related recommendations are not included.

The CPT manual characterizes a comprehensive history and exam in the context of a preventive visit as "age and gender appropriate" and "not** synonymous with the 'comprehensive' examination required in Evaluation and Management codes 99201-99350."

†Consistent with U.S. Preventive Services Task Force grade A/B preventive recommendations.

††Consistent with Centers for Disease Control and Prevention 2012 immunization schedule.

Family Practice Management®

Developed by Timothy Owolabi MD, CPC, Summit Physician Services, Chambersburg, Pa., and Isac Simpson, DO, Phoenix Baptist Hospital Family Medicine Residency, Phoenix, Ariz. Copyright © 2012 AAFP. Physicians may photocopy or adapt for use in their own practices; all other rights reserved. http://www.aafp.org/fpm/2012/0700/p12.html. Updated 11/2016.

FIGURE 5-2. Adult preventive care schedule. (From Owolabi T, Simpson I. Documenting and coding preventive visits: a physician's perspective. *Fam Pract Manag*. 2012;19[4]:12–16. http://www.aafp.org/fpm/2012/0700/p12.html. Copyright © 2012 American Academy of Family Physicians.)

factors for osteoporosis are white race, slight build, and family history of osteoporosis. Modifiable risk factors for osteoporosis include smoking, menopause, sedentary lifestyle, heavy alcohol and coffee consumption, and low calcium intake.

A concise adult preventive care schedule that describes the preventive recommendations by age, gender, and risk factors for adults over the age of 18 is presented in Figure 5-2. A web-based or smart phone application is also available at https://epss.ahrq.gov/PDA/index.jsp that allows for customizing patient screening recommendations.

RECOMMENDED SCREENING BY AGE GROUP AND RISK STATUS

USPSTF recommends screening for hypertension, tobacco use and cessation, HIV infection, alcohol misuse, depression, and obesity for adult men and women starting at age 18. Screening for hepatitis B and C, syphilis, and sexually transmitted disease is recommended for adult men and women after the age of 18 if at high risk. The American Academy of Family Physicians also recommends screening obese adults over age 40 for type 2 diabetes. For those individuals at high risk for coronary artery disease, daily aspirin is indicated when the benefits outweigh the risks.

RECOMMENDED SCREENING BY GENDER

Screening for lipid disorders is recommended for men over the age of 30 years. Earlier screening starting at age 20 is recommended for men at higher risk for cardiovascular disease.

Screening for intimate partner violence is recommended for all women over the age of 18. A Pap smear is recommended every 3 years starting at age 21, or every 5 years with human papillomavirus testing starting at age 30. Women should be counseled about adequate calcium intake and supplemented if needed, and those who desire pregnancy can be counseled about supplementation with folate to prevent birth defects.

CANCER SCREENING

For those ages 50 to 75, one of the following screenings is recommended:
- Colonoscopy every 10 years
- Computed tomography (CT) colonography every 10 years
- Flexible sigmoidoscopy every 5 years
- Fecal occult blood test

Many family physicians recommend a colonoscopy because it looks at the entire colon. Those with a family history (first-degree relative) of colorectal cancer or adenomatous polyps should begin screening at age 40 or 10 years before the youngest case in the immediate family, with a colonoscopy every 5 years.

Annual lung cancer screening (including CT) is recommended for adults ages 55 to 80 who have a 30-pack-a-year smoking history and currently smoke or quit smoking within the past 15 years.

Additional screening for women includes annual or biennial mammography for breast cancer beginning at age 40 as well as Pap smear screening for cervical cancer as noted earlier.

KEY POINTS

- The most common causes of death in adults aged 19 to 40 years are accidents, homicides, and suicides.

- Screening for cardiovascular risk factors and malignancy becomes a focus of health care visits for individuals over age 40.

6 | Preoperative Evaluation

Each year more than 27 million Americans undergo various types of surgery. Family physicians are often asked to evaluate these patients preoperatively. This evaluation is not just to "clear" patients but to identify and to intervene when appropriate in higher risk patients requiring surgical procedures. The physician must understand the risk factors associated with the surgical procedure and incorporate this information into the evaluation and treatment recommendations for such patients.

At least one surgical complication occurs in 17% of patients undergoing surgery. Surgical morbidity and mortality generally fall into one of the three following categories: cardiac, respiratory, or infectious complications. These complications increase for certain populations of patients. Identification of at-risk patients and preparation helps reduce the risks of surgery.

RISK FACTORS

Patients with angina, recent myocardial infarction (MI), arrhythmias, congestive heart failure (CHF), and diabetes are at significantly higher risk for perioperative MI, heart failure, or arrhythmias. An increased risk for cardiac complications is also present in elderly patients and those with abnormal electrocardiograms (ECGs), low functional capacity, history of stroke, and uncontrolled hypertension.

Surgeries may be classified as high-, intermediate-, or low-risk procedures. Those posing a high risk for cardiac complications (>5% cardiac risk) include vascular surgeries, emergency surgeries, and surgeries associated with increased blood loss or large fluid shifts. Intermediate-risk surgeries (1% to 5% cardiac risk) include most intrathoracic, intraperitoneal, and orthopedic procedures. Low-risk procedures (<1% cardiac risk) include cosmetic procedures, cataract operations, and endoscopies.

Patients at risk for pulmonary complications include those with lung disease—for example, asthma or chronic obstructive pulmonary disease (COPD)—obesity, a history of smoking, obstructive sleep apnea, and undiagnosed cough or dyspnea. Procedures that increase the risk of pulmonary complications are primarily abdominal or thoracic surgeries, with the rule being that the closer the surgery is to the diaphragm, the higher the risk of complications.

The most common causes of postoperative fever can be remembered by the mnemonic of the 5 "Ws" and include wound infections, wind (pneumonia), water (urinary tract infections), weins (deep venous thrombosis [DVTs]), and wacky drugs. Diabetes and vascular disease are patient factors associated with an increased risk of wound infections. Surgeries with potential spillage of infectious material, such as abscess drainage or gastrointestinal surgery, pose a higher risk of postoperative infections. Instrumentation of the urinary tract, as occurs during bladder catheterization or genitourinary surgery, increases the risk of developing a urinary tract infection.

CLINICAL EVALUATION

Preoperative evaluation consists of a thorough history and physical examination and a risk assessment, which then directs preoperative testing and perioperative medical management based on the urgency of the surgery. Urgency of surgery is categorized into emergency (within 6 hours), urgent (within 6 to 24 hours), time sensitive (within 1 to 6 weeks), and elective (up to 1 year). Risk associated with the procedure is considered either low (<1% risk of a perioperative cardiac complication) or elevated (>1%). Low-risk procedures include dermatologic procedures, cataract surgery, ambulatory surgery, breast surgery, and endoscopic procedures. If possible, the preoperative evaluation for elective surgery should take place within 1 month of the scheduled procedure but also allow time to correct any conditions that might preclude surgery. For example, if the preoperative examination revealed a previously undiagnosed atrial fibrillation, the condition could be stabilized before surgery, thus avoiding rescheduling.

The history should include information about the patient's current condition requiring surgery, past surgical procedures, bleeding/clotting disorders, and previous experience with anesthesia. It is important to assess the patient's exercise tolerance or functional level. In children, past medical history—including birth history, perinatal complications, congenital chromosomal or anatomic malformations, and recent infections, particularly upper respiratory infections or pneumonia—are important elements of the preoperative evaluation. The physician must inquire about any chronic medical conditions, particularly those involving the heart and lungs. Medications, including over-the-counter medications and herbals, must be noted. Medication dosing may have to be adjusted in the perioperative period. Aspirin, other nonsteroidal anti-inflammatory drugs (NSAIDs), herbals, and omega-3 fatty acids should generally be discontinued 1 week before surgery to avoid excessive bleeding (Table 6-1).

During the evaluation, immunization status can be assessed and updated as necessary. A history of tobacco, alcohol, and drug use should be elicited; ideally, the patient should quit smoking 8 or more weeks preoperatively to minimize the risk of pulmonary complications. A functional assessment should be made, and the physician should review the patient's social supports and potential need for assistance after hospital discharge. For example, a patient undergoing hip replacement who has only limited assistance available at home may require home services or temporary placement in a rehabilitation facility. Planning for these needs can be done before hospitalization.

The physician should pay particular attention during the physical examination to the bedside cardiopulmonary assessment. More than 20% of patients undergoing elective surgery have some form of cardiovascular disease. Key features that may warrant further evaluation include elevated blood pressure, heart murmurs, chest pain, signs of CHF, shortness of breath, and lung disease (most commonly obstructive lung disease). After the assessment or therapy, patients with identified cardiopulmonary disease may warrant a second examination just before hospitalization and surgery, especially if they have a history of moderate valvular stenosis/regurgitation,

TABLE 6-1. Perioperative Medication Management	
Medication	**Perioperative Recommendation**
Calcium channel blocker	Continue
Beta blocker	Continue
ACE/ARB	Hold for 10 hours before procedure
Insulin	Hold short acting the day of surgery; continue long acting at ½ the normal dose
Metformin	Stop 24 hours prior to procedure
Sulfonylureas	Hold on the day of surgery
Thiazolidinediones, DPP-4 inhibitors, GLP-1 agonists	Hold on the day of surgery
Aspirin, Prasugrel	Hold for 7 days prior depending on indication for therapy
Clopidogrel, Ticagrelor	Hold 5 days before procedure
Diuretic	Consider holding
Statins	Continue, consider adding in those with CV risk and high-risk or vascular surgery
Levodopa/carbidopa	Hold on the day of surgery
Estrogen	Hold on the day of surgery, resume when patient ambulatory

ACE, angiotensin-converting enzyme; ARB, angiotensin receptor blocker; DPP-4, dipeptidyl peptidase-4; GLP-1, glucagon-like peptide-1.

cardiac implantable electronic devices, pulmonary hypertension, congenital heart disease (CHD), or severe systemic disease. In children with recent upper respiratory infections, a second visit to assess the current state of the infection can allow the clinician to identify persistent fever, wheezing, or significant nasal discharge; this may, after consultation with the surgeon, result in postponement of the surgery.

DIAGNOSTIC EVALUATION

Clinical studies during the last 15 years have led to changes in preoperative screening. Although preoperative laboratory tests once routinely included a complete blood count (CBC), chemistry profiles, a urinalysis (UA), prothrombin time (PT), partial thromboplastin time (PTT), an ECG, and chest x-rays, recent studies demonstrate that extensive testing does not reduce morbidity and mortality. Among the small percentage of patients with unexpected abnormal results, patient management was rarely affected. Current recommendations call for selective ordering of laboratory tests based on patient-specific indications.

Generally, preoperative testing will include hemoglobin, UA, and—in patients over age 40—a serum glucose, and ECG. However, routinely obtaining a preoperative EKG has unproven benefits and potential risks. Urine pregnancy tests should be considered in women of childbearing age, and a chest x-ray, blood urea nitrogen (BUN), creatinine, and CBC in patients over 75 years of age. Other testing should be directed by specific indications prompted by the history and physical examination.

Patients with risk factors for cardiac complications undergoing elective or semielective surgeries may require preoperative cardiac evaluation (Fig. 6-1). Those requiring emergency surgery will need a postoperative cardiac assessment and management. In addition to an ECG, an echocardiogram may be useful for evaluating murmurs, left ventricular (LV) function, hypertrophy, and wall motion abnormalities. Although evaluation of LV function is not warranted in all patients, it is reasonable to assess it in patients with dyspnea of unknown etiology, those with current or prior heart failure (if not assessed within 12 months or if symptoms have worsened), and those with a history or examination findings suggesting systolic dysfunction. Patients with major clinical predictors—such as decompensated CHF, unstable angina, recent MI, severe valvular disease, or arrhythmias—warrant cardiology consultation, pharmacologic stress testing, and possibly angiography, especially when left main

coronary disease is suspected. For the remainder of patients, assessing functional capacity assists with decision making. A commonly used term to express the energy cost of a physical activity is a metabolic equivalent of task or MET, with one MET approximating a person's resting energy expenditure. Patients with good functional capacity can perform activities requiring four METs such as climbing two flights of stairs, walking up a hill effortlessly, or walking four or more blocks easily. Patients with poor functional capacity are limited to activities such as personal care, walking indoors around the house, or walking slowly on level ground. Patients with intermediate predictors (history of MI, angina, compensated CHF, diabetes, and renal disease) and poor functional capacity should have stress testing performed, as should patients with intermediate predictors undergoing high-risk procedures, such as vascular surgery. For patients with minor clinical predictors, only those with poor functional capacity who are undergoing high-risk procedures require stress testing. Those with positive stress test results warrant cardiologic consultation before proceeding with surgery.

A baseline chest x-ray may be helpful in patients at risk for pulmonary complications. Although published guidelines for preoperative pulmonary testing have not been shown to be predictive of complications, pulmonary function testing can still be helpful in diagnosing and assessing disease severity. A FEV_1 <1.5 liters is associated with an increased risk of pulmonary complications, and an FEV_1 <1.0 liter with an increased risk of prolonged intubation. Arterial blood gases (ABGs) may be helpful in patients with CO_2 retention, COPD, or restrictive lung disease. Other than for lung resection surgery, there are currently no preoperative guidelines that absolutely define prohibitive lung function. Preoperative evaluations should include the use of a preoperative risk calculator including the Revised Cardiac Risk Index (RCRI) or the American College of Surgeons National Surgical Quality Improvement Program (ACS NSQIP) Surgical Risk Calculator (https://riskcalculator.facs.org/RickCalculator/). RCRI is based on the type of surgery, presence/absence of ischemic heart disease, history of stroke, serum creatinine >2.0 mg/dL, current insulin-dependent diabetes, and CHF.

PROPHYLACTIC THERAPIES

Prophylaxis against postoperative infections, namely, wound or surgical site infections includes administering antibiotics 30 minutes before starting

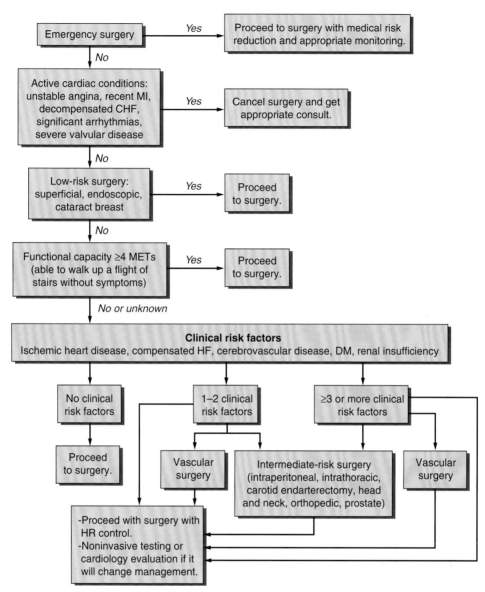

FIGURE 6-1. Preoperative cardiac evaluation. CHF, congestive heart failure; DM, diabetes mellitus; HF, heart failure; MET, metabolic equivalent of task; MI, myocardial infarction. (From Domino FJ, Baldor RA, Golding J, et al. *5-Minute Clinical Consult 2018*. 26th ed. Alphen aan den Rijn, The Netherlands: Wolters Kluwer; 2017.)

surgery and, for prolonged procedures, may include additional doses of antibiotics during the procedure. The administration of postoperative antibiotics is controversial, although many surgeons give one additional postoperative dose of antibiotic. Further doses should generally be reserved for those with suspected or documented infection. Antibiotic selection depends on the type of surgery. For most surgeries, cefazolin or vancomycin is used because these antibiotics cover skin flora, specifically *Staphylococcus aureus,* which is commonly responsible for wound infections. Gram-negative coverage is

recommended for gastrointestinal, oral, head and neck, and genitourinary surgeries, and anaerobic coverage should be provided for gastrointestinal and oral surgeries. Cefoxitin is commonly used for gastrointestinal surgeries and ciprofloxacin for genitourinary procedures; the combination of gentamicin and clindamycin is commonly recommended for head and neck surgeries.

Endocarditis prophylaxis may be indicated for selected individuals. Newer guidelines reflect a consensus that only people at greatest risk for bad outcomes from infective endocarditis (IE) should receive short-term preventive antibiotics before routine dental and medical procedures. Table 6-2 lists conditions associated with highest risk. Because prophylaxis prevented only an extremely small number of cases of IE, the emerging consensus is that preventive antibiotics in lower-risk situations do more harm than good because of the associated risks of antibiotic side effects, allergic reactions, and increasing antibiotic resistance. Not all dental procedures require antibiotic prophylaxis. For example, prophylaxis should be considered for procedures involving the manipulation of gingival tissue, the periapical region of teeth, or perforation of the mucosa and is not indicated for routine injection or placement of orthodontic appliances. Routine prophylaxis of genitourinary (GU) or gastrointestinal (GI) endoscopic procedures in those without active infection is not indicated. Table 6-3 lists dental regimens.

TABLE 6-2. Cardiac Conditions Associated with Highest Risk of Adverse Outcome from Endocarditis for Which Prophylaxis with Dental Procedures is Reasonable

Prosthetic cardiac valve or prosthetic material used for cardiac valve repair

Previous infective endocarditis

Congenital heart disease (CHD)

Unrepaired cyanotic CHD, including palliative shunts and conduits

Completely repaired congenital heart defect with prosthetic material or device, whether placed by surgery or by catheter intervention, during the first 6 months after the procedure[a]

Repaired CHD with residual defects at the site or adjacent to the site of a prosthetic patch or prosthetic device (which inhibit endothelialization)

Cardiac transplantation recipients who develop cardiac valvulopathy

[a]Prophylaxis is reasonable because endothelialization of prosthetic material occurs within 6 months after the procedure.
Source: From Wilson W, Taubert KA, Gewitz M, et al. AHA Guideline: prevention of infective endocarditis. *Circulation*. 2007;116: 1736–1754. Copyright © 2007, American Heart Association, Inc. Used with permission.

TABLE 6-3. Regimens for a Dental Procedure

Situation	Agent	Regimen: Single Dose 30–60 Minutes Before Procedure	
		Adults	**Children**
Oral	Amoxicillin	2 g	50 mg/kg
Unable to take oral medication	Ampicillin **OR**	2 g IM or IV	50 mg/kg IM or IV
	Cefazolin **OR**	1 g IM or IV	50 mg/kg IM or IV
	Ceftriaxone		
Allergic to penicillin or ampicillin–oral	Cephalexin[a,b] **OR**	2 g	50 mg/kg
	Clindamycin **OR**	600 mg	20 mg/kg
	Azithromycin **OR**	500 mg	15 mg/kg
	Clarithromycin		
Allergic to penicillin or ampicillin and unable to take oral medication	Cefazolin **OR**	1 g IM or IV	50 mg/kg IM or IV
	Ceftriaxone[b] **OR**	600 mg IM or IV	20 mg/kg IM or IV
	Clindamycin		

[a]Or other first- or second-generation oral cephalosporin in equivalent adult or pediatric dosage.
[b]Cephalosporins should not be used in an individual with a history of anaphylaxis, angioedema, or urticaria with penicillin or ampicillin.
IM, intramuscular; IV, intravenous.

Planning for surgery should also include DVT prophylaxis and efforts to maximize the patient's pulmonary function. Prophylaxis to prevent venous thromboembolism and pulmonary embolism should be provided to most surgical patients. The risk of developing DVT is approximately 15% to 30% in the general surgical patient and increases to 50% to 60% for patients undergoing hip surgery. Risk factors for developing DVT include age over 40, obesity, orthopedic surgery, CHF, prior or family history of DVT, stroke, malignancy, immobilization, trauma, and estrogen use. Accepted prophylactic therapies for lower-risk patients include early ambulation, gradient compression stockings, pneumatic compression stockings, and low-dose subcutaneous unfractionated or low-molecular-weight heparin. For high-risk patients, either low-molecular-weight heparin or warfarin should be considered. In cases where the risk of bleeding may be too high to permit the use of anticoagulants (e.g., certain neurosurgical procedures), pneumatic compression stockings are generally used. Maximizing preoperative pulmonary function in at-risk patients (e.g., those with COPD) may include treatment of any apparent infections and the use of bronchodilators, with or without corticosteroids, in those with reversible airway disease.

High-risk patients should be trained in the use of incentive spirometry before surgery.

Statin therapy started 2 weeks before surgery may reduce cardiac complications and acute kidney injury in appropriate patients. Current recommendations are that beta blockers should be continued in patients currently receiving beta blockers for coronary artery disease, symptomatic arrhythmias, and hypertension. Starting beta blockers is also indicated for patients undergoing vascular surgery who are at high cardiac risk (e.g., those with evidence of ischemia on preoperative testing or the presence of coronary heart disease), who are undergoing high-risk or intermediate-risk surgery. However, they should be started 2 to 7 days before surgery and **not** on the day of surgery. The usefulness of beta blockers for patients undergoing vascular surgery without clinical risk factors or for those undergoing intermediate-risk procedures or vascular surgery with a single risk factor remains uncertain. Contraindications to beta blockers include asthma, heart block greater than first degree, and bradycardia, and caution should be exercised in patients with heart failure. Ideally, beta blockers should be started a couple of days or weeks before surgery, and the dosage adjusted to achieve a resting heart rate of 60 beats/minute.

KEY POINTS

- Routine preoperative evaluation includes a thorough history and physical examination, with additional testing based on patient characteristics.

- Cardiac and pulmonary examination of patients are the major focus.

- New or unstable problems should be resolved before surgery.

- Risk factors for cardiac disease, the type of surgery, and the patient's functional status determine the need for cardiac evaluation.

- Patients scheduled for low-risk procedures (surgical risk <1%) who are stable do not require preoperative testing and can proceed to surgery.

- Incentive spirometry and smoking cessation can help limit pulmonary complications.

- Laboratory testing for the otherwise healthy patient includes a hemoglobin and urinalysis and in those over age 40, a serum glucose and ECG.

- Antibiotic prophylaxis is warranted for procedures with high infection rates, those involving implantation of prosthetic devices, and those in which the consequences of infection are particularly serious.

- DVT prophylaxis is warranted for most surgical patients.

7 | Family Violence: Awareness and Prevention

Family violence poses serious public health risks and manifests itself in various forms, including child abuse, violence between intimate partners (IPV), and elder abuse or neglect. Violence is often cyclical, and intervening to stop the cycle at any point will be beneficial to the survivors of family violence.

EPIDEMIOLOGY

INTIMATE PARTNER VIOLENCE

IPV may be physical, sexual, or psychological and can occur between heterosexual and same-sex couples, with the abuser exerting control over the victim. In most cases of IPV, men are the perpetrators of abuse and women the victims. IPV causes a spectrum of health risks, particularly for women, ranging from minor injuries to death. Recent studies estimate that 2 to 4 million women each year suffer an IPV-related injury and more than 1 million seek medical attention for such injuries. One in four women report experiencing IPV in their lifetime, and approximately 30% of all female homicides in the United States result from domestic violence. The highest risk occurs when a woman contemplates leaving their partner or immediately following a separation. In about 50% of the cases of IPV, child abuse also occurs.

CHILD ABUSE

In the United States, approximately one in four children is a victim of abuse or neglect at some time, with one in seven children experiencing abuse within the past year. Approximately 702,000 victims of childhood sexual and physical abuse and neglect were *reported* in 2014. The number of actual cases is likely much higher because many cases of child abuse go unreported. Intentional injury is the leading cause of injury-related death among children <3 years of age. Children who have been physically or sexually abused are more likely to suffer from improper brain development and impaired cognition (learning ability), lower language development; underdeveloped or aberrant socio–emotional (social and emotional) skills; blindness; cerebral palsy from head trauma; and experience a higher risk of heart, lung and liver diseases, obesity, cancer, high blood pressure, high cholesterol, anxiety, smoking, alcoholism, and drug abuse. In addition, approximately 25% of abuse survivors are at risk for delinquency, teen pregnancy, being arrested as juveniles, and are less likely to graduate high school.

ELDER ABUSE

Elder abuse and neglect is becoming more prevalent as more people are living longer than ever before. Around 62 million Americans are expected to be over the age of 65 by 2025 , and more than 7 million >85 years of age. Due to factors such as patient denial and underreporting by patients, caregivers, and physicians the full extent of elder mistreatment in the United States remains uncertain. The CDC defines elder abuse as ". . . an intentional act, or failure to act, by a caregiver or another person in a relationship involving an expectation of trust that causes or creates a risk of harm to an older adult. (An older adult is defined as someone age 60 or older.)" In a national study by the National Institute of Justice, 1 in 10 elders reported experiencing at least one form of elder abuse within the past year, and it is estimated that more than 2.5 million older adults are mistreated each year. Abusers are most likely to be caregivers such as adult children or a spouse. Neglect is the most common form of elder mistreatment, followed by physical abuse, financial exploitation, and emotional and sexual abuse.

PATHOGENESIS

Survivors of IPV are more likely to be young women between the ages of 12 and 35 years; from a lower income group; single, separated, or divorced; have not attended college; experienced abuse as children; and have a partner that abuses alcohol or drugs. The single most common risk factor in IPV is whether the victim witnessed parental violence as a child or as an adolescent. This risk factor is consistently associated with being a victim of violence from a spouse. Ongoing IPV results from one partner's need to achieve dominance and control. Many abusers were abused as children and continue the cycle of abuse in their intimate relationships with family members. Typically, a cycle of violence ensues in which an assault is followed by a time when the batterer is remorseful and often loving. Following this is a tension-building period, which then culminates in another episode of abuse. Over time, the episodes become more frequent and severe. IPV is also associated with poorer pregnancy outcomes. Up to one-third of pregnant women are abused during pregnancy, making battery more common than the combined incidence of rubella, Rh, and ABO (blood type) incompatibility; hepatitis; and gestational diabetes. Battered pregnant women are more likely to register late for prenatal care, suffer preterm labor or miscarriage, and have low-birth-weight infants.

The power and control wheel provides an understanding of the mechanics of abuse. Figure 7-1 summarizes the factors that increase the risk of domestic violence.

CLINICAL MANIFESTATIONS

HISTORY

Identifying victims of abuse is challenging in all but the most obvious cases. The chief complaint can be related to an injury or extend to any organ system. In many cases, abused patients may present with nontraumatic diagnoses, such as upper respiratory tract symptoms or abdominal pain.

Many studies identify provider barriers to recognizing IPV survivors, including a lack of knowledge or training, time limitations, inability to offer lasting solutions, and fear of offending the patient. Health care providers may have personal experiences that contribute to their reluctance to broach the issue of abuse. Class elitism, racial prejudice, and sexism may also act as barriers to the proper identification and treatment of victims of domestic violence.

PHYSICAL EXAMINATION

Certain types of injury patterns suggest family violence. These include injuries to the face, abdomen, and genitals. Injuries that can be hidden under clothing and multiple injuries in various stages of healing suggest possible abuse. Because many women seen in the emergency room for trauma are victims of abuse, there should be a high index of suspicion for any acute injury that does not have a clear cause. Burns in children are often a tip-off for abuse, particularly burn patterns that suggest an immersion injury or a cigarette burn. Weight loss in the elderly is a sign of malnutrition and may be an indicator of neglect. Other signs of elder abuse may be multiple bruises or fractures, welts, bite marks, burns, pressure ulcers, poor hygiene, and a generally unkempt appearance. Poor cognition is a strong risk factor for mistreatment and should be assessed.

SCREENING

SCREENING FOR VIOLENCE

The U.S. Department of Health and Human Services endorses the Institute of Medicine's recommendations that screening all patients for IPV and counseling is a core element of a woman's health visit. Screening at multiple times is important because some women do not disclose abuse the first time they are asked. Health care providers should receive adequate training and education to improve skills and confidence.

- Screen for IPV in a private and safe setting with the woman alone and not with her partner, friends, family, or caregiver.
- Use professional language interpreters and not someone associated with the patient.
- At the beginning of the assessment, offer a framing statement to show that screening is done universally and not because IPV is suspected. Also, inform patients of the confidentiality of the discussion and exactly what state law mandates that a physician should disclose.
- Incorporate screening for IPV into the routine medical history by integrating questions into intake forms so that all patients are screened whether or not abuse is suspected.

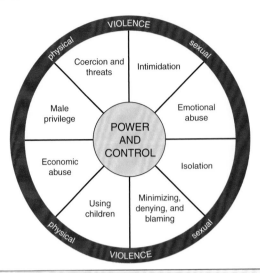

Coercion and threats	• Threatening to leave • Making the other person drop charges • Making the other person do illegal things
Intimidation	• Smashing things • Destroying the other person's property • Abusing pets • Displaying weapons
Emotional abuse	• Making the other person feel bad about themselves • Calling names • Making the other person think they are "crazy" • Playing mind games; inducing paranoia • Humiliating the other person • Making the survivor feel guilty
Isolation	• Controlling what the other person does, who they see and talk to, what they read, and where they go • Surveilling the survivor by texting, verifying with others • Limiting outside involvement • Using jealousy to justify actions
Minimizing, denying, and blaming	• Minimizing the abuse and not taking the survivor's concerns about violence seriously • Saying the abuse didn't happen • Shifting responsibility for the violence to the survivor • Saying the other person caused it
Using children	• Making the other person feel guilty because of the children • Using the children to relay messages • Using visitation to harass the other person • Threatening to take the children away
Male privilege (if the abuser is male and the victim is female)	• Treating her like a servant • Making all of the big decisions • Acting like the "master of the home" • Being the one to define male and female roles
Economic abuse	• Preventing the other person from getting or keeping a job • Making them ask for money • Giving the other person an allowance • Taking their money • Not letting the other person know about or have access to the family income

FIGURE 7-1. The power and control wheel. (Adapted from Domestic Abuse Intervention Programs, 202 East Superior Street, Duluth, MN 55802, www.theduluthmodel.org.)

- Establish and maintain relationships with community resources for women affected by IPV.
- Keep printed take-home resource materials such as safety procedures, hotline numbers, and referral information in privately accessible areas such as restrooms and examination rooms. Posters and other educational materials displayed in the office can also be helpful (Box 7-1).
- Ensure that staff training receives training about IPV and that training is regularly offered.

INTIMATE PARTNER VIOLENCE SCREENING

The following should prompt an assessment for IPV: seeking care for chronic problems such as abdominal pain, muscle and joint pain; or signs of depression, substance abuse, mental health problems, and requests for repeat pregnancy tests when the patient does not wish to be pregnant; new or recurrent sexually transmitted infections (STIs), asking to be tested for an STI, or expressing fear when negotiating condom use with a partner. Studies demonstrate that direct questioning of patients at risk for IPV yields better information than a written questionnaire. Frame the screening by telling the patient that you screen all women for IPV. Three important questions to ask are:

- Have you been hit, kicked, punched, or otherwise hurt by someone within the past year? If so, by whom?
- Do you feel safe in your current relationship?
- Is there a partner from a previous relationship making you feel unsafe now?

The first question regarding physical violence is nearly as sensitive and specific as the combination of all the three questions. Thus, the problem of identifying women involved in abusive relationships may be simplified by the use of routine screening tools such as the foregoing questions.

CHILD ABUSE SCREENING

Screening for child abuse during the interview is difficult, and standardized questions have not been shown to be sensitive or specific in detecting child abuse. However, open-ended questions about parenting and discipline may be useful in eliciting evidence of child abuse. For example, the health care provider may ask, "What do you do when he or she misbehaves? Have you ever been worried that someone was going to hurt your child?" Box 7-2 lists clues for suspecting

BOX 7-1. Intimate Partner Violence National Resources

Hotlines
- National Domestic Violence Hotline 1-800-799-SAFE (7233)
- Rape Abuse & Incest National Network (RAINN) Hotline 1-800-656-HOPE (4673)

Web Sites
- Futures Without Violence (previously known as Family Violence Prevention Fund) www.futureswithoutviolence.org
- National Coalition Against Domestic Violence www.ncadv.org
- National Network to End Domestic Violence www.nnedv.org
- National Resource Center on Domestic Violence www.nrcdv.org
- Office on Violence Against Women (U.S. Department of Justice) www.usdoj.gov/ovw

A current listing of state laws on elder abuse can be found at: https://ncea.acl.gov/resources/state.html

BOX 7-2. Clues to Child Abuse

The story given by the parents does not seem to explain the injury
The explanation given by the parent or caretaker is inconsistent or contradictory
There is a long interval between the injury and seeking care
The parent's reaction to the injury is inappropriate

The parent's interaction with the child seems inappropriate

that an injury has been caused by abuse. Neglect is another type of abuse and can take the form of medical, physical, or emotional neglect. Poor supervision, such as leaving a young child alone without adequate adult oversight, is another type of abuse.

ELDER ABUSE SCREENING

Screening for elder abuse can also be difficult. The elderly patient may be unable to provide information because of cognitive impairment or may fear retaliation from the abuser or placement in a nursing home. Asking open-ended questions about the patient's perception of safety at home is a good way to begin an interview. More specific questions should focus on incidents of rough handling, confinement, withholding of food and/or medicine, improper touching, and verbal or emotional abuse. Other red flags are a history of delay in seeking medical care, conflicting or improbable accounts of events, and a history of similar or other suspicious events.

TREATMENT AND INTERVENTION

The most important and most easily provided intervention is the simple message that no one deserves to be hurt and that the victim is not to be blamed for the behavior of the perpetrator.

INTIMATE PARTNER VIOLENCE INTERVENTION

Survivors of IPV report that the most desirable behaviors by physicians with whom they interact include listening, providing emotional support, and reassuring them that being beaten was not their fault. Women in the same study reported that the most undesirable behaviors include treatment of physical injuries without inquiry as to how they occurred.

Once a patient has been identified as a survivor of abuse, it is important to address safety needs, such as ascertaining whether there are guns or other weapons in the house. Simply asking patients whether they feel safe in going home can yield valuable information. Questions about the safety of children are crucial, because as many as 70% of violence perpetrators also abuse children. Patients should be encouraged to begin making plans to be safe whether or not they plan to leave their relationship or home situation.

Referral to community services is an important part of treatment for IPV survivors. Shelters provide much more than refuge. Women can take advantage of child services, counseling, and legal and employment services. The physician can offer to contact the police unless required by law to do so; in that case, the patient should understand the physician's duty

to report. Victims should be informed that IPV is a crime throughout the United States and that help is available from the judicial system. Civil protection orders (stay-away orders) are available in every jurisdiction. In addition to barring contact between the perpetrator and the victim, these orders can include temporary custody of children and mandate rent or mortgage payments by the batterer even if he is not allowed to live in the home.

The worst thing the physician can do is nothing. Even if the patient refuses any help, it is still critical to acknowledge the patient's disclosure and assign responsibility to the perpetrator. Supportive statements emphasizing that this is not the patient's fault and that violence is not an acceptable means of conflict resolution can be helpful. It is important to remember that terminating an abusive relationship is often a long process. Continuous support, follow-up, and accessibility are critically important for those individuals who choose to remain in an abusive relationship.

CHILD ABUSE INTERVENTION

Intervention studies in child abuse have concentrated on primary prevention. Home visits to high-risk families early in a child's life have been shown to decrease the rate of child abuse and the need for medical visits. Unfortunately, most clinicians do not have the option of providing this level of intervention, much less extending this type of treatment for long periods of time. In up to 60% of cases, there may be recurrent abuse despite interventions.

ELDER ABUSE INTERVENTION

Effective interventions for elder abuse may also be limited, in large part because the abuser is often an overworked primary caregiver. The patient's cognition should be assessed; if he or she is competent, the patient should be an active participant in treatment. In some cases, nursing home placement may be the best or the only option, but often a multidisciplinary team approach can be taken. Members of such teams include geriatricians, social workers, case management nurses, and representatives from legal, financial, and adult protective services. Team members can work together with the patient and caregiver and come up with solutions to eliminate the abuse.

DOCUMENTATION

Medical records must document abuse accurately and legibly, because these records are readily admissible at civil and criminal trials. They can provide objective diagnoses that can substantiate a victim's assertion of harm. Records can be used even when the survivor is unable or unwilling to testify. Whenever possible, the patient's own words should be used. The relationship of the perpetrator to the victim should also be clearly stated. If possible, the record should include photographs, because these are particularly valuable as evidence. Areas of tenderness, even in the absence of visible injury, should be documented in writing as well as on a body map. Attention to detail is invaluable when one is attempting to recreate the circumstances of abuse for the criminal justice system. A well-documented medical record improves the likelihood of successful prosecution without testimony from the health care provider.

REPORTING

In all states, suspected cases of child abuse or neglect must be reported to local child protective services agencies. In most states, suspected elder abuse must also be reported. Almost all states mandate reporting injuries that result from the use of a gun, knife, or other deadly weapon. It is unknown whether mandatory reporting improves patient or victim outcomes. Nevertheless, health care providers must be familiar with local laws and comply with them. A few states now require that health care workers report cases of suspected domestic violence. The reporting of abuse is **not** a substitute for proper intervention and management of child abuse, domestic violence, or elder abuse.

PERPETRATORS OF ABUSE

Information on perpetrators of IPV is complex. This is particularly worrisome because the solution to the problem of abuse lies largely in identifying underlying behaviors leading to violent actions within families and changing perpetrator behavior. Current theories hold that the cycle of battery, particularly in intimate partner violence, revolves around the agent of abuse having total control of the target of abuse. The primary goal of intervention should be to break the cycle of family violence; however, more research is needed.

KEY POINTS

- Approximately 30% of all female homicides in the United States are the result of domestic violence.

- Children who have been abused physically or sexually are significantly more likely to be sexually active as teens, to abuse tobacco and alcohol, to attempt suicide, and to exhibit violent or criminal behavior.

- The most common form of elder abuse is neglect, followed by physical abuse, financial exploitation, emotional abuse, and sexual abuse.

- The chief complaint can be related to an injury; however, in many cases, abused patients may present with nontraumatic diagnoses, such as upper respiratory tract symptoms or abdominal pain.

- The most important and most easily provided intervention is the simple message that no one deserves to be hurt and that the victim is not to blame for the behavior of the perpetrator.

CLINICAL VIGNETTES

VIGNETTE 1

A 72-year-old woman with hypertension and diet-controlled diabetes is scheduled to have cataract surgery, and her ophthalmologist requested that you "clear" her for surgery. She is sedentary but can navigate two flights of stairs without symptoms. She denies having complaints other than vision symptoms.

Laboratory testing 1 month ago, including HgbA1c, was within normal limits. Physical examination reveals BP 128/70, HR 72 regular, RR 14, normal cardiac and pulmonary examinations, and no edema or focal neurologic findings.

1. What additional tests should be performed preoperatively on this patient?

a. No additional testing
b. EKG
c. Chest x-ray
d. Cardiac stress testing
e. CBC and BMP

2. Two years later, the same patient develops claudication and, as a result, is less active and can no longer tolerate ascending a flight of stairs without resting. Her diabetes and hypertension are being treated with metformin and lisinopril. She also takes one baby aspirin daily. Arterial studies indicate moderately severe obstruction. She plans to undergo vascular surgery for her leg pains. Before her procedure, which of the following measures is warranted?
   a. DEXA scan
   b. Beta blockers initiated at time of surgery
   c. Cardiac stress testing
   d. Aspirin and clopidogrel
   e. No additional testing

3. The stress testing is negative, and the patient returns for a follow-up to her preoperative evaluation. Which of the following is an additional prophylactic measure that may be helpful preoperatively?
   a. Pentoxifylline
   b. Cilostazol
   c. Atorvastatin
   d. Clopidogrel
   e. Warfarin

VIGNETTE 2

A 77-year-old woman presents to establish care with you. She has a history of hypertension but is otherwise well. She is a former 40 pack-year smoker but quit 10 years ago. She has not had a Pap smear since age 66, and all prior Pap smears were normal. She gets annual mammograms, and her last colonoscopy was also normal at age 67. She had a Tdap and pneumococcal 23 valent vaccine 7 years ago and gets annual influenza vaccines.

1. Which of the following vaccines is currently indicated?
   a. Pneumococcal 13 valent vaccine
   b. Pneumococcal 23 valent vaccine
   c. Meningococcal vaccine
   d. Td vaccine
   e. IPV

2. Which of the following screening tests are indicated?
   a. Chest CT
   b. Abdominal aortic ultrasound

c. Pap smear
d. Colonoscopy
e. Mammogram

3. Her 50-year-old son presents the next day for his annual checkup. He is healthy, active, symptom free, and takes no medications. He does not smoke and drinks moderately. He has had all his childhood vaccines, and his last Td was at age 35 years. He has not had any lab or diagnostic testing done. At this time, which of the following vaccinations would you recommend?
   a. Pneumococcal
   b. Td
   c. Tdap
   d. Meningoccal
   e. HPV

4. Which diagnostic tests would you recommend at this time?
   a. PSA
   b. Chest CT
   c. Colonoscopy
   d. Stress test
   e. Abdominal aortic aneurysm (AAA) screening with abdominal ultrasound

VIGNETTE 3

A mother brings her three children in for their well-child visits. Her children are all girls aged 12 years, 5 years, and 6 months. They are all current with their vaccinations, but at this visit they will need the appropriate vaccines for their current age.

1. Which of the following vaccine combinations would the 6-month-old child receive?
   a. Hepatitis B, DTap, IPV, Hib, PCV13
   b. MMR, DTap, IPV
   c. HPV, IPV, Hepatitis B, Hib
   d. Meningococcal, MMR, DTap, PCV13

2. At the 5-year-old child's visit, which of the following vaccines would be indicated?
   a. HPV, DTap, IPV
   b. DTap, IPV, MMR, varicella
   c. Meningococcal, IPV, DTap
   d. Hepatitis B, varicella, PCV13

3. Which of the following would be included in the 12-year-old's recommended vaccinations?
   a. Hepatitis B, DTap, PCV13
   b. MMR, varicella
   c. Tdap, meningococcal, HPV
   d. Meningococcal, HPV, MMR

ANSWERS

VIGNETTE 1 Question 1

1. Answer A:

Although the patient has risk factors of hypertension, diabetes, and sedentary lifestyle, the proposed surgery is very low risk with a <1% risk of cardiopulmonary complications. No additional testing would be indicated in this patient, who has an exercise tolerance of >4 METS (able to walk up two flights of stairs) and is currently asymptomatic.

VIGNETTE 1 Question 2

2. Answer C:

The patient now has an unknown activity tolerance because of her underlying vascular disease, which is also a risk factor for cardiovascular disease. Before surgery, she needs a cardiac evaluation, and additional medical management or procedural intervention may be warranted if she has significant cardiac disease. Because of her claudication, she will need a chemical stress test such as an adenosine, dipyridamole, or dobutamine thallium scan. The medication serves the purpose of increasing the heart rate when a patient might not be able to raise his or her heart rate sufficiently because of a physical limitation. Beta blockers could be an option to control heart rate in the perioperative period but should be started several days before surgery. There is no role for a DEXA scan, and starting aspirin and clopidogrel would increase the risks of bleeding without an indication for this treatment.

VIGNETTE 1 Question 3

3. Answer C:

Cilostazol and pentoxifylline are used to attempt to improve symptoms in patients being treated medically for claudication related to underlying vascular disease but would not play a role in perioperative management of the patient. Clopidogrel increases the risk of perioperative bleeding, as would warfarin. Both these medications would be held before surgery to decrease the risk of bleeding. Atorvastatin before surgery can lower perioperative risk for cardiac and renal complications.

VIGNETTE 2 Question 1

1. Answer A:

Meningococcal and IPV vaccines are not routinely indicated in this age group. Td is not indicated because she received Tdap <10 years ago. For patients over age 65, pneumococcal 13-valent vaccine followed 1 year later by pneumococcal 23-valent vaccines is indicated. For those who have already received the 23-valent vaccine, the 13-valent should be administered at least 1 year after the 23-valent vaccine. For those who have received the 13-valent vaccine, the 23-valent vaccine can be administered 1 year after and at least 5 years after any prior 23-valent vaccine.

VIGNETTE 2 Question 2

2. Answer A:

The USPSTF recommends annual Chest CT screening in smokers aged 55 to 80 years and a 30+ pack-year history of smoking. This applies to current smokers or those who have quit within the past 15 years. Another condition of testing is the current condition of the patient in terms of expected survival and the ability to withstand intervention if a cancer were detected. AAA ultrasound screening is indicated one time in males over age 65 who have ever smoked. Pap smears may be discontinued after age 65 if prior screening has been normal. Both mammography and colonoscopy can be discontinued at age 75 years.

VIGNETTE 2 Question 3

3. Answer C:

Tdap should be provided as a one-time vaccination to all adults in place of Td. Tetanus booster vaccination is recommended every 10 years, and thus Tdap would be recommended now. Pneumococcal vaccine would not be recommended at this age unless he had an underlying indication, such as immunocompromise, respiratory disease, or smoking that places him at above-average risk. Meningococcal vaccine and HPV would not be routinely provided at this age.

VIGNETTE 2 Question 4

4. Answer C:

Colon cancer screening is routinely recommended to start at age 50 for average risk individuals. If there is a family history of colon cancer in a first-degree relative, screening should begin 10 years before the age at which the relative was diagnosed. PSA testing is not routinely recommended but may be discussed and offered to individuals having symptoms or a significant desire for testing but also understanding the pros and cons of testing. Chest CT is recommended for lung cancer annually in those with >30 pack-year history between the ages of 55 and 80. Stress testing is not a routine screen and would generally be performed in those with symptoms suspicious for underlying cardiac disease. AAA screening is provided to males, ≥65 years, who have ever smoked.

VIGNETTE 3 Question 1

1. Answer A:

MMR, HPV, and meningococcal vaccines are not indicated until the child is older. The vaccines listed in choice "A" are all indicated and can be provided by using combination vaccines to limit the number of injections necessary.

VIGNETTE 3 Question 2

2. Answer B:

HPV and meningococcal are indicated at an older age, and because the child is up to date for her immunizations, she should already have completed the hepatitis B series and PCV13 vaccinations. The vaccines listed in selection "B" are correct and should be provided at this visit.

VIGNETTE 3 Question 3

3. Answer C

MMR, hepatitis B, and PCV13 will have been completed by this age because she is noted to be current with her immunization status. At age 12, meningococcal, HPV, and Tdap should be provided to ensure that she remains up to date.

8 | Allergies

The term "allergy" can be defined as an immunoglobulin E (IgE)–mediated hypersensitivity to an antigen. Type I hypersensitivity reactions include allergic rhinitis, atopic dermatitis, conjunctivitis, asthma, food allergies, and systemic anaphylaxis.

EPIDEMIOLOGY

Allergic rhinitis affects up to 20% of the population, and 10% to 20% of children suffer from atopic dermatitis. Asthma occurs in 5% to 7% of the population and is associated with significant morbidity and an increasing number of deaths. Allergic rhinitis and asthma often coexist, and more than half of the asthma cases in the United States can be attributed to seasonal allergies. In some cases, allergic rhinitis and asthma may be thought of as manifestations of the same disease. Food allergies, although less common, occur in a significant number of individuals (1% to 3% of Americans).

PATHOGENESIS

In allergic rhinitis, allergens bind to IgE on mast cells on the nasal mucosa of a sensitized individual. This causes mast cells to degranulate, releasing chemical mediators such as histamines, leukotrienes, and bradykinins, which cause vasodilatation, fluid transudation, and swelling. Common seasonal allergens include pollens from trees, grasses, and weeds. Perennial rhinitis, which occurs throughout the year, is caused primarily by indoor allergens such as house dust, animal dander, and molds.

IgE-mediated reactions can also trigger asthma. Environmentally important allergens leading to asthma include air pollution, dust mites, and cockroaches, which may explain the increasing prevalence of asthma in the inner city.

Cutaneous, respiratory, or gastrointestinal exposure to allergens may cause symptoms in the exposed organ system or produce more generalized symptoms. Common skin manifestations of allergies include urticaria and eczema. Gastrointestinal symptoms associated with allergen exposure include nausea, vomiting, diarrhea, and abdominal pain. Foods most commonly found to be allergenic among children are milk, eggs, peanuts, soy, wheat, tree nuts, fish, and shellfish. Among adults, peanuts, tree nuts, shellfish, and fish are the most common, as approximately 70% of individuals appear to "outgrow" milk and egg allergies.

A severe, life-threatening systemic allergic reaction called **anaphylaxis** can occur from food allergies (e.g., to peanuts), during blood transfusions, from medications, or from insect stings of the Hymenoptera order (bees, wasps, and ants).

CLINICAL MANIFESTATIONS (Table 8-1)

HISTORY

The symptoms of allergic rhinitis include runny nose (rhinorrhea), sneezing, nasal congestion, conjunctivitis, and itching of the ears, eyes, nose, and throat. Nonproductive cough, nasal congestion with headaches, plugged or itchy ears, diminished smell and taste, or sleep disturbances may all be symptoms of allergies. Timing of the symptoms is important. Tree pollens tend to affect people more in the early spring, grasses in mid-May to June, and ragweed from August until the first frost. Those who are allergic to pollens typically have worse symptoms during the day and improve at night. The common perennial allergens are house dust, feathers, animal dander, and molds. In these patients, the symptoms may be worse at night. Continual waxing and waning throughout the year suggest a combination of

TABLE 8-1. Clinical Symptoms Associated with Allergic Reactions

Anaphylaxis	Rapid onset
	Angioedema, urticaria
	Dyspnea, wheezing
	Hypotension, tachycardia
Respiratory	Cough, sneezing
	Dyspnea, wheezing
	Hypoxia, angioedema
	Hoarseness, rhinorrhea
Gastrointestinal	Abdominal pain
	Nausea, vomiting
	Diarrhea
Skin/eyes	Conjunctival injection, tearing
	Pruritis, urticarial rash
	Edema

perennial and seasonal allergies. Food allergies often affect the skin and the gastrointestinal system. Food allergies may present with urticaria, usually within an hour of ingesting the offending agent.

Patients should be asked whether they have ever experienced symptoms suggestive of severe or anaphylactic reactions. Genetic factors, association with prior exposures, family history of atopy, atopic dermatitis, and history of asthma are risk factors with asthma being the strongest associated factor. Manifestations of anaphylaxis include agitation, palpitations, paresthesias, pruritus, difficulty swallowing, cough, and wheezing. Patients with these symptoms need emergency care, because the initial symptoms may progress rapidly and even lead to cardiovascular collapse.

PHYSICAL EXAMINATION

The physical examination should focus on the eyes, nose, throat, lungs, and skin. Patients may have conjunctivitis and increased lacrimation. The nasal mucosa may appear swollen and pale. The turbinates should be inspected to rule out any nasal polyps, which are common in patients with allergies. The term "allergic shiners" describes the darkening of the infraorbital skin in people with chronic allergies. Some patients may have a nasal crease across the bridge of the nose because of the frequent nose rubbing ("allergic salute") to relieve itching. The

sinuses should be examined for tenderness and the lungs for wheezing.

Skin reactions such as eczema and urticaria are common in children with food allergies. Atopic dermatitis in infants and young children is usually an exudative eruption with oozing and crusting primarily occurring in the head and neck areas, diaper area, forearms, and wrists. In preschool and school children, the rash is typically drier and scalier. Similar to adults, the rash is often found in the large flexures and the skin is dry, thickened, and lichenified with frequent evidence of scratch marks. An abdominal examination should be performed in patients presenting with gastrointestinal symptoms so as to exclude other causes for their symptoms.

DIFFERENTIAL DIAGNOSIS

The differential diagnosis depends on the presenting complaint. In allergic conjunctivitis, it is important to differentiate among viral, bacterial, allergic, and irritant causes of conjunctivitis. Viral and bacterial conjunctivitis are discussed in Chapter 27. Allergic conjunctivitis is often seasonal and occurs during periods of high exposure. Patients may also develop red eyes because of irritants such as dust and smoke.

Rhinorrhea can be due to a common cold, vasomotor rhinitis, atrophic rhinitis, rhinitis medicamentosa, or sinusitis. In common cold, the mucosa is usually red with thickened discharge, whereas with allergies the nasal mucosa appears pale and boggy or bluish. In nonallergic rhinitis, there is no pruritus. Patients with vasomotor rhinitis present with chronic nasal congestion with watery rhinorrhea, which may be intensified by sudden changes in temperature, humidity, or odors. Atrophic rhinitis is a condition seen in elderly patients and is characterized by marked atrophy of the nasal mucosa, chronic nasal congestion, and a bad odor. Rhinitis medicamentosa is caused by chronic use of cocaine or topical nasal decongestants. In sinusitis, the nasal discharge may be purulent and accompanied by headaches, nasal congestion, facial pain, and tenderness over the sinuses. Other causes of rhinitis include foreign bodies, nasal polyps, tumors, and nasal congestion associated with hormonal causes such as pregnancy, the use of birth control pills, and hypothyroidism. Wegener granulomatosis, midline granuloma, and sarcoidosis are rare but serious causes of nasal discharge.

The symptoms of food allergies include skin reactions and gastrointestinal symptoms. Urticarial lesions, or hives, are characterized by pruritic erythematous raised lesions, which may be migratory. Atopic dermatitis is an eczematous rash that is flat, erythematous, pruritic, and scaly and can be confused with contact dermatitis or lichen simplex chronicus. On rare occasions, a skin biopsy is needed to exclude other conditions. Evaluation of any gastrointestinal symptoms requires a thorough history and physical examination as well as investigation of an association of symptoms with the suspected allergen and a trial of avoidance to see if symptoms remit.

DIAGNOSTIC EVALUATION

The diagnosis of allergic disease is usually made on the basis of the history and physical examination. In most patients, treatment may be started without any diagnostic tests; if the patient responds to therapy, no further testing is needed.

Eosinophils found on microscopic examination of nasal smears are characteristic of allergic rhinitis. However, this test is not commonly performed because of its poor sensitivity and specificity. In patients who do not respond to empiric therapy, allergy testing is helpful. The radioallergosorbent test (RAST) tests the blood for the presence of IgE to different allergens. The test is sensitive but not specific; thus, many individuals may be positive on the RAST but may not be having clinical symptoms from the allergen identified by it. Skin-prick testing involves injecting a small amount of allergen into the skin and observing for local responses. This test is more specific, but less sensitive than the RAST and is usually performed by an allergist. Identifying offending allergens is useful for directing avoidance therapy. If no allergens are identified and the patient continues to have symptoms, flexible nasolaryngoscopy may be performed to rule out any anatomic or pathologic abnormalities. In patients with food allergies, the history should help formulate a possible list of allergenic foods. Avoidance and challenge testing can assess for different food allergies.

TREATMENT

The first treatment for any allergic disorder is allergen avoidance. Examples include staying indoors during a high-pollen day or reducing household dust by frequent cleaning, vacuuming using a high-efficiency particulate air (HEPA) filter, and removing dust-collecting items such as books or shag rugs. Pharmacologic therapy includes antihistamines, oral and topical decongestants, intranasal and oral corticosteroids, antileukotriene therapy with a selective leukotriene receptor antagonist (LTRA) and intranasal cromolyn sodium. Antihistamines are the first-line therapy for allergic rhinitis and are also helpful for other forms of allergy. They block the H_1 receptors, preventing the release of histamine, and help reduce sneezing, rhinorrhea, and itching. The main side effect of these drugs is sedation. However, newer nonsedating antihistamines are now available. A topical antihistamine nasal spray (azelastine) is also available, but is expensive compared with generic oral antihistamines. Topical nasal decongestant sprays have a very limited role in allergic rhinitis because of the risks of tachyphylaxis and rebound nasal congestion. Oral decongestants, such as pseudoephedrine, can relieve nasal congestion but should be used with caution in patients with hypertension, thyroid disease, diabetes, and difficulty in urination.

Intranasal steroids are the treatment of choice for most patients with moderate-to-severe persistent allergic rhinitis because of their effectiveness and minimal side effects. Oral corticosteroids are potent medications but have significant long-term side effects; therefore, their use should generally be restricted to 3 to 7 days. Cromolyn, which stabilizes mast cells, is available as an over-the-counter nasal spray. Cromolyn is only moderately effective but is very safe and well tolerated. It is often the first line of treatment in children and pregnant women. Topical therapies or oral antihistamines may provide relief for allergic conjunctivitis. LTRAs are also used to reduce allergic symptoms and may also benefit those with concomitant asthma. They have an excellent safety profile, and because they come in tablet form, they are easier for some patients to use than nasally inhaled steroids. Intranasal anticholinergics may be helpful in cases of persistent rhinorrhea but have little effect on obstructive symptoms. Figure 8-1 presents an overview of treatment for allergic rhinitis.

For patients with allergic skin manifestations, oral antihistamines, topical steroids, and cool colloid baths may be helpful. Oral steroids can be used for acute urticaria but should not be used chronically. Moisturizing lotions and creams to avoid dryness and to repair the skin barrier may improve symptoms. As with other forms of allergy, avoidance of any known triggers should be advised as well as avoiding skin irritants such as woolen or abrasive clothing. Patients with food allergies should avoid the foods that bring on the symptoms.

Therapy for patients with asthma is outlined in Chapter 38. In cases of anaphylaxis, the treatment of choice is epinephrine. Antihistamines, corticosteroids,

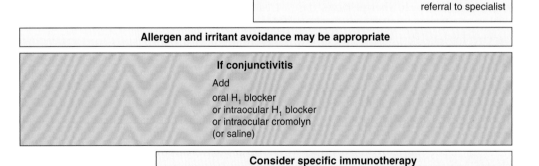

FIGURE 8-1. Algorithm for allergic rhinitis diagnosis and management. (Reprinted from Bousquet J, Khaltaev N, Cruz AA, et al. Allergic rhinitis and its impact on asthma (ARIA) 2008 update (in collaboration with the World Health Organization, GA(2)LEN and AllerGen). *Allergy*. 2008;63[suppl 86]:8–160, with permission.)

and nebulizer treatments are frequent adjunctive therapy to epinephrine. Patients with hypoxia and/or wheezing are provided oxygen and those with hypotension, intravenous fluids. Patients are frequently observed in a hospital setting for 12 to 24 hours following an anaphylactic reaction and released with antihistamine and corticosteroids as well as a close follow-up. Patients who have a history of anaphylaxis should carry injectable epinephrine. They should

wear an "alert" bracelet and have an emergency action plan that describes the signs and symptoms of anaphylaxis and emergency instructions.

In recalcitrant cases, immunotherapy may be tried. In this process, patients are exposed to the allergen by subcutaneous injections of increasing concentrations of allergens. The goal of immunotherapy is to induce a tolerance in the patient for the specific allergen triggering the symptoms.

KEY POINTS

- Allergies are common diseases in the population and their prevalence is increasing.
- Type I hypersensitivity reactions are mediated by antigen binding to IgE on mast cells and basophils; this causes the mast cells or the basophils to release mediators of the allergic response.
- Intranasal steroids are the treatment of choice for most patients with moderate-to-severe persistent allergic rhinitis.
- The first and definitive treatment for any allergic disorder is avoidance of the allergens.

9 | Back Pain

Approximately two-thirds of adults experience back pain at some time in their lives. It is the fifth most common reason for a healthcare provider visit in the United States and is the second most common complaint presenting in primary care. Approximately one-quarter of the U.S. adults report experiencing low back pain lasting at least 1 day over the past 3 months. Because of the self-limiting nature of acute back pain, many patients do not seek care. Even among those who are seeking care, symptoms typically improve rapidly and most patients resume normal activities within 1 month.

PATHOGENESIS

Ligaments, vertebral bones, facet joints, intervertebral disks, nerve roots, and muscles are all potential sources of back pain and it may be difficult to identify the exact source of mechanical back pain. The most common causes of back pain are muscular injuries and age-related degenerative processes in the intervertebral disks and facet joints. Muscle fibers of the paraspinal muscles may tear under strenuous activity such as twisting or heavy lifting. This results in bleeding and spasm, causing local swelling and tenderness. Obesity and poor conditioning contribute to the problem. Age-related degenerative changes in the intervertebral disks and facet joints are the result of chronic stress on the lumbosacral spine.

Weakening of the fibrous capsule can cause the disk to bulge or herniate beyond the interspace. Disk herniation is responsible for 95% of cases of nerve root impingement. The most common site of disk herniation is the L5–S1 level, followed by L4–L5. Table 9-1 reviews the symptoms and deficits associated with the different levels of nerve impingement. Back pain may also result from visceral structures near the spine such as the aorta, kidneys, pancreas, and gallbladder.

CLINICAL MANIFESTATIONS

HISTORY

The history should elicit the onset of pain as well as its severity, location, and character; aggravating and relieving factors; medical history and previous injuries; and psychosocial stressors. "Red flags" such as fever, night pain, weight loss, and bone pain suggest something other than mechanical low back pain and the need for further investigation. The presence of sciatica, a sharp pain that radiates down the back or side of the leg past the knee, is often a sign of disk herniation with nerve root irritation. Difficulty urinating, fecal incontinence, progressive weakness, and saddle anesthesia are symptoms of the cauda equina syndrome, a surgical emergency.

Spinal stenosis, a degenerative disease of the spine, is usually seen after age 50. Patients typically complain

TABLE 9-1. Impingement of Nerve Roots and Symptoms			
Level	Nerve Root	Deficits	Sciatica
L3–L4	L4	Patellar jerk (reflex) dorsiflexion of foot (motor) medial aspects of tibia (sensory)	Uncommon
L4–L5	L5	Extensor of great toe (motor) dorsum of foot/base of first toe (sensory)	Common
L5–S1	S1	Ankle jerk (reflex) plantar flexion (motor) buttock, post thigh, calf, lateral ankle, and foot (sensory)	Common

of back pain and may experience pseudoclaudication, or pain/paresthesias of the lower extremities or back, that worsens with standing or back extension.

The evaluation of a child with back pain requires the presence of a parent or caretaker. Sports participation may cause injuries. For example, back handsprings or walkovers in gymnastics and hyperextension in football are associated with spondylolysis and spondylolisthesis, which can cause pain. As a general rule, pain from spondylolysis, spondylolisthesis, Scheuermann disease, muscle disease, and overuse problems improves with rest. In contrast, tumor, infection, or inflammatory diseases can cause nighttime wakening due to pain and do not improve with bed rest.

The clinical manifestations of back pain are summarized in Table 9-2.

PHYSICAL EXAMINATION

A back examination should include (1) inspecting the back for deformity; (2) checking for leg-length discrepancy; (3) checking spinal motion; (4) palpating for focal tenderness suggestive of tumor, infection, fracture, or disk herniation; (5) performing a neurologic examination to identify motor or sensory deficits; and (6) testing straight leg raising (SLR). SLR is positive if sciatica is reproduced with elevation of the leg <60 degrees. Ipsilateral SLR is more sensitive for a herniated disk, whereas contralateral SLR (with the symptoms of sciatica in the

TABLE 9-2. Clinical Manifestations of Back Pain

Type	Onset	Trigger	Symptoms
Muscular	Acute	Heavy lifting	Lateralized back pain, pain in buttock and posterior upper thigh
Disk herniation	Recurrent	Trivial stress	Nerve root L5, S1 impingements, frequent sciatica
Spinal stenosis	Old age or congenital	OA[a] or congenital	Pseudoclaudication[a]
Spondylolisthesis[b]	Chronic	OA, spondylolysis	Nerve root L5, S1 impingement hyperextension activities
Compression fracture (fx)	Acute	Osteoporosis	Pain limited in middle-to-lower spine steroid use or myeloma
Neoplasms[c]	Insidious	Neoplasms	Night pain, not relieved with supine position
Cauda equina syndrome	Old age	Massive disk herniation	Overflow incontinence (90%), saddle anesthesia[d] (75%), decreased anal sphincter tone
Osteomyelitis	Acute	Back procedure	Fever, spinal tenderness
Inflammatory diskitis	Young age	*Staphylococcus aureus*	Refusal to walk, fever, signs of sepsis; disk space narrowing, sclerosis per radiograph
Ankylosing spondylitis	Young age	HLA-B27	Morning spinal stiffness, history of inflammatory bowel disease sacroiliitis, chest expansion <2.5 cm, "bamboo-spine" in radiograph
Spondylolysis	>10 years	Hyperextension	Back, buttock pain with lordosis with activity, tight hamstrings
Scheuermann disease	Young age	Fatigue	Round back, vertebral wedging, end plate irregularity per radiograph

[a]OA (osteoarthritis); pseudoclaudication is pain in the lower extremity worsened by walking and relieved by sitting down that mimics vascular insufficiency.
[b]Spondylolisthesis is forward subluxation of a vertebral body, usually in L4–L5 or L5–S1.
[c]Neoplasms include primary (i.e., multiple myeloma and spinal cord tumor) or metastatic to the spine (i.e., breast, lung, prostate, gastrointestinal, and genitourinary neoplasms).
[d]Saddle anesthesia is reduction in sensation over the buttocks, upper posterior thighs, and perineum.

leg opposite to the examined leg) is more specific for a herniated disk.

Examination of the abdomen, rectum, groin, pelvis, and the peripheral pulses is also important in patients with back pain. Other signs of systemic diseases are fever, breast mass, pleural effusion, enlarged prostate nodule, lymphadenopathy, and joint inflammation.

DIFFERENTIAL DIAGNOSIS

Box 9-1 lists the differential diagnosis of back pain. In general, the history and physical examination should help place patients with back pain into one of the following three broad categories: nonspecific low back pain, back pain associated with a radiculopathy or stenosis, and back pain associated with an underlying cause. Unfortunately, more than 85% of patients have nonspecific pain and cannot be given a definitive diagnosis. Often, they are classified as having a lumbar strain or mechanical low back pain. Only a small fraction of patients have a serious problem such as a fracture, malignancy, infection, or visceral disease as a cause of low back pain. Systemic diseases that may present as back pain include metastatic cancer, multiple myeloma, and osteoporosis.

DIAGNOSTIC EVALUATION

Box 9-2 lists indications for obtaining spinal x-rays. For most patients, x-rays are not recommended unless the pain persists beyond 6 weeks. Negative plain films do not rule out the possibility of significant disease.

Both magnetic resonance imaging (MRI) and CT are more sensitive than plain films for detecting spinal infections, cancers, herniated disks, and spinal

BOX 9-2. Indications for X-Rays in Patients with Back Pain

Age > 50
History of significant trauma
Neurologic deficit
Systemic symptoms
Chronic steroid use
Possible hereditary condition
History of drug or alcohol abuse
History of osteoporosis
Immunodeficient state
Pain persisting >6 weeks

stenosis; they have largely replaced myelography. Because these two tests are highly sensitive and frequently demonstrate "abnormalities" in normal individuals, the American College of Physicians and the American Pain Society discourage routine imaging in patients with nonspecific low back pain to avoid over diagnosis and unnecessary radiation exposure. They recommend imaging when there is strong suspicion of an underlying pathologic abnormality, when severe or progressive neurologic defects are present or if a patient is being considered for surgery or an epidural steroid injection. Electromyography and measurement of somatosensory-evoked potentials may help define the extent of neurologic involvement. Dual-energy x-ray absorptiometry scanning is indicated for those at risk for osteoporosis.

Blood tests are not necessary for most patients with back pain. A CBC, UA, calcium, phosphorus, erythrocyte sedimentation rate (ESR), and alkaline phosphatase may be considered in patients with suspected systemic disease, older individuals, and

BOX 9-1. Differential Diagnosis of Acute Low Back Pain

Mechanical Low Back Pain (97%)
Lumbar strain (70%), degenerative processes in the intervertebral disks and facet joints (10%), herniated disk (4%), compression fx (4%), spinal stenosis (3%), spondylolisthesis (2%), spondylolysis, trauma, congenital diseases

Nonmechanical Spinal Conditions (1%)
Neoplasia (0.7%), infections (0.01%), inflammatory arthritis (0.3%), Scheuermann disease, and Paget disease

Visceral Diseases (2%)
Diseases of pelvic organs (prostatitis, endometriosis, and chronic PID), renal diseases (nephrolithiasis, pyelonephritis, and perinephric abscess), aortic aneurysm, gastrointestinal disease (pancreatitis, cholecystitis, and penetrating ulcer)

those who fail conservative treatment. A CBC screens for infection, anemia associated with multiple myeloma or an occult malignancy. The ESR may be elevated in patients with malignancy, infection, or a connective tissue disease. Patients who may require long-term NSAIDs may require baseline renal and liver function tests.

TREATMENT

Serious nonmechanical causes of low back pain—such as infection, malignancy, or fracture—require treatment of the underlying problem. Patients with a progressive neurologic finding need hospital admission and prompt consultation.

Most patients with mechanical low back pain get better with conservative treatment consisting of pain control, education, reassurance, and appropriate activity. About 80% to 90% recover within 6 weeks and as a general rule the best therapies are those with the fewest harms and lowest costs. Bed rest is not recommended unless the pain is severe enough to preclude normal activities; even then it should be limited to 2 to 3 days because longer periods of bed rest result in deconditioning. During the acute phase of an attack, the patient should be encouraged to continue normal daily activities, including work, as tolerated, but told to avoid heavy lifting (>25 lb), twisting, prolonged sitting, driving for long periods, and heavy vibration. Traction and analgesic injection are usually not helpful in the acute stage. Although there are no well-controlled studies demonstrating the value of heat, ice, or massage, many clinicians and patients feel that these treatments are helpful and pose little risk.

First-line medications include acetaminophen and NSAIDs. While the 2017 ACP guidelines found no evidence that acetaminophen improves back pain, because of its low cost and safety many physicians view a therapeutic trial either alone or in combination with an NSAID as a reasonable option. NSAIDs can relieve pain and have an anti-inflammatory effect. However, they should be used with caution in patients with a history of gastritis, ulcers, hypertension, chronic renal failure, or CHF. For those at low risk of cardiovascular disease who cannot tolerate traditional NSAIDs, the cyclooxygenase-2 (COX-2) inhibitors such as celecoxib (Celebrex) have fewer GI side effects, although they still have the same adverse effects on the kidneys and on fluid balance. COX-2 inhibitors increase the risk of heart attack and stroke and so cautious prescribing is warranted for those with or at risk for cardiovascular disease. Opioid-containing analgesics, such as hydrocodone may be considered for moderate to severe pain unrelieved by NSAIDs and/or acetaminophen but their benefits need to be carefully weighed against their risks. Recent American College of Physicians (ACP) guidelines recommend that physicians consider NSAIDs as the first-line therapy and tramadol or duloxetine as the second-line therapy. Physicians should consider opioids only in patients who fail alternative treatments and only after a discussion of their substantial risks and realistic benefits with patients. For patients who fail to improve, nondrug interventions such as exercise, multidisciplinary rehabilitation, acupuncture, mindfulness-based stress reduction, tai chi, yoga, progressive relaxation, massage, cognitive behavioral therapy, or spinal manipulation may offer benefit.

The benefit of opioids for the long-term management of chronic low back pain remains questionable. Their benefit should be weighed against concerns related to long-term use including tolerance, medication misuse, hypogonadism, constipation, and hyperalgesia that paradoxically can cause an increase in pain over time.

Muscle relaxants are occasionally helpful for individuals in whom spasm plays a major role. However, they can cause dizziness, drowsiness, and may inhibit a return to normal activities. Comparison studies have not shown one agent to be superior to another. Patients with radicular low back pain may benefit from antiepileptic drugs such as gabapentin and those with chronic low back pain may benefit from tricyclic antidepressants. In contrast, selective serotonin reuptake inhibitors (SSRIs) do not appear to be effective for low back pain, and serotonin–norepinephrine reuptake inhibitors have not been studied. However, depression is common in patients with chronic low back pain and should be assessed and treated appropriately. Although prescribing steroids is a common practice, there is no evidence that systemic corticosteroids are more effective than placebo for back pain. Surgical treatment is indicated for cauda equina syndrome and for patients with intractable pain and worsening of neurologic deficits. For patients with herniated disks not responding after 4 to 6 weeks of conservative therapy, a diskectomy may be considered. For spinal stenosis, surgery may be of benefit to those who do not respond to conservative care and have disabling symptoms.

Patients with persistent or frequent recurrences of back pain merit referral. Physical therapy or epidural steroid injections benefit some patients, although evidence to support the use of spinal injections is limited. If the pain persists for more than 6 months, it is considered chronic and requires a different approach. Consultation with a physiatrist or chronic pain management specialist is often helpful and ensures that no remediable cause of back pain has been overlooked. Individuals who have not returned to work after 6 months due to back pain have only a 50% chance of ever being employed again.

KEY POINTS

- The majority of cases of acute low back pain are due to mechanical factors and resolve within 4 to 8 weeks with conservative treatment.

- SLR is positive if sciatica (not tightened hamstring) is reproduced with elevations of the leg <60 degrees.

- Surgical treatments are indicated for cauda equina syndrome and for patients with intractable pain, with worsening of neurologic deficits.

- "Red flags" such as fever, night pain, weight loss, and bone pain suggest something other than mechanical back pain.

10 | Chest Pain

The primary concern for patients with chest pain is to determine whether the pain is of cardiac origin. In addition to cardiac disease, chest pain may be due to pulmonary, GI, musculoskeletal, or psychological diseases. Emergent causes of chest pain include MI, aortic dissection, pulmonary embolus (PE), and pneumothorax. Patients with these diagnoses usually present to the emergency room, but may on occasion present in the outpatient setting. Chest pain in the office setting is most commonly due to musculoskeletal, GI, and cardiac causes. Approximately 15% of patients with chest pain do not fit into any diagnostic category and remain undiagnosed despite evaluation.

PATHOGENESIS

Chest pain may emanate from inflammation or injury to the structures in and around the thoracic cavity. Muscular chest pain is common and may occur when there is inflammation from overuse or injury to the muscles of the chest wall. The costochondral joints may also become inflamed from overuse or injury or in association with viral illnesses. Rib fractures may produce significant pain and are generally due to trauma, but they may also occur as a result of metastatic cancer.

Gastroesophageal reflux disease (GERD) and esophageal motility disorders are common causes of chest pain. The reflux of acidic gastric contents into the lower esophagus may produce esophagitis and chest pain that is indistinguishable from cardiac chest pain. The symptoms of gastritis and peptic ulcer disease may also be perceived by some patients as a substernal pain. Cholelithiasis and cholecystitis, which usually cause right-upper-quadrant pain, may also produce substernal pain.

Cardiac chest pain results from an insufficient oxygen supply to myocardial tissue, usually from coronary artery disease. The initial step in the development of atherosclerotic heart disease is the fatty streak. Over time, the fatty streak can enlarge into a calcified plaque, eventually narrowing the vessel lumen and impairing blood flow. If the plaque ruptures, lipids and tissue factors are released from the plaque, triggering a series of events that ultimately result in intravascular thrombosis and MI. If the plaque does not rupture, a gradual narrowing of the lumen can cause anginal chest pain. This is typically brought on by exertion as the myocardial oxygen demand exceeds the supply.

Because lung tissue does not have pain fibers, inflammation or irritation of the parietal pleura is responsible for the chest pain from pulmonary diseases such as pneumonia or PE.

Other causes of chest pain include psychological and neurologic diseases, such as herpes zoster and cervical or thoracic radiculopathies. Patients with herpes zoster may experience pain before the rash appears. Disk herniation or osteoarthritic narrowing of the cervical or thoracic foramen may result in nerve compression and chest pain following a radicular pattern. Patients with psychological disease, such as anxiety and panic disorder, may present with a variety of chest symptoms—including palpitations, dyspnea, and chest pain—as part of their symptom complex.

CLINICAL MANIFESTATIONS

HISTORY

Patients with chest pain should be asked about its severity, quality, location, and duration; aggravating factors; relieving factors; radiation of pain; and other associated symptoms. Myocardial pain is often described as substernal chest tightness or pressure that radiates to the left arm, shoulders, or jaw. Patients may also complain of diaphoresis, shortness of breath, nausea, and vomiting. Anginal pain is typically brought on by exercise, eating, or emotional excitement. The pain usually lasts from 5 to 15 minutes and disappears with rest or nitroglycerin. Pain that lasts <1 minute or >30 minutes should not be considered anginal. Pericardial pain is often persistent, sharp, severe, and relieved by sitting up. Breathing, lying back, or coughing may aggravate the pain. The pain of aortic dissection is anterior and severe; it often has a ripping or tearing quality, with radiation to the back or the abdomen.

Tracheobronchitis may cause a burning pain in the upper sternal area associated with a productive cough. Pain with pneumonia commonly occurs in the overlying chest wall and is aggravated by breathing and coughing. In pneumothorax, the pain is of sudden onset, sharp, unilateral, pleuritic, and associated with shortness of breath. Pleurisy is a sharp pleuritic chest pain, often in association with a preceding viral illness.

GERD causes a burning pain that radiates up the sternum. It is worsened by large meals and lying down. Antacids may relieve the pain. The pain of esophageal spasm, which is usually associated with swallowing, may be indistinguishable from cardiac pain. Because nitroglycerin relaxes smooth muscle, it may relieve the pain.

Musculoskeletal pain from costochondritis can often be reproduced on palpation. Patients are also reluctant to take a deep breath, because this aggravates the pain.

Patients with generalized anxiety often complain of chest pain. However, this pain is nonspecific. Associated symptoms include overwhelming fear, palpitations, breathlessness, and tachypnea.

PHYSICAL EXAMINATION

Vital signs help assess the urgency of the patient's complaints. Hypotension can occur with myocardial ischemia, pericardial tamponade, PE, and GI bleeding. Tachycardia may indicate severe illness, and arrhythmias can occur with cardiac or pulmonary causes of chest pain. The presence of fever suggests an infectious cause such as pneumonia. Inspection and palpation may reveal ecchymosis from an injury, the rash of shingles, crepitus associated with rib fractures, and the sharply localized tenderness of intercostal muscle pain or costochondritis.

A thorough cardiopulmonary examination is warranted for all patients with chest pain. Patients with myocardial ischemia may have an audible S_4 or

signs of congestive heart failure such as an S_3 and pulmonary rales. Pericarditis may cause a friction rub and pulsus paradoxus. Beck triad—consisting of jugular venous distention, muffled heart sounds, and decreased blood pressure—suggests cardiac tamponade, which may be seen in severe cases of pericarditis. In aortic dissection, patients may have hypotension, absence of peripheral pulses, and a murmur of aortic insufficiency. Patients with pneumonia have crackles on inspiration, dullness to percussion, and egophony, indicating consolidation. Signs of pneumothorax include hyperresonance to percussion, tracheal deviation, decreased breath sounds, and decreased tactile and vocal fremitus. Patients with pulmonary embolism likely have normal auscultatory findings, but may be tachycardic, tachypneic, and have lower extremity edema.

Patients with acute cholecystitis may have right-upper-quadrant abdominal tenderness. GERD and gastritis often cause epigastric pain on deep palpation. Esophageal spasm and psychogenic chest pain typically do not produce abnormal physical findings.

DIFFERENTIAL DIAGNOSIS

Common causes of chest pain are presented in Box 10-1. In the outpatient setting, musculoskeletal disease is present in more than one-third of patients with chest pain. GI disease occurs in approximately 20% of patients seen in the office with chest pain, followed in frequency by cardiac, psychogenic, and pulmonary causes. Cardiac and pulmonary diseases, although not the most common in the outpatient setting, should be considered in any patient presenting with chest pain because of the potentially life-threatening diseases these represent.

DIAGNOSTIC EVALUATION

The history and physical examination help classify the chest pain into cardiac, pulmonary, GI, musculoskeletal, or psychogenic causes. An ECG is a critical element for evaluating chest pain. Although an ECG can be normal in patients with heart disease, ST-segment elevation or depression is indicative of myocardial ischemia (Fig. 10-1). Diffuse ST-segment elevation is consistent with pericarditis, while Q waves can indicate an old or recent MI. Cardiac markers such as creatine phosphokinase (CPK), troponin, and myoglobin are intracellular macromolecules that diffuse from damaged cardiac myocytes into the circulation. These markers are sensitive tests for

BOX 10-1. Causes of Chest Pain

Cardiac
Myocardial infarction
Angina pectoris
Pericarditis
Aortic dissection

Pulmonary
Pulmonary embolus
Pneumothorax
Pneumonia
Tracheobronchitis

Musculoskeletal
Costochondritis
Muscular strain

Gastrointestinal
GERD
Esophageal spasm
Cholelithiasis

Psychogenic
Somatization disorders
Anxiety disorders (including panic disorder)

Neurogenic
Herpes zoster
Cervical or thoracic disease

determining whether myocardial injury or infarction is present. Troponins increase within 3 hours of onset and remain elevated for 5 to 14 days. They are the most sensitive and specific for MI. The MB fraction of CPK-MB serves as another sensitive test; it begins to rise within 4 hours, peaks at 24 hours after an MI and returns to baseline within 48 hours. CPK-MB is most useful in detection of reinfarction within 2 weeks of a prior MI. It is important to obtain serial cardiac markers, because the first set of cardiac markers is negative in 25% to 50% of patients with an acute MI. However, by 8 hours after the onset of symptoms, up to 95% of patients test positive. A negative troponin between 6 and 72 hours after the onset of chest pain is strong evidence against MI and acute coronary syndrome, particularly if the ECG is normal or near normal.

In stable patients with suspected cardiac disease, outpatient exercise stress testing is indicated. Patients should have a baseline ECG to detect abnormalities such as a conduction defect or strain pattern that make interpreting a stress test difficult. Patients with baseline ECG abnormalities or a positive exercise stress test should undergo radionuclide testing, a stress echocardiogram, and/or coronary angiography. If an individual is unable to exercise, then a chemical stress test using either adenosine or dobutamine to achieve a target heart rate may be necessary.

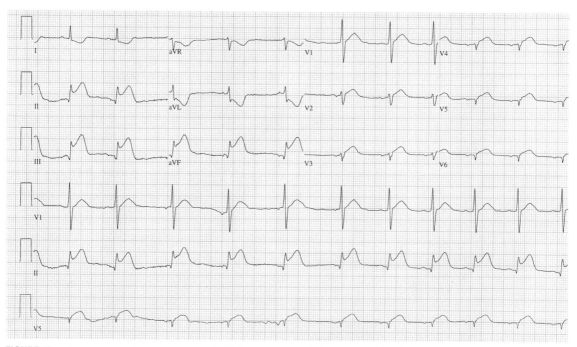

FIGURE 10-1. ST-segment elevation myocardial infarction. (From Rimmerman CM. *Electrocardiography Review: A Case-Based Approach*. Philadelphia, PA: Lippincott Williams and Wilkins; 2012.)

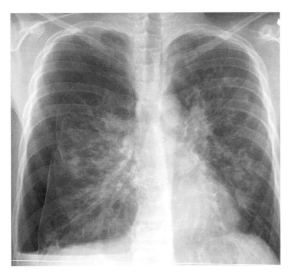

FIGURE 10-2. Pneumothorax. (From Collins J, Stern EJ. *Chest Radiology: The Essentials*. 3rd ed. Alphen aan den Rijn, The Netherlands: Wolters Kluwer; 2015.)

An echocardiogram can detect wall motion abnormalities in areas damaged by ischemic myocardial disease, pericardial effusions, and valvular heart disease. If the cause of pericarditis is not evident, an antinuclear antibody, blood urea nitrogen, creatinine, thyroid-stimulating hormone (TSH), and tuberculosis skin test are indicated.

A chest x-ray can detect pneumonia, pneumothorax (Fig. 10-2), or other lung pathology. If PE is suspected, a ventilation/perfusion scan or a spiral CT scan is generally indicated. Spiral CT scanning is the preferred test in those with abnormal chest x-ray findings due to underlying diseases such as COPD. Algorithms for assessing patients with possible pulmonary embolism utilize testing blood levels of D-dimer. A totally normal D-dimer level in a low-risk patient is strong evidence against a pulmonary embolism. Patients with suspected PE should also have a venous Doppler to rule out DVT.

Patients suspected of having musculoskeletal chest pain might not require any diagnostic testing. Evaluation for GI causes is discussed in Chapter 17.

TREATMENT

Any patient with suspected MI, unstable angina, or PE should be hospitalized for evaluation. Patients who present with MI should be stabilized initially with oxygen, nitroglycerin, and morphine for pain control. Aspirin alone has been shown to reduce the mortality from acute MI by more than 20%, and all patients with suspected MI should receive aspirin as soon as possible. In patients allergic to aspirin, clopidogrel may be used. Other drugs used to treat an acute MI include beta blockers, heparin, nitrates, angiotensin-converting enzyme (ACE) inhibitors, and thrombolytics. Ideally, the systolic blood pressure should be maintained at 100 to 120 mmHg (except in patients with previously severe hypertension) and the heart rate kept at about 60 beats/minute. Thrombolytics should be considered in patients <75 years of age with ST-segment elevation and a history consistent with an acute MI who present within 6 hours of the onset of chest pain. Studies suggest that treatment within 12 hours after the onset of pain may still be beneficial for older patients. Contraindications for thrombolytics include active internal bleeding, history of intracranial hemorrhage, recent surgery, intracranial neoplasm, arteriovenous malformation, aneurysm, bleeding diathesis, or severe uncontrolled hypertension. Percutaneous transluminal coronary angioplasty is emerging as an alternative to thrombolytic therapy in institutions that can provide emergent catheterization. Glycoprotein inhibitors are useful when added to heparin in patients with unstable angina and non-Q-wave infarctions.

Patients with stable angina may be treated in the outpatient setting and started on daily aspirin and sublingual nitroglycerin for anginal episodes. Beta blockers reduce the frequency of symptoms, increase anginal threshold, and reduce the risk of a subsequent MI in patients with a previous MI. Long-acting nitrates reduce anginal pain but do not increase longevity and require a daily nitrate-free period to avoid tolerance. For patients who continue to have angina despite maximal therapy with beta blockers and nitrates, calcium channel blockers, or ranolazine may aid in controlling symptoms. Aggressive treatment of risk factors such as hypertension, inactivity, and lipids is also an important component of long-term management. Guidelines for lipid lowering now target four groups of patients based on the presence of cardiovascular disease, diabetes, LDL-cholesterol >190 mg/dL, and cardiovascular 10-year risk of >7.5% (Box 10-2).

Aortic dissection is an emergency and requires hospitalization and surgical consultation. Pericarditis may improve with aspirin or other NSAIDs. Steroids should be considered in severe cases. PE requires anticoagulation. Warfarin is started concomitantly with heparin; once the international normalized

BOX 10-2. Target Groups for Lipid Lowering with Statins

Risk Factor(s)	Recommended Treatment
LDL-cholesterol ≥ 190 mg/dL	High-intensity statin
Diabetes mellitus and LDL-cholesterol 70–190 mg/dL	CV risk > 7.5%, high-intensity statin CV risk < 7.5% moderate-intensity statin
Known cardiovascular disease	Age < 75 years, high-intensity statin Age > 75 years, moderate-intensity statin
No diabetes or known cardiovascular disease, but cardiovascular risk of 7.5% for event within 10 years (http://www.cvriskcalculator.com/)	Moderate or high-intensity statin
Moderate-intensity statins: Atorvastatin 10–20 mg daily Rosuvastatin 5–10 mg daily Simvastatin 20–40 mg daily Pravastatin 40–80 mg daily	High-intensity statins: Atorvastatin 40–80 mg daily Rosuvastatin 20–40 mg daily

ratio (INR) reaches the therapeutic level, heparin may be discontinued. A smaller pneumothorax (<30%) in a stable individual can be managed conservatively; a larger pneumothorax requires chest tube insertion. Treatment for patients with pneumonia or bronchitis is outlined in Chapter 29. Costochondritis is treated with NSAIDs. The management of chest pain owing to GERD and GI causes is outlined in Chapter 17. Psychogenic disorders are discussed in Chapter 31.

KEY POINTS

- Chest pain can be due to pulmonary, GI, cardiac, musculoskeletal, or psychological causes.
- The most common emergent causes of chest pain include MI, unstable angina, aortic dissection, PE, and pneumothorax.
- Cardiac chest pain that lasts more than 30 minutes is most probably secondary to infarction.
- Beck triad—jugular venous distention, muffled heart sounds, and decreased blood pressure—indicates cardiac tamponade.
- Signs of pneumothorax include hyperresonance to percussion, tracheal deviation, decreased breath sounds, and decreased tactile and vocal fremitus.
- A patient who presents with MI should be stabilized initially with oxygen, nitroglycerin, and morphine for pain control.
- Contraindications to thrombolytics include active internal bleeding, history of cerebrovascular disease, recent surgery, intracranial neoplasm, arteriovenous malformation, aneurysm, bleeding diathesis, and severe uncontrolled hypertension.

11 | Constipation

Constipation is a common complaint in both adults and children. It occurs most often in the young and the elderly. Because most individuals eating an average diet will pass at least three stools per week, a clinically useful definition of constipation is the passage of less than three stools per week. Functional constipation is defined as any two of the following features: straining, lumpy, hard stools, sensation of incomplete evacuation, use of digital maneuvers, sensation of anorectal obstruction or blockage with 25% of bowel movements, and decrease in stool frequency (less than three stools per week).

PATHOGENESIS

Bowel movements depend on stool volume, colonic motility, and patency of the colon's lumen. Defecation involves a complex interaction between the central nervous system and the muscles that increase intra-abdominal pressure, relax the sphincter, and open the canal. Alteration of any one of these components can cause constipation. Anorectal disorders such as anal fissures or thrombosed hemorrhoids can cause constipation because patients may avoid defecation because of pain. Mechanical obstruction—as seen in cancer, strictures, or external compression—is another cause of constipation.

Patients with diminished fluid and fiber intake have decreased stool volume and can experience constipation. Colonic motility can be inhibited by a variety of medical conditions including hypothyroidism, hypercalcemia, hypokalemia, scleroderma, diabetes, and neurologic disorders such as multiple sclerosis, Parkinson disease, and paraplegia. Medications such as calcium channel blockers (e.g., verapamil), narcotics, and anticholinergics inhibit colonic motility. Irritable bowel syndrome (IBS) is characterized by abnormal colonic motility and in some patients causes delayed colonic transit followed by periods of more frequent and looser stools. Constipation is a common problem during pregnancy, thought to be due to increased progesterone, which can slow down the passage of fecal matter through the colon. A sedentary lifestyle or bed rest (e.g., postoperative patients) can also inhibit intestinal movement.

CLINICAL MANIFESTATIONS

HISTORY

Because many patients have misconceptions regarding normal stool patterns, the frequency of bowel movements and consistency of stool must be accurately determined. It is important to inquire about symptoms such as pain with defecation, abdominal distention, gas, nausea, emesis, abdominal discomfort, and the presence of blood in the stool. A dietary history should include questions about the type and quantities of liquid, fruits, vegetables, and fiber as well as any recent change in diet.

Past medical history, previous surgeries, exercise habits or recent immobility, and family history should be elicited. A review of medications, including over-the-counter medications, may identify the underlying cause. The review of systems should include questions about weight loss, fatigue, depression, and anxiety.

Alarm signs and symptoms, such as acute onset (especially in elderly), fever, nausea and/or vomiting, hematochezia, anemia, melena, unintentional weight loss of more than 10 lb, a change in stool caliber, family history of colon cancer, or inflammatory bowel disease, should be specifically noted and further diagnostic testing may be indicated.

PHYSICAL EXAMINATION

The physical examination begins with a general assessment of nutritional status, weight, and vital signs. The thyroid gland should be examined for abnormalities and the skin assessed for pallor or signs of scleroderma. The abdominal examination should note the frequency and pitch of bowel sounds, the presence of any distension or masses, and focal tenderness. The abdomen should be examined for any previous surgical scars. Rectal examination is useful for determining stool consistency, detecting occult blood, and ruling out rectal abnormalities such as fissure, ulcers, masses, or hemorrhoids as well as detecting impaction. A neurologic examination may detect signs of dementia, Parkinson disease, or neuropathy.

DIFFERENTIAL DIAGNOSIS

Box 11-1 lists the differential diagnosis for constipation. Causes can be related to colonic disease, structural abnormalities, anorectal disease, extracolonic disease, medications, diet, and psychological factors. In the outpatient setting, dietary factors (particularly inadequate fiber), medications, IBS, and poor fluid intake are common causes of constipation.

DIAGNOSTIC EVALUATION

The history and physical examination determine the need for further testing. For younger persons with a reasonable explanation for constipation and the absence of alarm symptoms, management can be instituted without further evaluation. Further testing is indicated in cases refractory to treatment, in older adults with new-onset constipation, in cases where the etiology is uncertain, or if the history and clinical evaluation reveal any alarm signs or symptoms. Laboratory evaluation should include a CBC, serum electrolytes, TSH, and calcium level. Anoscopy is helpful if there is concern about anal pathology such as internal hemorrhoids and fissures.

Abdominal x-rays are of limited value unless obstruction or fecal impaction is suspected. Further evaluation using flexible sigmoidoscopy, coupled with a barium enema or colonoscopy, may be necessary to detect strictures, masses, polyps, or diverticular disease. A full colonoscopy is indicated in patients with anemia, weight loss, heme-positive stools, or other situations in which a malignancy

BOX 11-1. Causes of Constipation

Insufficient dietary fiber
Inactivity

Medications
Opiates
Calcium channel blockers
Anticholinergics
Tricyclic antidepressants
Diuretics
Antacids
Clonidine
Levodopa
Laxative abuse

Metabolic Abnormalities
Hypokalemia
Hypercalcemia
Hypothyroidism
Scleroderma
Amyloidosis
Pregnancy

Neurologic Disorders
Parkinson disease
Paraplegia
Prior pelvic surgery
Diabetes mellitus
Irritable bowel syndrome
Hirschsprung disease

GI/Perianal Disorders
Colonic mass
Fissure
Hemorrhoids
Rectocele
Rectal prolapse
Diverticular disease

is suspected. During colonoscopy, biopsies of the mucosa can be performed to rule out amyloidosis, Hirschsprung disease, and cancer. The absence of neurons on a rectal biopsy demonstrates the presence of Hirschsprung disease.

TREATMENT

Disorders causing constipation such as hypothyroidism, bowel obstruction, or anal fissure should be treated accordingly. Some patients may only require education and reassurance that their bowel pattern is normal. In cases of functional constipation, dietary modification is recommended as initial management.

Patients should drink at least eight 8-oz glasses of water daily and consume large amounts of bran, fresh fruit, vegetables, beans, and whole grains. For those with limited fiber intake, dietary fiber should be increased gradually over a 2- to 3-week period in order to minimize adverse effects with a target of consuming 20 to 25 g daily. If possible, medications suspected to be causing or contributing to constipation should be discontinued or changed.

Patients may also benefit from "bowel retraining." Colonic motor activity is more prominent following a meal; therefore, encourage patients to have a bowel movement within the first 2 hours after waking and after breakfast. Specifically, patients should spend 10 to 15 quiet and unhurried minutes each day on the commode. Bowel retraining often requires 2 to 3 weeks to become effective and should become a part of the patient's daily routine.

If these modalities fail to alleviate the patient's symptoms and bowel obstruction has been ruled out, medications may be required. Numerous medications are available to treat constipation and some have significant side effects (Table 11-1). However, with adequate knowledge of the mechanism of action and risks, most medications for constipation can be administered safely.

BULK-FORMING AGENTS

These agents are effective in increasing stool frequency and softening the consistency of stool with minimal side effects.

Bulk-forming agents are high in fiber and increase stool volume by absorbing water. Examples include psyllium (Metamucil), methylcellulose (Citrucel), and polycarbophil (FiberCon). Common side effects include bloating and flatulence; if these agents are not taken with enough water, they may paradoxically worsen constipation.

OSMOTIC LAXATIVES

Osmotic laxatives should be considered in patients not responding to bulking agents.

Osmotic laxatives are nonabsorbable solutes that draw fluid into the intestinal lumen by creating an osmotic gradient. Examples include lactulose, magnesium salts (milk of magnesia), and polyethylene glycol (MiraLax). Side effects include bloating, increasing flatulence, and abdominal cramping. Magnesium salts are contraindicated in patients with renal failure.

STIMULANT AGENTS

Stimulants work by altering mucosal permeability and stimulating the activity of intestinal smooth muscle. Examples include phenolphthalein (Ex-Lax) and bisacodyl (Dulcolax). Chronic abuse of these may

TABLE 11-1. Medications for Constipation	
Medications with Adult Dosage	**Side Effects**
Bulk agents	
Psyllium (Metamucil), 1 tablespoon qd to tid	Bloating, impaction
Methylcellulose (Citrucel), 1–3 tablespoons qd	Fluid overload, impaction
Calcium polycarbophil (FiberCon), 1 tablet qd to tid	Fluid overload, impaction
Softeners	
Docusate sodium (Colace), 1–2 capsules qd	Skin rashes, hepatotoxicity
Stimulants	
Bisacodyl (Dulcolax), 1–2 tablets or suppositories qd	Gastric or rectal irritation
Senna (Senokot), 1–3 teaspoons, 2–3 tablets qd	Degeneration of myoneural plexuses
Senna/docusate (Peri-Colace), 1–2 tablets qd	Degeneration of myoneural plexuses, skin rashes, hepatotoxicity
Osmotics	
Lactulose (Cephulac), 1–2 tablespoons qd	Bloating
Magnesium (milk of magnesia, magnesium citrate)	Magnesium toxicity (with renal failure)
Polyethylene glycol, 17 g po qd	Bloating, cramping, increased flatulence

po, orally; qd, every day; qhs, every night; tid, three times daily.

lead to melanosis coli and constipation secondary to enteric nervous system damage. Another stimulant, senna, used in combination with fiber, has been found to improve stool consistency, frequency, and ease of stool passage in the geriatric population.

STOOL SOFTENERS

Stool softeners, suppositories, and enemas are used widely but have limited clinical efficacy.

Docusate sodium (Colace), a commonly prescribed stool softener, is often used for patients complaining of hard stools that are difficult to pass. It decreases surface tension and allows water and fat to mix in the stool. To work optimally, stool softeners must be taken with plenty of fluid.

ENEMAS AND SUPPOSITORIES

Warm tap-water enemas and suppositories work by distending and stimulating the rectum, which then leads to evacuation. These are primarily used only for persistent constipation in older adults and are especially useful in bedridden patients and those with stool impaction. Adverse effects include rectal mucosal damage. In patients with severe idiopathic constipation, surgeries such as hemicolectomy with ileorectal anastomosis may be a last resort.

KEY POINTS

- Constipation is commonly defined as less than three stools per week.
- Poor fluid intake and a lack of fiber are common causes of constipation in the primary care setting.
- A minimum daily fiber intake of 20 to 25 g/day is recommended for treatment and prevention of constipation.
- Patients should be advised to defecate after meals, taking advantage of increased colonic motility.

- Indications for laboratory testing include refractory constipation, recent onset of constipation in an older individual, heme-positive stools, and situations in which the etiology is unclear or the clinical evaluation suggests underlying pathology.
- Laxative use should be in the following order: bulk laxatives (if not responsive to lifestyle and dietary modifications), then use of osmotic laxatives (lactulose, sorbitol), followed by stool softeners and suppositories (glycerin, bisacodyl).

12 | Cough

Cough is among the most common complaints in family practice. It is defined as a sudden reflex expulsion of air from the glottis in an attempt to clear the airways of secretions and inhaled particles. This maneuver helps protect the lungs against aspiration and harmful irritants. Common causes of cough include viral or bacterial infections of the upper respiratory tract, irritant exposure, allergies, COPD, cancer, cardiac diseases, asthma, and psychological factors.

PATHOGENESIS

Ciliated pseudostratified columnar epithelium and mucus-producing goblet cells line the trachea and bronchi. These two types of cells are responsible for filtering particles in inspired air. Certain irritants and viral infections can damage the cilia lining of the airways, impairing the filtering process, and allowing microscopic particles to reach the lungs. These particles and thermal or chemical stimulants may irritate afferent receptors in the airways and trigger the cough reflex. The cough reflex is a complex interaction mediated peripherally by the vagus, trigeminal, glossopharyngeal, and phrenic nerves. The cough center is located in the medulla.

With upper respiratory tract infections (URIs), inflammation and increased mucous secretions stimulate the cough receptors in the upper airway. Common viral causes of infection include influenza, parainfluenza, adenovirus, respiratory syncytial virus, and rhinovirus. Bacterial causes include *Streptococcus pneumoniae*, *Mycoplasma pneumoniae*, and *Haemophilus influenzae*. A chronic cough is also a common presenting complaint in tuberculosis (TB) and cancer. The most common irritant associated with cough is cigarette smoke. Cancers and foreign bodies elicit the cough reflex by direct stimulation.

CLINICAL MANIFESTATIONS

HISTORY

A complete history of cough should include the timing, quality, associated symptoms, past medical history, smoking history, and medications. Knowing when the cough started is essential, because a chronic cough is defined as lasting more than 8 weeks. Patients who have a seasonal pattern may have a cough secondary to allergic rhinitis. Nocturnal coughing may indicate asthma, GERD, postnasal drip, or CHF. If symptoms occur with meals, aspiration should be considered. Exercise- or cold-induced cough indicates asthma. Cough and dyspnea on exertion suggest a cardiac etiology.

The quality of the cough is also important. A productive cough can be seen in infections such as bronchitis and pneumonia. A dry cough is common in postnasal drip and asthma. Furthermore, patients with postnasal drip feel an itching sensation in the throat and therefore, cough in an attempt to clear the throat. Hemoptysis is often seen in TB and cancer, and the acute onset of chest pain, dyspnea, tachycardia, and hemoptysis suggests a pulmonary embolus.

Patients should also be asked about other symptoms such as fever, chills, night sweats, weight loss, and hoarseness. Patients with weight loss and a chronic cough should be investigated for cancer.

Patients who present with cough and a medical history of CHF may have worsening CHF. Weight gain, due to fluid retention, may be an associated symptom. Postnasal drip is a common cause of cough in patients with allergies or a recent URI.

Certain medications, such as an ACE inhibitor, may cause a chronic nonproductive cough. In patients with asthma, beta blockers may exacerbate the asthma and cause a cough. Chronic use of nitrofurantoin can cause a cough secondary to interstitial fibrosis.

PHYSICAL EXAMINATION

The physical examination should focus on the ears, nose, throat, neck, and chest. Ears plugged with cerumen can result in a reflex cough (Arnold reflex). Patients with allergies often have a pale, boggy nasal mucosa with swollen turbinates. A purulent discharge from the nose may indicate sinusitis. In pharyngitis, the tonsils appear swollen and hyperemic. The posterior pharynx should be checked for increased secretions, which are often seen in patients with postnasal drip. Palpable cervical lymph nodes support the diagnosis of an infectious cause. During the chest examination, close attention should be paid to the lung and heart sounds. Murmurs and an S3 or gallop suggest a possible cardiac cause. Crackles may indicate an inflammatory process or worsening CHF. Diminished or bronchial breath sounds can occur with pneumonia. Wheezing may be heard with foreign body aspiration, CHF, COPD, or asthma.

DIFFERENTIAL DIAGNOSIS

The common causes of cough include URIs, irritants, allergies, asthma, COPD, cancer, and GERD. Viral infections, the most common cause of acute cough, occur more frequently in the winter months. Following a viral infection of the respiratory tract, a cough may persist for up to 8 weeks. Bacterial infections of the respiratory tract are also common causes of acute cough; they include sinusitis, pharyngitis, bronchitis, and pneumonia (Fig. 12-1). Cigarette smokers often have a chronic cough because of chronic irritant exposure. However, cancer should be ruled out in smokers with a persistent cough. Allergies may present with a chronic cough, usually due to a postnasal drip. A child who presents with a chronic cough lasting more than 8 weeks should be suspected of having asthma and/or allergies. Typically, the cough seen in asthma is dry and may worsen at night or after exercise. Cold air may also exacerbate a cough due to asthma. Patients with COPD or bronchiectasis may present with a chronic cough.

In individuals presenting with weight loss, night sweats, hemoptysis, and chronic cough, lung cancer or TB should be considered. GERD can cause a cough that is worsened by lying down; this may be associated with substernal burning or a sour taste in the mouth. Patients who cough when eating should be evaluated for aspiration. Individuals with an acute cough, dyspnea, and a swollen leg should be evaluated for possible PE. Certain medications such as ACE inhibitors, amiodarone, and nitrofurantoin can cause a dry cough. Finally, psychogenic cough may be a possibility. However, all the organic causes should be ruled out before this disorder is diagnosed.

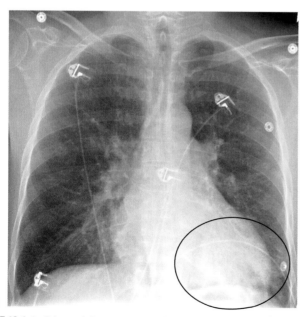
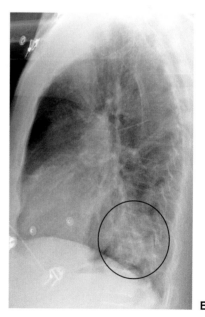

FIGURE 12-1. Left lower lobe pneumonia (encircled areas represent identified areas of infiltrate). (**A**) Posterior-anterior (PA) view of the chest x-ray (CXR). (**B**) Left lateral view of the CXR. (From Collins J, Stern EJ. *Chest Radiology: The Essentials*. 3rd ed. Philadelphia, PA: Lippincott Williams & Wilkins, 2015.)

DIAGNOSTIC EVALUATION

The diagnostic approach to cough begins with a good history and physical examination (Fig. 12-2). When viral infections of the respiratory tract are suspected, no further workup is necessary as long as the cough resolves in 6 to 8 weeks. If sinusitis is suspected, a patient may be started on antibiotics and monitored for resolution of the symptoms. If a cough is due to the use of an ACE inhibitor, discontinuing it should result in improvement within 4 weeks.

A CXR is necessary in most patients without an upper airway abnormality who have a new cough, persistent cough, or hemoptysis. The CXR can detect pulmonary infections, masses, pleural effusion, CHF, interstitial lung disease, bronchiectasis, and hilar lymphadenopathy. While not diagnostic, a CXR may show changes consistent with COPD. The CXR may be normal in some patients with neoplasm, pulmonary embolus, and sinus disease. If these diseases are suspected, further testing with CT scanning, bronchoscopy, a ventilation/perfusion (V/Q) scan, or an echocardiogram is indicated.

In immunocompetent patients with a persistent cough and a normal CXR, occult bronchospasm, allergies, GERD, or a combination of these are the most likely causes. Spirometry or an empiric trial of bronchodilator therapy may be helpful. Rarely, patients may require a methacholine challenge or postexercise spirometry to confirm the diagnosis of asthma. In patients with symptoms of reflux or for those who fail therapy for bronchospasm, empiric treatment for GERD or an upper-GI series may be helpful. Chronic cough that remains undiagnosed and persists despite therapy merits consultation.

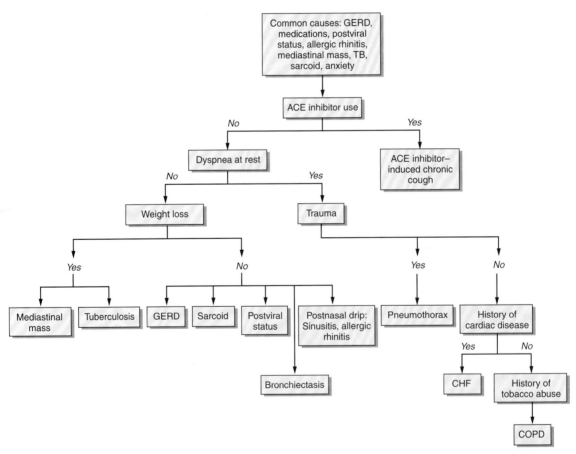

FIGURE 12-2. Chronic cough algorithm. ACE, angiotensin-converting enzyme; CHF, congestive heart failure; COPD, chronic obstructive pulmonary disease; GERD, gastroesophageal reflux disease; TB, tuberculosis. (From Domino FJ, Baldor RA, Grimes JA, et al. *The 5-Minute Clinical Consult Standard 2015.* 23rd ed. Alphen aan den Rijn, The Netherlands: Wolters Kluwer; 2014.)

TREATMENT

Cough is a symptom; therefore, treatment should focus on the underlying disease process as outlined in the respective chapters of this book. For example, treatment of GERD, elimination of an irritant such as smoking or passive exposure to smoke, bronchodilator therapy, or discontinuation of an ACE inhibitor would be appropriate. However, if the cough is significant enough that the patient seeks medical attention, symptomatic treatment with an antitussive may be warranted. For example, the postinfectious cough from a viral illness may last up to 8 weeks, and cough suppression may provide some symptom relief. Antitussive medications may be classified as either centrally or peripherally acting medications. Centrally acting drugs include codeine and dextromethorphan. Codeine is a narcotic that binds to the opiate receptors and suppresses the medullary cough center. Sedation is a common side effect. Dextromethorphan, a nonnarcotic centrally acting agent, is available in many over-the-counter (OTC) preparations. Although both codeine and dextromethorphan are commonly used, studies examining their effectiveness are often of poor quality and demonstrate conflicting results. In children younger than 2 years, treatment trials have not established their benefit and serious side effects may occur. In 2008, the U.S. Food and Drug Authority recommended against the use of OTC cough preparations in children younger than 2 years and advised caution in prescribing to older children. For an acute cough due to a common cold, a first-generation antihistamine plus a decongestant offers some modest decrease in the severity of cough. Studies have shown that gabapentin or the anti-inflammatory drug naproxen may also favorably affect cough.

Peripherally acting drugs such as benzonatate anesthetize the respiratory passages and the pleural stretch receptors, but are of questionable value. Mucolytic agents (guaifenesin) and fluids increase the volume and decrease the viscosity of secretions, which may help clear secretions from the respiratory tract more easily.

KEY POINTS

- In immunocompetent patients with a persistent cough and a normal CXR, occult bronchospasm, allergies, GERD, or a combination of these are the most likely diagnoses.

- Postnasal drip is a common cause of cough in patients with allergies or a recent viral infection of the upper respiratory tract.
- Centrally acting antitussive medications include codeine and dextromethorphan.

13 | Diarrhea

Diarrhea is defined as an increase in stool weight to more than 200 g/day. Clinically, diarrhea is defined as the passage of more than three abnormally loose stools per 24 hours. Acute diarrhea lasts <3 weeks, whereas chronic diarrhea is a persistent or recurring condition that lasts >3 weeks.

PATHOGENESIS

Fluid balance in the GI system represents a dynamic flux between absorption and secretion. Conditions that either increase fluid secretion or decrease absorption lead to diarrhea. Inflammation, hormones, or enterotoxins may trigger increased fluid secretion. A functional or anatomic decrease in the absorptive capacity of the bowel may cause diarrhea. Osmotically active solutes that retain fluid in the intestinal lumen may also increase stool volume. Altered bowel motility can impair absorption, either by decreasing the contact time of intestinal contents with the bowel mucosa or preventing the effective mixing of intestinal contents. Although the basic mechanisms of diarrhea are straightforward, more than one mechanism may contribute to diarrhea in a patient. For example, in a patient with Crohn disease, an abnormal ileum may cause decreased fluid absorption and increased secretion due to diffuse inflammation.

CLINICAL MANIFESTATIONS

HISTORY

Acute diarrhea has two common clinical presentations: either a watery, noninflammatory diarrhea or an inflammatory diarrhea with the presence of either blood or white blood cells (WBCs) in the stool. Symptoms may be mild, with no change in the patient's level of physical activity; moderate, with some limitation in physical activity; or severe, where patients are confined to bed.

It is important to ask patients with acute diarrhea about exposure to others with similar symptoms, recent travel, and whether they are taking antibiotics or other medications. A diet history is important, because excessive caffeine or alcohol intake and sorbitol-containing foods can all cause transient diarrhea. Overindulgence in milk or milk products in a lactose-intolerant individual can cause bloating, cramps, and diarrhea. Antibiotic use within 2 weeks suggests that diarrhea may be caused by either an alteration in bowel flora or a *Clostridium difficile* infection. Severe abdominal pain in an elderly individual accompanied by acute diarrhea suggests the possibility of ischemic colitis.

Watery stools accompanied by a low-grade fever, headache, and nausea or vomiting and achiness are consistent with a viral gastroenteritis. Traveler's diarrhea, due to toxigenic *Escherichia coli*, presents similarly to viral gastroenteritis. Bacterial infections—such as those due to *Shigella*, *Salmonella*, and *Campylobacter*—present with a prodrome of fever, headache, anorexia, fatigue, and stools that may initially be watery before becoming bloody. Salmonellosis is usually a self-limited infection acquired by ingesting contaminated poultry or eggs. *Campylobacter* infection is more common than either Shigellosis or salmonellosis and is usually acquired from ingesting contaminated poultry. *E. coli* O157:H7 accounts for up to one-third of cases of bloody diarrhea. Its presentation ranges from mild, crampy, watery diarrhea to life-threatening hemorrhagic colitis complicated by hemolytic uremic syndrome or thrombocytopenic purpura.

Diarrhea from food poisoning usually occurs several hours after eating contaminated food. Illness in several individuals exposed to a common food source and an absence of other associated symptoms are characteristic findings. *Staphylococcus aureus* commonly contaminates custard-filled pastries, whereas *Clostridium perfringens* is especially common in foods warmed on a steam table.

Chronic diarrhea can be either persistent or recurrent. Irritable Bowel Syndrome (IBS) typically affects young or middle-aged adults, with a 2:1 female-to-male predominance. It can present as diarrhea alternating with constipation or chronic recurring diarrhea. Other symptoms include abdominal pain relieved by defecation, fecal urgency, bloating, the need to strain to pass stool, and occasionally having a small amount of mucus in the stool. This condition may wax or wane over years. Any rectal bleeding that occurs in patients with IBS is usually due to anal trauma from passing a hard stool. In the active phase of an inflammatory bowel disease (IBD), a collective term for ulcerative colitis and Crohn disease, diarrhea is associated with abdominal pain, bloody stools, and fever. Extraintestinal manifestations include arthritis, liver disease, uveitis, and skin lesions. Flushing and wheezing associated with persistent diarrhea suggests carcinoid syndrome as a cause. Foul, greasy, and bulky stools characterize malabsorption syndromes causing diarrhea. Associated symptoms such as weight loss or neuropathy may result from malabsorption.

Giardiasis, amebiasis, and *C. difficile* can present with acute, intermittent, or chronic symptoms. *Giardia* is the leading cause of parasitic diarrhea. The organism is endemic to areas such as the Rocky Mountains and Russia. However, no natural water(e.g., river or lake) supply in North America should be considered free of giardia. It is also common in areas such as third-world countries where the water supply may be contaminated.

PHYSICAL EXAMINATION

Generally, the physical examination is more helpful for assessing the severity of the disease than determining a specific cause. Vital signs should be checked and the patient assessed for indications of significant dehydration, such as dry mucous membranes, tachycardia, and orthostatic changes in blood pressure and pulse. The abdomen should be carefully examined and a rectal examination performed, checking for occult blood.

DIFFERENTIAL DIAGNOSIS

Viral gastroenteritis is the most common cause of acute diarrhea. Rotavirus is the most common virus in children, whereas the Norwalk virus is

BOX 13-1. Common Medications Associated with Diarrhea

Alpha-glycoside inhibitors (e.g., acarbose)
Antacids
Antidepressants (SSRIs)
Antibiotics
Colchicine
Lactulose
Laxatives
Loop diuretics
Protein pump inhibitors
Quinidine
Theophylline
Thyroxine

most common in adults. Food poisoning from staphylococcal toxins, clostridial toxins, and the ingestion of *Campylobacter*, *Salmonella*, *Shigella*, and enteropathogenic *E. coli* are common bacterial causes of diarrhea. Parasites such as *Giardia* and amebiasis are less frequent causes of diarrhea in the United States. Traveler's diarrhea is usually due to *E. coli* but can be caused by other bacterial diseases. Dietary indiscretion, alcohol, caffeine, and drug side effects are common noninfectious causes (Box 13-1). In the outpatient setting, the most common causes for persistent diarrhea are IBS, IBD, lactose intolerance, and chronic or relapsing GI infections such as giardiasis, amebiasis, and *C. difficile*.

Microscopic colitis is increasingly becoming recognized as a relatively common and important cause of chronic intermittent watery diarrhea in middle-aged and elderly adults. It consists of two separate but related diseases, collagenous colitis and lymphocytic colitis, which are similar clinically but differ in histologic appearance.

Celiac disease or gluten-sensitive enteropathy is another relatively common disorder, affecting about 0.5% to 1% of the population. It is a chronic disorder in which ingesting gluten damages the small intestinal mucosa in genetically susceptible individuals. Although increasing awareness of the disease and better screening tests have led to more individuals being diagnosed, it is still under-recognized. Classically, patients experience diarrhea, malabsorption, and weight loss. The diagnosis is confirmed by observing typical mucosal changes on biopsy, which then improve following gluten restriction. Box 13.2 lists causes of chronic diarrhea.

BOX 13-2. Causes of Chronic Diarrhea

Increased Secretion
Clostridium toxin
Cholera toxin
Noninvasive microbial gastroenteritis (e.g., viral gastroenteritis, *Campylobacter*)
Carcinoid syndrome
Vasoactive intestinal peptide secreting tumors
Villous adenoma

Increased Osmotic Load
Sorbitol ingestion (dietetic candy)
Bile salt malabsorption
Pancreatic insufficiency
Lactose intolerance
Malabsorption
Postgastrectomy syndrome
Magnesium containing laxatives

Inflammation
Ulcerative colitis
Crohn disease
Radiation-induced colitis
Invasive microbial gastroenteritis (e.g., *Shigella*)

Altered Motility
Thyrotoxicosis
Irritable bowel syndrome
Autonomic neuropathy (e.g., diabetic associated enteropathy)

DIAGNOSTIC EVALUATION

Most cases of acute diarrhea are self-limited, and diagnostic tests are usually not indicated. Signs of more severe disease—such as significant dehydration, more than six stools per 24 hours, bloody stools, high temperatures, severe abdominal pain, and failure to improve after 48 to 72 hours—suggest a need for a more detailed evaluation. The threshold for evaluating immunocompromised or elderly individuals should be lower.

Examination of a stool specimen for leukocytes and occult blood is a useful first test in patients with acute diarrhea. A stool specimen with less than three to four WBCs per high-power field (HPF) usually indicates a noninflammatory, self-limited process. If there is blood in the stools or an inflammatory process is suspected, a stool culture should be sent and an assay for *C. difficile* toxin ordered for those patients with recent antibiotic exposure. The acute onset of bloody stools merits

testing for Shiga toxin, along with cultures specifically for *E. coli* O157:H7. Patients at risk for *Giardia* or other parasitic infections—such as those who have traveled to a high-risk area (e.g., tropical Africa, Asia, or Latin America), attend day care, are HIV-positive, or have had possible exposure to contaminated water—should have their stools evaluated for ova and parasites.

The diagnostic evaluation for chronic diarrhea should be individualized. The history should help focus the approach (Figure 13-1). Box 13-3 lists signs suggestive of a serious underlying disorder. For patients whose history and PE suggest a benign illness, only a limited evaluation is needed. For example, a patient with suspected lactose intolerance who responds to a lactose-free diet needs no further testing. About 5% of cases of chronic diarrhea are due to medications, and no further evaluation is needed in individuals who respond to either stopping or decreasing a medication known to cause diarrhea. For patients with chronic diarrhea whose cause is not readily apparent, an initial evaluation may consist of a CBC, ESR, and checking stools for occult blood, leukocytes, ova, and parasites, as well as an assay for *C. difficile* toxin for patients with recent antibiotic exposure. Tissue transglutaminase (tTG) antibody and endomysial antibody (EMA) are blood tests that screen for celiac disease and have replaced the antigliaden antibody test because of its poor sensitivity and specificity. A Sudan stain can detect the presence of excess stool fat in patients with suspected malabsorption.

For patients with associated left-lower-quadrant pain or bloody diarrhea, a sigmoidoscopy is indicated; this procedure can detect mucosal ulcerations, friability, and masses. Suspected IBD may be confirmed by biopsy. A biopsy can also detect less common diseases, such as amyloidosis and microscopic colitis, where the colon can appear normal both visually and radiographically. In individuals with suspected

BOX 13-3. Symptoms Suggestive of a Serious Underlying Etiology for Diarrhea

New onset in patients aged >40 years
Nocturnal symptoms
Aggressive course
Weight loss
Rectal fissures
Anemia
Elevated erythrocyte sedimentation rate

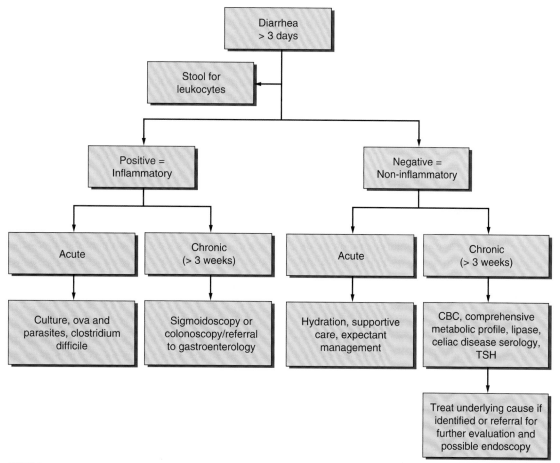

FIGURE 13-1. Basic approach to evaluation of diarrhea. CBC, complete blood count; TSH, thyroid-stimulating hormone.

IBS, a limited evaluation, including sigmoidoscopy, may be sufficient to exclude more serious disorders. Often patients with chronic diarrhea of unclear etiology or suspected IBD may need referral to a gastroenterologist for evaluation.

TREATMENT

Most patients with acute diarrhea can be managed with an alteration in diet and fluid therapy. Oral rehydration is sufficient unless the patient is severely dehydrated. Commercial rehydration solutions, such as Pedialyte or Rice-Lyte, designed to replace fluids and electrolytes, are most commonly used for infants and children. Sports drinks, fruit drinks, and flat soft drinks supplemented with crackers, soup, or bland foods are usually adequate for treating older children and adults.

Boiled starches such as rice, noodles, or potatoes and avoiding milk products or caffeine-containing foods are usually recommended for patients with acute diarrhea. For children, a BRAT diet (*b*ananas, *r*ice, *a*pplesauce, and *t*oast) is traditionally used despite limited evidence demonstrating its efficacy. Preparations containing kaolin and pectate are available OTC but are of uncertain value. Bismuth subsalicylate (Pepto-Bismol) is also used for diarrhea and may have an antisecretory effect. The antimotility drugs such as loperamide are considered the drugs of choice for nonspecific treatment. They should not be used in febrile patients with inflammatory or infectious diarrhea.

Specific management depends on the cause of the diarrhea. The decision to use antibiotics in patients with bacterial diarrhea depends on the infective organism, health of the individual, and systemic symptoms. All cases of Shigella should be treated with a fluoroquinolone or, if the organism is sensitive, with trimethoprim/sulfamethoxazole (TMP/SMX). *Salmonella* infections causing mild to moderate symptoms should generally not be treated because antibiotics may prolong the carrier state. Patients with salmonellosis who have severe symptoms or those at risk for bacteremia (immunocompromised individuals or elderly patients) should be treated with a fluoroquinolone.

If symptoms are still present when the culture results become available, erythromycin or a fluoroquinolone shortens the duration of a *Campylobacter* infection. Invasive *E. coli* with bloody diarrhea should be treated with a fluoroquinolone or TMP/SMX. Traveler's diarrhea due to toxigenic *E. coli* responds to a short course of a fluoroquinolone or TMP/SMX. Azithromycin is the antibiotic of choice for traveler's diarrhea among children and pregnant women and for areas in which quinolone-resistant campylobacter is endemic.

C. difficile infections should be treated with metronidazole (an alternative is oral vancomycin). *Giardia* is treated with metronidazole.

For lactose-intolerant patients, a 1- to 2-week trial of a lactose-free diet is usually sufficient to decrease symptoms. Lactase-containing capsules taken orally before consuming dairy products are also effective. Antimotility agents such as loperamide may provide relief for IBS patients with significant diarrhea. Antispasmodics, such as dicyclomine, can benefit patients with crampy abdominal pain, and antidepressants have been shown to relieve pain and may be effective in low doses. Alosetron and eluxadoline are indicated for women with severe diarrhea-dominant disease, and lubiprostone and linaclotide are indicated for those with constipation as the dominant symptom. A high-fiber diet and/or a psyllium fiber supplement (e.g., Metamucil) may be helpful for IBS patients with alternating diarrhea and constipation.

Management goals for IBD are to control active disease, monitor stool frequency and amount, detect complications, and refer for surgery when appropriate. Commonly used medications are sulfasalazine and corticosteroids. Other medications include cyclosporine and tumor necrosis factor (TNF) or integrin inhibitors (e.g., infliximab, natalizumab). Patients are generally managed conjointly with a gastroenterologist.

Microscopic colitis is usually treated stepwise, first with nonspecific therapy followed by bismuth and either cholestyramine or 5-aminosalicylic acid. Budesonide is indicated for those not responding to these initial therapies, and cases resistant to budesonide may require oral corticosteroids or immune modifiers. Similar to IBD, patients are generally managed conjointly with a gastroenterologist.

Celiac disease responds to diet, and patients should be referred to a dietician knowledgeable about gluten-free diets.

KEY POINTS

- Most cases of diarrhea are due to infectious agents, particularly viruses.
- A bacterial infection, IBD, ischemic colitis, or malignancy can all cause bloody diarrhea.
- The most common viral pathogens causing diarrhea are the Norwalk virus, rotavirus, and enterovirus.
- Fluoroquinolones are active against *Salmonella*, *Shigella*, and *E. coli*.

14 | Dizziness/Vertigo

Dizziness, or vertigo, is a vague symptom often described by patients as a sensation of abnormal movement (either motion of self or motion of the environment spinning around them). Many underlying conditions present with this symptom, and a careful history is critical to differentiate true vertigo from other causes of dizziness.

PATHOGENESIS

Patients who experience true vertigo have a problem affecting either the peripheral or the central vestibular systems.

The peripheral vestibular apparatus is located bilaterally in the semicircular canals. Vertigo can occur when this apparatus is subjected to inflammation, stimulation, or destruction of the hair cells of the eighth cranial nerve. For example, in benign positional vertigo (BPV), particulate matter or otoliths form in the semicircular canal (analogous to renal stone formation). When these otoliths become dislodged and stimulate the sensory hair cells in the semicircular canals, vertigo results. Other causes of vestibular dysfunction that can cause vertigo include acute labyrinthitis, vestibular neuronitis, and viral infection of the semicircular apparatus. Ménière disease, a condition of undetermined etiology, occurs when endolymphatic hydrops results in increased pressure within the semicircular canals and damage to the sensory hair cells. Finally, direct damage to the eighth cranial nerve may result from ototoxic medications or from an acoustic neuroma. An acoustic neuroma is a tumor (schwannoma) of the eighth cranial nerve that gradually grows and compresses the eighth cranial nerve and eventually the brainstem.

Vertigo may result from central vestibular pathway dysfunction because of vascular insufficiency or hemorrhage, demyelination, brain tumors, or medications. Centrally, the vestibular pathways are located in the brainstem that communicate and coordinate position with the cerebellum and cerebral cortex. Typically, patients with central vertigo have other brainstem or cranial nerve findings in association with the vertigo. Vertigo may occur in association with migraine as a result of vascular spasm in the vertebrobasilar artery system. Multiple sclerosis (MS) is a demyelinating disease that may affect the brainstem and disrupt the vestibular pathways. Finally, medications may affect the brainstem nuclei or cranial nerve eight, causing vertigo.

CLINICAL MANIFESTATIONS

HISTORY

The patient's description of what they mean by dizziness is the most important initial step and helps distinguish vertigo from dizziness. True vertigo is suggested when the patient uses terms such as "spinning," "weaving," or "rocking" to describe the sensation. Vertigo is frequently associated with head movements, can occur both in the supine or upright position, and is often accompanied by nausea and vomiting. In contrast, symptoms that occur only with change in position from the supine to upright positions suggest dizziness and not vertigo caused by problems such as dehydration or anemia.

Medical history should note prior occurrence of similar symptoms, the presence of other medical diseases, and medication use. Some characteristic associations in the patient's presentation and history:

- BPV generally occurs as an isolated symptom and is short-lived, recurrent, and associated with particular head movements. BPV recurs in up to 30% of patients in 2 to 3 years following an episode.

- Ménière disease usually presents with the cardinal features of vertigo, tinnitus, and hearing loss. The vertigo and hearing loss may initially present as fluctuating symptoms, and can last from 30 minutes to 12 hours. If untreated, the hearing loss may become permanent.
- Vestibular neuritis is a viral illness that causes vertigo. When accompanied by hearing loss, it is called labyrinthitis. However, the nomenclature for vestibular disease is ill defined and terms such as "vestibular neuronitis," "neurolabyrinthitis," and "unilateral vestibulopathy" are often used interchangeably. Vertigo in association with a viral illness generally resolves in 2 to 10 days.

The presence of other cranial nerve symptoms, cerebral, or cerebellar neurologic symptoms suggests vertebrobasilar insufficiency, neoplasm, stroke, MS, or acoustic neuroma as a cause.

- Medication side effect: Loop diuretics and aminoglycoside antibiotics are drugs associated with vertigo from damage to the eighth cranial nerve. Phenytoin may affect the brainstem nuclei. Diuretics and antihypertensive medications may lead to orthostatic symptoms through volume depletion or blood pressure–lowering effects. High-dose salicylates may also cause vertigo.
- Vertebrobasilar insufficiency may present acutely as a transient ischemic attack or stroke. Patients usually have a history of hypertension or smoking (increasing risk for atherosclerosis and subsequently vertebrobasilar insufficiency).
- Vertigo with MS may present as a flare of the underlying disease. MS patients typically have symptoms that wax and wane with disease activity, but usually have other symptoms in association with vertigo.
- Acoustic neuromas generally have an insidious onset and slowly progressive symptoms including vertigo, tinnitus, and hearing loss.

PHYSICAL EXAMINATION

The physical examination should include neurologic examination, assessment of orthostatic blood pressure, and cardiovascular examination. Carotid bruits should be noted. The neurologic examination should include a hearing assessment and examination of the cranial nerves. Hearing loss suggests a peripheral cause, whereas brainstem abnormalities (ataxic gait, double vision, vomiting, slurred speech, and incoordination) suggest a central process. The presence and direction of nystagmus should be noted. Bidirectional or vertical nystagmus and nystagmus lasting >1 minute suggests a brainstem origin for the vertigo. Nystagmus <1 minute duration and fatiguing with repetition suggest a peripheral cause. Provocative maneuvers for the symptoms should be included in the examination. For example, true vertigo is brought on by head movement and by the Barany (Dix-Hallpike) maneuver (Fig. 14-1). During the Barany maneuver, the patient is seated with the head turned to the right and is quickly lowered to the supine position with the head over the edge of the examination table 45 degrees below horizontal. The test is then repeated with the head turned to the left. The test is positive if symptoms are reproduced with an 80% sensitivity for BPV. Nystagmus is also typically seen during this maneuver. Orthostatic positional changes that bring on symptoms suggest dehydration, anemia, or cardiac causes. Symptoms brought on by hyperventilation suggest anxiety or other psychogenic causes.

DIFFERENTIAL DIAGNOSIS

True vertigo is due to either central or peripheral vestibular disease and has a narrower differential diagnosis. In assessing for central versus peripheral causes of vertigo, important distinguishing features are the presence of isolated vertigo with or without hearing loss, which suggests peripheral disease, and associated brainstem or other neurologic symptoms, which suggest a central disease (Box 14-1). Of note, dizziness in the elderly is usually multifactorial in its etiology (including vertigo, physical deconditioning, polypharmacy, cardiovascular disease, visual difficulties, vasovagal, and hypoglycemia); making it important to obtain an accurate medication history and review of systems to ensure complete assessment.

DIAGNOSTIC EVALUATION

The history and physical examination direct any further evaluation and the treatment approach. For those patients in whom the diagnosis is unclear or if it is uncertain whether the vertigo is central

BOX 14-1. Differential Diagnosis for Vertigo

Peripheral Vestibular Disease
Benign positional vertigo
Acute labyrinthitis
Vestibular neuronitis
Ménière disease
Acoustic neuroma

Central Vestibular Disease
Vertebrobasilar insufficiency or hemorrhage
Multiple sclerosis
Brain tumor (e.g., glioblastoma or metastatic disease)

Other Medical Diseases
Cerebellar disease (e.g., degeneration, infarcts)
Peripheral neuropathy (e.g., diabetic)
Ophthalmologic disease (e.g., cataracts, macular degeneration)
Hypoglycemia
Psychiatric disease (e.g., panic disorder, anxiety)

Polypharmacy

or peripheral, further testing with electronystagmography and audiometry may be helpful. Audiometry is useful for diagnosing Ménière disease (low-frequency hearing loss) and may suggest the need for further evaluation for acoustic neuroma (asymmetric hearing loss).

Additional testing helpful in evaluating central causes of vertigo and to identify acoustic neuromas include magnetic resonance imaging (MRI) and brainstem auditory evoked response (BAER) testing. MRI may reveal scattered areas of demyelination, suggesting MS, or may show evidence of prior stroke or masses, suggesting vertebrobasilar insufficiency or brain tumors as causes. BAER testing can distinguish cochlear from retrocochlear hearing loss, thus helping to distinguish peripheral disease from more central disease. To identify posterior circulation atherosclerotic disease, magnetic resonance angiography (MRA) can be performed.

TREATMENT

Treatment of vertigo is differentiated by treatment directed at the underlying cause and treatment focused on symptom management. When a central cause is suspected, aggressive evaluation and therapy directed at the underlying disease are warranted. Peripheral causes of vertigo are usually acute and self-limited, although empiric therapy often helps control symptoms. Medications used to treat labyrinthitis, vestibular neuronitis, and BPV include antihistamines (meclizine), dimenhydrinate, antiemetics (prochlorperazine and metoclopramide), and benzodiazepines (e.g., lorazepam). These medications do not treat the underlying cause but may reduce symptoms. Drowsiness is their primary side effect. Follow-up is essential to assure resolution of symptoms and assess the need for further workup.

Other treatments include the Epley maneuver for BPV, which is performed by rotating the patients through a series of positions in an attempt to relocate the debris in the semicircular canal into the vestibule of the labyrinth (Fig. 14-1). It has a success rate approaching 80%. Vestibular exercises wherein a patient performs a Barany maneuver to reproduce his or her symptoms and holds the position until the symptoms are extinguished are also useful. This exercise is repeated several times daily and the time to extinction of symptoms should progressively grow shorter with an increasing performance of the exercise.

Ménière disease is a chronic condition that can lead to permanent hearing loss. These patients require chronic therapy directed at the underlying disease, not just symptomatic therapy. Diuretics, in particular acetazolamide or hydrochlorothiazide, have been found to be helpful in managing Ménière disease. Salt restriction is also considered an important adjunct to the use of diuretics.

Vertigo associated with central vestibular disease is also often chronic. Vestibular exercises and gait training may be beneficial to these patients, along with therapy directed at the underlying disease. For example, in patients with vertebrobasilar vascular disease, blood pressure should be controlled, lipid levels lowered, and aspirin or warfarin prescribed to help prevent additional events. Acoustic neuroma is managed surgically and requires referral to an otolaryngologist. Elderly patients with multifactorial dizziness may require generalized approach such as lowering dose of antihypertensive medications, physical therapy, and glycemic control.

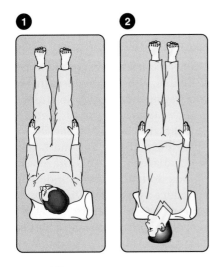
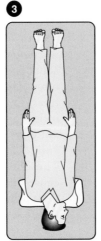
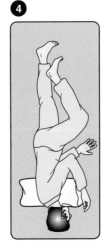
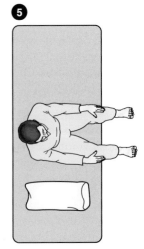

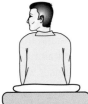
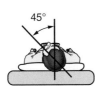
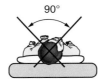
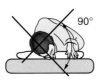

FIGURE 14-1. Barany and Epley maneuvers: step 1 is the Barany maneuver, reproducing the patients symptoms, followed by Epley maneuver in steps 2-5. (From Drislane FW, Acosta J, Caplan L, et al. *Blueprints Neurology*. 4th ed. Alphen aan den Rijn, The Netherlands: Wolters Kluwer; 2014.)

KEY POINTS

- True vertigo occurs due to disease in the central or peripheral vestibular system.

- BPV generally occurs as an isolated symptom; the vertigo is short-lived, recurrent, and associated with particular head movements.

- Vertigo, tinnitus, and hearing loss are the cardinal features of Ménière disease. The vertigo and hearing loss are initially fluctuating.

- In assessing for central versus peripheral causes for vertigo, important distinguishing

features are the presence of isolated vertigo with or without hearing loss, which suggests peripheral disease, and associated brainstem or other neurologic symptoms, which suggest a central disease.

- Peripheral causes of vertigo are characterized by the absence of brainstem signs and symptom. They are usually acute and self-limited.

- Medications used to treat labyrinthitis, vestibular neuronitis, and BPV include meclizine, dimenhydrinate, antiemetics, and benzodiazepines.

15 | Fatigue

Fatigue is defined as the subjective complaint of tiredness or diminished energy level to the point of interfering with normal or usual activities. It is one of the top 10 chief complaints leading to family practice office visits; surveys report that between 5% and 20% of the general population suffer from persistent and troublesome fatigue. It is a constitutional symptom with many etiologies that can lead to multiple diagnoses, extensive laboratory testing, and repeat office visits. Among the extensive causes of fatigue, organic etiologies account for a minority of cases.

PATHOGENESIS

The pathogenesis of fatigue is ill defined and varies depending on the underlying cause. For example, fatigue is associated with many psychiatric conditions and the majority of these patients have a psychological or functional basis for their fatigue. Fatigue associated with conditions such as CHF, COPD, and metabolic abnormalities may be due to altered oxygen and nutrient delivery peripherally. Fatigue associated with inflammatory conditions, such as connective tissue diseases and infectious diseases, may be due to factors released as part of the inflammatory response.

CLINICAL MANIFESTATIONS

An accurate history is crucial in differentiating a patient's source of fatigue. Characterizing the patient's complaint in terms of time course, exacerbating and alleviating factors, stressors, variability in symptoms, and associated symptoms help narrow the potential causes for the fatigue and direct the initial workup. Clarifying a patient's description of fatigue is also essential as muscle weakness, daytime sleepiness, or shortness of breath may be considered fatigue by the patient but would trigger the need for a different workup to a clinician. Preexisting medical conditions and medications should be noted as many medications such as muscle relaxants, benzodiazepines, and antidepressants may exacerbate symptoms. Fatigue should be described as acute (<1 month), prolonged (>1 month), or chronic (>6 months), and should be evaluated in the context of a comprehensive history including identifying red flags such as recent weight loss, dry skin, lymphadenopathy, or risky sexual behavior. Characteristic features of both psychogenic and organic disease are discussed below.

HISTORY

Psychogenic

Psychogenic causes include depression, anxiety, chronic fatigue syndrome (CFS; systemic exertion intolerance disease), substance abuse issues, and domestic abuse. Fatigue that is constant and does not worsen with activity or is not alleviated with rest is likely psychogenic. Patients with identifiable stressors, a stressful and nonsupportive family structure, or a primary mood disturbance suggest psychogenic fatigue. Frequently, patients with psychological disease have a sleep disturbance with either insomnia or early morning awakening. The fatigue associated with psychiatric causes is frequently worse in the morning and may be alleviated by activity. The patient may have multiple and nonspecific complaints along with a normal physical examination. As fatigue is strongly associated with psychiatric disorders, patients should be screened for behavioral etiologies such as depression.

Physiologic

Physiologic fatigue results from situations that would cause most people to be fatigued, such as not getting enough sleep. Physiologic fatigue is common in mothers of newborns, individuals who do shift work, athletes who overtrain, and among third-year medical students. Management of these patients should include encouraging good sleep hygiene, building an exercise routine, and encouraging patients to manage their time effectively and to adopt a balanced lifestyle.

Organic Disease

In contrast to psychogenic fatigue, fatigue from organic causes often presents more abruptly and shows a progressive course. Identifiable stressors are often absent, and the family structure may be supportive. Sleep disturbance may be present but is often related to the underlying disease process. A reactive or secondary depression may result when the patient recognizes that something is wrong. The fatigue is often noted to be less in the morning and worsened with activity. The patient may have fewer and more specific associated symptoms than seen in psychogenic fatigue, and the physical examination may suggest potential underlying causes. Sleep apnea, for example, should be suspected if the patient is obese, snores loudly at night, or describes excessive daytime somnolence. Thyroid abnormalities should be suspected in patients complaining of hot/cold intolerance, changes to skin, weight loss/gain, and patients found to have a goiter on physical examination.

PHYSICAL EXAMINATION

In patients presenting with a complaint of fatigue, a complete physical examination should be performed in an attempt to determine the etiology. The patient's general appearance and vital signs should be noted. A patient with fatigue from physical illness may look pale and sickly, with a slumping posture and a sagging face. Pallor suggests anemia, whereas darkening of the skin may point toward Addison disease as a potential cause. The thyroid gland should be palpated and signs of hyperthyroidism and hypothyroidism such as exophthalmos, skin changes, weight gain, and pretibial myxedema noted. Careful examination of all lymph nodes is essential, along with checking the individual's joints for signs of inflammation. Heart and lung examination may reveal the presence of murmurs, gallops, wheezing, or rales, suggesting a cardiopulmonary etiology. Stigmata of alcohol abuse and a urine drug screen should be sought. A thorough neurologic examination may identify neuromuscular disease as the cause.

DIFFERENTIAL DIAGNOSIS

The differential diagnosis for fatigue is extensive and includes psychiatric, infectious, connective tissue, endocrine, neurologic, oncologic, and cardiopulmonary causes (Box 15-1). By far the most common category

---

BOX 15-1. Common Conditions Leading to Fatigue, by System and Process

Psychogenic: depression, anxiety, adjustment reactions, situational life stress, sexual dysfunction, physical/sexual abuse, occupational stress, and professional burnout, drug or alcohol abuse

Endocrine: DM, hypothyroidism, hyperparathyroidism, hypopituitarism, Addison disease, electrolyte disorders, malnutrition

Hematologic: anemia, lymphoma, and leukemia

Renal: acute renal failure (ARF), chronic renal failure (CRF)

Liver: hepatitis, cirrhosis

Immunologic/connective tissue: AIDS or AIDS-related complex, sarcoid, mixed connective tissue disease, polymyalgia rheumatic

Neuromuscular: upper/lower motor neuron disease from stroke, neoplasm, demyelination, amyotrophic lateral sclerosis, poliomyelitis, disk herniation, myasthenia gravis, and muscular dystrophies

Pulmonary: infectious states (TB, pneumonia), COPD, sleep apnea

Cardiovascular: CHF, cardiomyopathy, valvular heart disease

Reproductive: pregnancy

Iatrogenic: medications

AIDS, acquired immune deficiency syndrome; CHF, congestive heart failure; COPD, chronic obstructive pulmonary disease; TB, tuberculosis.

BOX 15-2. Diagnostic Criteria for Chronic Fatigue Syndrome

The diagnosis is established by fulfilling major criteria plus 6 or more of the minor criteria plus 2 or more of the physical criteria, or 8 or more of the 11 minor symptom criteria.

Major Criteria
1. New onset of persistent or relapsing fatigue not previously present, sufficient to reduce daily activity by 50% or more, lasting at least 6 weeks.
2. Exclusion of other conditions that may produce similar symptoms (see Box 15-1).

Minor Criteria
1. Mild fever (37.5°C–38.6°C) or chills
2. Sore throat
3. Painful cervical or axillary lymph nodes
4. Unexplained generalized muscle weakness
5. Muscle discomfort or myalgias
6. Prolonged (>24 hours) generalized fatigue after previously tolerated exercise
7. Generalized headaches unlike previous cephalalgia
8. Migratory arthralgias without joint swelling or redness
9. Neuropsychiatric complaints, that is, photophobia, scotomata, forgetfulness, irritability, confusion, inability to concentrate, difficulty in thinking, depression
10. Sleep disturbances
11. Onset of main symptom complex in hours or a few days

Physical Criteria
A physician should document these on at least two occasions, at least 1 month apart.
1. Low grade fever
2. Nonexudative pharyngitis
3. Palpable or tender anterior or posterior cervical or axillary nodes (<2 cm in diameter)

of diagnosis among fatigued patients is psychiatric or psychological disorders, accounting for 60% to 80% of cases. Depression accounts for the majority of psychogenic cases. Medical causes account for up to 8% of such cases. The leading physical causes of fatigue are infections, metabolic disorders, and medications. Of the remainder, 4% meet the criteria for CFS, a disease of unknown etiology often attributed to a persistent mononucleosis infection from the Epstein–Barr virus (EBV) (Box 15-2). Despite exhaustive workup, many patients with fatigue remain undiagnosed.

DIAGNOSTIC EVALUATION

The history and physical examination help determine the likelihood of an organic versus a psychiatric etiology (Fig. 15-1). If the history points to a psychiatric cause, consider utilizing the Generalized Anxiety Disorder Assessment (GAD7), depression screening tool (PHQ9), or mood disorder questionnaire. In patients with characteristics suggesting an organic

cause, further evaluation should be directed at the suspected underlying cause. For example, in patients with suspected hyperparathyroidism, elevated levels of serum calcium and parathyroid hormone might confirm the diagnosis.

In patients with suspected organic disease but without an apparent diagnosis suggested by the history and physical screening, laboratory tests including a CBC (to rule out anemia), ESR (if symptoms are consistent with polymyalgia rheumatica), comprehensive metabolic profile (glucose, liver function tests, creatinine), UA, urine drug screen (UDAP), and thyroid function tests are recommended. Pregnancy testing should be considered in women of childbearing age and HIV testing for individuals at risk for this disease. A drug screen can occasionally be productive. Additional laboratory or imaging tests should be ordered based on findings in the history and physical examination. Examples of tests that may be helpful include a CXR to look for adenopathy, occult CHF, and primary lung tumors or metastatic

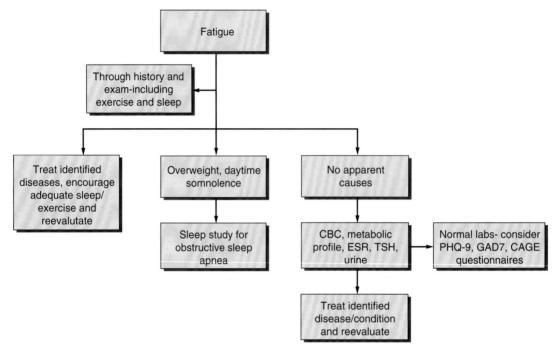

FIGURE 15-1. Algorithm for approach to fatigue. CBC, complete blood count; ESR, erythrocyte sedimentation rate; GAD7, Generalized Anxiety Disorder 7; PHQ-9, Patient Health Questionnaire-9; TSH, thyroid-stimulating hormone.

disease. An ECG may detect a silent infarction or ischemia. In patients at risk, Lyme titers and TB skin testing might be of benefit. Sleep studies may be helpful in excluding sleep apnea and other sleep disorders. Testing for autoimmune markers such as antinuclear antibody (ANA), rheumatoid factor, or celiac disease antibodies is not recommended unless patients are complaining of other specific symptoms related to these disorders.

TREATMENT

Psychiatric evaluation and treatment may be necessary for patients with persistent fatigue due to anxiety or depression. For patients with an identified medical condition, treatment of the underlying process is the recommended treatment for fatigue. There is no specific therapy for CFS, although data suggest that patients with CFS may benefit from cognitive behavioral therapy and graded exercise therapy. Additional therapy is targeted toward associated symptoms (e.g., NSAIDs for myalgias).

In individuals with persistent fatigue of unknown causes, therapy may consist of an empiric trial of antidepressants or withdrawal of a medication known to cause fatigue. Some patients also benefit from moderate levels of exercise and other efforts to reduce the stresses in their lives.

KEY POINTS

- Fatigue occurs in up to 20% of patients seeking care.
- Psychological causes should be at the top of the differential diagnosis for all patients presenting with fatigue, because the majority of cases have psychiatric causes.
- Medical history can help in determining a psychiatric versus organic cause and thus aid in directing the evaluation of fatigue.

16 | Headache

Headaches are one of the most common medical complaints encountered in primary care. Types of headaches include: migraine, tension-type, cluster, and chronic daily headache. Tension-type headache is the most common type of headache reported in the primary care setting.

More than 90% of adults experience headaches over a 1-year period and more than 15% of these consult a physician. Although most headaches seen in the outpatient setting are benign, it is important to identify those rare instances when a headache may be secondary to a life-threatening illness.

Clinical features such as sudden onset headache, no similar headache in the past, altered mental status, seizure, headache with exertion, onset after age 50, and associated visual disturbance are potential warning signs of a serious underlying case and the need for urgent medical attention.

PATHOGENESIS

Headache originates in either intracranial or extracranial structures. Intracranial pain-sensitive structures include the trigeminal, glossopharyngeal, vagus, and first three cervical nerves. In addition, the dura, arteries, and venous sinuses are pain-sensitive; however, the brain parenchyma is not. Disease processes that cause pressure or inflammation of pain-sensitive structures, distention of blood vessels, and obstruction of cerebrospinal fluid (CSF) can cause pain. For example, a mass lesion can cause headache by displacing a pain-sensitive structure, whereas a ruptured aneurysm can inflame the meninges.

The neurogenic inflammatory hypothesis is the most accepted theory explaining migraine headache. This theory views migraine as a primary neuronal event with subsequent changes resulting from the effects of neurotransmitters on the vasculature and the blood flow. Neuropeptides trigger the release of kinins and other bioactive substances that cause inflammation and vasodilation. Serotonin receptors are believed to be an important part of this process, which explains why serotonin analogs or agonists benefit patients with migraine.

Extracranial sources of headache include skin, muscles, blood vessels, skull periosteum, sinuses, and teeth. Clinical problems affecting the eyes, sinuses, cervical spine, temporomandibular joint, and cranial nerves can all cause headaches.

Tension headaches were traditionally thought to originate from scalp muscles. However, myographic recordings show that many but not all individuals with tension headaches have muscle contraction. Studies suggest that migraine and tension headaches may have similar pathophysiologic mechanisms but with different expression of symptoms. This overlap explains why some patients with tension headaches experience migraine-like symptoms.

CLINICAL MANIFESTATIONS

HISTORY

Medical history provides the most useful diagnostic information and physical examination helps exclude organic pathology. Relevant history includes location (unilateral vs. bilateral), severity (worst headache of my life), quality (throbbing, squeezing), duration, frequency, associated neurologic symptoms, aggravating or alleviating factors (foods, rest, menstruation, and OTC medications), and associated symptoms (nausea, emesis, fever, and visual changes). Other relevant information includes caffeine intake, because caffeine withdrawal is a known cause of headaches, and whether the headache awakens the patient from sleep. Foods such as chocolate, alcohol, nuts, and aged cheese may trigger migraines. Reviewing medications is important because a number of drugs such as indomethacin, nifedipine, cimetidine, captopril, nitrates, and oral contraceptives can trigger headaches. Family history is especially important when suspecting migraine headaches.

Migraine Headaches

These typically start between the ages of 15 and 45 years, with a 3:1 female predominance.

Migraine is an episodic disorder associated with severe headache and nausea and/or light and sound sensitivity. Migraine headaches require at least two of the following four headache characteristics for diagnosis: unilateral location, pulsatile quality, moderate-to-severe intensity, or aggravation by movement. They should also be associated with one of the following symptoms: nausea, vomiting, or photo- or phonophobia. Migraines last between 4 and 72 hours and may be accompanied by an aura. Migraine aura is experienced by 25% of people with migraine experience and usually the aura precedes the headache. Typical positive symptoms of aura include seeing bright lines, shapes or objects, tinnitus, noises, burning, pain, paresthesias, jerking, or repetitive movement. Negative symptoms of migraine aura include absence or loss of function, such as loss of vision, hearing, and feeling or ability to move a part of the body. A family history of migraine is present in more than 80% of those who suffer from migraines and is a useful diagnostic criterion.

Exacerbating factors for migraine include lack of or irregular sleep, hunger, stress, menstruation, visual stimuli, weather changes, fasting, sleep disturbances, lights, exercise, sexual activity, and certain foods. The diagnosis of migraine is based on history, physical examination, and meeting the diagnostic criteria set by the *International Classification of Headache Disorders*, 3rd edition (ICHD-3). Although neuroimaging is not required for diagnoses, it can be helpful to exclude other diseases.

Tension Headaches

Tension-type headache is the most common headache in the general population. Tension-type headache is usually diagnosed based on clinical presentation and diagnostic criteria according to the ICHD-3. Typical tension-type headache presents with two of the following: mild-to-moderate intensity, bilateral, nonthrobbing headache located in the bilateral occipital and/or frontal areas and not brought on by activity.

The headache is usually described as dull or band-like, often lasts for hours, and is frequently associated with stress and mental tension. Tension headaches usually do not awaken patients from sleep and are not generally associated with vomiting or neurologic symptoms. Headaches can also be classified by frequency: non-episodic <1 day per month or episodic from 1 to 14 days per month. Chronic tension-type headaches are defined as more than 15 days of headaches per month. Unlike migraine headaches, hereditary factors play a minor role in tension-type headaches.

Cluster Headaches

These headaches are severe, unilateral, localized to the periorbital/temporal area, and usually accompanied by one of the following symptoms: lacrimation, rhinorrhea, ptosis, miosis, nasal congestion, and eyelid edema. These headaches occur in "clusters," with one to eight daily attacks lasting 15 to 90 minutes for a period of 4 to 6 weeks. These episodes are followed by pain-free intervals lasting 3 to 6 months. Cluster headaches are more common in men (8:1 ratio), but overall are far less common than tension or migraine headaches.

Analgesic Headaches

These headaches are seen in patients who chronically use analgesic or antimigraine drugs, especially those containing caffeine. Daily use of low-dose analgesics is much riskier for analgesic headaches than occasional use of large doses. The headache initially worsens when the analgesics are discontinued, but improves after a few weeks.

New-Onset Headaches

These headaches merit close attention. A subarachnoid hemorrhage (SAH) should be considered in any patient who does not usually have headaches and presents with the "worst headache of my life." An acute headache with ataxia, profuse nausea, and vomiting is consistent with a cerebral hemorrhage. Fever with frontal or maxillary tenderness is suggestive of acute sinusitis.

PHYSICAL EXAMINATION

Physical examination should include vital signs, funduscopic and cardiovascular assessment, palpation of the head and neck, and a thorough neurologic evaluation. The examination is important to help identify secondary or organic causes of headache. A neurologic examination is essential because a neurologic deficit is an important sign of intracranial pathology. Neurologic examination should include mental status evaluation, cranial nerve examination, fundoscopy, otoscopy, and motor, reflex, cerebellar and sensory testing. Some types of headaches can be associated with specific abnormalities. Patients with muscle contraction headaches may demonstrate muscle tightness or trigger points over the posterior occiput in several areas. Temporal artery tenderness in an elderly patient raises the possibility of temporal arteritis, whereas sinus tenderness, congestion, and fever are most consistent with sinusitis. Headache accompanied by a stiff neck may indicate an SAH or meningitis. Headache with abnormal physical signs—such as a high blood pressure, a focal neurologic deficit, or papilledema—may indicate the presence of a mass lesion or malignant hypertension.

DIFFERENTIAL DIAGNOSIS

Headaches may be classified as primary or secondary. Primary headaches have no underlying organic disease and include migraine, tension headaches, and cluster headaches. Secondary headaches result from an underlying disorder such as intracranial mass, infection, cerebrovascular accident (CVA), head trauma, drug withdrawal, or metabolic disorders (Box 16-1 gives a complete list). Although primary headaches are not life threatening, they are often very debilitating to patients.

BOX 16-1. Causes of Secondary Headaches

Subarachnoid hemorrhage
Intracranial mass
Posttraumatic
Infection
Glaucoma
Sinus disease
Drug withdrawal
Benign intracranial hypertension (pseudotumor cerebri)
Hypoxia
Hypercapnia
Postlumbar puncture
Neuralgias

DIAGNOSTIC EVALUATION

The objectives in evaluating a headache patient are to (1) identify patients with life-threatening conditions, (2) identify those with secondary headaches such as sinusitis, and (3) provide symptom relief to those with primary headache.

Patients presenting with an acute onset of severe headache, especially in the presence of meningeal signs, high fever, or evidence of increased intracranial pressure, need urgent evaluation. A CT scan is helpful in detecting an SAH or intracerebral bleed. If the CT scan is negative in a patient with a suspected SAH, a lumbar puncture is indicated because a CT scan is normal in 10% of patients with SAH. A lumbar puncture can also help detect significant disease in patients with meningeal signs and provide fluid for identifying the cause of meningitis. Because of the risk of brainstem herniation, a lumbar puncture is contraindicated when increased intracranial pressure is suspected. In general, blood tests play a limited role in the evaluation of headache patients. A CBC may be helpful in assessing a patient with suspected meningitis, and a normal ESR is helpful for ruling out temporal arteritis.

Neuroimaging may also be performed in patients exhibiting focal neurologic signs or symptoms, onset of headache with exertion, cough, or sexual activity. Other indications for imaging may include the presence of an orbital bruit, new-onset headache after age 40 years, recent change in headache pattern, frequency, or severity of headaches, and progressive worsening of headache despite appropriate therapy.

Box 16-2 lists indications for neuroimaging.

BOX 16-2. Indications for Neuroimaging

Headache of recent onset (<6 months)
Headache beginning after 50 years of age
Worsening headaches
Headache that does not fit primary headache pattern
Associated seizure
Focal neurologic signs or symptoms
Personality change
Severe headaches unresponsive to therapy
History of significant trauma
New headache in a cancer patient

TREATMENT

Treatment for tension headaches includes avoiding the stress associated with these headaches or improved stress management. Biofeedback, relaxation, and deep-breathing exercises are often effective. In addition, non-narcotic analgesics such as NSAIDs (e.g., ibuprofen 400 to 600 mg three times a day) or acetaminophen (650 mg four times a day) usually alleviate symptoms and are generally the first line of pharmacologic therapy. Low doses of antidepressants such as amitriptyline (10 to 75 mg PO daily) can be effective for reducing the number and severity of chronic tension headaches. If these measures fail to improve the headache significantly or if the headache is associated with neurologic symptoms, the diagnosis of tension headache should be questioned and further evaluation pursued.

Primary treatment of migraine headaches includes avoiding headache triggers, withdrawal from stressful environments (often by lying down in a dark, quiet bedroom with a cool washcloth placed on the forehead), and rest. A lifestyle that encourages a regular schedule of sleep, meals, and physical activity as well as avoidance of stress, alcohol, caffeine, tyramine (found in aged cheeses and red wine), nitrates (found in cured meats), and artificial sweeteners is often helpful.

Serotonin receptor agonists are available in a variety of forms and are the primary medications to abort an attack. Triptans are one of the most commonly used agents among this class and are available as injections, nasal sprays, and tablets and may be administered in multiple doses until the patient's symptoms resolve. All the triptans have similar chemical structures and mechanisms of action. Although there are subtle differences among them, there is no clear therapeutic advantage to one over another. If one triptan is poorly tolerated or does not work on at least two occasions, a different triptan should be tried. Antiemetics including metoclopramide, prochlorperazine, and chlorpromazine can be used along with triptans. Due to their vasoconstrictive properties, the triptans are contraindicated in patients with coronary artery disease (CAD), peripheral vascular disease (PVD), and uncontrolled hypertension.

Ergotamine is another serotonin receptor agonist that also has dopamine and adrenergic receptor activity. It is available as an oral, sublingual, or suppository medication and is maximally effective when administered early in the course of a migraine. Because it has vasoconstrictive properties, ergotamine is contraindicated in patients with CAD or PVD.

Dihydroergotamine (DHE) can be given parenterally and can be useful in the treatment of acute migraine in the emergency room setting. Table 16-1 lists medications for treatment of acute migraines.

Depending on patients' symptoms, NSAIDs, acetaminophen, antiemetics, narcotics, and caffeine are frequently prescribed. Physicians should use caution when using mild analgesics alone to treat migraines, as their limited duration of effectiveness may result in "rebound" symptoms. As a result, patients may take higher than recommended doses. In patients who suffer from migraines more than twice a week, beta blockers, calcium channel blockers, antidepressants, and antiseizure medications (e.g., divalproex sodium) can provide effective prophylactic therapy (Table 16-2). Prophylactic therapy should also be considered in patients in whom abortive agents are ineffective, poorly tolerated, or contraindicated. Patients with menstrual migraines may benefit from a brief course of NSAIDs taken for several days before and after menses. Prophylactic therapy is selected according to a patient's age and comorbidities—for example, trying an antidepressant first in someone with concomitant depression.

Patients with cluster headaches should be counseled to avoid known precipitants. Breathing 100% oxygen at 7 to 10 L/minute for 10 to 15 minutes via a tight-fitting mask may abort an acute attack. If the patient has no cardiac risk factors, sumatriptan 6 mg SC with an additional 6 mg given 1 hour later is helpful. Alternatively, dihydroergotamine mesylate 1 mg IM or IV may improve symptoms. Prednisone starting at 60 to 80 mg/day followed by a 2- to 4-week taper can shorten the duration of episodes and diminish the frequency and intensity of symptoms. Other medications commonly used to treat or prevent cluster headache include verapamil, NSAIDs, propranolol, amitriptyline, and lithium. Patients in whom these therapies do not help may benefit from referral to a neurologist or major headache center.

Temporal arteritis should be considered in older patients who have pain on palpation of the temporal artery. Although these patients often have an elevated erythrocyte sedimentation rate, definitive diagnosis requires biopsy of the temporal artery. Patients with temporal arteritis should be started on steroids promptly, as a delay in treatment may result in blindness.

TABLE 16-1. Medications for Acute Treatment of Migraines

Nonspecific Medications	Dose	Adverse Reactions
Nonsteroidal anti-inflammatory drugs		
Ibuprofen	400–800 mg q6h	GI upset, bleeding disorder, G6PD
Naproxen	275–550 mg q2–6h	deficiency
Aspirin	650–1000 mg q4–6h	
Analgesics plus caffeine		
Acetaminophen, aspirin, caffeine	250–500 mg acetaminophen and aspirin, 65–130 mg caffeine q4–6h	As above plus palpitations, anxiety
Isometheptene/dichloralphenazone/acetaminophen (Midrin)	Two with onset, 1qh, maximum five per episode	Hypertension, dizziness, caution renal/liver disease, hypertension, cardiac disease, or MAOI use
Narcotics		
Hydromorphone	2–4 mg PO q3–4h 0.5–2 mg IV q1–2h	Sedation, respiratory depression
Butorphanol nasal	One spray, repeat in 60–90 minutes; may repeat sequence in 3–4 hours	As above
Antiemetics		
Prochlorperazine	5–10 mg orally or 25 mg rectally as adjunct to other treatments	Sedation, hypotension dystonic reactions
Metoclopramide	10 mg as adjunct to other treatments	Sedation, dystonic reaction
Migraine-Specific Medications		
Triptans		
Sumatriptan	6 mg SC; 25–100 mg PO or 1–2 sprays nasally; may repeat SC dose in 1 hour, oral and nasal in 2 hours	Nausea, vomiting, chest pain; contraindicated with ergot or MAOI use; caution with CAD
Rizatriptan	5–20 mg orally, may repeat in 2 hours	As above
Zolmatriptan	2.5–5 mg orally, may repeat in 2 hours	As above
Ergotamine	1–2 mg orally every hour up to three doses in 24 hours	Arrhythmia, vasospasm, nausea, vomiting
Ergotamine plus caffeine	Two tablets orally, then one every 30 minutes to maximum of six per attack and 10 per week	As above plus myocardial infarct, pulmonary fibrosis
Dihydroergotamine	1 mg parenterally every hour to maximum of 2 mg IV and 3 mg SC/IM; intranasal one spray in each nostril with repeat dose in 15 minutes; maximum four sprays per day	Hypertension, CVA, cardiac ischemia, arrhythmia, nausea, vomiting

CAD, coronary artery disease; CVA, cerebrovascular accident; G6PD, glucose-6-phosphate dehydrogenase; IM, intramuscular; MAOI, monoamine oxidase inhibitor; PO, by mouth; SC, subcutaneous.

TABLE 16-2. Medications for Migraine Prophylaxis

Class	Dose Range	Cautions
Beta blockers		
Propranolol	40–320 mg/day	Heart block greater than first degree; congestive heart failure; asthma/reactive airways
Atenolol	50–150 mg/day	As above
Metoprolol	50–300 mg/day	As above
Tricyclic antidepressants		
Amitriptyline	10–300 mg/day	Cardiac conduction abnormalities; glaucoma; urinary retention; seizure disorder
Nortriptyline	10–150 mg/day	As above
Imipramine	10–200 mg/day	As above
Calcium channel blockers		
Verapamil	120–720 mg/day	Heart block greater than first degree; congestive heart failure; hypotension
Diltiazem	90–360 mg/day	As above
Anticonvulsants		
Divalproex sodium	250–1500 mg/day	Pregnancy, liver disease
Topiramate	25–200 mg/day	Fatigue, nausea, anorexia common
Serotonin antagonists		
Cyproheptadine	4–16 mg/day	Elderly, glaucoma, MAOI use, urinary outflow obstruction
Methysergide	2–8 mg/day	Hypertension, heart disease, pulmonary disease, collagen vascular disease, vascular disease, renal or hepatic insufficiency, pregnancy
Monoamine oxidase inhibitors		
Phenelzine	30–90 mg/day	Dietary and food restrictions necessary, congestive heart failure, liver disease

MAOI, monoamine oxidase inhibitor.

KEY POINTS

- Headache originates in either intracranial or extracranial structures. Intracranial pain-sensitive structures include the trigeminal, glossopharyngeal, vagus, and the first three cervical nerves.

- The neurogenic inflammatory hypothesis is the most widely accepted theory explaining migraine headache. This theory views migraine as a primary neuronal event with subsequent changes resulting from the effects of neurotransmitters on the vasculature and blood flow.

- Headache accompanied by a stiff neck may indicate a subarachnoid hemorrhage or meningitis.

- The objectives in evaluating a headache patient are to (1) identify patients with life-threatening conditions; (2) identify those with secondary headaches, such as sinusitis; and (3) provide symptom relief to those with primary headaches.

- Serotonin receptor agonists are available in a variety of forms and are the primary medications used to abort a migraine headache.

- Temporal arteritis should be considered in older patients who have pain on palpation of the temporal artery.

17 | Heartburn

The most common causes of heartburn symptoms are GERD, peptic ulcer disease, gastritis, and nonulcer dyspepsia.

EPIDEMIOLOGY

Heartburn from GERD is experienced daily by 7% of the population, weekly by 15%, and at least monthly by up to 40%. Peptic ulcer disease is present in 1.5% of the population and has a lifetime incidence of about 10%. Duodenal ulcers occur more commonly than gastric ulcers and at a young age. Peptic ulcer affects men slightly more than it affects women. Nonulcer dyspepsia occurs in up to 25% to 30% of the population at some point over their lifetime.

PATHOGENESIS

Gastroesophageal reflux occurs when gastric contents reflux or enter the esophagus. Decreased lower esophageal sphincter (LES) pressure or increased intra-abdominal pressure plays a significant role in this process. Exposing the esophagus to the low pH of the gastric contents can cause inflammatory changes leading to esophagitis. Long-term acid exposure may also result in the metaplastic transformation of the squamous cells lining the esophagus to adenomatous cells (Barrett esophagus). Patients with Barrett esophagus are at a higher risk (30- to 40-fold) for developing esophageal cancer. Continued inflammatory reaction can also lead to esophageal scarring, stricture formation, and dysphagia. However, there is a correlation between the severity of symptoms and the degree of esophageal damage.

Peptic ulcer disease and gastritis have similar causes and risk factors. Typically, the gastric and duodenal mucosa are resistant to any damage from acid secretion. Peptic ulcers and gastritis occur when the defense mechanisms are compromised or less commonly when acid secretion is sufficient to overwhelm the defenses.

Helicobacter pylori infection is the most significant risk factor for peptic ulcer disease. In 10% to 20% of infected individuals, gastric or duodenal ulcers develop. Exactly why peptic ulcers develop in some individuals and not in others remains unclear. Infection with *H. pylori* is also associated with an increased risk of gastric adenocarcinoma and gastric lymphoma.

NSAIDs contribute to gastritis and ulcer formation by blocking cyclooxygenase-1 production of prostaglandins that maintain mucosal blood flow, secretion of mucus, and bicarbonate. Without these protective factors, acid-induced inflammation and ulcers may result. Stress-induced gastritis and ulcers are thought to occur due to impaired mucosal defenses resulting from vasoconstriction and resultant tissue hypoxia.

Nonulcer dyspepsia is a poorly understood disease with symptoms such as those of GERD and peptic ulcer disease. The pathophysiology is thought to be related to altered GI motility, GI contractile patterns, and transit of food.

CLINICAL MANIFESTATIONS

HISTORY

Initial evaluation of individuals with heartburn includes the patient's detailed description of the episodes along with assessing the risk for other diseases with heartburn as a presenting symptom.

GERD is characterized by burning pain in the epigastric, sternal, and throat accompanied by a sour taste in the mouth, and is aggravated by lying down or bending over. Increases in abdominal pressure, as occurs with pregnancy, may worsen esophageal reflux. Burning, aching, or gnawing pain in the epigastric region or upper quadrants of the abdomen is typical of peptic ulcer disease. Chest tightness and pain brought on by exertion and relieved by rest are more typical of cardiac disease. Colicky upper abdominal pain is more consistent with cholecystitis, nephrolithiasis, irritable bowel syndrome (IBS), or nonulcer dyspepsia as possible causes.

Esophageal reflux may be alleviated by antacids or food, but frequently recurs within 1 to 2 hours. The pain of peptic ulcer disease is more intense and may awaken patients in the middle of the night, the middle of the night; is typically mid-epigastric and relieved by eating. Eating usually aggravates cholecystitis and sometimes gastric ulcers. The pain of nephrolithiasis is independent of ingestion of food. The pain of nonulcer dyspepsia is more variable but often related to eating.

GERD can cause respiratory symptoms such as cough, wheezing, sore throat, and laryngitis. GERD is a common cause of chest pain, but heartburn associated with shortness of breath or activity should raise concerns about a cardiac etiology for the patient's symptoms.

Motility disorders associated with connective tissue and neuromuscular disease can cause esophageal symptoms. Medications such as theophylline and calcium channel blockers can precipitate or exacerbate symptoms associated with GERD. NSAIDs are associated with gastric and duodenal ulcers as well as heartburn. The patient should also be asked about medications used to alleviate symptoms, particularly with the availability of OTC H_2 blockers and proton pump inhibitors (PPIs).

Smoking worsens gastroesophageal reflux and is a risk factor for peptic ulcer disease. Dietary factors associated with lowering LES pressure include consumption of coffee, chocolate, mints, fatty foods, and alcohol. There are no specific dietary correlates for peptic ulcer disease. However, alcohol can cause gastric irritation with resultant gastritis.

PHYSICAL EXAMINATION

Physical examination generally cannot distinguish among gastritis, peptic ulcer disease, nonulcer dyspepsia, and GERD. All these typically have minimal physical findings other than epigastric tenderness. A positive test for fecal occult blood makes the presence of peptic ulcer disease and erosive gastritis or esophagitis more likely diagnoses than simple gastroesophageal reflux.

Cardiac findings such as S_3, S_4, pulmonary rales, or an irregular rhythm signify underlying cardiac disease. Abdominal tenderness with pancreatitis is typically periumbilical, whereas the tenderness with cholecystitis occurs in the right upper quadrant and is associated with a positive Murphy sign. Nephrolithiasis typically presents no physical findings other than possible costovertebral angle tenderness. Palpation of a mass suggests the presence of a neoplasm.

DIFFERENTIAL DIAGNOSIS

Table 17-1 presents a comprehensive differential diagnosis for patients complaining of heartburn. Differential diagnosis also includes infections (e.g., *Candida* or herpes), pill-induced esophagitis, biliary

TABLE 17-1. Differential Diagnosis of Heartburn

Condition	Typical Symptoms
Gastroesophageal reflux disease	Regurgitation, dysphagia
Peptic ulcer disease	Gnawing epigastric pain, nausea, vomiting, bloating
Gastritis	Same as peptic ulcer disease
Nonulcer dyspepsia	Upper abdominal/epigastric pain, bloating, belching, flatulence, nausea
Coronary artery disease/angina	Chest pressure, nausea, diaphoresis, palpitations
Cholelithiasis	Colicky right upper quadrant pain with meals, radiation to scapular region
Pancreatitis	Severe constant midabdominal pain, radiation to the back
Infectious esophagitis	Dysphagia, associated immunocompromised condition
Medication or chemical esophagitis	Dysphagia, associated ingestion
Scleroderma/polymyositis with secondary gastroesophageal reflux	Associated signs of connective tissue disease, potential risk of stricture/dysphagia

disease, motility disorders, and CAD. No specific etiology is found for about 50% to 60% of patients with heartburn.

Nonulcer dyspepsia is a poorly understood disease with symptoms overlapping GERD, peptic ulcer disease, and gastritis. Patients may have symptoms consistent with GERD, peptic ulcer disease, and gastritis, or may present with dysmotility symptoms such as abdominal bloating or cramping. This is generally considered a diagnosis of exclusion. If the initial laboratory evaluation (CBC, testing stools for occult blood, and *H. pylori* serology) is normal in patients below age 45, empiric therapy can be initiated based on the patient's predominant symptoms. Patients presenting after age 45 require more aggressive evaluation, because organic disease becomes more prevalent as patients grow older.

Regurgitation is a classic symptom of reflux in children. Almost half of healthy infants regurgitate daily. Symptoms such as failure to gain weight, apnea, wheezing, or recurrent pneumonia should prompt further investigation.

DIAGNOSTIC EVALUATION

No single test is accepted as the standard for diagnosing GERD. However, several tests are useful in evaluating patients with heartburn. Early diagnostic evaluation is indicated when complications such as weight loss, vomiting, or bleeding are present, or when a patient fails to respond to therapy.

Esophagogastroduodenoscopy (EGD) is the diagnostic tool most frequently used in evaluating the symptoms of heartburn or dysphagia and assessing the upper GI tract in patients with GI blood loss. EGD detects esophagitis, erosions, ulceration, malignancies, webs, diverticuli, and strictures; it can also be therapeutically useful in treating ulcer disease and strictures. EGD is indicated in patients more than age 45 with new-onset heartburn; patients with evidence of GI bleeding, early satiety, and vomiting; and individuals whose symptoms persist despite therapy.

Barium studies, such as the barium swallow or upper GI series, can reveal anatomic abnormalities such as esophageal spasm and may detect reflux. However, barium studies have a lower sensitivity than EGD for detecting ulceration, erosions, and tumors, and they do not allow tissue diagnosis.

Ambulatory esophageal pH monitoring can be useful for patients with suspected GERD who have normal endoscopy and have either atypical symptoms or are refractory to therapy. A thin pH probe is placed through the patient's nose into the esophagus 5 cm above the LES. The percentage of time the esophageal pH is below 4 in conjunction with the patient's symptoms provides diagnostic information. The reported sensitivity and specificity of this test are $\sim 95\%$.

Esophageal manometry involves monitoring of LES pressures and esophageal peristalsis. Its primary role is to evaluate patients for motility disorders.

***H. pylori* testing** can be useful in assessing patients with heartburn. Currently, there are four different tests: the rapid urease test, histologic staining, serologic and fecal antigen tests, and urea breath tests.

The rapid urease test analyzes tissue samples obtained during endoscopy for the presence of urease, a marker of *H. pylori* infection. This test has a sensitivity of about 90% and a specificity of 98%. The test itself is inexpensive and can be performed quickly, but obtaining samples is expensive because of the costs associated with endoscopy. If the rapid urease test is negative in a patient with ulcers or gastritis, a separate sample can be sent for histologic staining for *H. pylori*.

Histologic staining is very sensitive and specific for *H. pylori*; however, results are less readily available, and this procedure is more expensive than the urease test.

Serologic and fecal antigen tests have the advantage of being noninvasive, inexpensive, and highly sensitive and specific (>90%). The disadvantages are that serology remains indefinitely positive; a positive test can indicate a prior infection and not necessarily current activity; and patients in their 20s are rarely positive, whereas more than 50% of those in their 60s are positive. Serologic testing is most useful in younger populations and for diagnosing *H. pylori* in radiographically diagnosed duodenal ulcers. Fecal antigen testing suffers from the inconvenience of collecting a stool sample, but is inexpensive and can be used to test for cure.

Urea breath tests involve having the patient ingest urea labeled with radioactive carbon. If *H. pylori* is present, urease hydrolyzes the urea, and the patient exhales labeled carbon dioxide. The test is both sensitive and specific, but can be expensive and may not be readily available.

TREATMENT

Table 17-2 outlines common heartburn treatments. Typical GERD symptoms of heartburn and regurgitation

TABLE 17-2. Treatments for Common Causes of Heartburn

Disease	Treatments	Example
GERD	Behavioral changes	• Avoid fatty foods, spicy foods, chocolate, mints, citrus • Avoid alcohol, caffeine • Avoid large meals and reclining after meals
	Medications	
	• H_2 blockers	Cimetidine, ranitidine, famotidine, nizatidine
	• Proton pump inhibitors	Omeprazole, lansoprazole, dexlansoprazole, esomeprazole, pantoprazole, rabeprazole
Peptic ulcer disease/gastritis		
• *H. pylori*-positive	Medications	
	• Antibiotics	Clarithromycin, amoxicillin, metronidazole
	• Proton pump inhibitors	Omeprazole, lansoprazole, dexlansoprazole, esomeprazole, pantoprazole, rabeprazole
• *H. pylori*-negative	Medications	
	• H_2 blockers	Cimetidine, ranitidine, famotidine, nizatidine
	• Proton pump inhibitors	Omeprazole, lansoprazole, dexlansoprazole, esomeprazole, pantoprazole, rabeprazole
Nonulcer dyspepsia	Behavioral changes	Avoid offending foods
		Reassurance
Dysmotility symptoms	Medications	Metoclopropamide
Ulcer-like or reflux	Medications	
	• H_2 blockers	Cimetidine, ranitidine, famotidine, nizatidine
	• Proton pump inhibitors	Omeprazole, lansoprazole, dexlansoprazole, esomeprazole, pantoprazole, rabeprazole

can be treated empirically with lifestyle modifications, although most patients with significant reflux require acid-suppressive therapy using H_2 blockers or PPIs. New recommendations advocate step-down therapy from a PPI to a less-intense regimen that remains effective, such as a lower dose of the PPI, an H_2 blocker, antacids, or lifestyle management. Lifestyle modifications include elevating the head of the patient's bed, losing weight if an individual is obese, avoiding foods that lower the tone of the LES, eliminating the use of aspirin and other NSAIDs,

and stopping tobacco use. Patients with symptoms persisting beyond 6 weeks merit a referral for diagnostic evaluation, such as an endoscopy.

The rate of recurrence with GERD is high because the underlying pathophysiologic process is unchanged when therapy is discontinued. Moderate-to-severe esophagitis and atypical symptoms, particularly respiratory symptoms, may require long-term treatment. Nonetheless, attempts to step-down therapy should be made after 8 weeks of symptom control. Some patients may require only intermittent therapy along with continued lifestyle modifications. Severe esophagitis, Barrett esophagus, and stricture are markers of severe reflux and require long-term treatment, even in the absence of symptoms, to reduce the risk of esophageal carcinoma, bleeding, and stricture.

Therapy for peptic ulcer disease and gastritis depends on whether *H. pylori* is present. If it is, therapy directed against this organism is indicated. Regimens include triple therapy with combinations of omeprazole (a PPI), clarithromycin, and amoxicillin or metronidazole for 7 to 14 days. Triple-therapy regimens have cure rates of $\sim$ 90%. Alternative regimens or for those failing initial therapy include H_2 blockers, bismuth subsalicylate combined with a fluoroquinolone, tetracycline, or other antibiotic options. After the antibiotic regimen has been completed, PPIs are generally continued for 4 to 8 weeks for duodenal ulcers and for 6 to 12 weeks for gastritis or gastric ulcers. EGD is recommended to document healing of gastric ulcers because they pose a higher risk of cancer.

Patients with NSAID-related ulcers are generally treated with acid-suppression therapy and discontinuing the NSAID. If NSAIDs must be used, options include switching the patient to a nonacetylated salicylate such as salsalate (Disalcid) or a COX-2 inhibitor, using an enteric-coated preparation and prescribing the lowest effective dose. If NSAIDs must be used in patients with a history of ulcer, misoprostol (Cytotec), or a PPI can help prevent recurrence.

Therapy for nonulcer dyspepsia involves avoiding foods or medications that aggravate symptoms, reassurance regarding the absence of a serious disease, and medications directed at the predominant symptoms. In patients with ulcer-like or reflux symptoms, acid-suppressing agents are helpful, whereas dysmotility-related symptoms—such as nausea, bloating, or early satiety—respond better to motility agents. If treatment is initially successful, 4 weeks of continuous therapy is followed by a trial off medication. Some patients need only intermittent therapy, whereas others may require continuous treatment. In such cases, periodic attempts to wean the patient off medication should be attempted to see whether symptoms recur.

KEY POINTS

- Heartburn is a common symptom, affecting 40% or more of the population monthly.
- GERD, peptic ulcer disease, gastritis, and nonulcer dyspepsia are the major causes of heartburn symptoms.
- Atypical symptoms of dysphagia, early satiety, weight loss, or blood loss should trigger a GI workup.

- EGD is the most useful diagnostic tool for evaluating heartburn.
- *H. pylori* is a leading causative factor in peptic ulcer disease and gastritis.
- Antibiotic therapy, along with PPIs, is used to treat *H. pylori*-positive patients with peptic ulcer disease or gastritis.

18 | Hematuria

Hematuria can be either gross (visible to the naked eye) or microscopic. Microscopic hematuria is defined as more than three red blood cells (RBCs) per HPF. Often hematuria is an incidental finding. However, it should be evaluated, especially in adults, because up to 10% of cases have a serious underlying cause.

PATHOGENESIS

Causes of hematuria include systemic illness and intrarenal (glomerular) and extrarenal diseases. Glomerular disease can cause leakage of RBCs into the renal tubules, resulting in both RBCs and RBC casts in the urine. Urinary cancers, stones, or infections can all cause hematuria.

CLINICAL MANIFESTATIONS

HISTORY

A careful medical history can suggest causes such as menstruation, viral infection, recent exercise, trauma, and sexual activity. Males can determine if, in the case of gross hematuria, whether the blood was visible at the onset of the void, throughout the stream, or at the end of the void. Initial hematuria implies a urethral etiology, whereas terminal hematuria suggests a prostatic etiology. Table 18-1 lists risk factors associated with more serious disease.

Flank pain may point to pyelonephritis, kidney infarction, or a kidney mass. Flank pain radiating into the groin suggests a kidney stone. Urgency, frequency, and dysuria occur with inflammation of the lower urinary tract from conditions such as cystitis.

Fever is common with pyelonephritis, but is also present in up to 90% of patients with renal cell carcinoma. Painless hematuria may be a presenting sign of a urinary tract malignancy. It is the most common presenting symptom of bladder cancer

TABLE 18-1. Risk Factors for Hematuria

Age >35
Male
Smoker
Occupational exposure to chemicals or dyes
History of gross hematuria
Urologic disease
Analgesic abuse

and is present in approximately 40% to 66% of the patients diagnosed with renal cancer.

Menstrual bleeding may be mistaken for hematuria. Trauma increases the likelihood of a kidney, ureteral, or urethral injury as the cause for hematuria. A recent streptococcal infection may be a clue for poststreptococcal glomerulonephritis, whereas exposure to TB increases the risk of a TB infection. A recent URI may cause hematuria in a patient with IgA nephropathy (Berger disease). A previous history of kidney stones, nephritis, cystitis, or bladder cancer suggests recurrence as a possible cause of hematuria. Valvular heart disease in association with recent dental work or a history of intravenous drug use increases the risk of bacterial endocarditis as a possible cause of microhematuria. Hemoptysis combined with hematuria is a symptom of pulmonary-renal (Goodpasture) syndrome.

Medication history is important. Interstitial nephritis can result from several medications, including NSAIDs, cephalosporins, proton pump inhibitors, and ciprofloxacin. Interstitial nephritis may cause hematuria, fever, and/or a skin rash. Chemotherapeutic agents, such as cyclophosphamide, can cause hemorrhagic cystitis. Several medications (e.g., pyridium and rifampin) discolor the urine and may be mistaken for hematuria.

Family history may suggest familial causes of hematuria including sickle cell disease or trait, benign familial hematuria, polycystic kidney disease, or Alport syndrome (autosomal recessive and associated with deafness).

PHYSICAL EXAMINATION

Costovertebral angle tenderness is common with pyelonephritis and tumors that stretch the renal capsule. Kidney stones may cause severe pain such that patients find it difficult to sit still.

An abdominal mass may be present with polycystic kidney disease or renal cell carcinoma. Suprapubic tenderness occurs with cystitis, and urethral discharge suggests urethritis.

In men, a rectal examination may reveal an enlarged smooth prostate gland, consistent with benign prostatic hypertrophy (BPH), or a nodular hard prostate, as is found in prostate cancer. A tender, boggy prostate is a sign of prostatitis. A pelvic examination in a woman may reveal a pelvic source of the bleeding.

Hypertension and peripheral edema are common findings with glomerulonephritis. Patients with atrial fibrillation are at risk for developing emboli and kidney infarction. In children and young adults, palpable purpura, arthritis, and abdominal pain are signs of Henoch–Schönlein purpura.

DIFFERENTIAL DIAGNOSIS

Lesions involving the kidneys, ureters, bladder, prostate, and urethra can all present with hematuria. Gross hematuria is usually associated with infection, stones, and neoplasm. Up to 5% of patients with microscopic and up to 30% to 40% with gross hematuria have a malignancy. In children, benign familial hematuria, glomerular disease, hypercalciuria, infection, and perineal irritation or trauma are the most common etiologies. In young adults, the most likely causes are infection, stones, trauma, or a urinary tract tumor. In older age groups, bladder cancer and prostate disease increase in prevalence. Systemic lupus erythematosus (SLE) may present with hematuria. Blood disorders such as sickle cell, coagulopathies, and leukemia are rare causes of hematuria and as noted earlier, drugs may cause hematuria. Individuals on anticoagulants who have hematuria should be evaluated because underlying lesions are frequently found. Box 18-1 lists the differential diagnosis for hematuria.

BOX 18-1. Differential Diagnosis of Hematuria

Hematologic
Coagulopathy, sickle cell hemoglobinopathies

Kidney/Glomerular
Glomerulonephritis, benign familial hematuria, multisystem disease (systemic lupus erythematosus, Henoch–Schönlein purpura, hemolytic uremic syndrome, polyarteritis nodosa, Wegener granulomatosis, Goodpasture syndrome)

Kidney/Nonglomerular
Renal vein or artery embolus, tuberculosis, pyelonephritis, polycystic kidney disease, medullary sponge kidney, acute interstitial nephritis, tumor, vascular malformation, trauma, papillary necrosis, exercise

Postrenal
Stones, tumor of ureter/bladder/urethra, cystitis, tuberculosis, prostatitis, urethritis, Foley catheter placement, exercise, benign prostatic hypertrophy

DIAGNOSTIC EVALUATION

The quantity of bleeding, the clinical setting, and other associated findings on the UA determine the extent of the evaluation (Fig. 18-1). Dipstick testing may be too sensitive and lacks specificity. For example, the presence of myoglobin or hemoglobin may be read as positive for blood on the dipstick and a positive urine dipstick result should be confirmed by microscopic examination. Identifying the presence or absence of dysmorphic RBCs such as RBC casts, or proteinuria, is important, because RBC casts and proteinuria suggest bleeding from a glomerular source. In interstitial nephritis, proteinuria and eosinophiluria may be present.

In the presence of hematuria *and* pyuria, a urine culture should be obtained. Pyuria, defined as more than four or five WBCs per HPF, points to infection as the cause. A repeat UA is indicated after successful treatment of the infection. If normal, no further treatment or evaluation is indicated in healthy individuals younger than 35 to 40 years. Similarly, a repeat UA to confirm the presence of hematuria in an individual suspected of having a benign cause,

Urinalysis with RBC > 3/HPF	
History and physical exam with apparent cause: treat and repeat. If negative after treatment, routine follow-up	Casts or proteinuria: work-up for glomerular causes, ultrasound; consider nephrology referral

Persistant hematuria not consistent with glomerular causes	
CT urography; ultrasound in pregnant patients	CBC, basic metabolic profile

High risk (Table 18-1)	Low risk
Positive CT: treatment and follow-up; referral for cystocopy	Negative evaluation: consider urology evaluation Postive CT: treatment and follow-up

FIGURE 18-1. Workup of hematuria. CBC, complete blood count; CT, computed tomography; HPF, high-power field; RBC, red blood cell.

such as menstrual bleeding or vigorous exercise, is helpful before embarking on an extensive workup.

Persistent hematuria or hematuria in individuals more than 35 years of age merits further investigation. In the absence of significant proteinuria ($>2+$ proteinuria), dysmorphic RBCs, or infection, hematuria usually indicates a nonglomerular cause. Routine blood tests include a CBC, BUN, and creatinine. Voided urine cytology is no longer recommended because of low sensitivity and specificity. For patients with evidence of glomerular bleeding such as RBC casts or heavy proteinuria (>3 or $4+$), a more extensive laboratory workup is indicated. Tests include an ESR, ANA test, cryoglobulin assay, antistreptococcal enzyme tests (ASO, anti-DNAse B), and an antineutrophil cytoplasmic antibody (ANCA) test to screen for granulomatosis with polyarteritis or vasculitis. Plasma complement levels should be tested, with low levels associated with SLE and poststreptococcal glomerulonephritis. Other useful tests include checking for eosinophiluria in patients with suspected interstitial nephritis and TB cultures in cases of persistent sterile pyuria. A hemoglobin electrophoresis can detect sickle cell disease and other hemoglobinopathies. Serum IgA levels are helpful in patients suspected of having Berger disease or Henoch–Schönlein purpura. Serum antiglomerular basement membrane antibodies can be positive in Goodpasture syndrome, and serum and urine immunoelectrophoresis can help diagnose multiple myeloma and other monoclonal gammopathies.

In recent years, CT urography has replaced an intravenous pyelogram (IVP) as the initial test to evaluate the upper urinary tract. Multiphasic CT urography can detect hydronephrosis, calculi, masses, as well as pyelonephritis and kidney abnormalities. A downside to CT urography is the amount of radiation a patient receives. IVP is a cost-effective and widely available alternative, but it may miss small masses or require additional testing to characterize lesions.

An ultrasound (US) study can safely rule out obstruction, evaluate kidney size, and identify masses or cysts. In the patient with suspected glomerular disease, a US is the initial study of choice. In pregnant women, a US and retrograde pyelography are recommended for evaluation. Rarely, renal arteriography is needed to evaluate a traumatic injury, a suspicious kidney mass, or an arteriovenous malformation.

Cystoscopy is the best way to evaluate the lower urinary tract and is indicated for all patients with risk factors for malignancy. This procedure can detect bladder neoplasm, bladder stones, BPH, urethral strictures, and cystitis. The value of cystoscopy is less clear in younger individuals and left to the discretion of the urologist.

TREATMENT

Management depends on the underlying cause. The presence of a defined lesion or the need to undergo cystoscopy merits referral to a urologist. Poststreptococcal glomerulonephritis therapy is generally limited to treating the associated hypertension. Rapid or progressive deterioration of kidney function, hematuria associated with proteinuria (>2+), or suspected glomerulonephritis merit consultation to a nephrologist for evaluation and consideration of kidney biopsy.

Despite an extensive evaluation, no cause of hematuria can be found in 8% to 10% of patients. These individuals require follow-up with monitoring of the UA and blood pressure for 2 to 3 years.

KEY POINTS

- Asymptomatic microscopic hematuria is defined as more than three RBCs per HPF.
- Common causes for hematuria include glomerulonephritis, UTI, stones, trauma, and neoplasm of the urinary tract.
- Important risk factors for malignancy as a cause for hematuria are age >35 years, prior urologic disease, smoking, and environmental exposures.
- Familial causes of hematuria include benign familial hematuria, sickle cell disease or trait, polycystic kidney disease, Alport syndrome, and familial hypercalciuria.

19 | Jaundice in Adults

Jaundice (icterus) is yellow staining of the sclera, skin, and other tissues due to hyperbilirubinemia. Total serum bilirubin in a healthy person is normally 0.2 to 1.2 mg/dL and consists of both conjugated and unconjugated bilirubin. Jaundice usually becomes clinically evident when the bilirubin level reaches 2.0 to 2.5 mg/dL. Increased levels of bilirubin can be due to overproduction, impaired uptake by the liver, or impaired excretion. In adults, jaundice occurs most often due to liver disease or obstruction of the common bile duct.

EPIDEMIOLOGY

Hepatitis accounts for up to 75% of the cases of jaundice in young adults. Hereditary disorders such as Gilbert and Crigler–Najjar syndromes are less common causes of jaundice. Gilbert syndrome is a benign, lifelong condition, and is often diagnosed early in life. It affects 3% to 5% of the population. Crigler–Najjar syndrome is a rare disorder that is also diagnosed early in life. For patients more than age 45 years, 60% of cases of jaundice result from obstruction and slightly more than half of these cases are related to gallstones. An underlying malignancy accounts for most of the remaining cases.

PATHOGENESIS

Bilirubin is the major breakdown product of hemoglobin. Bilirubin binds to albumin and is transported to the liver for conjugation with glucuronic acid to form bilirubin diglucuronide (conjugated bilirubin or direct bilirubin). After conjugation, bilirubin is excreted through the biliary system into the small intestine. In the intestine, bacteria convert bilirubin to stercobilinogens, which gives stools its brown color. Because unconjugated bilirubin is not water soluble, it does not pass through the glomerular membrane,

and as a result does not appear in the urine. However, conjugated bilirubin (bilirubin diglucuronide) is water soluble and can be confirmed by finding bilirubin (bilirubinuria) in the urine. Bilirubinuria is typical of hepatocellular or cholestatic jaundice and results in a positive urine dipstick test for bilirubin and a characteristically dark tea-colored urine.

An elevated serum bilirubin can either be unconjugated or conjugated. The causes of unconjugated hyperbilirubinemia are secondary to overproduction, hemolysis, or defects in bilirubin conjugation. Overproduction of bilirubin can be seen in diseases such as thalassemia, sideroblastic anemia, and vitamin B_{12} deficiency, all of which result in ineffective erythropoiesis. Gilbert, Dubin–Johnson, and Crigler–Najjar syndromes are characterized by a defect in the liver's ability to conjugate bilirubin, causing an increase in unconjugated hyperbilirubinemia. Decreased hepatic uptake of bilirubin, secondary to sepsis or right heart failure, can also elevate unconjugated bilirubin.

Impaired excretion of bilirubin from the liver causes conjugated hyperbilirubinemia. This can occur at the cellular level due to hepatocellular disease, in the ductule due to medication exposure (e.g., phenothiazines or estrogens), or in the septal ducts due to primary biliary cirrhosis. In addition, obstruction of the common bile duct by gallstones or pancreatic cancer can cause conjugated hyperbilirubinemia.

CLINICAL MANIFESTATIONS

HISTORY

The presence of right-upper-quadrant pain suggests a hepatobiliary cause. Nausea and vomiting accompanied by flu-like symptoms preceding jaundice may indicate hepatitis. Other questions in the history of present illness should include the presence of pruritus, urine discoloration, increased abdominal

TABLE 19-1. Risk Factors for Hepatitis

Travel to an endemic area
Living or working in an institution with long-term residents, e.g., prison, long-term care facility
Working in daycare
Having blood transfusions
Getting a tattoo or body piercing
Sharing needles, razors, or toothbrushes
Hemodialysis
IV drug use
Participating in anal sex
Eating raw shellfish

girth (ascites), fever, and weight loss. Patients should be asked about risk factors for hepatitis such as intravenous drug use, alcohol consumption, contact with hepatitis patients, recent blood transfusions, recent travel, and prior history of immunizations (see Table 19-1). A family history of episodic jaundice in the setting of intercurrent illness is consistent with Gilbert disease. Current and past medications including any herbal or over-the-counter medicines should be noted. Drugs that may cause jaundice include acetaminophen, isoniazid, nitrofurantoin, methotrexate, sulfonamides, oral contraceptives, chlorpromazine, and phenytoin.

Patients with hereditary cholestatic syndromes or intrahepatic cholestasis may present with pruritus, light-colored stools, and malaise, or they may be totally asymptomatic. Patients with hepatitis may have malaise, anorexia, low-grade fever, and right-upper-quadrant pain. Also, the urine may appear tea-colored because of the excretion of conjugated bilirubin. Patients who present with right-upper-quadrant pain without fever may have an obstruction of the common bile duct, resulting in jaundice. In patients who present with Charcot triad (high fever, right-upper-quadrant pain, and jaundice), cholangitis should be ruled out. Jaundice and weight loss are findings associated with carcinoma of the head of the pancreas.

PHYSICAL EXAMINATION

Physical examination should focus on signs of liver disease, such as spider angiomas, gynecomastia, and palmar erythema. The abdominal examination should assess for liver size, abdominal tenderness, and masses. Splenomegaly is common when hemolysis causes jaundice. A palpable gallbladder (Courvoisier sign) indicates gallstones as a cause of jaundice. Viral hepatitis usually causes a mildly tender liver with slight-to-moderate enlargement. Findings such as a small liver, ascites, splenomegaly, spider angiomas, gynecomastia, palmar erythema, and other stigmata of cirrhosis suggest advanced hepatocellular disease. The eyes should be checked for Kayser–Fleischer rings, which indicate Wilson disease. On rare occasions, carotenemia from excessive consumption of carotene-rich foods such as carrots and sweet potatoes can cause a harmless yellow pigmentation of the skin, especially of the hands and soles. In carotenemia, the sclera is not discolored.

DIFFERENTIAL DIAGNOSIS

Box 19-1 lists the causes of jaundice grouped by pathophysiology. Causes range from nonserious conditions such as Gilbert syndrome to potentially fatal diseases such as pancreatic cancer. Obstruction, intrahepatic cholestasis, and hepatocellular disease cause the majority of cases of jaundice. In young patients, hepatitis is the most common cause of jaundice. In older individuals, obstruction from stones or tumors is more common.

DIAGNOSTIC EVALUATION

The diagnostic approach begins with the history and physical examination, which should provide clues as to the etiology of the patient's jaundice. Testing usually begins with a CBC, UA, and a liver panel test, including transaminases, total bilirubin, alkaline phosphatase, and albumin. An elevated conjugated bilirubin level and urine dipstick positive for bilirubin indicate obstruction, cholestasis, or hepatocellular injury. If the urine dipstick is negative for bilirubin, the cause is more likely a hemolytic process or Gilbert syndrome, the most common type of hereditary hyperbilirubinemia. Gilbert syndrome is characterized by a mild, recurrent elevation of bilirubin precipitated by fasting or mild illness without systemic symptoms or other liver test abnormalities. Anemia with an elevated reticulocyte count, increased lactate dehydrogenase, fragmented RBCs on peripheral smear, and a low serum haptoglobin suggests hemolysis. In patients with elevated conjugated bilirubin, the pattern of

BOX 19-1. Differential Diagnosis for Adult Jaundice

Unconjugated Hyperbilirubinemia
Increased production
Hemolytic anemia secondary to ineffective erythropoiesis
Thalassemia
Sideroblastic anemia
Pernicious anemia
Genetic hemolytic anemias, e.g., sickle cell, spherocytosis, G6-PD deficiency
Acute hemolytic diseases
Impaired uptake of bilirubin
Gilbert syndrome
Crigler–Najjar syndrome

Conjugated Hyperbilirubinemia
Hereditary cholestatic syndromes
Faulty excretion of bilirubin
Dubin–Johnson syndrome
Rotor syndrome
Hepatocellular dysfunction
Biliary epithelial damage
Hepatitis
Cirrhosis
Intrahepatic cholestasis
Drugs
Biliary cirrhosis
Sepsis
Biliary obstruction
Choledocholithiasis
Biliary atresia
Carcinoma of biliary duct
Sclerosing cholangitis
Pancreatic cancer

the liver enzyme elevations provides clues to the cause of the jaundice. Transaminases elevated out of proportion (more than five times the normal) to the alkaline phosphatase suggest liver dysfunction. Conversely, an obstructive enzyme pattern is characterized by an elevated alkaline phosphatase (more than three times the normal level) out of proportion to the rise in transaminases (less than four to five times the normal). Gamma glutamyl transpeptidase usually parallels the rise in alkaline phosphatase. This test is useful for confirming that an elevated alkaline phosphatase is caused by liver disease, because increases in alkaline phosphatase can also occur in bone disease. A low serum albumin concentration suggests chronic liver disease.

If liver disease is suspected as the cause of jaundice, the following tests should be performed, as indicated by the history and physical examination:

1. Hepatitis profile to screen for hepatitis A, B, and C;
2. Antimitochondrial antibody to screen for primary biliary cirrhosis;
3. Serum iron, transferrin saturation, and ferritin to screen for hemochromatosis;
4. Serum ceruloplasmin and urine copper levels to screen for Wilson disease;
5. Antismooth muscle and antinuclear antibodies to screen for autoimmune hepatitis.

Imaging tests are useful for patients with obstructive disease. Ultrasound (US) is a noninvasive test useful for detecting dilated bile ducts indicative of obstruction. The sensitivity and specificity of this test is in the range of 90% to 95%. Although an US can detect obstruction, it is less helpful in determining the site and the cause of the obstruction. A CT scan or magnetic resonance cholangiopancreatography is more likely to identify the site or cause of obstruction, but is more expensive than US.

If an obstruction is identified and additional anatomic detail is needed, endoscopic retrograde cholangiopancreatography (ERCP) can provide visualization. This test is also useful if obstructive jaundice is suspected, despite negative imaging procedures. Complications of ERCP include infection and pancreatitis.

TREATMENT

The treatment of jaundice depends on the underlying disease process. Any drug that may cause jaundice should be discontinued. If there is a complete resolution of laboratory abnormalities within 2 weeks of withdrawing the offending agent, no further workup or treatment is needed. Symptomatic pruritus can be treated with cholestyramine and antihistamines such as diphenhydramine. Pernicious anemia, which may cause a hemolytic anemia, can be treated with vitamin B_{12} replacement.

Patients with obstructive jaundice may have to be treated surgically. For patients with gallstones, either open or laparoscopic cholecystectomy is indicated.

In some cases of obstructive jaundice, an ERCP can be both diagnostic and therapeutic. Common bile duct stones may be removed via the endoscope or a stent placed to relieve the biliary obstruction, to reduce inflammation, and prepare a patient for surgery. Most patients with a neoplasm require surgery. This surgery can either be palliative or intended for definitive treatment. Patients with obstructive jaundice and fever with chills should be hospitalized and treated for possible cholangitis with intravenous antibiotics.

Hepatitis can usually be treated on an outpatient basis. However, patients with severe nausea and vomiting who become dehydrated should be hospitalized.

KEY POINTS

- Jaundice becomes clinically evident when the bilirubin level is >2.0 to 2.5 mg/dL.
- Hepatitis accounts for up to 75% of the cases of jaundice in younger adults.
- Biliary obstruction from gallstones or malignancy is more common in older patients.
- Drugs causing jaundice include acetaminophen, isoniazid, nitrofurantoin, methotrexate, sulfonamides, and phenytoin.
- Weight loss and painless jaundice are signs of pancreatic cancer.
- Low serum albumin in a jaundiced patient suggests a chronic process.

20 | Knee Pain

Knee pain is most often due to acute trauma or over-use, but can also be the result of degenerative disease, inflammatory arthritis, and crystalline arthropathies. Knowledge of the function and anatomy of the knee is essential in diagnosing and treating knee pain.

PATHOGENESIS

The knee is the largest joint in the body and performs a hinge-like motion. The lateral and medial tibiofemoral articulations are the weight-bearing portions of the knee, whereas the patellofemoral articulation acts as a fulcrum for added quadriceps strength. The meniscal cartilage provides cushioning between the bones and a smooth surface for movement. The lateral and medial collateral ligaments provide lateral and medial stability to the knee joint, whereas the anterior and posterior cruciate ligaments, located inside the joint, provide anterior-to-posterior stability. The knee also has multiple bursae that provide lubrication for the many dynamic components of the knee and allow for fluid movement.

Injury or inflammation to either the soft-tissue or the bony structures of the knee may cause pain. For example, inflammation of the bursae from either direct trauma or microtrauma associated with overuse can cause pain. Patellar tendonitis is another common cause of pain that results from overuse with activities, such as running or jumping. Twisting injuries place stress on the cartilage and may result in a meniscal tear, whereas sprains of the medial and lateral collateral ligaments usually result from a direct blow to the knee while the foot is planted.

Patellofemoral pain syndrome occurs with overuse in combination with biomechanical factors, such as muscle imbalance. These factors cause improper tracking of the patella, which normally rests in the patellofemoral groove of the femur. Overuse and repeated impact with the knee in flexion lead to increased pressure in this groove and discomfort.

Osgood–Schlatter disease is a common cause of anterior knee pain in adolescents. The pain is located on the anterior tibial tubercle and is thought to be due to activities that increase traction on the patellar tendon. This stress leads to microavulsions of the growth plate on the tibial tubercle where the patellar tendon inserts.

CLINICAL MANIFESTATIONS

HISTORY

Depending on the cause of the knee pain, patients may report swelling, erythema, limited range-of-motion, bruising, and decreased activity. If an injury causes knee pain, the mechanism of injury (e.g., direct impact to the lateral knee during full extension), occurrence of a "popping" sensation, degree of swelling, and ability to ambulate after the event are all relevant pieces of information. The sensation of an unstable knee (the feeling of giving way) suggests damage to a ligament. Locking of the knee is more consistent with a torn meniscus or a loose body that becomes trapped. Furthermore, useful history includes recent trauma, initiation of a new exercise regimen, duration of the knee pain, and a description of activities or positions that aggravate or alleviate the pain.

Sudden onset of severe knee pain and effusion in a middle-aged man without a history of trauma is most commonly due to gout. Often, there is a previous history of a gout attack. Although patients with gout may have a fever, an elevated temperature with a swollen, red joint is more consistent with septic arthritis. In younger individuals, gonorrhea is the most common infection; therefore, it is important to inquire about genitourinary symptoms such as a vaginal or penile discharge.

Up to 10% of the population over age 65 suffers from symptomatic osteoarthritis of the knee. Obesity is a major risk factor. The pain is chronic, often starting in the anterior and medial portions of the knee, but it can involve the whole knee joint. Mild stiffness in the morning lasting less than 30 minutes is common. Prolonged standing or walking may precipitate or worsen symptoms.

Prolonged morning stiffness and pain that is worse in the morning, improves with motion, and is associated with systemic symptoms such as fever suggests an inflammatory arthritis. In rheumatoid arthritis, multiple symmetric joint involvement is the rule, although patients may develop pain only in the knee. Pain behind the kneecap that is worsened by standing up or climbing stairs is consistent with patellofemoral pain syndrome.

PHYSICAL EXAMINATION

Examination should be performed with the patient in the supine position with both legs fully exposed. During general inspection, asymmetry, bruising, bony deformities, effusions, and erythema of the knee should be noted. Feet and hips should be examined for abnormalities contributing to, or causing the knee pain. A key part of the examination is to determine whether the pain is intra- or extra-articular. Pain on both active and passive ranges of motion suggests an intra-articular problem, whereas pain on active but not on passive motion of the joint suggests extra-articular disease. Palpation along the joint line and bony landmarks is followed by determining the degree of flexion and extension of both the healthy and injured knees. Pain during any segment of the examination provides clues as to which components of the knee may be injured. Varus and valgus stress test are used to assess the medial and lateral collateral ligaments, while maneuvering the knee between full flexion and full extension. Anterior-to-posterior laxity is assessed via the Lachman test. This maneuver is performed by flexing the knee at 20 to 30 degrees, holding the femur stable, and moving the tibia forward. The degree of laxity is assessed by comparison with a healthy knee and determines the competency of the cruciate ligaments. The McMurray test is used to evaluate the meniscus. This test is performed with the knee fully flexed and the foot rotated outward to test medial meniscus and inward to test lateral meniscus. The knee is then fully extended while rotating the foot in the opposite direction. A painful "click" is considered a positive test and indicates a possible meniscal injury.

DIFFERENTIAL DIAGNOSIS

Common diagnoses of knee pain include ligamentous injuries, meniscal injuries, bursitis (patellar, anserine), fractures, patellofemoral pain syndrome, Osgood–Schlatter disease, iliotibial band syndrome, Baker cyst, osteoarthritis, rheumatoid or other types of inflammatory arthritis, gout, pseudogout, and septic arthritis.

DIAGNOSTIC EVALUATION

Many patients can be diagnosed by history and physical examination alone. However, x-rays should be obtained in all patients who are thought to have a possible fracture and may help determine the degree of arthritis (Fig. 20-1). MRI is useful to diagnose rupture of the anterior cruciate ligament (ACL) and can often detect injury to the meniscus and collateral ligaments.

Laboratory testing may be helpful in evaluating patients with fever, rash, or involvement of other joints. An elevated ESR can be a clue to a systemic

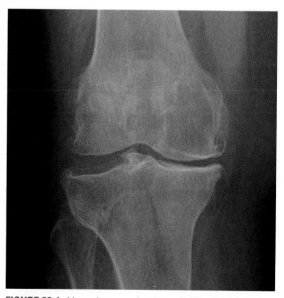

FIGURE 20-1. X-ray image of osteoarthritis of the knee. (From Moskowitz RW, Altman RD, Buckwalter JA, et al. *Osteoarthritis: Diagnosis and Medical/Surgical Management.* 4th ed. Philadelphia, PA: Lippincott Williams & Wilkins; 2007.)

TABLE 20-1. Characteristic Synovial Joint Fluid Findings with Different Causes for Knee Pain

Cause	Finding
Noninflammatory (e.g., osteoarthritis)	<2000 WBCs, clear, yellow
Inflammatory (e.g., gout, pseudogout, RA)	>2000 WBCs, cloudy, yellow
Infection/septic joint	>20,000 WBCs, cloudy, yellow
Trauma	Bloody, aspirate

RA, rheumatoid arthritis; WBCs, white blood cells.

process. A rheumatoid factor and an ANA help screen for rheumatoid arthritis and lupus. A CBC and UA levels may also be helpful.

Acute isolated knee pain with an effusion should be evaluated with an arthrocentesis (Table 20-1). The fluid should be sent for determination of cell count, glucose, Gram stain, culture, and examination for crystals. Uric acid crystals (negatively birefringent under polarized light) in the joint fluid are diagnostic of gout, whereas calcium pyrophosphate crystals (weakly positively birefringent) are seen in pseudogout. A bloody aspirate following trauma suggests a significant injury to the knee, and a rare finding of fat globules indicates a fracture. Diagnostic arthroscopy may be helpful in patients with persistent pain despite a normal x-ray and laboratory test results.

TREATMENT

Rest and NSAIDs or acetaminophen are sufficient to manage the majority of patients with knee pain. In patients with mild-to-moderate degenerative joint disease (DJD), weight loss, judicious use of exercise and rest, physical therapy, and medications control most symptoms. Glucosamine sulfate may help treat chronic symptoms of osteoarthritis in some patients. A series of intra-articular injections of hyaluronic acid for treatment of osteoarthritis can be useful for alleviating symptoms in patients with mild-to-moderate osteoarthritis. With severe DJD that is unresponsive to conservative therapy, referral to an orthopedist for possible surgery is appropriate.

Following a knee injury, acute pain usually responds to rest, ice, and NSAIDs. A knee immobilizer may provide support, reduce pain by restricting mobility, and prevent further injury. If there is suspicion of a more severe injury such as a meniscus or ligament tear, orthopedic referral is appropriate.

Treatment of patellofemoral pain syndrome is geared toward the perceived causes. In patients with overpronation, orthotics are often beneficial.

Relative rest, physical therapy, nonimpact activities, ice, and NSAIDs all benefit patients suffering from this disorder. Taping and patellar stabilizing braces may benefit patients with obvious lateral subluxation.

NSAIDs usually improve the pain of inflammatory arthritis. Most family physicians comanage individuals with rheumatoid arthritis along with a rheumatologist, especially patients requiring disease-modifying medications (e.g., methotrexate). Joint infection is a medical emergency and merits hospitalization, drainage, and intravenous antibiotics. Gout usually responds to NSAIDs. Patients with multiple attacks may benefit from prophylactic therapy with allopurinol, probenecid, or colchicine. Colchicine or prednisone may be used for acute attacks in patients unable to take NSAIDs.

Osgood–Schlatter disease and soft-tissue inflammatory conditions, such as patellar tendonitis, usually respond to treatment consisting of reducing activities that exacerbate the pain, application of ice, occasional use of NSAIDs, and range-of-motion and stretching exercises. Rarely, referral for surgical consultation and care is necessary.

A tear of the ACL is a more serious injury with long-term implications. Patients often report a "popping" sensation inside the knee, related to a sudden change in direction or direct trauma. Patients experience immediate pain, and a significant effusion typically develops within a few hours. In patients who want to remain active, surgical reconstruction is the preferred therapy. However, in older, less-active patients, physical therapy and use of a brace may suffice.

Tears of the meniscus typically result from a twisting motion, but a clear event causing the injury may not always have occurred. Treatment of meniscal tears is symptomatic with rest, ice, compression, and elevation. Many patients with persistent symptoms benefit from arthroscopic knee surgery to remove the torn piece, thus allowing for smooth tracking between the articulated surfaces.

KEY POINTS

- The feeling of the knee giving way suggests damage to a ligament. Locking of the knee is more consistent with a torn meniscus or loose body that becomes trapped.

- A sudden onset of severe knee pain and effusion in a middle-aged man in the absence of trauma is most commonly due to gout.

- Up to 10% of the population more than age 65 suffers from symptomatic osteoarthritis of the knee.

- Plain x-rays should be obtained in all the patients who are thought to have a possible fracture.

- MRI is used to diagnose rupture of the ACL and can often detect injury to the meniscus and collateral ligaments.

- Acute isolated knee pain with an effusion should usually be evaluated with an arthrocentesis.

- A knee injury usually responds to rest, ice, and NSAIDs. A knee immobilizer may provide support, reduce pain by restricting mobility, and prevent further injury.

- NSAIDs usually improve the pain of inflammatory arthritis.

21 | Lymphadenopathy

Lymphadenopathy is the enlargement of the lymph glands, usually larger than 1 cm. Two exceptions are inguinal or cervical lymph nodes (LNs), which are considered normal up to 1.5 cm, and epitrochlear, supraclavicular, or popliteal LNs, which are considered enlarged if larger than 0.5 cm. Generalized lymphadenopathy is defined as enlargement of LNs in three or more noncontiguous areas. Regional lymphadenopathy exists when the swelling is limited to a specific region, such as the cervical LNs.

PATHOGENESIS

Three mechanisms can produce enlarged LNs. First, LNs can increase in size due to reactive hyperplasia when cells within the gland respond to an antigen or inflammation. They can also increase in size if primary cells within the lymph gland transform into neoplastic cells and enlarge the gland as they proliferate. Finally, LNs may enlarge if there is an invasion of cells from outside the node, such as malignant cells from a metastatic cancer or from a benign infiltrating disorder, such as sarcoidosis.

CLINICAL MANIFESTATIONS

HISTORY

Lymphadenopathy usually causes no symptoms unless the nodes are acutely inflamed, large enough to cause lymphatic obstruction, or are pressing on a nerve or other structures. If symptoms are present, they usually relate to the underlying disease. Regional lymphadenopathy can be caused by a local infection or inflammation in the area drained by the LN. The history should focus on the area in question. For example, in the cases of cervical lymphadenopathy, asking about pharyngeal symptoms, dental problems, and hoarseness is appropriate.

Generalized lymphadenopathy requires a thorough history, because it is seen in a wide spectrum of diseases, including infections as well as immunologic, metabolic, and malignant disorders. Onset is important, because acute infection becomes a less likely cause as time passes and new onset (<2 weeks) or long-standing (>12 months) lymphadenopathy is less likely to be malignant. Constitutional symptoms such as fever and weight loss suggest cancer, systemic infection, or connective tissue disease. Recent rashes, arthralgias, pharyngeal symptoms, or pet exposure may suggest a specific diagnosis, such as connective tissue disease, viral illness, or cat scratch fever. Syphilis and AIDS should be considered in patients at risk for these infections. Lymphadenitis associated with lymphangitis is a common manifestation of bacterial infections in the extremities, and is usually associated with pain and tenderness. Systemic symptoms such as fever and chills are common.

Risk factors for less-common infections include contact with sheep (brucellosis), geographic locale (coccidioidomycosis or histoplasmosis), and animal bites (*Francisella tularensis* or *Pasteurella*).

PHYSICAL EXAMINATION

All LNs should be characterized by size, tenderness, texture, and consistency. Small, palpable cervical LNs (<1 cm) are common in children. Mild inguinal bilateral lymphadenopathy (<1.5 cm) is common throughout life. Although size alone is not a diagnostic factor, LNs larger than 3 cm in an adult suggest neoplasm. Box 21-1 lists characteristics associated with different etiologies and other clues on physical examination that may suggest a specific etiology. Red streaks extending from a cellulitis toward a swollen, tender LN is consistent with lymphangitis and lymphadenitis.

BOX 21-1. Lymphadenopathy Characteristics and Findings

Lymph Node Characteristics
Malignant: hard, matted, fixed, nontender, and usually >3 cm
Infectious: warm, erythematous, fluctuant
Reactive: discrete, rubbery, and freely mobile

Key Findings of Associated Disorders
Thyromegaly: hyperthyroidism
Arthritis: connective tissue disease and leukemia
Massive splenomegaly: cancer, infectious mononucleosis, storage diseases, leukemia, and lymphoma
Skin rash: viral exanthem, connective tissue disease, and Kawasaki disease

Generalized lymphadenopathy is usually characterized by multiple small and discrete LNs often associated with splenomegaly.

DIFFERENTIAL DIAGNOSIS

Generalized lymphadenopathy can be caused by infection, immunologic disorder, metabolic disease, malignancy, and miscellaneous inflammatory conditions. Common viral infections causing lymphadenopathy include infectious mononucleosis, cytomegalovirus (CMV), and HIV. Less-common infections include TB, syphilis, histoplasmosis, and toxoplasmosis. Immunologic disorders include connective tissue disease such as SLE or rheumatoid arthritis and reactions such as a drug reaction or serum sickness. Metabolic disorders include hyperthyroidism and, rarely, storage diseases such as Gaucher and Niemann–Pick diseases. Malignant causes of generalized lymphadenopathy include leukemia, lymphomas, metastatic carcinoma, and malignant histiocytosis. Additional causes include disorders such as Kawasaki disease and intravenous drug use.

Differential diagnosis of localized lymphadenopathy depends on the involved region. Cervical lymphadenopathy is the most commonly encountered form and is usually caused by infections, primarily upper respiratory tract infections (URIs). Box 21-2 lists the differential diagnoses of lymphadenopathy by region.

DIAGNOSTIC EVALUATION

Lymphadenopathy is common and usually indicates benign, self-limited disease. This is particularly true among children and young adults who are prone to reactive lymphadenopathy. Localized lymphadenopathy usually represents disease from the area of drainage. For example, cervical LNs are commonly enlarged by infections involving the pharynx, salivary glands, and scalp. If it appears that the patient has a benign cause of lymphadenopathy, close observation or limited testing (e.g., a mononucleosis spot test [Monospot or strep screen]) is indicated to confirm the suspected diagnosis. In contrast, in individuals whose initial assessment suggests a malignant disorder, such as an enlarged, hard, matted cervical LN in a patient with a history of smoking or alcohol abuse (both risk factors for head and neck squamous cell cancer), require more extensive testing and consideration of an LN biopsy.

If the diagnosis is uncertain, stepwise testing with a CBC and serology is appropriate. A markedly abnormal CBC revealing a severe anemia or malignant cells implies cancer and an urgent need for more complete evaluation, including bone marrow or LN biopsy. A CBC may also suggest infectious mononucleosis or a viral infection (atypical lymphocytes), pyogenic infection (granulocytes), or hypersensitivity states (eosinophilia). Serologic testing may be helpful, including a Monospot or EBV titers. Other serologic tests that may be helpful are those for CMV or toxoplasmosis titers, HIV antibodies, ANA, and rheumatoid factor. A CXR is indicated in the presence of pulmonary symptoms, in severely ill patients, or in those with supraclavicular lymphadenopathy. A CXR is also useful as a second level of evaluation for persistent undiagnosed lymphadenopathy. The presence of hilar lymphadenopathy suggests sarcoidosis, lymphoma, fungal infection, TB, or metastatic cancer. A positive TB skin test suggests mycobacterial infection. Urethral and cervical cultures can be helpful for determining

BOX 21-2. Differential Diagnosis of Lymphadenopathy by Region

Cervical

Upper respiratory infection
Bacterial infection of head and neck
Mononucleosis
CMV
Toxoplasmosis
Mycobacterial infection
Neoplasm—primary and metastatic
Kawasaki disease
Sarcoidosis
Reactive hyperplasia

Supraclavicular Lymphadenopathy

Tuberculosis
Histoplasmosis
Sarcoid
Lymphoma
Metastatic disease, particularly lung and gastrointestinal

Axillary

Upper extremity infection
Connective tissue disease
Cat scratch disease
Neoplasm

Epitrochlear

Hand infection
Secondary syphilis

Inguinal

Local or lower-extremity infection
Localized skin rash
Syphilis
Lymphogranularum venereum
Genital herpes
Chancroid
Cat scratch disease
Neoplastic disorders

Mediastinal Lymphadenopathy

Sarcoidosis
Tuberculosis
Histoplasmosis
Coccidioidomycosis
Lymphoma
Metastatic cancer

the cause of inguinal lymphadenopathy. Culturing LN tissue or aspirated fluid may also be of value. Special stains can detect cat scratch disease and mycobacteria. Rarely, blood cultures are required in the cases of suspected bacteremia or unusual diseases such as tularemia, plague, and brucellosis.

Imaging studies such as US, CT, or MRI of the involved area may be useful to differentiate lymphadenopathy from nonlymphatic enlargement. A CT scan is used for evaluating hilar LNs or to demonstrate the presence of abdominal LNs. Imaging may also identify a primary lesion that accounts for the regional lymphadenopathy. A bone marrow examination is indicated for patients with severe anemia, thrombocytopenia, or the presence of malignant cells on peripheral smear.

If there is clinical suspicion of a neoplasm or an illness such as TB or sarcoidosis, and a diagnosis cannot be established, LN biopsy should be considered. Clinical factors such as LN size and irregularity, the presence of weight loss, or an enlarged liver or spleen suggest a need for an early biopsy. Enlarged supraclavicular LNs are often associated with serious underlying disease and usually require early biopsy. During a follow-up for undiagnosed lymphadenopathy, LNs that remain constant in size for 4 to 8 weeks or fail to resolve within 8 to 12 weeks should be biopsied.

TREATMENT

Management is directed at the underlying cause. The treatment of viral infections is largely symptomatic. Cat scratch disease may benefit from antibiotics such as TMP/SMX. Nodes affected by atypical mycobacteria may need surgical excision combined with three antituberculosis drugs such as isoniazid, rifampin, and ethambutol. Initial therapy for acute unilateral cervical lymphadenitis consists of antibiotics active against *Streptococcus* and *Staphylococcus*, such as a cephalosporin, erythromycin, or semisynthetic penicillin such as dicloxacillin. Neoplastic disease should be referred to an oncologist for treatment.

KEY POINTS

- Generalized lymphadenopathy is defined as an enlargement of LNs in three or more noncontiguous areas. Regional lymphadenopathy exists when the swelling is limited to a specific region such as cervical LNs.

- Lymphadenopathy usually causes no symptoms unless the nodes are acutely inflamed, large enough to cause lymphatic obstruction, or are pressing on a nerve or other structure.

- Infection, immunologic disorder, metabolic disease, malignancy, and miscellaneous inflammatory conditions can cause generalized lymphadenopathy.

- Localized lymphadenopathy usually represents disease from the area of drainage.

22 | Nausea and Vomiting

Nausea is the sensation of having to vomit and often precedes or accompanies vomiting. Vomiting, which can be either voluntary or involuntary, is the forceful expulsion of gastric contents through the mouth. In most instances, in the family practice setting, the symptoms are caused by a self-limited illness, such as viral gastroenteritis. However, vomiting can be a presenting symptom for a more serious illness.

PATHOGENESIS

Vomiting is under the control of two central nervous system (CNS) centers, the vomiting center in the medullary reticular formation and the chemoreceptor trigger zone in the fourth ventricle. Vagal nerve irritation and impulses from the sympathetic nerves in the throat, head, abdomen, and GI tract can send impulses to the vomiting centers. Vestibular disturbances, drugs, and metabolic abnormalities can activate the chemoreceptor trigger zone and cause vomiting. Efferent impulses from the CNS then travel to the effector muscles, causing a stereotypical vomiting response that varies little regardless of cause.

CLINICAL MANIFESTATIONS

HISTORY

A thorough history is critical to effectively sorting out the many causes of nausea and vomiting. It is important to characterize the duration, timing, frequency, and type of vomiting. Acute symptoms lasting <1 week suggest an infection, intoxication, drug effect, metabolic abnormality, or visceral disease. Early-morning nausea and vomiting are common with pregnancy but are also typical of vomiting associated with uremia and adrenal insufficiency. The relationship of nausea to food can be helpful. Symptoms precipitated by eating are common with

GI disorders, such as acute gastritis, peptic ulcer disease, and gastric outlet obstruction, or can be associated with psychogenic factors. Vomiting several hours after eating can occur with diabetic gastroparesis, gastric outlet obstruction, or gastric malignancy, whereas vomiting immediately after meals suggests bulimia as a possible cause. Projectile vomiting may indicate pyloric stenosis in infants or can occur with CNS disease that causes increased intracranial pressure. Characterizing the type of vomitus can be helpful. The presence of bile indicates an open pylorus, whereas feculent vomitus is seen in patients with a lower GI obstruction or gastrocolic fistula. Bloody or coffee-ground emesis indicates bleeding from the esophagus, stomach, or duodenum. Less commonly, bloody vomitus is seen in patients with blood swallowed from bleeding in the mouth or nose.

Nausea and vomiting accompanied by fever, watery diarrhea, and abdominal cramps are typical for viral gastroenteritis. Food poisoning usually begins within 6 hours of eating the offending substance and resolves within 24 to 48 hours. Abdominal pain with nausea may indicate a surgical problem, such as appendicitis or cholecystitis. Cramps may be caused by gastroenteritis or an early obstruction. Visceral pain syndrome—seen with MI, renal colic, and pancreatitis—commonly causes nausea. Vestibular vertigo suggests an acute vestibular cause, such as labyrinthitis. Recurring vertigo, tinnitus, and vomiting are consistent with Ménière disease. Headache associated with vomiting is common with migraine.

The possibility of drug-induced nausea should always be considered. Common examples include macrolide antibiotics, metronidazole, opiates, NSAIDs, estrogen containing hormone preparations, digitalis, theophylline, and chemotherapeutic agents. The medical and surgical history often suggests possible causes. Diabetic ketoacidosis should always be considered in diabetic individuals with nausea and vomiting. A history of coronary artery disease or renal insufficiency raises the possibility of nausea and vomiting caused by one of these conditions. Previous abdominal surgeries increase the risk of obstruction.

PHYSICAL EXAMINATION

The physical examination includes an overall assessment of appearance, vital signs, and volume status. Infants and elderly individuals are most prone to significant dehydration and electrolyte imbalance. The abdominal examination can provide clues to the underlying etiology in patients with abdominal pain. Localized tenderness may indicate a specific cause. For example, a large, tender liver suggests hepatitis, and a positive Murphy's sign is consistent with cholecystitis. Tenderness with guarding, or rebound tenderness, occurs with peritoneal irritation. High-pitched bowel sounds are consistent with an early obstruction, whereas decreased or absent bowel sounds are consistent with peritonitis, ileus, or late obstruction.

With vestibular disorders, head movement will reproduce the patient's symptoms of vertigo, nausea, and vomiting in association with the physical finding of nystagmus. A neurologic examination can detect signs such as papilledema, indicating increased intracranial pressure; ataxia, indicating a cerebellar disorder; or a stiff neck, suggesting meningitis.

DIFFERENTIAL DIAGNOSIS

Nausea is a nonspecific symptom, and in addition to GI diseases, the list of diseases that can cause nausea and vomiting encompasses a wide range of conditions (Box 22-1). The most common causes of acute nausea and vomiting in the family practice setting are infection, gastroenteritis, food poisoning, metabolic disorders, and medication side effects. The acute onset of nausea with severe abdominal pain suggests a more severe cause, such as obstruction, peritoneal irritation, and pancreatic or biliary disease.

Chronic nausea and vomiting are frequently related to structural lesions in the upper GI tract, such as peptic ulcer disease, gastroparesis, and gastric outlet obstruction. Other causes include metabolic abnormalities such as uremia or chronic hepatitis. Psychological causes are more common in younger

BOX 22-1. Differential Diagnosis for Nausea and Vomiting

Gastrointestinal
Gastroenteritis
Food poisoning
Biliary/cholecystitis
Intestinal obstruction
Pancreatitis
Appendicitis
Diverticulitis
Gastritis/peptic ulcer disease

Metabolic
Hepatitis
Renal failure
Diabetes mellitus (poorly controlled)
Adrenal insufficiency

Medications
Hormones (estrogen/oral contraceptive pills)
Nonsteroidal anti-inflammatory
Macrolides
Metronidazole
Theophylline
Digitalis
Narcotics
Chemotherapy

Visceral
Myocardial infarction
Nephrolithiasis

Other
Pregnancy
Psychogenic
Migraines
Vestibular (Ménière, labyrinthitis)
Elevated intracranial pressure (e.g., pseudotumor cerebri, CNS malignancy)

individuals and in women. Persistent early-morning vomiting without another explanation such as pregnancy raises the possibility of increased intracranial pressure and an underlying neurologic disease.

DIAGNOSTIC EVALUATION

The history and physical examination often suggests the likely cause of nausea and vomiting, such as pregnancy, dietary indiscretion, labyrinthitis, gastroenteritis, food poisoning, or medications. In these instances, testing may be indicated only to confirm the diagnosis (e.g., pregnancy) or, in situations of more protracted vomiting, to check for electrolyte abnormalities. Significant volume depletion elevates the BUN and can cause hemoconcentration with a rise in hematocrit. Drug levels, such as a digoxin level, are useful in suspected drug toxicity. Liver function tests are useful when hepatitis is suspected. Visceral pain syndromes causing nausea, such as an MI or renal colic, usually have associated symptoms that indicate the need to investigate these possibilities. However, in diabetic individuals and the elderly, it is common for an MI to present primarily with nausea and vomiting. The threshold for obtaining an ECG in these individuals should be low.

Patients with nausea and vomiting may need imaging tests along with laboratory tests. Plain films can help rule out an acute obstruction. A US can detect gallstones and changes compatible with pancreatitis. Testing for *Helicobacter pylori* antibodies may be helpful, because ulcer disease is a common cause of persistent nausea.

Chronic nausea and vomiting are most commonly related to structural lesions affecting the upper GI tract. Endoscopy, gastric emptying studies or barium studies are helpful in identifying outlet obstruction and motility disorders. Evidence of extrinsic compression on a barium study may require a US or CT scan for further evaluation. Suspected gastroparesis can be confirmed with a nuclear gastric emptying study.

Persistent early-morning nausea in the absence of a pregnancy or metabolic disease raises the possibility of increased intracranial pressure; therefore, CT or MRI imaging of the head should be considered. Recurrent vomiting of unknown cause may be a result of a psychological problem. Indications of this include vomiting around mealtimes, inappropriate attention to body image, abnormal appetite, and a conflict-filled social environment.

TREATMENT

Management should be directed at the underlying cause. For most individuals with self-limited illnesses, simple dietary measures are sufficient. Typical dietary advice consists of advising clear liquids followed by small quantities of dry foods such as crackers. Nausea and vomiting resulting from medications are usually resolved by discontinuing the medication. If the drug is essential, decreasing the dosage of the medication or changing to an alternative medication may help reduce nausea.

Phenothiazines such as prochlorperazine (Compazine) and promethazine (Phenergan) are among the most commonly used drugs to treat nausea and vomiting; they are centrally acting agents that can control symptoms caused by drugs, metabolic diseases, or gastroenteritis. Their most common side effects include sedation, but they can also cause extrapyramidal symptoms, especially in children. The serotonin antagonists, such as ondansetron, are another useful category of medication that is commonly used, and are particularly helpful with chemotherapy-related nausea and vomiting. In patients with vestibular symptoms, the antihistamine meclizine (Antivert) is helpful. Other antihistamines such as dimenhydrinate (Dramamine) or diphenolate are also effective. Antihistamines can cause drowsiness; thus, patients should be cautioned about driving or operating machinery when taking these drugs.

Patients with gastroparesis may benefit from dietary modification along with a prokinetic agent such as metoclopramide (Reglan) or erythromycin. Side effects of metoclopramide include anxiety, extrapyramidal reactions, and, rarely, tardive dyskinesia. Scopolamine, an anticholinergic, is used primarily for the prophylaxis of motion sickness. It comes in the form of both a pill and a patch. Psychogenic vomiting is best managed with a psychiatric consultation.

Treatment of the nausea and vomiting of pregnancy depends on the severity of disease. Dietary manipulation, such as eating small, frequent meals that are bland, high in carbohydrates, and low in fat, may be helpful. Ginger, pyridoxine (vitamin B_6), and doxylamine may be useful in patients failing dietary therapy. If these treatments are ineffective, a trial of one of the phenothiazines (e.g., Compazine) is warranted.

Patients with evidence of significant dehydration or with a significant laboratory abnormality warrant intravenous fluids. Patients failing to benefit from intravenous fluids and medication may benefit from nasogastric suction to decompress the stomach.

KEY POINTS

- In most instances, patients seen in the family practice setting with nausea and vomiting have a self-limiting illness.

- Nausea and vomiting accompanied by fever, watery diarrhea, and abdominal cramps are typical of viral gastroenteritis.

- Common medications causing nausea include the macrolide antibiotics, metronidazole, opiates, NSAIDs, estrogen, digitalis, theophylline, and chemotherapeutic agents.

- Phenothiazines are commonly used centrally acting agents that help control nausea. Side effects include sedation and extrapyramidal symptoms, especially in children.

23 | Painful Joints

The key to evaluating joint pain involves three issues: (1) Are the symptoms related to the joint or the periarticular structures? (2) Is the problem monoarticular or polyarticular? (3) Is the process inflammatory or noninflammatory?

PATHOGENESIS

Arthritis can result from degenerative processes or inflammatory disease. A noninflammatory disease, such as osteoarthritis, usually stems from the breakdown of cartilage and can eventually cause mechanical joint problems.

Inflammatory disease is mediated by cellular and humoral factors, such as prostaglandins, leukotrienes, interleukin-1, and tumor necrosis factor (TNF). Neutrophils, macrophages, lymphocytes, and other cellular mediators of inflammation are involved. Infection, crystalline arthritis, and the autoimmune diseases (e.g., rheumatoid arthritis [RA]) are examples of inflammatory arthritis. Periarticular symptoms involve tendons and muscles, but may also present as joint pain.

CLINICAL MANIFESTATIONS

HISTORY

The number and location of joints involved are important. Monoarticular complaints make infection, gout, pseudogout, trauma, or toxic synovitis more likely. Multiple joint involvement suggests a connective tissue disease, osteoarthritis, or RA. Symmetric polyarthritis is consistent with RA. An acute onset of joint pain is most consistent with trauma, infection, or crystalline arthropathy, whereas a more prolonged course suggests osteoarthritis, RA, connective tissue disease, or fibromyalgia. RA and other connective tissue diseases are systemic diseases, and symptoms such as fatigue and malaise are common associated complaints.

Factors affecting the pain are also important. Nocturnal pain in a single joint in a younger individual raises the possibility of a tumor. Pain that increases with use is consistent with osteoarthritis and tendonitis, whereas pain that decreases with use is more consistent with RA. Morning stiffness that lasts more than 45 minutes suggests an inflammatory arthritis. Migratory patterns raise the possibility of rheumatic fever, disseminated gonococcemia, Reiter syndrome, and Lyme disease. Nonarticular pain usually does not produce loss of joint function and may cause pain only with movement in certain directions. In contrast, arthritic pain usually causes discomfort with all joint motions. Gout is characterized by the sudden onset of pain, erythema, limited range of motion, and swelling. The attack may be triggered by trauma, dietary or alcohol excess, or surgery.

Medications such as procainamide and isoniazid can cause a lupus-like syndrome. Clinical features such as fever, rash, oral ulcers, renal disease, and serositis suggest SLE. A complete review of systems is helpful to avoid overlooking symptoms such as dry eyes and dry mouth, which might suggest Sjögren syndrome or urethritis, which is associated with Reiter syndrome. Table 23-1 lists clues from the history that suggest certain diagnoses.

PHYSICAL EXAMINATION

Many causes of arthritis have systemic manifestations. Skin manifestations of SLE include malar rash or mouth ulcers. Other skin lesions and associated illnesses include nail pitting and psoriatic arthritis, erythema migrans and Lyme disease, papulovesicular pustular lesions and disseminated gonococcemia, tophi and gout, heliotropic eyelid rash with dermatomyositis and SLE, and rheumatoid nodules with RA.

TABLE 23-1. Diagnostic Clues for Arthritis	
Historical Clues	**Associated Disease**
Recent URI	Toxic synovitis
Recent sore throat, migratory arthritis, nodules, skin rash	Rheumatic fever
Deer tick bite	Lyme disease
Recent rubella immunization	Immunologic-related arthritis
Diarrhea	Inflammatory bowel disease
Podagra	Gout
Urethral discharge	Reiter disease or gonococcal arthritis
Dry mouth/dry eyes	Sjögren syndrome
Muscle weakness	Myositis
Photosensitivity	SLE
Heliotropic rash	Dermatomyositis
Low back pain	Ankylosing spondylitis
Conjunctivitis	Reiter syndrome
Uveitis	Inflammatory bowel disease
Older age	Gout, pseudogout
Younger age	Rheumatoid arthritis, SLE
Male	Gout, ankylosing spondylitis, Reiter disease, and hemochromatosis
Recurrent joint subluxation, family hx of joint hypermobility	Marfan or Ehlers–Danlos syndromes
Acute monoarticular arthritis with severe pain, effusion	Infection or crystalline arthropathy
Raised silver plaques	Psoriatic arthritis
Malar rash	SLE
Fever	Infection, gout, systemic inflammatory disorders, e.g., SLE
Raynaud phenomenon	SLE, mixed connective tissue disease

SLE, systemic lupus erythematosus; URI, upper respiratory tract infection.

Fingertip atrophy or ulcers along with calcinosis and telangiectasia are signs of scleroderma. Keratoderma blennorrhagia, a hyperkeratotic lesion on the palms and soles, and balanitis circinate, a shallow, painless ulcer on the penis, are signs of Reiter syndrome. Conjunctivitis and uveitis are suggestive of joint diseases associated with IBD. The cardiopulmonary examination may reveal signs of an effusion, pleuritis, or pericarditis, which can be seen in RA and SLE. Splenomegaly can also be found in individuals with RA and SLE.

An inflamed joint is usually diffusely tender, and there is often increased warmth, redness, and joint effusion. Noninflammatory joint disease usually has more focal tenderness and few signs of inflammation.

Range of motion and joint deformity should be noted. Irregular bony enlargements in the proximal and distal interphalangeal joints (Bouchard and Heberden nodes) are signs of osteoarthritis. A tender bony mass near a joint may be a sign of a tumor.

Examination of the periarticular tissues is important, because tendonitis, bursitis, and myositis can mimic joint pain.

DIFFERENTIAL DIAGNOSIS

Differential diagnosis can be approached by the number of joints involved, and whether the process is inflammatory. Table 23-2 lists the differential diagnosis of polyarticular arthritis.

TABLE 23-2. Differential Diagnosis of Polyarthritis

Inflammatory	Noninflammatory
Rheumatoid arthritis	Osteoarthritis
SLE	Amyloidosis
Gout	Sickle cell disease
Pseudogout	Hypertrophic pulmonary osteoarthropathy
Septic arthritis	Myxedema
Reiter syndrome	Hemochromatosis
Sarcoidosis	Paget disease
Lyme disease	
Gonococcemia	
Viremia	
Subacute bacterial endocarditis	
Psoriatic arthritis	
Scleroderma	

SLE, systemic lupus erythematosus.

TABLE 23-3. Joint Fluid Analysis

WBC (cells/mm^3)	Interpretation
<2000	Noninflammatory (e.g., osteoarthritis)
2000–50,000	Mild to moderate inflammation (e.g., rheumatoid arthritis, crystalline arthritis)
50,000–100,000	Severe inflammation (e.g., sepsis or gout)
>100,000	Septic joint until proven otherwise

The differential diagnosis of monoarthritis includes infection, crystal-induced arthropathies (gout and pseudogout), trauma, and osteoarthritis. Gonorrhea is the most common infection causing septic arthritis. Another cause of monoarticular arthritis is solitary joint involvement with a polyarticular arthritis, such as RA, presenting in a single joint. Reiter syndrome, ankylosing spondylitis, psoriatic arthritis, colitis-associated arthritis, and viral synovitis often present with monoarticular arthritis.

DIAGNOSTIC EVALUATION

Arthrocentesis is the definitive diagnostic procedure for patients with monoarticular arthritis and joint effusion. Cloudy fluid suggests infection or crystalline disease, whereas bloody joint fluid following trauma suggests internal derangement. Joint fluid examination should include leukocyte count, Gram stain, culture, glucose, and an examination for crystals using polarized microscopy. Calcium pyrophosphate crystals, which cause pseudogout, are positively birefringent, whereas uric acid crystals, which cause gout, are negatively birefringent. Table 23-3 shows guidelines for determining whether the fluid is inflammatory.

Early in the course of arthritis, x-rays may be normal. Radiographic changes in osteoarthritis include nonuniform joint space narrowing, changes in the subchondral bone, and osteophytes (Fig. 20-1).

Osteoarthritic changes may be seen in the absence of symptoms, and the severity of the x-ray does not correlate with the degree of symptoms. RA usually affects the hands and wrists (Fig. 23-1); x-rays of these joints can assist in establishing the diagnosis and assessing disease progression. Radiographic evidence of RA includes periarticular soft-tissue swelling, periarticular osteopenia, uniform loss of joint space (nonuniform loss is more consistent with osteoarthritis), and bony erosions, which generally occur only after several months of active disease (Fig. 23-2). Bony erosions can also be seen in septic arthritis and gout. MRI scanning is useful for diagnosing periarticular soft-tissue injury.

In suspected inflammatory disease, an ESR or C-reactive protein (CRP) are useful, but nonspecific measures of inflammation. Leukocytosis is common in patients with septic arthritis. RA is a clinical diagnosis, and there are no laboratory tests or histologic or radiologic findings are specific for RA. However, a rheumatoid factor is positive in about 85% of the

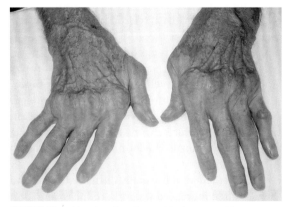

FIGURE 23-1. Hands of patient with rheumatoid arthritis. (From St. Clair EW, Pisetsky DS, Haynes BF. *Rheumatoid Arthritis*. Philadelphia, PA: Lippincott Williams & Wilkins; 2004.)

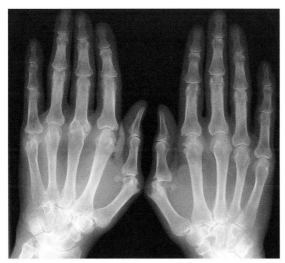

FIGURE 23-2. Radiograph of patient with rheumatoid arthritis. (From St. Clair EW, Pisetsky DS, Haynes BF. *Rheumatoid Arthritis*. Philadelphia, PA: Lippincott Williams & Wilkins; 2004.)

patients and helps establish the diagnosis in a patient with polyarthritis. Generally, the higher the rheumatoid factor titer, the more likely it is that the patient has RA. Up to 5% to 15% of normal individuals are rheumatoid factor-positive, but usually in lower titers. Anticyclic citrullinated peptide (anti-CCP) is 75% sensitive and 95% specific for RA, and is also a part of the diagnostic criteria in diagnosing RA. Box 23-1 lists criteria used for diagnosing RA.

ANA testing is sensitive for SLE but lacks specificity, and low titers are often falsely positive. Titers greater than 1:160 or more are falsely negative in only about 5% of individuals. If an ANA is positive, testing for antibodies to double-stranded DNA (dsDNA) and for

BOX 23-1. Criteria Used in Diagnosing Rheumatoid Arthritis

Morning stiffness >1 hour
Arthritis in three or more joints
Involvement of the wrist, metacarpophalangeal (MCP), or proximal interphalangeal (PIP) joints
Symmetric arthritis
Rheumatoid nodules
Positive rheumatoid factor or anticyclic citrullinated peptide
Increase erythrocyte sedimentation rate or C-reactive protein
Bony erosions on hand or wrist films
Symptoms present for >6 weeks

extractable nuclear antigens is indicated. Antibodies to dsDNA are present in about 70% of SLE patients, but when present are very specific. Antibodies to the Smith antigen are also very specific for SLE, but positive in only 30% of patients.

Routine chemistries are useful in assessing renal function and uric acid. A UA can screen for glomerular injury associated with connective tissue disease.

TREATMENT

Management depends on the underlying cause. The goals of treating arthritis are to alleviate pain, control inflammation, and prevent joint destruction. Regardless of the cause, physical therapy is often helpful for maintaining joint function, muscle strength, and mobility. In acute flares, it is important to protect the joint (e.g., splinting) to reduce pain and prevent future damage.

Septic arthritis requires appropriate antibiotics and drainage. The first line of pharmacologic therapy of osteoarthritis is acetaminophen. NSAIDs are effective but have more side effects. The symptoms of RA are treated with NSAIDs. Studies suggest that much of the joint damage seen in RA occurs early in the course of the disease, and most experts recommend consulting with a rheumatologist and starting disease-modifying drugs (Table 23-4) such as methotrexate early in the course of RA. Corticosteroids in RA may be used as a bridge therapy until other medicines take effect and may be given orally or in the form of a single joint injection. Biologic disease-modifying drugs are also approved for severe RA and are directed at interfering with cytokines. These drugs break the inflammation cascade by affecting the activity of TNF, interleukin-1, or other cytokines. Examples of biologic disease-modifying agents include infliximab, a monoclonal antibody against TNF, and entanercept, a soluble receptor for TNF. SLE is treated with NSAIDs, corticosteroids, antimalarials, or azathioprine. Gout may be treated with NSAIDs, colchicine, or corticosteroids. NSAIDs are first-line agents and are administered in high doses and then tapered over several days. If NSAIDs are contraindicated, either a short course of oral prednisone or an intra-articular injection of a corticosteroid is usually very effective. Colchicine exerts its effect by inhibiting the leukocyte phagocytosis of urate crystals. It is less favored than NSAIDs because of its slower onset and GI side effects. For patients with frequent attacks, allopurinol, which inhibits the formation of uric acid, or a uricosuric agent, such as probenecid, may be helpful. However, these agents should not be started during an acute attack.

TABLE 23-4. Disease-Modifying Drugs for Rheumatoid Arthritis

Drugs	Side Effects
Nonbiologic disease-modifying drugs	
Methotrexate	Bone marrow toxicity, hepatitis, and stomatitis
Sulfasalazine	Rash
Hydroxychloroquine	Retinopathy
Gold	Glomerular toxicity, proteinuria, rash
Penicillamine	Bone marrow toxicity, proteinuria, rash
Azathioprine	Immunosuppression
Leflunomide	Bone marrow toxicity, immunosuppression, hepatitis
Biologic disease-modifying drugs	
Etanercept, infliximab, adalimumab	Immunosuppression
Anakinra	Immunosuppression
Abatacept	Immunosuppression
Rituximab	Bone marrow suppression; arrhythmias, renal failure, hepatitis

KEY POINTS

- The key to evaluating joint pain involves three issues: (1) Are the symptoms related to the joint or to the periarticular structures? (2) Is the problem monoarticular or polyarticular? (3) Is the process inflammatory or noninflammatory?

- Morning stiffness that lasts >45 minutes suggests an inflammatory arthritis.

- The differential diagnosis of monoarthritis includes infection, crystal-induced arthropathies (gout and pseudogout), trauma, and osteoarthritis.

- Arthrocentesis is indicated in most cases of a new joint effusion to rule out infection or gout and to help distinguish between an inflammatory and noninflammatory process.

- Although RA is a clinical diagnosis, a rheumatoid factor is positive in about 85% of patients. Generally, the higher the rheumatoid factor titer, the more likely the patient has RA.

- Regardless of the cause, physical therapy is often helpful for maintaining joint function, muscle strength, and mobility.

- The first line of pharmacologic therapy of osteoarthritis is acetaminophen. NSAIDs are effective, but may have more side effects.

24 | Palpitations

A patient with palpitations has an abnormal awareness of the heartbeat. He or she may describe the palpitations as a fluttering, skipping, pounding, or racing sensation. Most palpitations in the outpatient setting are benign, but it is essential to identify those that are life threatening.

PATHOGENESIS

Normally, individuals are unaware of the 60 to 100 heartbeats that occur each minute. Heartbeat awareness may occur when there are changes in the rate, rhythm, or contractility of the heart. Palpitations may occur as a result of cardiac or endocrine disease, an increase in sympathetic tone, or medications. Patients with an underlying cardiac disease, such as valvular heart disease or a cardiomyopathy, may have an altered conduction within the cardiac chambers or an increased automaticity of foci within the heart, leading to tachycardias such as atrial fibrillation or flutter. Disease within the conduction system may alter conduction of the cardiac impulses, resulting in either bradycardia or tachycardia. If impulses are blocked, a bradycardia results. If a reentrant circuit is present, then a tachycardia may occur.

Hyperthyroidism causes a hyperkinetic state, and palpitations or tachycardias are common. Pheochromocytoma is a rare adrenal disorder with excess circulating catecholamines that can cause sympathetic overstimulation and tachycardia and palpitations. Psychiatric conditions—such as anxiety, panic disorder, and depression—are also associated with increased sympathetic tone. Other noncardiac medical causes of palpitations include anemia and dehydration or hypovolemia.

Medications can affect cardiac conduction. Common medications associated with palpitations include theophylline, digoxin, beta agonists, antiarrhythmic medications, and OTC stimulants such as pseudoephedrine. Alcohol, tobacco, and illicit drugs such as cocaine can also cause palpitations.

CLINICAL MANIFESTATIONS

HISTORY

The patient's description of symptoms and associated complaints such as lightheadedness, dizziness, or syncope is important. Patients with palpitations and dizziness, near-syncope, or syncope may warrant hospitalization, monitoring, and aggressive evaluation. The onset and duration of symptoms may give clues to the cause. Paroxysmal episodes that begin and resolve abruptly are characteristic of paroxysmal arrhythmias such as atrial fibrillation or supraventricular tachycardia. Isolated extra or pounding beats are characteristic of premature ventricular contractions (PVCs) or premature atrial contractions (PACs). The duration of symptoms as well as provocative or palliative factors may help in determining the cause. For example, sinus tachycardia and supraventricular tachycardias may be associated with exertion or emotional upset, whereas benign PACs or PVCs often disappear with exertion. Medication use should be reviewed for possible toxicity or side effects. Diabetics may experience palpitations with hypoglycemic reactions. Patients taking stimulants by prescription or illicitly may experience palpitations as side effects. Alcohol use is associated with supraventricular tachycardia and atrial fibrillation. A review of systems should include assessment for other cardiac symptoms, pulmonary disease, abnormal bleeding, and symptoms suggestive of either thyroid or adrenal disease.

PHYSICAL EXAMINATION

Physical examination should include assessment of orthostatic changes. The pulse rate and any heart rhythm irregularity or extra beats should be noted. Pallor suggests anemia, and exophthalmos or goiter may indicate hyperthyroidism. Special attention should be paid to the cardiopulmonary examination, including not only the rate and rhythm but also the presence of rubs, murmurs, clicks, and gallops that may indicate structural heart disease. A mental status examination—looking for signs of anxiety disorders, depression, or substance abuse—may provide clues to noncardiac etiologies.

DIFFERENTIAL DIAGNOSIS

Box 24-1 lists the differential diagnosis for palpitations, and includes both cardiac and noncardiac etiologies. The majority of patients seen in the family practice setting do not have a cardiac etiology. Generalized anxiety disorder and panic disorder are the psychiatric disturbances most commonly associated with palpitations. Panic disorders are frequently associated with other psychiatric disorders such as agoraphobia, major depression, and substance abuse. However, it should not be assumed that an underlying behavioral issue is the cause of palpitations, because a nonpsychiatric cause is seen in up to 13% of such patients. Predictors of a cardiac etiology include male sex, report of irregular heartbeat symptom duration of >5 minutes, palpitations affecting sleep, and a history of heart disease. Isolated extra heartbeats or skipping of heartbeats suggest PACs or PVCs as the cause (Fig. 24-1). Sudden onset and cessation of palpitations suggest paroxysmal supraventricular tachycardia (Fig. 24-2). A less-abrupt onset and cessation of palpitations are more common with stimulant or medication use. Sustained symptoms can be seen with fever, dehydration, hyperthyroidism, or anemia. Some patients experience an exaggerated perception of sinus rhythm or palpitations. These patients are more likely to be female, have a fast heart rate, report palpitations during normal examination, and engage in lesser amounts of physical activity.

BOX 24-1. Causes for Palpitations

Cardiac
PVCs
PACs
Paroxysmal supraventricular tachycardia/atrial fibrillation/atrial flutter
Multifocal atrial tachycardia
Frequent PVCs/PACs
Ventricular tachycardia
Mitral valve prolapse
Sick sinus syndrome (tachycardia–bradycardia syndrome)
Cardiomyopathy
Prolonged QT interval syndrome
Ischemic heart disease
Wolff–Parkinson–White syndrome

Noncardiac
Exertion
Anxiety
Hypoglycemia
Hyperthyroidism
Pheochromocytoma
Anemia
Electrolyte imbalance
Dehydration
Fever
Pregnancy
Panic disorder
Somatization
Hyperventilation
Medications:
  Theophylline
  Beta agonists
  Pseudoephedrine
  Antiarrhythmic drugs
  Tricyclic antidepressants
  Phenothiazines
  Stimulants/cocaine
Alcohol
Tobacco
Caffeine

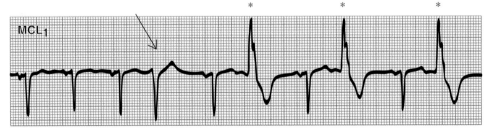

FIGURE 24-1. Premature beats. (From Wagner GS. *Marriott's Practical Electrocardiography*. 12th ed. Philadelphia, PA: Lippincott Williams & Wilkins; 2014.) MCL, modified chest lead; arrow indicates premature beat originating from right ventricle; each asterisk indicates premature beat originating from left ventricle.

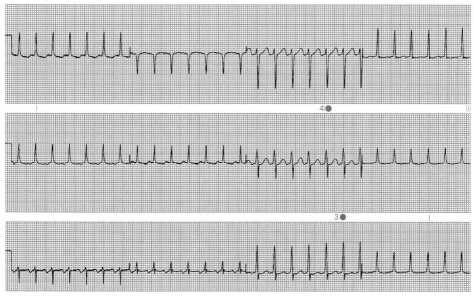

FIGURE 24-2. Supraventricular tachycardia. (From Wagner GS. *Marriott's Practical Electrocardiography*. 12th ed. Philadelphia, PA: Lippincott Williams & Wilkins; 2014.)

DIAGNOSTIC EVALUATION

Initial laboratory testing should include a hemoglobin, electrolytes, and TSH. Patients on medications such as digoxin that can affect cardiac rhythm should have serum levels checked. Blood glucose should be checked in diabetic patients. In selected patients, screening for a pheochromocytoma by measuring urine and serum catecholamines may be warranted.

Cardiac evaluation begins with a 12-lead ECG, which may detect an arrhythmia or abnormalities associated with arrhythmias. For example, a short PR interval and a delta wave occur with Wolff–Parkinson–White syndrome, which is associated with paroxysmal supraventricular tachycardias. Abnormalities in atrial or ventricular voltages and Q waves may signify the presence of an underlying cardiac disease.

Further, cardiac evaluation often includes echocardiography to assess cardiac anatomy. Information can be gained about atrial and ventricular size, valvular abnormalities, ventricular systolic function, and whether hypertrophic subaortic stenosis or wall motion abnormalities are present. A 24-hour Holter monitor records the cardiac rhythm for 24 hours and can detect an arrhythmia. During this period, the patient keeps a log of symptoms, and correlation with the monitor recording shows the heart's rhythm at the time of symptoms. For patients who do not have daily symptoms or who did not have symptoms while the monitor is being worn, an event monitor may

be an effective tool. Event monitors can be carried for 30 days or more and are patient-activated at the time of symptoms. The event recording can be transmitted by telephone to a monitoring station.

Stress testing should be considered for patients who have symptoms in association with exercise or who complain of chest pain or pressure. Finally, an invasive electrophysiologic study should be considered in syncopal or near-syncopal patients with heart disease and those with suspected ventricular tachycardia or heart block. Electrophysiologic study may document the abnormality and direct therapy.

TREATMENT

Therapy is directed by the underlying cause of the palpitations. Patients with panic disorder may benefit from treatment with tricyclic antidepressants or SSRIs. SSRIs have a slow onset of action and either bridge therapy with anxiolytics or beta blockers may be needed for 4 to 6 weeks until antidepressant therapy becomes effective. Patients with anemia need further evaluation for its cause. Treatment of underlying hyperthyroidism, anxiety, infection, and dehydration usually resolve symptoms in patients affected with these diseases. For many patients, adjustment of medication or insulin dosages and avoidance of stimulants such as caffeine may resolve symptoms.

Treatment of supraventricular tachycardias may include the use of medications (beta blockers or calcium channel blockers) or catheter ablation of any identified bypass tracts. Patients with chronic or intermittent atrial fibrillation usually merit anticoagulation with warfarin or other oral anticoagulants (thrombin or factor Xa inhibitors) to prevent thromboembolism. Younger, low-risk patients with atrial fibrillation and no history of hypertension, CHF, coronary artery disease, or history of transient ischemic attacks (TIAs) or a CVA may be treated with aspirin.

Isolated PVCs or PACs are common and can occur in healthy people without an underlying heart disease. In those without an underlying heart disease, the prognosis is good. Reducing alcohol intake, caffeine and other stimulants, tobacco cessation, adequate sleep, and stress reduction often resolve symptoms. They do not require treatment, but beta blockers may be considered for symptom relief in those with bothersome symptoms who fail to respond to lifestyle changes.

Individuals with PVCs and an underlying heart disease (e.g., abnormal stress test or echocardiogram) should be referred to a cardiologist. Malignant ventricular arrhythmias may merit antiarrhythmic therapy along with implantation of an automatic implantable cardiac defibrillator. If an antiarrhythmic drug is used, consultation with a cardiologist is often helpful, because therapy can be complex, and arrhythmia is a side effect of many of these drugs. Angioplasty or bypass surgery may be required for individuals with severe coronary artery disease.

Long QT syndrome is characterized by a prolonged QT interval on EKG. In addition to palpitations, these individuals are at an increased risk for cardiac arrest, and consultation with a cardiologist is helpful. Several medications, such as fluoroquinolones, macrolides, SSRIs, TCAs, phenothiazines, antiarrythmics, and antihistamines are associated with long QT syndrome and should be stopped when possible. Beta blockade is indicated in some forms and an implantation of a cardiac defibrillator should be considered in those at high risk of sudden death.

KEY POINTS

- The patient with palpitations has an abnormal awareness of the heartbeat, in terms of either the rate or intensity of the perceived heartbeat.

- Palpitations may occur due to the presence of cardiac or endocrine disease, increase in sympathetic tone, fever, dehydration, or medications.

- Cardiac evaluation should include a 12-lead ECG, echocardiography, monitoring (Holter, event monitor), and, in selected patients, stress testing or electrophysiologic study.

- Therapy is directed by the identified underlying cause.

25 | Pharyngitis

Sore throat, or pharyngitis, is a common reason for visits to family physicians' offices. There are many potential causes for pharyngitis, including viral and bacterial infections, allergies, gastroesophageal reflux, thyroiditis, smoking, and other irritants. A careful history and physical examination can help determine the patients who need further evaluation. Appropriate laboratory investigations can help identify the cause of these symptoms.

PATHOGENESIS

Bacterial and viral pathogens are responsible for causing most cases of infectious pharyngitis, and are spread by inhalation of airborne particles or by exposure to respiratory or oral secretions. Winter and early spring are peak seasons for sore throat. The incubation period for symptoms to develop may be as short as 24 to 72 hours.

The most common etiologic viral agents are respiratory viruses, such as adenovirus, parainfluenza virus, and rhinovirus. Pharyngitis associated with these agents is usually part of a broader upper respiratory tract infection with rhinorrhea, cough, and often conjunctivitis. Herpangina, characterized by tonsillar and palatal ulcerations, is caused by Coxsackievirus. Infectious mononucleosis caused by EBV may present with pharyngitis alone or with fever, posterior cervical lymphadenopathy, and malaise. The herpesvirus can also cause a pharyngitis or stomatitis.

Streptococcus pyogenes (group A strep) pharyngitis accounts for about 10% of infectious cases in adults and as many as 35% in children. It typically presents with fever and sore throat that is self-limited. Immunologically mediated complications of streptococcal infection include acute rheumatic fever and self-limited glomerulonephritis. Rheumatic fever

can lead to long-term valvular heart disease, such as mitral stenosis, and a strep pharyngitis should be treated within 10 days of onset to prevent this complication. Local complications of Streptococcus pharyngitis include peritonsillar and retropharyngeal abscesses that can progress to deeper infections and airway compromise.

Other bacteria that can cause self-limited pharyngitis, either alone or as part of a respiratory infection, include *Mycoplasma, Chlamydia, Hemophilus*, and *Corynebacterium*. Fungal pharyngitis may occur in immunocompromised patients, and *Gonococcal* pharyngitis may occur as a sexually transmitted disease through oral sex.

Noninfectious causes of pharyngitis include sleep apnea, GERD, and cigarette smoke through its irritant effects. Allergies can also lead to pharyngeal irritation and may present with throat itchiness, lymphoid hyperplasia, nasal obstruction, and postnasal drip.

CLINICAL MANIFESTATIONS

HISTORY

Streptococcal infection most commonly occurs in children from 5 to 15 years of age and is rare in children less than age 3. Mononucleosis is classically a disease of teenagers, known as the *"kissing disease."* The history should include associated symptoms and known exposures to illness. For example, <25% of patients with positive strep cultures have rhinorrhea and cough. The presence of these symptoms and a low-grade fever suggests a viral etiology. The classic symptoms for streptococcal infection are fever higher than 101°F (38.3°C) in association with a sore throat, but few other respiratory symptoms. The chronicity of the disease is also helpful in determining its cause. Viral and uncomplicated bacterial infections resolve in about 1 week, whereas noninfectious causes are more persistent. Early-morning sore throat without fever or other associated symptoms suggest(s) a noninfectious cause such as GERD or postnasal drip.

Medical history may suggest potential causes or lead to consideration of less-common etiologies. For example, patients with a history of allergies may experience a sore throat secondary to seasonal or environmental allergies. Immunocompromised patients may develop fungal infections or complications with bacterial infections (e.g., peritonsillar abscess). Greenish exudates and dysuria or urethral discharge combined with pharyngitis suggest gonococcal pharyngitis. Patients with sandpaper-like exanthems and a "strawberry tongue" may have scarlet fever, which is associated with group A beta-hemolytic streptococci. Pharyngitis in patients with a history of rheumatic fever warrants evaluation for recurrence of streptococcal disease. Group A streptococcus may lead to rheumatic fever or rarely poststreptococcal glomerulonephritis. Other complications include peritonsillar abscess, retropharyngeal abscess, meningitis, pneumonia, bacteremia, otitis media, sinusitis, cervical lymphadenitis, and scarlet fever. About one in four patients with Group A streptococcus report a recent exposure.

PHYSICAL EXAMINATION

Vital signs and an examination of the ears, nose, throat, and lungs are essential parts of the evaluation. The throat in classic group A strep infection is erythematous with tonsillar exudates. There are often palatal petechiae, and there may be a "strawberry tongue" appearance with prominent red papillae on a white-coated tongue. Tender cervical lymphadenopathy and an elevated temperature (>100.4°F) increases the likelihood of a Group A streptococcal infection. Physical examination should also include a lung examination, because many patients also exhibit respiratory symptoms. Patients with a history of a previous streptococcal infection may present with symptoms and signs of rheumatic fever, such as joint swelling, pain, subcutaneous nodules, erythema marginatum, or a heart murmur. Mononucleosis, gonococcal infection, and on occasion other bacterial or viral infections may, on pharyngeal examination, be indistinguishable from streptococcal pharyngitis. About half of the patients with mononucleosis have splenic enlargement on abdominal examination. Vesicular lesions suggest either herpesvirus or coxsackievirus infection, whereas adenovirus often causes an accompanying conjunctivitis and diarrhea. Diphtheria is characterized by an adherent gray membrane, low-grade fever, tonsillitis, and tender cervical lymphadenopathy. Kawasaki disease affects children who are <5 years of age. Signs and symptoms include conjunctivitis, a strawberry tongue, cracked red lips, unexplained prolonged fever ≥5 days, and a desquamating rash involving the palms and soles.

DIFFERENTIAL DIAGNOSIS

Most patients with an acute pharyngitis have either a viral or a bacterial infection. The goal is to identify and to treat strep infection to avoid complications, yet to avoid the risk and expense of unnecessary antibiotic treatment. Table 25-1 lists the differentiating features of viral versus bacterial pharyngitis. Common viruses include adenovirus, parainfluenza virus, rhinovirus, coxsackievirus, herpes, CMV, and EBV. In addition to group A strep, other streptococcal bacteria (groups C and G) may cause pharyngitis, but are not associated with the complications of group A. Other bacteria causing pharyngitis including *Gonococcus*, *Chlamydia*, *Mycoplasma*, *Corynebacterium*, and less commonly pneumococci, staphylococci, fusobacteria, and *Yersinia*. Fungi may cause infection in immunosuppressed patients. An unusual but important cause of pharyngitis is the retroviral syndrome (HIV).

Noninfectious causes of pharyngitis should be suspected in patients without fever and with persistent or recurring symptoms. Common noninfectious causes of pharyngitis include sleep apnea, gastroesophageal reflux, allergies, and referred pain from primary otologic or dental disease. Uncommon, but important noninfectious causes include malignancy, aplastic anemia, lymphoma, and leukemia.

TABLE 25-1. Characteristics of Viral versus Bacterial Pharyngitis

Signs and Symptoms	Viral	Bacterial
Conjunctivitis	More common	Less common
Malaise and fatigue	More common	Less common
Hoarseness of voice	More common	Less common
Low-grade fever	More common	Less common
High-grade fever	Less common	More common
Diarrhea	More common	Less common
Abdominal pain	More common	Less common
Rhinorrhea	More common	Less common
Cough	More common	Less common

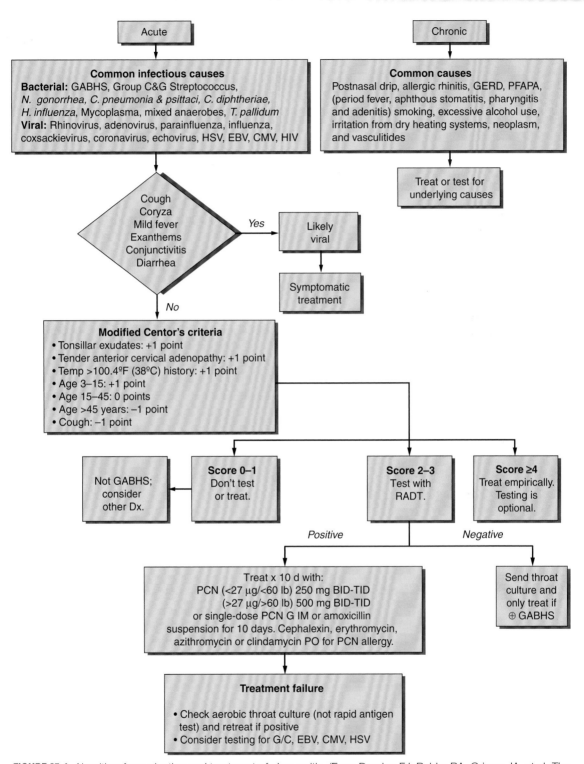

FIGURE 25-1. Algorithm for evaluation and treatment of pharyngitis. (From Domino FJ, Baldor RA, Grimes JA, et al. *The 5-Minute Clinical Consult Standard 2015*. 23rd ed. Alphen aan den Rijn, The Netherlands: Wolters Kluwer; 2014.)

DIAGNOSTIC EVALUATION

Physical examination alone cannot accurately determine whether a bacterial infection is present. Options in testing for Group A strep include a rapid antigen detection test (RADT) and throat culture. Throat culture is the "gold standard" test and is considered definitive. RADT is a common in-office test that is reported to have a sensitivity of 70% to 90% and a specificity of more than 90%. The Centor criteria are a commonly used clinical decision tool to identify patients who need diagnostic lab testing or antibiotic therapy to diagnose Group A Strep. Figure 25-1 depicts a testing and treatment algorithm for pharyngitis with application of modified Centor criteria. Testing for gonococcal pharyngitis requires a throat swab inoculated in Thayer–Martin medium. Fungal infection may be identified by the use of a slide prepared with KOH stain or may be detected on routine throat cultures. Patients with a history of rheumatic fever or who have symptoms and exposure to a documented case of Group A streptococci may be treated without culture or testing.

Infectious mononucleosis is usually suspected in patients with typical symptoms of fatigue, lymphadenopathy, splenomegaly, and/or sore throat combined with testing results. Heterophile antibody testing, also known as the **Monospot test**, is commonly performed in many offices. Although the Monospot test may be positive as early as 5 days into the infection, it can take up to 3 weeks to convert to a positive test. Alternatively, EBV IgM antibodies may be elevated as early as 2 weeks after infection. In patients presenting with suspected mononucleosis and an initial negative test, repeat testing may be necessary.

TREATMENT

Streptococcal pharyngitis should be treated to prevent rheumatic fever, suppurative complications, and to decrease person-to-person spread of the infection. The treatment of choice for strep throat is penicillin, either as a 10-day oral course or a single intramuscular injection of benzathine penicillin. For patients allergic to penicillin, clindamycin, erythromycin, or a newer macrolide such as azithromycin may be used. For treatment failures, amoxicillin–clavulanic acid or clindamycin are commonly used. Although Groups C and G streptococci may be cultured and can cause pharyngitis, antibiotic therapy has not been shown to be beneficial. Treatment for viral pharyngitis is largely supportive and symptomatic. Lozenges and warm saltwater gargles may provide topical relief. Analgesic drugs such as acetaminophen or ibuprofen can help reduce pain. The treatment of gonococcal infections is covered in Chapter 53.

KEY POINTS

- There are many potential causes of pharyngitis, including viral and bacterial infections, allergies, and irritants.
- Evaluation and testing for infectious etiologies is largely targeted toward identification of Group A strep infection because of its association with complications such as rheumatic fever.
- The treatment of choice for strep throat is penicillin, whereas treatment for the other causes of pharyngitis is largely supportive care.

26 | Proteinuria

Proteinuria in adults is defined as protein excretion >150 mg per 24 hours; in children, proteinuria varies with the child's age and size. Nephritic-range proteinuria is defined as daily excretion of between 150 mg and 3.5 g, whereas nephrotic-range proteinuria is defined as the daily excretion of more than 3.5 g of protein over 24 hours. The causes of proteinuria range from benign conditions such as orthostatic proteinuria to life-threatening conditions such as glomerular nephritis with rapidly progressive kidney failure. Proteinuria is often first identified as an incidental finding on UA during a routine office visit.

PATHOGENESIS

The glomerulus is a filter that allows the elimination of water and waste, while preventing the loss of large proteins to excretion. Each day, a normal glomerular filtrate contains between 500 and 1500 mg of low-molecular-weight proteins. Most of these proteins are resorbed and metabolized by the renal tubular cells. Because urine testing may turn positive at a concentration of 100 mg/mL, normal individuals may test trace-positive for proteinuria on an office dipstick.

Significant proteinuria may occur from glomerular damage and increased filtration of normal plasma proteins, renal tubular diseases that affect resorption, or overflow proteinuria. Glomerular disease can be either primary or secondary. Primary glomerular diseases include minimal change disease, focal segmental glomerulosclerosis, membranoproliferative glomerulonephritis, membranous nephropathy, and IgA nephropathy. Secondary causes include infections, systemic diseases, or drug-related effects on the glomerulus (see Table 26-1).

Overflow proteinuria occurs when there is production of abnormal proteins that pass through

TABLE 26-1. Systemic Illnesses Causing Proteinuria

Amyloidosis

Carcinoma

Cryoglobulinemia

Diabetes mellitus

Drugs/toxins

Goodpasture syndrome

Henoch–Schönlein purpura

HIV-associated nephropathy

Leukemia

Lymphoma

Multiple myeloma

Polyarteritis nodosa

Preeclampsia

Sarcoidosis

SLE

Transplant nephropathy

Infections:
  Subacute bacterial endocarditis (SBE)
  Syphilis
  Post-streptococcal glomerular nephritis
  CMV
  EBV
  HIV
  Hepatitis B and C
  Malaria
  Toxoplasmosis

Medications:
  Antibiotics
  Analgesics
  Anticonvulsants
  ACE inhibitors
  Antimetabolites
  Heavy metals

the glomerulus. The type of protein found in the urine differs depending on the cause. (For example, Bence–Jones proteins seen in multiple myeloma). Glomerular disease usually results in significant albumin excretion, whereas tubular disease that may affect the resorption of excreted protein is associated with an array of low-molecular-weight proteins. Immunoglobulin-related proteins are found in multiple myeloma or monoclonal gammopathy.

Functional proteinuria may occur in association with fever, strenuous exercise, seizures, abdominal surgery, epinephrine administration, and heart failure without evidence of intrinsic kidney disease. Proteinuria is related to changes in renal hemodynamics that result in increased glomerular filtration of plasma proteins. Functional proteinuria usually resolves within several days of the inciting event and is not associated with progressive disease.

Proteinuria can be either transient or persistent. Persistent proteinuria is defined as the presence of proteinuria on at least two separate occasions. Orthostatic, postural, or daytime proteinuria accounts for 60% of patients with asymptomatic proteinuria. Typically, patients are <30 years old and have protein excretion of <2 g/day; and the proteinuria occurs when the patient is in the upright position and normalizes in the supine position. Nephrotic-range proteinuria (>3.5 g/24 hours) is usually the consequence of glomerular damage.

CLINICAL MANIFESTATIONS

HISTORY

Proteinuria can be idiopathic or due to underlying renal or systemic diseases. Patients with glomerulonephritis usually present with hematuria, RBC casts, and mild-to-moderate hypertension. These patients typically have proteinuria and edema, but not as prominently as patients with nephrotic syndrome. Nephrotic syndrome consists of massive proteinuria, hypoalbuminemia, hyperlipidemia, lipiduria, and edema, usually in the absence of hematuria and RBC casts.

The focus of the history is to determine the possible causes of proteinuria and assess the severity of the condition. Dependent edema suggests nephrotic-range proteinuria, and hypertension indicates the possibility of significant kidney disease. History may reveal the presence of systemic illnesses that are associated with proteinuria, such as long-standing diabetes mellitus, SLE, CHF, multiple myeloma,

and amyloidosis. A detailed review of medications is important. Dysuria and frequency along with a fever indicate a possible UTI.

PHYSICAL EXAMINATION

Skin changes such as malar rashes, vasculitis, and purpura can be signs of a connective tissue disease. Diabetic retinopathy is strongly associated with proteinuria, and the fundi should be carefully examined. Looking for lymphadenopathy, heart failure, abdominal masses, hepatosplenomegaly, ascites, labial or scrotal edema, and peripheral edema, along with assessing blood pressure are important. Fever may be present in infectious causes.

DIFFERENTIAL DIAGNOSIS

The differential diagnosis for proteinuria is extensive. Benign transient proteinuria is a common problem that resolves spontaneously and is most often seen in children or young adults. Exercise, CHF, fever, UTI, and orthostatic proteinuria are common causes of transient proteinuria in patients without a significant kidney disease.

Although individuals may have isolated proteinuria without other urinary symptoms or disease, persistent isolated proteinuria suggests underlying glomerular or tubular disease. Primary kidney diseases include acute kidney injury, acute tubular necrosis, acute or chronic glomerulonephritis, and polycystic disease. Systemic illnesses causing proteinuria are listed in Table 26-1. Diabetes, in particular, is an important cause of proteinuria. About one-third of type 1 and one-fourth of type 2 diabetics have persistent proteinuria, which is a clinical precursor to advanced diabetic nephropathy. Drugs and toxins can cause proteinuria, as can certain infections. About 50% to 75% of the cases of nephrotic-range proteinuria are due to intrinsic kidney disease. The remaining causes are most often due to systemic illnesses such as diabetes, SLE, amyloidosis, or one of the several rheumatologic diseases that cause glomerular injury.

DIAGNOSTIC EVALUATION

A urine dipstick is a simple, readily available screening tool for proteinuria. A 1+ protein level usually represents ∼ 30 mg/dL of protein excreted. A 4+ usually indicates >1000 mg/dL. The common urine dipstick reagents react to albumin and can fail to detect other abnormal proteins such as Bence–Jones proteins. A sulfosalicylic acid test measures the total concentration of proteins, including Bence–Jones proteins. False-positive dipstick results can be seen with dehydration, gross hematuria, UTI, recent exercise, or highly alkaline urine.

If the patient has two or more positive dipstick tests, a 24-hour urine protein collection is indicated, along with a urine creatinine clearance determination. Alternatively, because of the difficulties in obtaining a true 24-hour collection, a spot urine specimen can be used to calculate the protein to creatinine ratio, which is an accurate proxy for 24-hour urine collection.

If orthostatic proteinuria is suspected, an orthostatic test may be performed. The patient is instructed to urinate and discard the first morning urine before a collection. A 16-hour daytime collection should stop before bedtime, followed by an overnight specimen collection. Patients with true orthostatic proteinuria have elevated proteinuria during the day that returns to normal at night. Alternatively, obtain a urine sample first thing in the morning while the patient is still recumbent and check the protein–creatinine ratio. If the result is normal, the diagnosis is established.

A total 24-hour protein excretion exceeding 1 g suggests significant kidney involvement. Urine analysis and microscopy may help narrow the differential. The presence of RBC casts in the urine indicates glomerular disease. WBC casts may be seen in pyelonephritis and interstitial nephritis. Oval fat bodies, if present, are due to lipiduria, as seen in nephrotic syndrome. A qualitative urine protein electrophoresis (UPEP) or immunofixation electrophoresis (IFE) to rule out a monoclonal component is indicated. Further evaluation includes, a chemistry panel (including a BUN, creatinine, albumin, and total protein), lipid profile, ESR, antistreptolysin O (ASO) titer, and a C3–C4 complement level. A chemistry panel identifies electrolyte imbalances, serum protein levels, and assesses kidney function. The CBC identifies a normocytic normochromic anemia, as seen in chronic kidney disease or multiple myeloma. Serum complement levels are low in some acute glomerulo-nephritides and lupus nephritis. An ESR screens for connective tissue diseases and other inflammatory states. ASO titers indicate whether there has been a recent streptococcal infection.

An ANA, hepatitis panel, rapid plasma reagin (RPR) test, HIV testing, and serum protein electrophoresis (SPEP) should be ordered selectively based on the history, physical examination, or previous laboratory results. An ultrasound is helpful in determining the kidney size, ruling out polycystic kidney disease or masses, and detecting an obstructive nephropathy.

TREATMENT

Treatments for proteinuria depend on the underlying cause. Transient proteinuria is very common in children and young adults and disappears with repeat testing. Long-term studies indicate that both transient proteinuria and orthostatic proteinuria are benign conditions that require no treatment.

Patients with chronic kidney disease, nephrotic-range proteinuria, hematuria or RBC casts, or an uncertain underlying cause should be referred to a nephrologist. Patients with nephrotic syndrome are also more susceptible to atherosclerosis, thrombotic processes, and infection by encapsulated bacteria. They require pneumococcal vaccine (Pneumovax) and treatment for dyslipidemia. A nephrologist may perform a kidney biopsy to rule out treatable forms of glomerulonephritis, such as membranous glomerulonephropathy, which may respond to steroids or immunosuppressive therapy. ACE inhibitors benefit patients with diabetes and proteinuria. Asymptomatic patients with low-range proteinuria may be observed with periodic blood pressure monitoring and an annual assessment of kidney function. Referral to a nephrologist should be considered if chronic kidney disease or hypertension develops.

KEY POINTS

- Proteinuria in adults is protein excretion >150 mg per 24 hours. Nephrotic range proteinuria is the excretion of more than 3.5 g of protein over 24 hours.

- Patients who suffer glomerulonephritis generally present with hematuria or RBC casts, and mild-to-moderate hypertension. Nephrotic syndrome consists of massive proteinuria, hypoalbuminemia, hyperlipidemia, lipiduria, and edema.

- Diabetes is an important cause of proteinuria. About one-third of those with type 1 and one-fourth of those with type 2 diabetes have persistent proteinuria.

- A total 24-hour protein excretion exceeding 1 g suggests significant kidney involvement.

- Patients with reduced glomerular filtration rate, nephrotic range proteinuria, hematuria or RBC casts, or proteinuria of uncertain etiology should be referred to a nephrologist.

27 | Red Eye

A red eye is the most common ophthalmologic complaint encountered by family physicians, accounting for 1% of all visits. Most cases are benign, self-limited conditions that can be treated by the family physician. However, a few conditions that cause red eye are sight-threatening, such as corneal ulceration, iritis, and glaucoma. The family physician should recognize these and, if necessary, refer the patient to an ophthalmologist.

PATHOGENESIS

A red eye may be caused by pathology in the conjunctiva, corneal, uveal tract, eyelids, or orbit. Infection or occlusion of glandular structures—namely, the meibomian glands, glands of Zeis, or nasolacrimal duct—can cause swelling and redness of the eyelid or periorbital structures. Infection of the meibomian glands is termed internal hordeolum, whereas an external hordeolum or stye is an infection of the glands of Zeis. Sterile inflammation of the meibomian gland due to glandular occlusion is termed a chalazion. Blepharitis is an infection, inflammation, and scaling of the eyelid margins. Occlusion of the nasolacrimal duct with secondary infection is referred to as dacryocystitis. Infection may also spread to the orbital or periorbital region from sinus infections, leading to orbital or periorbital cellulitis.

The conjunctiva is a thin, transparent vascular tissue that lines the inner aspect of the eyelids (palpebral conjunctiva) and extends over the sclera (bulbar conjunctiva) before terminating at the limbus, where it is continuous with the corneal epithelium. A healthy conjunctiva is the first barrier to infection, which is why external infections of the eye commonly cause an inflammation or hyperemia of the subconjunctival vessels giving the conjunctiva an erythematous and injected appearance, hence the term "red eye."

Other ocular inflammatory conditions, such as iritis or glaucoma, can also manifest as a red eye due to hyperemia of the ciliary vessels of the sclera through the transparent conjunctiva. Another cause of red eye is a subconjunctival hemorrhage, which is a benign condition that results from bleeding in the small fragile vessels of the conjunctiva, usually in response to minor trauma or straining. However, conjunctivitis is by far the most common cause of red eye.

CLINICAL MANIFESTATIONS

HISTORY

The history should include a thorough ocular, medical, and medication history, including a complete review of systems evaluating for autoimmune diseases (arthralgias, diarrhea, melena, hematochezia, and rash), upper respiratory illness, or urinary tract infection. The ocular history should focus on the type of discomfort, changes in vision, presence of discharge, duration of symptoms (acute, subacute, or chronic), unilateral or bilateral involvement, contact with anyone having similar ocular symptoms, and any specific environmental or work-related exposure. In addition, particular attention should be given to the following ocular symptoms: pain, visual changes (blurred vision/photophobia), and the type of discharge.

The degree of discomfort helps determine the need for urgent referral to an ophthalmologist. Pain suggests a more serious ocular pathology, such as acute angle-closure glaucoma, iritis, keratitis, scleritis, uveitis, corneal ulceration, or orbital cellulitis. Discomfort associated with conjunctivitis is often described as burning, tearing, or irritating. Itching is the hallmark of allergic conjunctivitis, but can also be present in viral or bacterial conjunctivitis. Visual changes suggest serious ocular disease and are not seen with conjunctivitis or subconjunctival hemorrhage. Discharge is a common finding in patients with conjunctivitis, and the type of discharge, purulent or mucoid, may help in distinguishing bacterial from viral or allergic causes of conjunctivitis. A history of trauma or a gritty feeling in one eye associated with pain may suggest a foreign body or corneal abrasion.

PHYSICAL EXAMINATION

The eyelids and periorbital region should be checked for erythema and inflammation. Next, examine the conjunctiva for a pattern of any redness detected. Conjunctival erythema may be due to subconjunctival hemorrhage, conjunctival hyperemia, or the presence of a "ciliary flush." Subconjunctival hemorrhage is a collection of blood under the conjunctiva and is bright red, with distinct borders. Conjunctival hyperemia is diffuse erythema of the conjunctival lining with no borders and involves both the bulbar and palpebral conjunctiva. The term "ciliary flush" refers to a violaceous hyperemia of the vessels surrounding the cornea, and along with photophobia and a sluggishly reactive pupil is a sign of iritis.

Note the presence, quality, and quantity of any discharge. Examine each pupil, look for any irregularities in shape or size in comparison with the other pupil, presence of hypopyon or hyphema, and its reactivity to light. Evaluate the intraocular movement and then, with the ophthalmoscope, inspect the cornea for opacities, surface irregularities, or foreign bodies. Assess the optic disk for an increase in the cup–disk ratio, which may signify the presence of glaucoma. An important part of the examination is checking visual acuity with a Snellen eye chart.

DIFFERENTIAL DIAGNOSIS

The most common causes for red eye include hordeolum, chalazion, blepharitis, corneal abrasion, subconjunctival hemorrhage, and conjunctivitis. One should also be familiar with the signs and symptoms of glaucoma and iritis, so that a prompt referral for therapy can be provided. These diseases are described in Table 27-1. Other less-common causes of red eye include scleritis, episcleritis, anterior uveitis, and keratitis, all of which require ophthalmologic referrals.

DIAGNOSTIC EVALUATION

Initial assessment involves a thorough ophthalmoscopic examination. Presence of pain, discharge, and photophobia are important historical findings,

and assessing papillary reactivity, visual acuity, and fluorescein testing are important (Fig. 27-1). When a patient presents with ocular pain, corneal ulceration or laceration should be ruled out by a fluorescein dye test. To perform this test, apply fluorescein dye to the lower eyelid (drops or impregnated strip) and view the cornea under a cobalt-blue light (Wood lamp) searching for disruptions of the corneal epithelium (ulcers or lacerations).

Conjunctivitis is the most common cause of a red eye, and typically there is a discharge with the eyelids crusted together in the morning and the absence of pain or visual changes. Most cases of conjunctivitis are self-limited and the cost–benefit ratio for culturing the eye discharge precludes its routine use. The conjunctiva has a bacterial flora composed of many species, including *Staphylococcus aureus* and, less commonly, *Corynebacterium* and *Streptococcus* species. Some healthy patients may also harbor *Pseudomonas* and fungi as a part of their normal conjunctival flora, especially contact lens wearers who do not properly clean their lenses. Infectious conjunctivitis is usually due to a viral infection, but in about 5% patients it is bacterial. In severe cases, in the very young, or in patients who do not respond to therapy, cultures may be useful. A Gram stain of the discharge may help identify a bacterial agent. Multinucleated giant cells are suggestive of a herpes infection. Tonometry to measure intraocular pressure is useful in a suspected case of acute glaucoma. In a patient with suspected serious orbital or periorbital cellulitis, a CBC and imaging, such as an orbital CT scan, may be indicated.

TREATMENT

Therapy for blepharitis generally involves measures aimed at eyelid hygiene. Specifically, the use of a mild soap, such as a baby shampoo, diluted with water to scrub the lids, is recommended. Additional measures may include the use of warm compresses and a topical antibiotic ointment.

The inflammation and pain from a hordeolum or chalazion may respond to the use of warm compresses. A hordeolum may also respond to topical antibiotic therapy. If an associated cellulitis is present, systemic antibiotics that are active against *S. aureus*, the most common pathogen, are indicated. A chronic chalazion may require intralesional steroid injections or surgical drainage for resolution. Hordeola rarely require incision and drainage for treatment.

TABLE 27-1. Differential Diagnosis of Red Eye

Disease	Description	Other
Blepharitis	Chronic lid margin erythema, scaling, loss of eyelashes	Associated with staphylococcal infection, seborrheic dermatitis
Hordeola/chalazion	Painful nodules on or along lids	Hordeola associated with staphylococcal infection; chalazion-sterile
Conjunctivitis	Burning, itching, discharge, lid edema	
Viral	Unilateral at first, then spread to the other eye within days clear, mucoid discharge, preauricular adenopathy common	Associated with upper respiratory infection; very contagious; occurs primarily in the summer
Hyperacute bacterial	Copious purulent discharge	Potentially sight-threatening; associated with gonorrhea, sexually transmitted disease (STDs), neonates
Acute bacterial	Bilateral moderate purulent discharge with morning matting of eyelids	*Hemophilus influenza*, staphylococcal, *Streptococcus pneumonia*; occurs primarily in the winter
Inclusion conjunctivitis	Persistent watery discharge	Chlamydia; neonates and young adults, associated with STDs
Allergic	Itching, tearing	Associated with other allergy symptoms
Subconjunctival hemorrhage	Nonblanching red "spot," painless without visual changes or discharge	Associated with trauma, cough, or Valsalva (e.g., straining)
Corneal abrasion/foreign body	Pain, "foreign body" sensation	Abrupt, associated with incident or work exposure
Iritis	Pain, photophobia, papillary constriction, cloudy cornea, and anterior chamber	Associated with connective tissue diseases, ocular injury
Acute angle-closure glaucoma	Pain, tearing, dilated pupil, shallow anterior chamber, halos around lights	Ocular emergency, more common among patients >age 50

Treatment recommendations for conjunctivitis are presented in Table 27-2. For hyperacute bacterial conjunctivitis, prompt, aggressive treatment is necessary to avoid sight-threatening complications. Viral conjunctivitis is self-limited, lasting 7 to 10 days. Although many clinicians prescribe antibiotic drops for these infections, there is only modest evidence that this practice shortens the duration of symptoms. Ninety-five percent of patients shed the virus for up to 10 days after the onset of symptoms. All patients should receive advice regarding hygiene, such as avoiding eye–hand contact, good hand-washing habits, and using a personal face cloth and towel to limit the spread of the infection. Bacterial conjunctivitis requires topical antibiotic treatment and occasionally systemic antibiotic treatment (amoxicillin–clavulanate), particularly if there is concomitant acute otitis media, as is frequently the case with nontypable *H. influenza*.

Subconjunctival hemorrhage requires no treatment and usually resolves over several days. Treatment for a foreign body includes removal with the help of a topical anesthetic for the eye and a moistened cotton swab. If the foreign body cannot be removed, an ophthalmology referral is indicated.

Patients with iritis and acute glaucoma need urgent referral to an ophthalmologist. After thorough ophthalmologic examination, therapy for iritis often involves the use of cycloplegic and anti-inflammatory (e.g., topical steroids) medications. Acute medical treatment for glaucoma usually involves acetazolamide 500 mg and topical 4% pilocarpine ophthalmic solution to constrict the pupil. Patients with apparently benign conditions whose symptoms persist or recur should also be referred to an ophthalmologist.

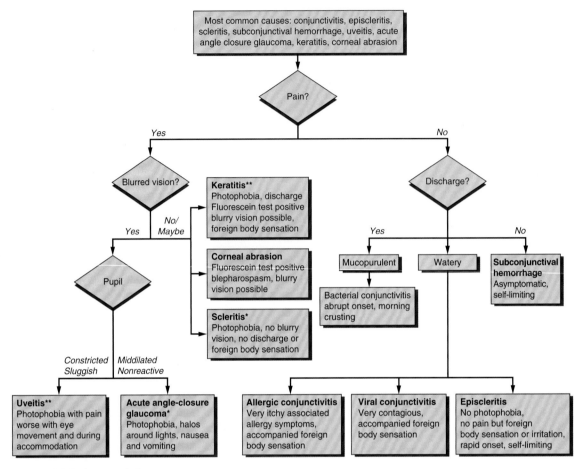

FIGURE 27-1. Algorithm with an approach to the red eye. (From Domino FJ, Baldor RA, Golding J, et al. *5-Minute Clinical Consult 2018*. 26th ed. Alphen aan den Rijn, The Netherlands: Wolters Kluwer; 2017.)

TABLE 27-2. Therapy for Conjunctivitis

Etiology	Treatment
Viral	Local measures: cool compresses
Herpes	±Oral antiviral, topical antiviral (e.g., acyclovir) ophthalmology referral
Bacterial	Local measures; ophthalmic erythromycin ointment, fluoroquinolone ophthalmic drops, or TMP-SMX ophthalmic drops; Gonococcal conjunctivitis requires systemic antibiotics (e.g., IV or IM ceftriaxone); Chlamydial conjunctivitis requires 2–3 weeks of oral therapy (e.g., erythromycin or doxycycline)
Allergic	Local measures for allergen avoidance, topical or systemic antihistamines (e.g., loratadine)

IM, intramuscular; IV, intravenous; TMP-SMX, trimethoprim/sulfamethoxazole.

KEY POINTS

- The most common cause of red eye is conjunctivitis.
- The most common etiology of conjunctivitis is viral; this is a self-limited but extremely contagious condition.
- In conjunctivitis, a purulent discharge usually indicates a bacterial infection, whereas a watery discharge is more consistent with an allergic or viral etiology.
- Itching is the hallmark of allergic conjunctivitis.
- Acute angle-closure glaucoma should be considered in patients more than 50 years of age with a painful red eye.
- Suspected corneal ulceration, iritis, and glaucoma are sight-threatening and should be referred to an ophthalmologist.

28 | Respiratory Infections

Respiratory tract infections are the leading cause of illness among children and adults. Clinically, it is useful to distinguish between upper and lower respiratory tract infections. URIs consist of infections affecting the respiratory structures above the larynx. Lower respiratory tract infections (LRIs) encompass the trachea, bronchi, and pulmonary structures.

EPIDEMIOLOGY

URIs include the common cold, sinusitis, and pharyngitis. Adults average two to four colds per year. Although most individuals with these conditions do not seek medical care, they are still among the most common reasons for family physician visits. Rhinoviruses account for 30% to 50% of the cases of the common cold; coronaviruses represent another 10% to 20%. The remaining cases are either due to an unidentifiable virus or a host of viruses including influenza, parainfluenza, respiratory syncytial virus, and adenovirus. Laryngitis is viral in origin in 90% of the cases, most commonly due to influenza, rhinovirus, adenovirus, or parainfluenza virus. The etiologic agents of pharyngitis and otitis media are described in Chapters 25 and 73, respectively.

LRIs include bronchitis and pneumonia. Bronchitis is an inflammation of the lining of the bronchial tube. Viral infections cause approximately 95% of bronchitis cases in healthy adults. Nonviral causes include chemical irritation, *Mycoplasma*, and *Chlamydia*.

Pneumonia is defined as inflammation of the lung parenchyma. In the United States, there are more than 4.5 million cases of community-acquired pneumonia (CAP) each year; about one-third of these require hospitalization. Pneumonia is the sixth leading cause of death.

PATHOGENESIS

Most URIs are caused by viruses, which replicate in the nasopharynx and cause inflammation as well as edema, erythema, and nasal discharge. Transmission occurs primarily by hand contact with the infecting agent.

Sinusitis is an infection that occurs when inflammation and swelling of the mucosal membranes block the ostia draining the sinuses, thus allowing pooling of mucus and bacterial proliferation. Sinusitis may also occur if anatomic abnormalities such as polyps obstruct the ostia. Occasionally, sinusitis results from a dental abscess. Bronchitis is characterized by edematous mucosal membranes, increased bronchial secretions, and diminished mucociliary function. Acute exacerbations of chronic bronchitis are frequently precipitated by a viral infection, but bacteria colonizing the airway also play a role in infections.

Pneumonia is an inflammation of the terminal airways, alveoli, and lung interstitium, usually from infection. The primary mechanism by which pneumonia occurs is through the aspiration of oropharyngeal secretions colonized by respiratory pathogens. Aspiration of gastric contents and hematogenous spread are less common. Factors that predispose an individual to develop pneumonia are abnormal host defenses (e.g., malnutrition, immunocompromise), altered consciousness (which can lead to aspiration), ineffective cough (as is seen in patients with neuromuscular diseases or following surgery), and abnormal mucociliary transport (which is seen in smokers, COPD patients, and following a viral bronchitis).

CLINICAL MANIFESTATIONS

HISTORY

The clinical symptoms of a cold are well known and typically begin with a scratchy sore throat followed by sneezing, nasal congestion, and rhinorrhea. General malaise, fever, hoarseness, cough, low-grade fever, and headache are also frequent symptoms. The acute syndrome usually resolves in about 1 week; however, a cough may persist for several weeks.

Persistent purulent nasal discharge, facial pain exacerbated by leaning forward, and maxillary or frontal pain are symptoms of sinusitis. Many patients with acute sinusitis may experience "double sickening," with improvement in their cold symptoms followed by a relapse with increased pain and nasal discharge.

Acute bronchitis usually presents with a productive cough and is often accompanied by URI symptoms. Low-grade fever and fatigue are common.

Pneumonia may present with symptoms very similar to those of bronchitis. However, patients with pneumonia are more likely to have a high fever, experience dyspnea and chills, have chest pain, and develop complications such as hypoxia or cardiopulmonary failure. Common organisms for CAP in previously healthy adults are *Streptococcus pneumoniae, Hemophilus influenzae, Mycoplasma pneumoniae,* and *Chlamydia pneumoniae.*

In patients with suspected pneumonia, it is important to inquire about underlying diseases such as diabetes mellitus, COPD, asthma, alcohol abuse, and HIV. It is also important to inquire about recent travel, seizures, and environmental or occupational exposures. HIV positivity increases the likelihood of an opportunistic infection, with organisms such as *Pneumocystis carinii,* CMV, fungus, or *Mycobacterium tuberculosis.*

PHYSICAL EXAMINATION

The history and physical examination are often sufficient to make the diagnosis. Important examination elements include measuring vital signs; an ear, nose, and throat (ENT) examination; palpation of the neck and sinuses; and a thorough cardiopulmonary examination.

Patients with URIs usually have a swollen, red nasal mucosa. Fever accompanied by purulent nasal discharge, facial tenderness, and a loss of maxillary transillumination suggest sinusitis. Although most patients with bronchitis have clear lungs, some may have rhonchi, hoarse rales, or wheezing. Patients with pneumonia are more likely to have abnormal vital signs such as fever, tachypnea, tachycardia and they tend to appear ill. The vital signs and general appearance are also important in assessing the degree of illness. Marked abnormalities of the vital signs and poor general appearance suggest the need for hospitalization. Although the lungs may

be clear in patients with pneumonia, usually there are abnormalities such as localized rales, bronchial breath sounds, wheezing, or signs of consolidation such as dullness to percussion.

DIFFERENTIAL DIAGNOSIS

The diagnosis of a cold is usually self-evident. Occasionally, allergic or vasomotor rhinitis can be confused with a URI. Influenza should be differentiated from the common cold, because specific treatment may be effective. The differential diagnosis of acute sinus pain includes dental disease, nasal foreign body, and migraine or cluster headache. Table 28-1 lists some clinical features that help distinguish between pneumonia and bronchitis.

Although most patients with fever, cough, and patients exhibiting an infiltrate on CXR have an infection, noninfectious causes should also be considered. These include cardiac disease, pulmonary embolus, atelectasis, and malignancy. Generally, the presentation of noninfectious causes tends to be more insidious and the patient is afebrile.

DIAGNOSTIC EVALUATION

Most patients with URIs are diagnosed clinically. Blood testing or imaging is not required for patients with acute sinusitis unless they appear toxic or have a complication of sinusitis, such as orbital cellulitis or cavernous thrombosis. CT is the imaging procedure of choice and is also indicated in patients with chronic sinusitis, recurrent sinusitis, poor response to therapy, those with a possible tumor, and those planning to undergo surgery.

If pneumonia is suspected on history and physical examinations, a CXR is indicated (Figs. 28-1 and 28-2). This can distinguish between bronchitis and pneumonia,

TABLE 28-1. Distinguishing Features of Lower Respiratory Tract Infections

Bronchitis	Pneumonia
Antecedent upper respiratory tract infection	Acute onset of cough, fever, and tachypnea
Cough	
No or low-grade fever	Chest pain
Clear lungs or coarse rhonchi	Leukocytosis Rales
Normal chest x-ray	Pulmonary infiltrate on chest x-ray

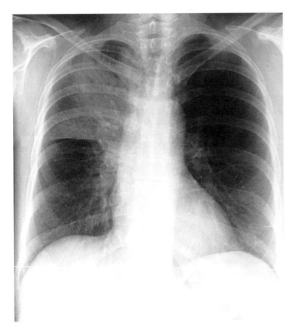

FIGURE 28-1. Posteroanterior (PA) chest x-ray depicting pneumonia. (From Müller NL, Franquet T, Lee KS, et al. *Imaging of Pulmonary Infections*. Philadelphia, PA: Lippincott Williams & Wilkins; 2007.)

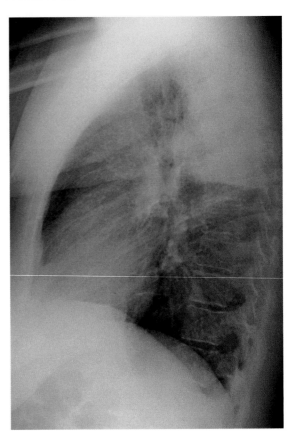

FIGURE 28-2. Lateral chest x-ray depicting pneumonia. (From Müller NL, Franquet T, Lee KS, et al. *Imaging of Pulmonary Infections*. Philadelphia, PA: Lippincott Williams & Wilkins; 2007.)

assess the extent of disease, detect pleural effusions, and help distinguish between infectious and non-infectious causes. Laboratory tests for suspected pneumonia include a CBC, electrolytes, BUN, creatinine, pulse oximetry, sputum for Gram stain and culture, and liver function tests. Patients admitted to the hospital should have blood cultures and—based on the clinical evaluation—HIV and serology testing (e.g., *Legionella testing*) may be indicated. Urinary antigen testing (e.g., *S. pneumoniae* and *Legionella*) can help guide treatment decisions.

TREATMENT

UPPER RESPIRATORY TRACT INFECTIONS

Fluids, rest, and either NSAIDs or acetaminophen help relieve pain and fever and URI symptoms. Sympathomimetics such as pseudoephedrine can reduce nasal congestion. Topical decongestants (e.g., phenylephrine) have fewer systemic side effects than oral decongestants, but their use should be limited to 3 to 4 days to avoid tolerance and rebound congestion. Ipratropium bromide nasal spray is an anticholinergic agent that reduces rhinorrhea, but is of limited benefit in reducing congestion. Vitamin C and zinc supplementation may shorten the duration of symptoms. The treatment of sinusitis should be directed toward improving drainage and

eradicating pathogens. Decongestants, hydration, analgesics, warm facial packs, humidification, and sleeping with the head of the bed elevated are useful adjunctive measures. Mucolytics such as guaifenesin may be of benefit. Most patients with a URI have some element of sinusitis that is self-limited and resolves with symptomatic care. If symptoms persist for more than a week, antibiotics are usually started and administered for 10 to 14 days. Amoxicillin or doxycycline is suitable for initial therapy. For patients allergic to these medications, clindamycin, or quinolones may be substituted. Most individuals respond within 5 days of initiating treatment. Macrolides and TMP/SMX are generally not recommended due to high rates of resistance by *S. Pneumoniae*. Box 28-1 summarizes the initial treatment of rhinosinusitis.

For patients who fail to respond, a broader-spectrum antibiotic is indicated. The antibiotic used in a patient experiencing a treatment failure should be different from the antibiotic used as initial therapy. For individuals whose symptoms persist despite therapy, a CT scan and ENT referral is appropriate.

BOX 28-1. Initial Treatment of Rhinosinusitis

Hydration with increased fluid intake, saline nasal spray
Over-the-counter decongestants, analgesics
Topical nasal decongestants for no more than 3–4 days
Guaifenesin may provide some benefit
For symptoms persisting longer than 7–10 days or other signs or symptoms of bacterial infection, consider antibiotics.
First-line: amoxicillin, cefuroxime, doxycycline
Penicillin allergy: levofloxacin, clindamycin
Second-line: amoxicillin/clavulanic acid, levofloxacin, moxifloxacin

BOX 28-2. Indications for Hospitalization

Systolic blood pressure <90
Pulse rate greater than 140
PO_2 less than 90% or 60 mm Hg
Presence of abscess or pleural effusion
Marked metabolic abnormality
Concomitant disease such as:
  CHF
  Renal failure
  Malignancy
  Diabetes mellitus
  COPD
Age >65
Unreliable social situation

In toxic-appearing patients or those with suspected complications such as osteomyelitis, orbital cellulitis, or intracranial disease, urgent hospitalization and consultation are indicated.

LOWER RESPIRATORY TRACT INFECTIONS

Treatment for bronchitis includes symptomatic care with fluids, decongestants, smoking cessation, and cough suppressants. Multiple studies indicate that antibiotics are almost never helpful for acute bronchitis and can often be harmful. Although controversial, some authorities advocate using antibiotics for severe or persistent cases of bronchitis.

In patients with pneumonia, an important consideration is the locus of care. Box 28-2 lists some indications for hospitalization. For patients suitable for outpatient therapy, antibiotics are administered and are closely monitored. If possible, therapy is guided by the sputum Gram stain results. However, these stains are often impractical or unobtainable in the outpatient setting, so that most family physicians start empiric antibiotic therapy. For healthy adults <60 years old, erythromycin or a newer extended-spectrum macrolide such as azithromycin is a suitable choice. Doxycycline is an acceptable, less-expensive alternative. For patients over age 60, a fluoroquinolone with good activity against *Pneumococcus* (e.g., levofloxacin), a newer extended-spectrum macrolide, or a second-generation cephalosporin is a good choice for empiric therapy. Because infection with an atypical pathogen is unlikely in children 2 months to 5 years of age, the recommended outpatient treatment for them is high-dose amoxicillin (80 to 90 mg/kg/day) for 7 to 10 days. Older children should be treated with a macrolide because of the increased incidence among them of *Mycoplasma* and *C. pneumoniae* infections.

KEY POINTS

- Adults average two to four colds per year. Rhinoviruses account for 30% to 50% of the cases of the common cold; coronaviruses for another 10% to 20%.

- Common organisms for CAP in previously healthy adults are *Streptococcus pneumoniae*, *Hemophilus influenzae*, *Mycoplasma pneumoniae*, or *Chlamydia pneumoniae*.

- A CXR can distinguish between bronchitis and pneumonia, assess the extent of disease, detect pleural effusions, and help distinguish between infectious and noninfectious causes.

- Blood tests or imaging is not required for patients with acute sinusitis unless they appear toxic or have a complication of sinusitis, such as orbital cellulitis or cavernous thrombosis.

- Erythromycin or a newer extended-spectrum macrolide (e.g., azithromycin) or doxycycline is a suitable choice for healthy adults <60 years old with pneumonia. For patients over age 60, a fluoroquinolone with good activity against *Pneumococcus* (e.g., levofloxacin), a newer macrolide, or a second-generation cephalosporin is suitable for empiric pneumonia therapy.

29 | Shortness of Breath

Dyspnea, defined as a sensation of difficult or uncomfortable breathing, is a common complaint associated with a variety of different underlying causes. Presentations vary from acute dyspnea, associated with MI or PE, to chronic dyspnea, associated with CHF or COPD. The manner and location in which a patient presents can also vary. For example, the patient with acute dyspnea is more likely to present to an acute care setting, such as the emergency room, whereas patients with chronic dyspnea are more likely to present in an office setting for evaluation and care. This chapter discusses acute dyspnea briefly and focuses more on chronic causes.

PATHOGENESIS

Dyspnea may be caused by one of several different mechanisms. In general, dyspnea occurs when the perceived demand for oxygen or respiration is not being met or when the work of breathing is increased. For example, with a pneumonia or PE, the lung's ability to provide sufficient oxygen to the peripheral and central chemoreceptors is diminished and the patient experiences dyspnea. Other causes associated with limitations in respiration or oxygen delivery include CHF, interstitial lung disease, pulmonary hypertension, and severe anemia. With obstructive lung disease, such as asthma, the patient may have a normal or near-normal PO_2 and decreased PCO_2 and yet experience dyspnea due to the increased work of breathing. Mechanical causes of dyspnea include obesity, pleural effusion, ascites, and kyphoscoliosis. Finally, anxiety may cause the patient to hyperventilate and perceive this increased respiratory effort as dyspnea.

CLINICAL MANIFESTATIONS

HISTORY

The onset, progression, associated diseases, and symptoms of dyspnea direct the patient's evaluation.

Patients presenting with acute and rapidly progressive symptoms should be questioned about chest pain, history of cardiopulmonary disease, fever, and recent surgery or travel. Table 29-1 summarizes some historical features and their associated conditions for acute dyspnea. These patients should generally be sent to the emergency room setting, where they can be monitored and promptly evaluated for cardiopulmonary causes such as pneumonia, MI, and PE.

Patients with chronic dyspnea, a gradually developing course, or episodic dyspnea may be evaluated in the outpatient setting. The patient should be asked about any past history of cardiac or respiratory disease. Patients with a history of asthma, COPD, or CHF may be experiencing exacerbations of their underlying disease. Associated symptoms should be noted. For example, substernal chest pressure in association with dyspnea occurs with angina. A patient who complains of a swollen leg in association with dyspnea may be experiencing a PE. Patients with a history of melena or dysfunctional uterine bleeding may be experiencing dyspnea due to severe anemia. Inquiries about stress and symptoms of perioral

TABLE 29-1. Historical Clues for Acute Dyspnea

Historical Features	Etiologies
Cough	Bronchospasm, pneumonia
Sputum production	Pneumonia
Pleuritic chest pain	PE, pneumothorax, pneumonia
Substernal chest pain	CHF, MI
Hemoptysis	PE, pneumonia
Recent travel	DVT with PE

CHF, congestive heart failure; DVT, deep venous thrombosis; MI, myocardial infarction; PE, pulmonary embolus.

numbness and paresthesias help assess whether anxiety is the cause of the symptoms.

PHYSICAL EXAMINATION

The physical examination should assess the patient's vital signs and focus on the heart and lungs. Heart examination should note the rate and rhythm of the heart in search of arrhythmias, such as atrial fibrillation, which may trigger dyspneic symptoms. The presence of an S_3 and jugular venous distention suggests CHF. Peripheral edema may be a sign that fluid overload is contributing to the patient's symptoms. Pursed lip breathing and prolonged expiration are consistent with COPD.

The lung examination should note respiratory rate and effort as indicated by the use of the accessory muscles. Inspection should note the chest and abdominal contours, looking for the barrel-chested appearance of COPD or the stigmata of cirrhosis and ascites. Percussion should be performed to detect possible pleural effusions. Auscultation for the presence of rales, wheezing, rubs, or diminished breath sounds should be performed in the assessment for cardiopulmonary causes.

DIFFERENTIAL DIAGNOSIS

Differential diagnosis can be divided into acute and chronic dyspnea. Box 29-1 presents some of the common causes for dyspnea. Anxiety or cardiopulmonary causes account for the majority of patients with dyspnea; asthma, COPD, pneumonia, and CHF are the most frequent cardiopulmonary causes.

DIAGNOSTIC EVALUATION

The critical initial factor in evaluating the patient with dyspnea is to assess its severity and whether the patient requires immediate intervention. Pulse oximetry is available in many offices, and along with the history and physical examination, can assess oxygenation and help determine where and how to further evaluate the patient. Reviewing vital signs for fever, tachycardia, tachypnea, and hypertension or hypotension help assess the degree of illness and unstable patients require evaluation in the emergency room setting. A CXR should be obtained for most patients with a complaint of dyspnea. X-ray findings may show an infiltrate typical of pneumonia, vascular engorgement, or pulmonary edema (characteristic

BOX 29-1. Common Causes for Dyspnea

> **Acute Dyspnea**
> Bronchospasm
> Pulmonary edema
> Pulmonary embolism
> Pneumothorax
> Pneumonia
> Myocardial infarction
> Acute anxiety attack/panic disorder
> Anemia
> Upper airway obstruction
>
> **Chronic Dyspnea**
> Congestive heart failure
> Chronic obstructive pulmonary disease
> Asthma
> Interstitial lung disease
> Pulmonary hypertension
> Pleural effusion
> Obesity
> Ascites
> Kyphoscoliosis
> Anemia
> Anxiety
> Lung mass

of CHF), or reveal hyperinflation and flattened diaphragms characteristic of obstructive lung disease. A CXR can also demonstrate pleural effusions, a pneumothorax, a lung mass, or increased interstitial lung markings and the characteristic honeycomb appearance of interstitial lung disease. Patients with MI, PE, and acute anxiety may have normal CXRs. Chest CT may help determine the etiology when signs or symptoms point to an underlying malignancy, chronic infection, pulmonary embolus, interstitial lung disease or when the diagnosis remains uncertain.

In most cases, history and physical examinations are sufficient to diagnose the cause. In general, symptoms such as chronic cough, sputum production, occupational exposure, or heavy smoking point to a pulmonary rather than a cardiac cause. However, without prominent pulmonary complaints it may be hard to distinguish cardiac from pulmonary disease. Pulmonary function testing may be helpful in diagnosing obstructive or restrictive lung disease as the cause (Fig. 29-1). In addition, arterial blood gases may be indicated to document respiratory status.

An ECG can help assess those with acute dyspnea. In addition to detecting arrhythmia, acute

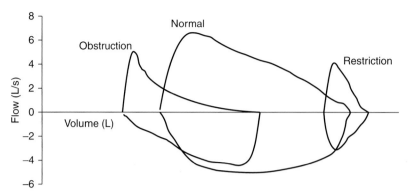

FIGURE 29-1. Pulmonary function tests. (From Morris TA, Ries AL, Bordow RA. *Manual of Clinical Problems in Pulmonary Medicine*. 7th ed. Philadelphia, PA: Wolters Kluwer; 2014.)

ST-segment changes suggest angina or MI and the need for hospitalization. An echocardiogram can assess systolic function and detect the systolic or diastolic dysfunction that may underlie pulmonary congestion and CHF. The echocardiogram can also detect pulmonary hypertension. Exercise stress testing may be helpful in the evaluation of cardiac abnormalities as well as for exercise-induced asthma.

A CBC is indicated to determine the WBC and hemoglobin. An elevated WBC may suggest an underlying infectious process, such as pneumonia, as the cause for dyspnea. Anemia, especially acute anemia, can cause dyspnea and if present, requires further workup to determine its cause (see Chapter 36). Blood levels of brain natriuretic peptide (BNP) are sometimes helpful for distinguishing CHF from a pulmonary cause of dyspnea in the acute setting. BNP is a neurohormone originating in the cardiac ventricles and is elevated in CHF.

Patients should be asked about hemoptysis. If present, it raises the possibility of malignancy, infection, bronchiectasis, or pulmonary embolism.

In patients with episodic symptoms and a normal cardiopulmonary evaluation, GERD with secondary bronchospasm should be considered. Empiric therapy may be a diagnostic, if symptoms are relieved. For still undiagnosed patients, pulmonary referral should be considered. Finally, consideration of psychiatric causes such as anxiety and panic disorder is warranted for patients with a normal cardiopulmonary evaluation.

In pediatric patients, CAD and pulmonary embolism are rare, whereas foreign-body aspiration or upper airway obstruction is more common than in adults. Other common conditions in the pediatric population include asthma and respiratory tract infections such as pneumonia and bronchiolitis.

TREATMENT

Management of dyspnea depends on the underlying cause. For example, patients with PE require hospitalization and anticoagulation. Patients diagnosed with pneumonia may be treated with antibiotics on an inpatient or outpatient basis, depending on the severity of the disease. Those with bronchospasm require bronchodilators. CHF may be treated acutely with diuretics followed by long term management, as outlined in Chapter 41. Therapies for COPD, asthma, obesity, anxiety, anemia, and pneumonia are outlined in their respective chapters.

KEY POINTS

- The most common causes for dyspnea are cardiopulmonary diseases.
- Acute dyspnea can result from life-threatening conditions such as MI, pulmonary embolism, pneumothorax, or pneumonia.
- Chronic dyspnea in adults is most commonly caused by CHF or COPD.

- CXRs should be obtained in most patients with dyspnea.
- Anemia, anxiety, obesity, ascites, and kyphoscoliosis are other potential causes of dyspnea.
- Asthma and respiratory tract infections such as pneumonia and bronchiolitis are common causes of dyspnea in the pediatric population.

30 | Shoulder Pain

Shoulder pain affects people of almost all ages, but is most prevalent in individuals of middle to older ages.

PATHOGENESIS

Normal shoulder motion requires smooth articulations between the glenohumeral, acromioclavicular (AC), sternoclavicular, and scapulothoracic joints. The head of the humerus articulates with the glenoid labrum in a "ball and saucer" fashion (vs. the "ball and socket" articulation of the hip). A shallow articulation allows for a wide range of shoulder motion and also explains why the shoulder is the most commonly dislocated joint. The four muscles of the rotator cuff (supraspinatus, infraspinatus, teres minor, and subscapularis) help stabilize the joint by holding the head of the humerus firmly against the glenoid. The subdeltoid and subacromial bursae are located above the muscles and tendons of the rotator cuff and facilitate fluid movement. Superficial to these bursae are the trapezius, serratus anterior, and rhomboid muscles, which provide scapular stability. All these structures should function in concert to create a smooth motion. Trauma or chronic stress to any single structure can lead to global dysfunction and pain.

The degenerative process that results in bursitis, tendonitis, and shoulder impingement often begins in the supraspinatus or bicipital tendons, which have a poor blood supply and are often under stress. The rotator cuff tendons can become inflamed from being compressed between the humeral head and the acromion. Degenerative changes usually occur in individuals over 50 to 60 years of age and can ultimately involve other tendons, bursae, and sometimes the entire capsule.

CLINICAL MANIFESTATIONS

HISTORY

A complete history includes age, dominant hand, medications, medical history, type of work, and activity level. It is important to determine whether the pain is acute or chronic and to inquire about associated trauma, swelling, redness, laxity, catching, and decreased range of motion.

Patients with rotator cuff problems usually present with an aching shoulder, which becomes acutely painful with overhead activity. Discomfort while abducting the arm past 90 degrees is characteristic of rotator cuff tendonitis. Complete tears of the rotator cuff usually follow trauma, such as a fall, and rarely occur before middle age. Bicipital tendonitis often occurs in combination with rotator cuff tendonitis and is less common as an isolated condition. The pain can be severe and often radiates down the anterior aspect of the humerus.

Determining what activities increase pain provides clues to the underlying problem. For example, pain with activities such as throwing, swimming, or serving a tennis ball suggests rotator cuff tendonitis, whereas chronic pain and stiffness with limited motion suggests adhesive capsulitis (frozen shoulder). A frozen shoulder is most common in middle age and more prevalent in women than in men. It generally follows a period of immobilization from injury or some other medical condition.

Most dislocations and subluxations occur secondary to trauma. Patients often complain of a popping sensation in their shoulder, along with weakness and intermittent pain. Pain from cervical radiculopathy may result in shoulder pain and often radiates to the elbow. Referred pain to the shoulder can occur in a variety of conditions, such as gallbladder disease, subdiaphragmatic inflammation, pulmonary infarction, and intra-abdominal perforation.

PHYSICAL EXAMINATION

The physical examination should include inspection of the shoulder for asymmetry, surgical scars, deformity, or muscle atrophy. Palpation should be performed to pinpoint the areas of tenderness, such as in the AC joint or the bicipital groove. A deformity may be evident in AC separations, fractures, and dislocations. If a fracture or an AC separation is not visually evident, palpation may reveal it.

Range-of-motion testing is critical in evaluating shoulder pain and should be done for both shoulders to allow for comparison. Pain with both active range of motion (AROM) and passive range of motion (PROM) suggests joint or ligament involvement, whereas pain with AROM but not PROM suggests muscular and/or tendon injury. The performance of range-of-motion movements against resistance helps determine the etiology of the pain. For example, patients with rotator cuff injuries often have pain accompanied by weakness when they abduct the fully extended arm against resistance with the thumbs pointing down. This maneuver compresses the tendons of the rotator cuff against the coracoacromial arch and elicits pain when there is inflammation of the rotator cuff or subacromial bursa. Pain with this maneuver is often called a positive "empty can" sign and indicates inflammation of the compressed structures (Fig. 30-1).

Another method for examining the rotator cuff is via the "drop-off" test. This test is performed by passively abducting the patient's shoulder and then

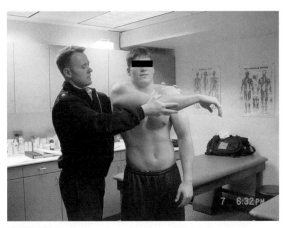

FIGURE 30-2. Crossed-arm test for AC joint pathology. (From Krishnan SG, Hawkins RJ, Warren RF. *The Shoulder and the Overhead Athlete*. Philadelphia, PA: Lippincott Williams & Wilkins; 2004.)

observing him or her lower the hand to the waist level. A sudden drop of the arm toward the waist indicates a rotator cuff tear.

Cross-arm testing is performed by having the patient raise the arm to 90 degrees and then actively adducting the arm (thus bringing the tested arm across the body) (Fig. 30-2). Pain with this maneuver at the AC joint suggests pathology in that region and is therefore useful in differentiating between impingement and AC joint pathology.

Patients with a suspected shoulder dislocation or subluxation should have *stability testing* of the tested shoulder. The apprehension test measures anterior instability; it is performed by abducting the arm to 90 degrees, rotating it externally, and then applying anterior traction to the humerus (Fig. 30-3). Any pain or apprehension evinced

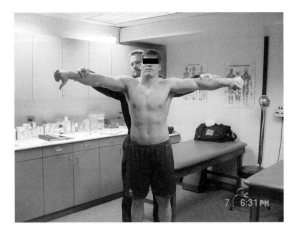

FIGURE 30-1. Empty can test (Jobe's test). (From Krishnan SG, Hawkins RJ, Warren RF. *The Shoulder and the Overhead Athlete*. Philadelphia, PA: Lippincott Williams & Wilkins; 2004.)

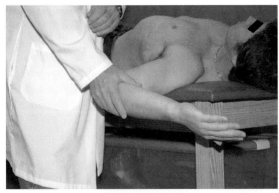

FIGURE 30-3. Apprehension test. (From Krishnan SG, Hawkins RJ, Warren RF. *The Shoulder and the Overhead Athlete*. Philadelphia, PA: Lippincott Williams & Wilkins; 2004.)

by the patient indicates anterior glenohumeral instability. Pushing the humeral head posteriorly and feeling for increased laxity when the arm is abducted to 90 degrees and the elbow flexed to 90 degrees assesses posterior instability of the glenohumeral joint.

Tenderness just lateral to the acromion suggests subacromial bursitis. Cervical root compression can sometimes be differentiated from intrinsic shoulder pain by reproducing the pain with the neck movement.

DIFFERENTIAL DIAGNOSIS

Extrinsic disease can sometimes present as shoulder pain. Examples include cervical radiculopathy, diaphragmatic irritation, and MI. Box 30-1 lists causes of shoulder pain.

Intrinsic shoulder pain is far more common than extrinsic shoulder pain and includes disorders such as osteoarthritis, fracture, dislocation, rheumatoid arthritis, gout, and osteonecrosis. In the absence of trauma, soft-tissue diseases such as rotator cuff tendonitis, bursitis, and bicipital tendonitis are the most common causes of shoulder pain. Less common are rotator cuff tears, biceps tendon rupture, and adhesive capsulitis.

BOX 30-1. Causes of Shoulder Pain

Extrinsic
Cervical disk disease
Thoracic outlet syndrome
Gallbladder disease
Myocardial infarction
Diaphragmatic irritation

Intrinsic
Bone/joint abnormalities
Dislocation/subluxation
Arthritis
Infection
AC joint sprain
Fractures
Osteonecrosis
Soft-tissue abnormalities
Bicipital tendonitis
Impingement syndrome
Bursitis (subacromial)
Rotator cuff tendonitis/tear
Adhesive capsulitis (frozen shoulder)
Subdeltoid bursitis

DIAGNOSTIC EVALUATION

The history and physical examination are often sufficient to suggest the diagnosis. In patients with bursitis, tendonitis, and rotator cuff syndromes, no diagnostic workup is indicated unless the pain persists for more than 4 to 6 weeks. If the clinical evaluation suggests cervical disease, x-ray films of the cervical spine and possibly a CT or MRI scan are indicated. History and physical examination are usually sufficient to indicate whether evaluation is necessary to rule out conditions causing referred pain.

In patients with trauma or persistent shoulder pain, x-rays can detect conditions such as fracture, dislocation, arthritis, metastatic disease, or avascular necrosis. In soft-tissue syndromes, x-rays are usually unremarkable except in cases with calcific tendonitis. Calcium deposits in the areas of the bicipital tendon or in the supraspinatus tendon where it inserts in the greater tuberosity of the humerus may be present. MRI is a useful and noninvasive means of assessing the presence of rotator cuff tendonitis or complete tears of the rotator cuff.

TREATMENT

The mainstay of treatment for soft-tissue inflammation is NSAIDs, combined with ice or heat, and brief periods of rest followed by physical therapy. Physical therapy helps preserve normal motor function before severe weakness and decreased range of motion compound the problem. Basic principles of physical therapy include maintaining range of motion, flexibility, and strength. Treatment progresses from passive range-of-motion exercises to assisted active exercises, isometrics, and finally active strength building. Most inflammatory conditions resolve with conservative care in 6 to 8 weeks. In cases where the inflammation of the tendons is very severe or in acute calcific tendonitis, a steroid injection is often helpful.

A completely torn rotator cuff does not heal spontaneously and may require surgery. However, many people with partial or small tears respond to symptomatic care and an exercise program.

Adhesive capsulitis may be difficult and frustrating to treat. Active exercise to increase the range of motion is the cornerstone of nonoperative therapy. Occasionally, surgery may be indicated. Therapy for arthritis consists primarily of acetaminophen or NSAIDs and exercise. Steroid injections may also provide some relief. AC sprains are treated with NSAIDs and a sling until the pain resolves. Third-degree separations or those involving significant displacement of the clavicle should be referred to an orthopedist. Fractures, rotator cuff tears, advanced arthritis, dislocations, or joint instability and persistent symptoms without improvement are other common indications for orthopedic referral.

KEY POINTS

- Rotator cuff tendonitis, bursitis, and bicipital tendonitis are the most common causes of shoulder pain.
- Traumatic causes of shoulder pain include AC separation, shoulder dislocation, and fractures.
- X-ray testing should be reserved for patients with a history of traumatic injury or persistent pain despite therapy.
- Management for soft-tissue etiologies of shoulder pain commonly involves the use of NSAIDs and physical therapy.

31 | Somatic Symptom Disorder

Somatic symptom disorder is broadly defined as emotional or psychological distress that is experienced and expressed as physical complaints. Somatic symptom disorder replaces the former terminology of "somatization" and can occur in the presence of physical illness, with symptoms either unrelated to the illness, or out of proportion to objective findings. It is important to understand that patients with somatic symptom disorder are not faking their symptoms; the pain, distress, and other problems they experience are real and can be disabling even when no physical cause can be found.

Approximately half of all family practice patients have at least one medically unexplained physical symptom (MUPS). Patients often view physical symptoms as a more acceptable entry into the medical care system than an emotional complaint, and about 70% of patients with emotional disorders present with a somatic complaint as the reason for their office visit.

PATHOGENESIS

The pathophysiology of somatic symptom disorder is not well understood. Multiple theories have been proposed, but no single underlying theory explains somatic symptom disorder. Genetic factors may play a role because somatic symptom disorder is much more common in females and familial patterns have been reported. One theory is that the CNS, specifically the amygdala, regulates sensory information abnormally, resulting in symptoms. Behavioral theories suggest that somatic symptom disorder is a learned behavior in which the environment reinforces the illness behavior. Somatic symptom disorder is also thought by some to be a defense mechanism.

Precipitating factors include stressful life events, which can either be positive (such as marriage) or negative (such as a death in the family). Interpersonal conflict either at work or home is a common risk factor. Somatic symptom disorder can lead to symptoms in several ways. Patients may amplify symptoms of an acute or chronic problem or alternatively give several physical complaints while de-emphasizing psychological problems such as depression. Some patients experience physiologic disturbances, such as palpitations or an irritable bowel, which may be mediated through the autonomic nervous system. On rare occasions, patients can experience conversion symptoms that may serve a symbolic function, such as "hysterical blindness" or "pseudoseizures" (non-epileptiform seizure-like activity). Conversion symptoms typically do not conform to any known physiologic mechanisms.

CLINICAL MANIFESTATIONS

HISTORY

The symptoms of somatic symptom disorder range from occasional functional complaints to a full-blown syndrome that meets the criteria of the *Diagnostic and Statistical Manual of Mental Disorders*, fifth edition (DSM-V), for a somatic symptom disorder. The most common of these entities is somatic symptom disorder, which is characterized by at least one somatic symptom that results in significant disruption of daily life; significant actions, thoughts, or feelings about the symptoms; somatic symptom actions, thoughts, or feelings that are excessively time-consuming or out of proportion to the degree of seriousness, and/or accompanied by a high level of anxiety for at least 6 months. DSM-V criteria no longer require the presence of four pain symptoms, two GI symptoms, one sexual symptom, and one pseudoneurologic symptom that are medically unexplained. Rather, the new criteria focus on how somatic symptoms are disproportionate compared with physical findings or illness. Of note, the presence of a medically explained symptom versus a medically unexplained symptom does not predict differences in disability, healthcare utilization, patient satisfaction, or mood; however, the number of symptoms predicts greater healthcare utilization and poorer health status. Other related disorders include conversion disorder, psychological factors affecting a medical condition, factitious disorder, and other nonspecific somatic symptom disorders. The prevalence of somatic symptom disorder is <0.1% in males, 2% in the general female population, 12% in the general medical clinical population, 9% among tertiary hospital inpatients, and up to 20% of first-degree female relatives of affected patients. Individuals with a history of physical or sexual abuse are more likely to have somatic symptom disorder and most patients are diagnosed before age 30.

A thorough history is important in assessing patients with suspected somatic symptom disorder. Unfortunately, the presence of a physical illness or abnormalities discovered on physical examination does not eliminate somatization. Clues that should raise suspicion for somatic symptom disorder are listed in Box 31-1. Pain is the most frequent complaint. Symptoms often cluster around the cardiovascular system, such as atypical chest pain, palpitations, racing heart, and shortness of breath; the nervous system, such as headache, memory loss, dizziness, lightheadedness, and paresthesias; GU, with sexual or menstrual problems, or the GI system, with complaints such as heartburn, gas, and indigestion.

PHYSICAL EXAMINATION

A careful and thorough physical examination is useful for eliminating organic disease. Several diseases, such as hyperparathyroidism, HIV, and systemic lupus erythematosis, can present with what appear to be somatization complaints. Psychiatric examination usually describes a mildly anxious and/or depressed mood with a normal affect.

DIFFERENTIAL DIAGNOSIS

Differential diagnosis includes anxiety, depression, post-concussion syndrome, schizophrenia, and malingering.

Medical disorders that affect multiple systems or produce nonspecific symptoms that are either transient or recurring can be confused with somatization. Box 31-2 lists some other illnesses that masquerade as somatization.

DIAGNOSTIC EVALUATION

A thorough history and physical examination are essential. Not only an unsuspected illness may be diagnosed, but a normal examination is also critical for providing effective reassurance and avoiding unnecessary testing. Unless there is evidence suggesting a specific disorder, extensive testing should be avoided. For further evaluation of somatic symptom burden, the PHQ-15 (Fig. 31-1) and SSS-8 are useful tools.

BOX 31-1. Clues to Somatic Symptom Disorder

Complaints that are inconsistent with known pathophysiology
Multiple and vague symptoms: description of symptoms can be inconsistent or bizarre
Symptoms persist despite adequate medical treatment
Symptoms that exceed objective findings
Illness begins with a stressful event
The patient "doctor shops"
History of numerous workups with insignificant findings
The patient refuses to consider psychological factors or discuss issues other than medical concepts
There is evidence of an associated psychiatric disorder
The patient has a hysterical personality
Demanding yet disparaging of the physician
The patient uses graphic and emotional language
Unreasonable demands for treatment and drugs
Dwelling on symptoms and proud of suffering

BOX 31-2. Differential Diagnosis of Somatic Symptom Disorder

Chronic fatigue syndrome
Dementia
Fibromyalgia
Substance abuse
Sarcoidosis
Metastatic cancer
Leukemia
Multiple sclerosis
Hyperthyroidism/Hypothyroidism
Lyme disease
Malaria
Tuberculosis
Syphilis

PHYSICAL SYMPTOMS (PHQ-15)

During the <u>past 4 weeks</u>, how much have you been bothered by any of the following problems?

	Not bothered at all (0)	Bothered a little (1)	Bothered a lot (2)
a. Stomach pain	☐	☐	☐
b. Back pain	☐	☐	☐
c. Pain in your arms, legs, or joints (knees, hips, etc.)	☐	☐	☐
d. Menstrual cramps or other problems with your periods **WOMEN ONLY**	☐	☐	☐
e. Headaches	☐	☐	☐
f. Chest pain	☐	☐	☐
g. Dizziness	☐	☐	☐
h. Fainting spells	☐	☐	☐
i. Feeling your heart pound or race	☐	☐	☐
j. Shortness of breath	☐	☐	☐
k. Pain or problems during sexual intercourse	☐	☐	☐
l. Constipation, loose bowels, or diarrhea	☐	☐	☐
m. Nausea, gas, or indigestion	☐	☐	☐
n. Feeling tired or having low energy	☐	☐	☐
o. Trouble sleeping	☐	☐	☐

For office coding: Total Score T_____ = _____ + _____)

Developed by Drs. Robert L. Spitzer, Janet B.W. Williams, Kurt Kroenke and colleagues, with an educational grant from Pfizer Inc. No permission required to reproduce, translate, display or distribute.

FIGURE 31-1. Physical symptoms (PHQ-15). Severity score: low, 5-9; medium, 10-14; high, 15-30.

TREATMENT

An important step is to legitimize and acknowledge the complaints, share the patient's frustrations, and express continued interest and hope. The treatment should focus mainly on restoring and maintaining function. An explanation of symptoms should be presented in functional or physiologic terms, if possible. One approach is to alert the patient that although a thorough examination and testing did not reveal a life-threatening illness, there is still a problem and it is not uncommon to see patients with problems that are not completely explained. Although no cure exists, there are interventions that should help them feel better than they do now. Most importantly, do not tell a patient "it's all in your head." Writing a consultation letter to other medical professionals describing somatic symptom disorder may be of benefit. This intervention focuses away from polypharmacy and a rule out/find-and-fix approach while emphasizing rehabilitation, recovery, and behavioral/lifestyle management.

A well-defined program should be initiated and presented to the patient. Treatments should be time-limited and expectations set. Even if the treatment consists of reassurance and symptom control, definitive information about what to expect and instructions for follow-up can help reduce anxiety.

For example, a physician might say, "We will try this medicine for 4 weeks. Although it may not relieve your symptoms entirely, you should improve enough to participate in your weekly book club meeting. We will know how this is working by whether you miss any meeting dates. I will see you in 4 weeks so we can see how you are managing." Often, engaging the patient in behavioral methods, such as keeping a diary, helps. Consultation with a psychologist or a mental health counselor can help by confirming the diagnosis and recommending effective treatments, such as cognitive behavioral therapy (CBT). Goals of behavioral therapy include relieving stress, developing better coping mechanisms for physical symptoms, and reducing preoccupation with symptoms. While over testing should be avoided, one should also keep in mind that patients with somatic symptom disorder also develop organic disease, and prevention, screening, and evaluation of new or changing symptoms should be part of the overall treatment plan.

Antidepressants with or without antipsychotics can benefit patients with physical symptoms even without comorbid major depression or an anxiety disorder. However, medication should be used sparingly and in low doses. Patients with somatic symptom disorder often have a poor tolerance for side effects. There is rarely an indication for using narcotics or long-term benzodiazepine use in this population.

KEY POINTS

- Somatic symptom disorder is defined as emotional or psychological distress that is experienced and expressed as physical complaints.

- A thorough history and physical examination are essential to eliminate the possibility of organic disease.

- Unless there is evidence suggesting a specific disorder, extensive testing should be avoided.

- An important step in management is to legitimize and acknowledge the complaints, share the patient's frustrations, and express continued interest and hope.

- Pharmaceuticals can benefit patients with major depression or an anxiety disorder that presents with somatic symptoms.

32 | Swelling

Edema is swelling caused by excess fluid trapped in tissues; edema may be localized or generalized and most commonly develops in dependent parts of the body, such as the legs. Leg edema is commonly encountered in family practice, occurring in about 15% of healthy subjects over age 65. The importance of leg edema is its frequent association with illnesses such as DVT, CHF, or renal failure, which can cause significant morbidity and mortality.

PATHOGENESIS

Edema results from an imbalance of factors affecting the distribution of fluid between the intravascular and extravascular spaces. Edema forms when the production of interstitial fluid exceeds its removal through the venous or lymphatic system. Factors contributing to edema are:

1. Increased capillary hydrostatic pressure;
2. Reduced intravascular oncotic pressure;
3. Increased capillary permeability;
4. Reduced lymphatic drainage from the interstitial space.

As a result of gravity, edema occurs most commonly in the lower extremities.

CLINICAL MANIFESTATIONS

HISTORY

Most patients with edema complain of leg swelling, but other symptoms include weight gain, tightness of shoes or clothing, puffiness in the eyes or face—especially in the morning—and an increase in abdominal girth. Patients with associated pulmonary edema may complain of exertional dyspnea, orthopnea, and paroxysmal nocturnal dyspnea. Inquiring about signs of sleep apnea, such as excessive snoring, daytime sleepiness, and fatigue, may lead to a diagnosis of obstructive sleep apnea with associated pulmonary hypertension and edema. It is important to review medications, because NSAIDs and vasodilators, such as nifedipine or prazosin, can cause fluid retention. ACE inhibitors can cause localized facial edema. A history of diurnal variations of 4 to 5 lb/day in healthy young women suggests idiopathic cyclic edema.

PHYSICAL EXAMINATION

A rapid increase in weight over a short period of time is one of the cardinal signs of edema. Generalized edema suggests renal or hepatic disease. The examination should focus on the cardiopulmonary, abdominal, and pelvic examinations. Neck vein distension along with peripheral edema and rales suggest CHF or pulmonary hypertension. Findings such as palmar erythema, spider telangiectasia, and ascites point to cirrhosis. The presence of a prostatic or pelvic mass and inguinal adenopathy raises the possibility of lymphatic obstruction. Obesity, previous episodes of phlebitis, and peripheral neuropathy all predispose individuals to chronic edema. Chronic venous insufficiency can cause leg edema and is associated with the physical examination findings of stasis dermatitis and venous varicosities.

The degree of edema and whether it is unilateral or bilateral should be noted. Differences in calf circumference of > 3 cm with tenderness along the deep veins suggest possible DVT. The knee should also be checked because a ruptured Baker cyst can also cause acute calf pain and swelling mimicking a DVT. The edema should be tested to see how easily it pits (leaves an indention behind when the skin is pressed) and whether the area is tender (Fig. 32-1). Nonpitting leg edema where the indentation made by pressure does not persist may be a sign of hypothyroidism. Localized nonpitting edema is common in patients with lymphedema.

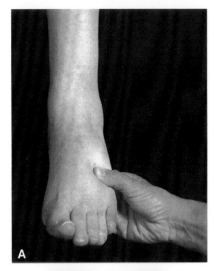

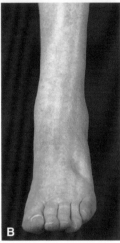

FIGURE 32-1. Pitting edema. (From *Stedman's Medical Dictionary for the Health Professions and Nursing.* 7th ed. Philadelphia, PA: Lippincott Williams & Wilkins; 2011.)

DIFFERENTIAL DIAGNOSIS

The most common causes of generalized edema are hypoalbuminemia (<2.5 g/100 mL), CHF, cirrhosis, nephrotic syndrome, and renal insufficiency. Obesity and obstructive sleep apnea are other common associated diseases. Although bilateral leg edema is associated with systemic diseases, in the family practice setting it is more commonly due to chronic venous insufficiency. Regional edema is usually due to increased capillary pressure from causes such as venous insufficiency or obstruction. Venous obstruction can be due to infection, trauma, thrombophlebitis, or immobility. It can also be a result of external obstruction due to fibrosis, radiation, surgery, neoplasm, or lymph nodes. Box 32-1 lists the causes of leg edema.

BOX 32-1. Causes of Leg Edema

Bilateral or Generalized Edema
CHF
Pulmonary hypertension from lung disease
Cirrhosis
Hypoalbuminemia
Renal disease
Chronic renal failure
Glomerulonephritis
Nephrotic syndrome
Medications
Myxedema (hypothyroidism)
Idiopathic edema
Allergic reaction

Unilateral Leg Edema
Acute
Cellulitis
Deep vein thrombosis
Hematoma or soft-tissue injury
Baker cyst
Chronic
Venous insufficiency
Lymphedema
Extrinsic compression
Neoplasm
Lymphoma

DIAGNOSTIC EVALUATION

Routine laboratory tests for patients with generalized edema include a chemistry panel, a CBC, a UA, and a CXR. The chemistry panel assesses renal function, albumin levels, and electrolytes. A UA provides important information about the presence of renal disease and can detect nephrotic-range proteinuria. Hypoalbuminemia occurs with malnutrition, nephrotic syndrome, or liver disease. CXR can detect pulmonary congestion and effusions, assess heart size, and provide clues to the presence of pericardial disease. A TSH can rule out hypothyroidism in cases of suspected myxedema. Further cardiac testing such as an ECG and echocardiogram is indicated for patients with CHF or suspected obstructive sleep apnea.

For patients with unilateral leg edema, a US can test for a DVT. Failure of the vein to compress and impaired venous flow correlate with the presence of a DVT. One strategy for detecting DVT is to combine D-dimer testing and a pretest risk assessment with US testing. In patients considered at low to intermediate risk for a DVT, D-dimer testing in conjunction with prerisk probability assessment, such as the Wells score, can help determine the need for a US and reduce the need for testing. A negative test in a low-risk patient has a strong negative predictive value. A positive test in a low-risk patient is associated with about a 15% chance of a DVT and indicates a need for further evaluation. A CT scan of the abdomen and pelvis is indicated in cases of suspected obstruction from a mass.

TREATMENT

Treatment of the underlying cause is important. For example, lymphedema may resolve with treatment of an underlying malignancy. Nephrotic syndrome may respond to corticosteroids. Diuretics and ACE inhibitors can relieve edema associated with CHF. Nasal CPAP and therapy for pulmonary hypertension may help with edema associated with obstructive sleep apnea. Edema due to a medication usually responds to withdrawal of the medication.

Nonpharmacologic measures such as leg elevation, compression stockings, and salt restriction are useful. Patients with leg edema should routinely avoid prolonged sitting with their knees bent and may benefit from sleeping with a pillow under their legs. Support stockings or custom-made pressure gradient hose can reduce dependent edema. Stockings above the knee may work better, but are often poorly tolerated. Compressive stockings are contraindicated in patients with arterial insufficiency. Initial salt restriction consists of eliminating added salt and avoiding high-sodium foods. Pneumatic compression stockings may be beneficial for patients with venous insufficiency or lymphedema that is refractory to other therapies.

Diuretics should be used cautiously as an adjunct to nonpharmacologic therapy. Lymphedema and edema due to chronic venous insufficiency do not typically respond to diuretics. Patients receiving diuretics should be monitored to avoid over-diuresis. Symptoms of excessive diuresis are nonspecific and may include weakness, fatigue, lethargy, and confusion. Monitoring includes following the patient's weight, checking orthostatic blood pressure, and measuring electrolytes and renal function periodically to detect common metabolic abnormalities—such as hyponatremia, hypokalemia, metabolic alkalosis, and prerenal azotemia—associated with diuretics.

KEY POINTS

- Leg edema is a common problem in family practice, occurring in about 15% of healthy subjects over age 65. The importance of leg edema is its frequent association with illnesses such as CHF or renal failure, which can cause significant morbidity and mortality.

- Generalized edema is usually a result of hypoalbuminemia or cardiac, renal, or hepatic disease.

- Nonpharmacologic measures for treating edema—such as leg elevation, compression stockings, and salt restriction—are useful.

- Diuretics should be used cautiously as an adjunct to nonpharmacologic therapy. Lymphedema and edema due to chronic venous insufficiency do not typically respond to diuretics.

33 | Weight Loss

Unintended weight loss is a worrisome finding that may indicate the presence of a significant underlying physical or psychological illness. It can occur in people of all ages and has many potential causes.

PATHOGENESIS

Unintended weight loss results when caloric intake is less than caloric expenditure. This may result from diminished intake, malabsorption, excessive loss of nutrients, or increased caloric expenditure.

Diminished caloric intake may be due to decreased interest in food, inability to obtain food, attenuated awareness of hunger, pain associated with the ingestion of food, and early satiety. Malabsorption of calories can occur with hepatic, pancreatic, and intestinal disorders. Loss of nutrients may result in the body being unable to maintain caloric homeostasis. Examples include recurrent vomiting or diarrhea, glucosuria, and significant proteinuria. Increased nutrient demand is the result of any process that increases basal metabolic rate. Chronic infection, hyperthyroidism, excessive exercise, and malignancy are common causes of increased metabolic rate. Cachexia is commonly noted in association with ongoing diseases such as cancer or AIDS and is associated with increased nutrient demands and a systemic inflammatory response. Unlike malnutrition, cachexia cannot be reversed nutritionally and disproportionately affects muscle mass, leading to increased weakness.

CLINICAL MANIFESTATIONS

HISTORY

The first step in evaluating a patient with weight loss is to determine the degree of weight loss and the period of time over which it occurred. Because many older patients may not recognize a significant weight loss,

a decline in serial weight measurements is often the presenting sign. If a previous weight measurement is unavailable, asking about changes in waist size or how clothing fits may be helpful. Once significant weight loss is confirmed, a thorough review of systems helps direct the physical examination and laboratory testing.

Questions about daily food intake, alterations in appetite, pain with swallowing, early satiety, episodes of emesis, and changes in bowel habits are important. Foul-smelling, greasy, bulky stools suggest malabsorption. Especially in young women, attitudes toward food and body image should be assessed. A distorted body image may suggest the presence of an eating disorder.

Patients should be asked about fever, cough, shortness of breath, alterations in patterns of urination, abdominal pain, melena, hematochezia, rash, headaches, and other neurologic symptoms. Signs of depression such as difficulty concentrating, changes in sleeping patterns, social isolation, and recent losses should be elicited. In the case of cognitively impaired patients, family members and caregivers should be interviewed. The past medical history, previous surgeries, medications, tobacco use, alcohol intake, family history, and HIV risk factors should be reviewed. A social history is important to identify issues such as poverty, isolation, or an inability to shop or cook, which may lead to weight loss.

PHYSICAL EXAMINATION

The physical examination begins with measuring height, weight, and vital signs to detect the presence of fever or tachycardia. General inspection should note stigmata of systemic disease, including hair loss, temporal wasting, pallor, poor hygiene, bruising, jaundice, and diminished orientation.

Evaluation of the oropharynx should assess dentition, presence of oral thrush, and petechiae. Neck examination should note any thyromegaly or lymphadenopathy.

Lungs should be examined for decreased breath sounds, crackles, wheezes, and evidence of consolidation. The heart should be examined for irregular rhythm, murmurs, gallops, and the presence of a pericardial effusion. Abdominal examination should note surgical scars, the quality of bowel sounds, and the presence of organomegaly, ascites, tenderness, or masses. Rectal examination is important for evaluating the prostate and checking for occult blood and stool consistency. In women, breast and pelvic examinations should be performed to evaluate for malignancy. Neurologic examination should assess memory, concentration, posterior column function, and focal abnormalities. Psychiatric evaluation may provide evidence of a mood disorder or anorexia nervosa.

DIFFERENTIAL DIAGNOSIS

Table 33-1 lists some important causes of weight loss. It is useful to organize the differential diagnosis by the categories of decreased intake, impaired absorption, nutrient loss, and increased demand. For many conditions, such as cancer or end-stage CHF, weight loss occurs long after diagnosis. In COPD, about 35% of patients experience weight loss as the disease progresses. In contrast, weight loss is an early finding in illnesses such as anorexia nervosa, pancreatic cancer, malabsorption, apathetic hyperthyroidism, diabetes, Alzheimer disease, and HIV. A physical cause for weight loss can be found in about 65% of patients and a psychiatric cause in another 10%. Depression is the most common psychiatric cause, and along with substance abuse may present with profound weight loss. Anorexia nervosa is seen primarily in adolescent females and young adults. The diagnosis is based on weight loss leading to a body weight 15% below normal combined with a distorted body image, fear of weight gain, and, in females, the absence of at least three consecutive menstrual cycles. Other psychiatric and medical illness must be excluded. In approximately 25% of individuals with weight loss, no identifiable cause is found.

DIAGNOSTIC EVALUATION

Unintended weight loss exceeding 5% in 1 month or 10% in 6 months deserves evaluation. Since weight loss is usually a late symptom of disease, the cause may be identified through information gathered by the history and physical examinations combined with conventional laboratory testing, such as a CBC, serum electrolytes, BUN, creatinine, calcium, glucose, liver function tests, albumin, TSH, UA, CXR, ESR, C-reactive protein

TABLE 33-1. Differential Diagnosis of Weight Loss

Decreased Intake

Alcohol/substance abuse

Anorexia nervosa

Congestive heart failure

Depression

Dementia

Hepatitis

Medications (e.g., digitoxin toxicity)

Ulcer disease

Uremia

Splenomegaly

Bowel obstruction

Poverty/social isolation

Poor dentition

Malabsorption

Gastric bypass

Pancreatic insufficiency

Inflammatory bowel disease

Celiac sprue

Cholestasis

Protein-losing enteropathy

Nutrient Loss

Significant proteinuria

Diabetes (uncontrolled)

Chronic emesis

Fistula

Chronic diarrhea

Increased Demand

Chronic infection (e.g., tuberculosis)

Malignancy

Hyperthyroidism

Excessive exercise

Infection (e.g., parasites)

(CRP), and stool test for occult blood. In patients without obvious symptoms or abnormalities on initial testing, continued support and observation are warranted because the yield of further testing is extremely low.

However, for patients with symptoms or suspected causes based on initial assessment, further testing should be pursued. In patients with GI symptoms, upper endoscopy, colonoscopy, abdominal US, abdominal CT, lipase, amylase, and stool analysis may be warranted. HIV antibody testing and TB skin testing should be performed in all individuals with risk factors. In patients in whom malabsorption is suspected, a D-xylose test can distinguish between pancreatic and small bowel disease. Antitissue transglutaminase antibodies should be measured if there is concern about celiac sprue. In alcoholics and those with a macrocytic anemia, vitamin B_{12} and folate levels should be measured.

TREATMENT

Patients with an obvious cause for weight loss—such as peptic ulcer disease, gallstones, infection, diabetes, hyperthyroidism, or cancer—should be treated accordingly. Weight loss associated with depression typically responds well to antidepressant therapy. Mirtazapine is an antidepressant that is frequently used to stimulate appetite. In patients with dementia, one-to-one feeding support along with nutritional supplements often helps reverse weight loss. The use of an instant breakfast powder in whole milk is a less costly alternative to commercially available supplements (e.g., Ensure) in lactose-tolerant individuals. Megestrol acetate, cyproheptadine, and dronabinol are sometimes used as appetite stimulants in patients with cancer or AIDS.

Patients with anorexia nervosa need psychiatric referral and very close follow-up. The goal is restoration of normal body weight and resolution of psychological difficulties. Treatment programs conducted by experienced teams in the outpatient setting are often helpful; but in severe or recalcitrant cases, admission to the hospital for bed rest, supervised meals, and intense behavioral and psychotherapy are indicated because between 2% and 6% of patients die from complications of the disorder or commit suicide. Patients with severe malnutrition may require enteral or parenteral feeding.

In the setting of pancreatic insufficiency, oral pancreatic enzyme preparations and fat-soluble vitamin supplements (vitamins A, D, E, and K) should be instituted. Alcoholics and those suffering from malabsorption need vitamin B_{12} and folate supplementation. Finally, observation along with frequent follow-up is considered appropriate management in patients with a normal history, physical examination, and laboratory evaluation.

KEY POINTS

- A weight loss >5% of total body weight over a period of 6 months is generally considered abnormal and warrants further investigation.
- Unintended weight loss may be the result of diminished intake, malabsorption, excessive loss of nutrients, or increased caloric expenditure. Cancer and chronic disease are common causes for both decreased intake and increased caloric expenditure.
- A physical cause for weight loss can be found in about 65% of patients and a psychiatric cause in another 10%.

CLINICAL VIGNETTES

VIGNETTE 1

A 30-year-old, slender, nonsmoking male presents with pain in his left leg following a 5-hour plane trip across the country. He hiked up mountains a lot on his trip but recalls no specific injury. Examination reveals normal skin coloration, no edema, and slight tenderness with active use of and palpation over the mid gastrocnemius.

1. Testing to evaluate this patient's leg pain would include which of the following?
   a. Tibia-fibula x-ray
   b. D-dimer
   c. Venous duplex scan
   d. CT scan of the chest

2. The 68-year-old father of the above patient, who also was on this trip, presents with shortness of breath and pleuritic right-sided chest pain. He is modestly obese with chronic 1+ leg edema in association with stable, mild CHF and hypertension that are being treated with furosemide, carvedilol, and lisinopril. His vital signs reveal a HR of 110, regular rhythm, respiratory rate of 28, and BP 120/76. Lung examination reveals clear breath sounds without rales or wheezing. Next step in evaluation of this patient would include which of the following?
   a. CXR
   b. D-dimer
   c. Chest CT scan
   d. Echocardiogram

3. Chest CT scan reveals the presence of bilateral pulmonary emboli. Which of the following treatments is indicated for this condition?
   a. Low-molecular-weight heparin (LMWH) and warfarin
   b. LMWH alone
   c. Warfarin alone
   d. Clopidogrel
   e. Aspirin

VIGNETTE 2

A 28-year-old, slender, nonsmoking male with no significant past medical history presents with shortness of breath while walking to work from the train. He also noted pleuritic chest pain associated with his breathing problems. Vital signs are RR 24, HR 105, BP 110/80, and O_2 saturation 95%. His lung examination reveals breath sounds diminished on the right side and tympany to percussion. His CXR is shown below.

1. Initial treatment of this patient should include which of the following?
   a. NSAID therapy and outpatient follow-up
   b. Cardiac consultation for catheterization/PCI
   c. Oxygen and needle aspiration of the right chest
   d. Antibiotic therapy for 10 days
   e. No therapy is indicated

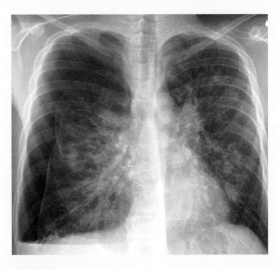

VIGNETTE 3

A 56-year-old male accountant presents with onset this morning of substernal chest pressure while working. He complains of being short of breath with some mild nausea and diaphoresis. He is a former smoker and is being treated for hypertension. His examination reveals a regular pulse at about 70 beats/minute, RR 16, and BP 120/70. His heart examination is RRR without murmur, he has no edema, and the lungs are clear. His EKG is shown below.

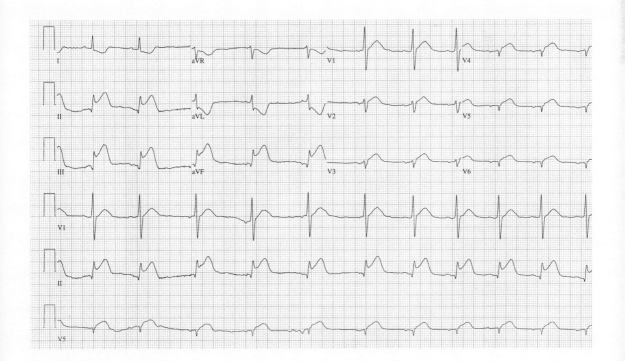

1. Laboratory testing that would confirm your diagnosis would include which of the following?
   a. Arterial blood gases
   b. Cardiac enzymes
   c. D-dimer
   d. ESR

2. The patient undergoes percutaneous angioplasty and stenting and is now ready for discharge. Appropriate therapy on discharge would include which of the following?
   a. Aspirin, clopidogrel, a statin, and beta blocker
   b. Hydralazine, aspirin, and diltiazem
   c. Aspirin and beta blocker
   d. Beta blocker and a statin

ANSWERS

VIGNETTE 1 Question 1

1. Answer B:

The long plane trip raises the possibility of DVT. In this low-risk active patient without swelling or other clinical features suggesting a DVT a normal D-dimer test eliminates the need for further testing. If there was a history of trauma or bone tenderness, then a tibia-fibula x-ray may be warranted to assess for potential fracture. Venous duplex scanning to rule out a DVT is warranted in higher risk patients or in this case if the D-dimer is elevated. A chest CT can detect pulmonary embolus or other lung/chest wall lesions but would not be indicated in this patient who has no respiratory symptoms or chest pain.

VIGNETTE 1 Question 2

2. Answer C:

This patient has underlying medical diseases including obesity and congestive heart failure that increase his risk for venous thromboembolic disease. Though his symptoms may be due to these underlying diseases, the increased risk and recent travel make ruling out thromboembolic disease a priority. D-dimer levels increase with age and heart disease, and testing has less clinical utility in those with a high pretest probability of venous thromboembolic disease. A CXR may be useful in assessing for pulmonary edema or pneumonia, but is not a good diagnostic test for pulmonary emboli. An echocardiogram may show an increase in pulmonary artery pressure with a pulmonary embolus, but is generally not the initial test of choice in cases of suspected pulmonary emboli. A spiral chest CT scan or V/Q nuclear scan is the preferred test.

VIGNETTE 1 Question 3

3. Answer A:

Patients with venous thromboembolic disease and pulmonary embolus generally require therapy for 6 to 12 months following an initial event under conditions that are reversible. Patients with recurrent disease and those with a predisposition to venous thromboembolic disease that is not reversible may require treatment indefinitely. Anticoagulation with heparin or LMWH followed by oral warfarin is the most common and traditional therapy for most patients. Administer LMWH for a minimum of 5 days to overlap with warfarin until the PT INR is therapeutic for 2 days. Warfarin is then continued after the LMWH is stopped with ongoing monitoring of PT INR. Pregnant women cannot take warfarin and thus require heparin or LMWH. Other oral agents that are available include Factor Xa inhibitors as well as direct thrombin inhibitors. These newer medications offer the advantage of a fixed dose regimen without the need for monitoring the INR. They also have fewer food and drug interactions than warfarin. Trials are in progress to establish the role of these agents in treating PE.

VIGNETTE 2 Question 1

1. Answer C:

The patient has a right-sided pneumothorax on the x-ray consistent with his physical examination findings of decreased breath sounds and tympany to percussion. Therapy may include aspiration and observation or chest tube placement depending on the symptoms and size of the pneumothorax. Antiinflammatory therapy may help with the pleuritic chest pain but would not be sufficient treatment. The patient's symptoms are not consistent with cardiac disease, and the presentation and x-ray do not indicate a pneumonia that would require antibiotic treatment.

VIGNETTE 3 Question 1

1. Answer B:

This EKG reveals ST elevation consistent with a myocardial infarction in the inferior leads (II, III, aVF). Cardiac enzymes are indicated to support this diagnosis. Myoglobin generally rises first (2 to 4 hours), but is not specific for cardiac muscle. CPK-MB (4 to 6 hours) and troponin (3 to 12 hours) rise next. Serial enzymes are generally ordered, and the degree of troponin elevation has been associated with mortality and adverse events. Arterial blood gases and D-dimer might be of benefit in addressing patients with suspected pulmonary embolus. ESR is a nonspecific indicator of inflammation and may be elevated in patients with pericarditis. EKG findings of pericarditis include more diffuse ST elevation in association with an elevated ESR and sharp pleuritic chest pain exacerbated by lying flat.

VIGNETTE 3 Question 2

2. Answer A:

Beta blocker, statin, and aspirin therapies are the mainstays of post-MI therapy, often along with ACE inhibitors as well. In patients with a new stent, clopidogrel is often prescribed in conjunction with aspirin to prevent stent thrombosis. The optimal duration of dual platelet inhibition remains uncertain but is usually continued for at least 6 to 12 months. Diltiazem and hydralazine do not have significant roles in ischemic heart disease. Hydralazine is an effective antihypertensive agent and when combined with nitrates can be useful in treating congestive heart failure. Diltiazem is a mild antihypertensive that has a role in heart rate control with atrial fibrillation.

34 | Acne

Acne is the most common chronic skin condition treated by physicians; it affects more than 85% of adolescents and young adults and about 15% of affected individuals seek treatment. Although most commonly seen in teenagers, acne may occur transiently in neonates and may persist beyond puberty into the third and fourth decades of life. Acute acne can cause physical pain, low self-esteem, increased social and emotional anxiety, whereas long-term sequelae include scarring and hyperpigmentation.

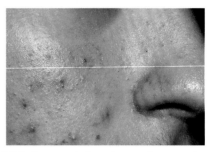

FIGURE 34-1. Open and closed comedones and pustules. (From Goodheart HP. *Goodheart's Photoguide of Common Skin Disorders*. 2nd ed. Philadelphia, PA: Lippincott Williams & Wilkins; 2003.)

PATHOGENESIS

The pathogenesis of acne is multifactorial. It includes hyperkeratosis with resulting blockage of the pilosebaceous canal, increased growth of *Propionibacterium acnes*, overproduction of sebum, and inflammation. Androgen production stimulates the sebaceous gland, causing an increase in cell turnover, an increase in sebum production, and cohesiveness of keratinocytes in the pilosebaceous canal. This alteration in keratinization makes the keratinous material in the follicle stickier, causing a blockage of the canal. The blocked pilosebaceous gland produces a small cystic swelling resulting in a raised area of the follicular duct just below the epidermis, referred to as a microcomedone. If the duct dilates with stratum corneum cells, causing an opening of the follicular mouth, it is referred to as an open comedone or "blackhead"; if the mouth remains closed, it is referred to as a closed comedone or "whitehead" (Fig. 34-1).

The combination of sebum, desquamated cells, and obstruction of the follicular opening creates an environment conducive to the overgrowth of the gram-negative anaerobic diphtheroid bacteria, *P. acnes*. This bacterium is part of the normal skin flora and secretes a low-molecular-weight chemotactic factor and lipase enzymes that break down the triglycerides of sebum into free fatty acids. This breakdown irritates the follicular wall,

leading to the formation of an erythematous papule on the skin. Neutrophils release hydrolases, which may further disrupt the integrity of the follicular wall, causing rupture and leakage into the underlying dermis, leading to the formation of a pustule. If this inflammatory process continues, it eventually leads to the formation of a nodule and subsequently a cyst.

Androgens are a primary stimulus of sebaceous gland proliferation and increased sebum production, which explains why acne often develops during puberty. Because girls reach puberty earlier than boys, the peak of acne in girls is reached between 14 and 17 years of age, compared to ages 16 to 19 in boys. Neonatal acne is caused by maternal androgens that stimulate the sebaceous glands, which have not yet involuted to their childhood state of immaturity. Neonatal acne is usually mild and can be observed during the second to fifth months of life, after which the pilosebaceous units involute, only to reemerge again near puberty.

CLINICAL MANIFESTATIONS

HISTORY

The history should include onset and distribution of skin lesions and any associated aggravating or alleviating factors. The patient should be asked about aggravating foods, smoking, recent stressors, depression, suicidal ideation, skin care practices (scrubbing, picking, squeezing), association with menses, whether temperature affects the skin, and if there are seasons of the year during which the lesions are worse. Cosmetics, topical skin preparations, or exposure to heavy oils or greases may contribute to follicular plugging. Medications such as corticosteroids, androgens, anticonvulsants, and lithium may contribute to acne. Patients should be asked about other symptoms of androgen excess, such as voice change and change in hair growth and distribution. The sudden onset of widely distributed, severe acne may be associated with androgen excess, either from an androgen-secreting tumor or from the ingestion of exogenous androgens.

PHYSICAL EXAMINATION

The physical examination focuses on characterizing and localizing the skin lesions. Acne lesions usually develop in areas with the greatest density and size of sebaceous glands. The face is usually involved. Other commonly affected areas are the chest, shoulders, and upper back. Additional note should be made of hair pattern, and in cases of suspected virilization, a genital examination should be performed to assess for pelvic masses or clitoromegaly.

The prime focus of the examination is to characterize and classify the acne. Acne lesions are classified into either **comedonal** (whiteheads, blackheads) or **inflammatory** (papules/pustules, nodules/cysts). Most cases of acne are pleomorphic and include comedones, papules, pustules, and nodules. Patients with mild acne usually have whiteheads and blackheads, a few papules, and some pustules. Moderate acne consists of many papules and pustules and a few nodules. Severe acne, also referred to as nodulocystic acne, consists of many papules, pustules, and nodules or cysts. In women, localization of acne on the jaw line is most likely hormonally mediated.

DIFFERENTIAL DIAGNOSIS

Common conditions that mimic the lesions of acne vulgaris include acne rosacea, folliculitis, hidradenitis suppurativa, and perioral dermatitis. Acne rosacea is a chronic vascular inflammatory disorder affecting mainly adults between the ages of 30 and 50 years. It is characterized by a vascular component (redness, telangiectasia, flushing, blushing) and an eruptive component (papules and pustules) affecting only the face. Patients are extremely sensitive to facial vasodilatory factors such as exposure to extreme heat or cold, excessive sunlight, and ingestion of alcohol, spicy foods, hot liquids, and highly seasoned food. Folliculitis is the infection of hair follicles from the epidermal surface

by *Staphylococcus*, often from shaving. Hidradenitis suppurativa consists of the appearance of inflammatory cystic lesions, typically in the axilla and groin of obese individuals. Perioral dermatitis is an eruption around the mouth, nose, and eyes affecting young women; it is thought to have a bacterial etiology. These patients have papules and pustules resembling folliculitis, there are no whiteheads or blackheads, and there is a clear zone around the vermilion border. Androgen excess, such as polycystic ovarian syndrome (PCOS), and medications can cause acne.

DIAGNOSTIC EVALUATION

No special tests are required in the evaluation of acne other than skin examination. In those women with suspected androgen excess, serum testosterone, androstenedione, sex hormone binding globulin, prolactin, 17-hydroxyprogesterone, serum cortisol, LH/FSH ratio, fasting/postprandial insulin, and dehydroepiandrosterone sulfate levels may help in guiding further evaluation and therapy.

TREATMENT

The principle of acne therapy is to disrupt the cycle of follicular plugging and increased sebum production and to reduce bacterial colonization and inflammation. Evidence suggests that diets with high glycemic loads and dairy intake, to a lesser extent, may affect acne and that in some instances adjusting dietary intake may help. Cleaning products such as Neutrogena, Dove, and Cetaphil may help. It is important that providers stress patience with a treatment regimen because most therapies take at least 8 to 12 weeks to show improvement.

Topical agents such as tretinoin (Retin-A) are often the first line of therapy. Tretinoin increases cell turnover and reduces the cohesion between keratinocytes, helping to unplug the follicle. The medication usually causes some redness, burning, and peeling of the skin within the first 3 to 4 weeks of treatment. This may make the comedones more visible, causing many patients to believe that they are worsening and to stop using their medication prematurely. To increase tolerability and medication adherence, use milder products (a lower concentration or cream rather than gels), gradually increase application frequency from twice weekly to every other day to daily use, and use combination products (such as adapalene/benzoyl peroxide) with easy medication dispensers such as pumps. However, with continued use of tretinoin, most patients improve after the 6th week, with best results seen at 9 to 12 weeks of treatment. Retin-A also causes the skin to become much more sensitive to irritants such as sun exposure, wind, dryness, and cold temperatures; thus, it is recommended to use a noncomedogenic moisturizing ointment along with the tretinoin. Other, milder comedolytics include salicylic acid, sulfur preparations, and azelaic acid. Azelaic acid has antibacterial and keratolytic properties and is useful in patients with mild-to-moderate acne who cannot tolerate tretinoin. Matching the preparation vehicle to skin type may also aid tolerability. Typically, individuals with dry skin find creams or lotions less drying, whereas those with oily skin often do better with less greasy preparations such as gels or solutions.

The goal of treatment for mild-to-moderate acne is to reduce the follicular bacterial population by using topical antibiotics (erythromycin or clindamycin) and keratolytics. Benzoyl peroxide has bacteriostatic properties, which make it an effective treatment for mild inflammatory acne. Patients should be advised that this medication can dry the skin and can bleach clothes and pillowcases. Several topical preparations combine benzoyl peroxide with a topical antibiotic (Benzaclin, Benzamycin). Due to increasing resistance of *P. acnes* to topical erythromycin and even some cross-resistance to topical clindamycin, topical antibiotic agents should not be used alone. However, combination preparations, such as Benzamycin, do not appear to promote resistant strains of *P. acnes*. If topical retinoids are used in conjunction with a topical antibacterial, they should be applied at different times (i.e., antibacterial in the morning and retinoid in the evening because sunlight can inactivate the retinoid). If

lesions do not improve after 6 weeks of treatment, an oral antibiotic can be added to the regimen. Antibiotics should not be used indefinitely and their use limited to 6 months. The most effective antibiotics are tetracycline, doxycycline, minocycline, and erythromycin. In adolescent girls, combined oral contraceptives such as ethinyl estradiol with levonorgestrel, drospirenone, norgestimate, or norethidrone have the same efficacy as antibiotics after 6 months of treatment. The main effect of oral contraceptives is to suppress ovarian androgen production and thus reduce sebum production. Similarly, spironolactone, due to its antiandrogen effects, may be tried in recalcitrant cases.

If the combination of oral antibiotic and topical retinoid is insufficient, prescribing isotretinoin (Accutane) often helps treat moderate-to-severe acne. Accutane is associated with significant toxicity and requires close monitoring under the direction of an experienced clinician. It is extremely teratogenic and severe malformations occur in 25% to 30% of fetuses exposed to the drug. Female patients must commit to two forms of birth control for at least 1 month prior to therapy, during therapy, and 1 month after therapy. Other adverse effects include dry skin, elevated triglycerides, and depression. In patients with comedones larger than 1 cm, one may consider physical treatments such as comedone extractions and intralesional corticosteroid injections with triamcinolone. Other patients with primarily inflammatory lesions may benefit from chemical peels, phototherapy, or photodynamic therapy. Acne therapy is summarized in Table 34-1.

TABLE 34-1. Acne Treatment	
Severity	**Treatment**
Mild, noninflammatory	Topical retinoid at low strength, increase as needed or tolerated
Mild, minimal inflammation	Topical retinoid at night plus benzoyl peroxide alone or combined with topical antibiotic
Moderate, pustules, some nodules	Topical retinoid and oral antibiotic
Severe, numerous cysts, nodules, and inflammation	Isotretinoin alone or topical retinoid, oral antibiotic, and isotretinoin

KEY POINTS

- Acne vulgaris affects ~ 85% of adolescents.
- Overproduction of sebum and *P. acnes* are etiologic agents leading to the development of acne.
- Comedonal acne is treated with topical keratolytics (retinoids) and/or benzoyl peroxide.
- Inflammatory acne is treated with topical agents combined with oral antibiotics.

- Most treatment regimens take 8 to 12 weeks to show improvement.
- Isotretinoin (Accutane) is reserved for severe or moderate acne that is unresponsive to treatment.
- Isotretinoin is extremely teratogenic and requires close monitoring by an experienced clinician.

35 | Alcohol and Substance Abuse

Substance problems encompass a wide range of severity. Consequences can include legal problems, health problems, and recurrent social, work-related, or interpersonal problems.

EPIDEMIOLOGY

Alcohol and substance abuse are among the most serious social and medical problems in the United States. Americans use two-thirds of the world's illegal drugs and 80% of the world's opioid supply despite accounting for only about 5% of the world's population. Substance abuse affects all age groups, and each year there are approximately 100,000 deaths resulting from alcohol abuse; more than 40,000 deaths from opioid or heroin overdose (17,000 of which were related to prescription opioids), and another 20,000 deaths from the use of other illicit substances. An estimated 20% of adults in the United States are at risk for alcohol- and substance-related problems, with 13% meeting diagnostic criteria for substance abuse or dependence during their lifetimes. Approximately 10% of all drivers report driving under the influence of drugs or alcohol each year. Societal costs stem from lost productivity, costs of alcohol-related illness, unintended pregnancies, spread of infectious diseases, drug-related crime, interpersonal violence, premature death, and motor vehicle accidents (MVAs). Alcohol is associated with the three leading causes of death in adolescents (homicide, suicide, and MVAs). Among the elderly, up to 10% may be abusing alcohol at any given time. Fetal alcohol syndrome is the most common birth defect among newborns in the United States. Opioid use/abuse in pregnant women can lead to neonatal abstinence syndrome in neonates and potentially weeks to months of stays in a neonatal intensive care unit (NICU).

PATHOGENESIS

At-risk behavior occurs when an individual drinks or occasionally uses substances to the level of intoxication. The concern is the risk of progression to more frequent drinking, trauma, and accidents. A person who abuses substances is one who engages in intermittent, repetitive, and planned drinking or usage to levels of intoxication. Abuse becomes dependence when the patient loses control over his or her use despite persistent social, physiologic, occupational, and physical problems. Tolerance arises when a person requires more drugs to achieve the same "high" effect. These individuals experience withdrawal symptoms if use stops abruptly. The etiology of substance abuse is not completely understood but is likely multifactorial. Genetic factors appear to play a role. Individuals with an alcoholic parent have a three to four times greater risk of becoming dependent on alcohol, and identical twins have a greater concordance of alcoholism than fraternal twins.

Nongenetic factors also contribute: emotional or interpersonal stress may serve as an initiator and maintainer of alcohol abuse. Parental and peer values can contribute to substance abuse. Adults who grew up in dysfunctional families and/or are in dysfunctional family situations are at increased risk for alcohol abuse. Patients who have an underlying psychopathology, such as depression or anxiety, often abuse alcohol and other drugs as a form of self-medication. Age of first use of alcohol or other substances substantially influences future risk of abuse and dependence. Those individuals who first drank alcohol before age 15 years are four times more likely to become addicted to alcohol than someone who had their first drink after age 20. Nearly 70% of people who try an illicit drug before 13 years of age will become substance abusers over the next 7 years in comparison to just 27% who first try an illicit drug after 17 years of age.

CLINICAL MANIFESTATIONS

HISTORY

Symptoms of substance abuse vary greatly. Box 35-1 lists concerns or complaints that may be presenting symptoms of alcoholism or illicit drug use. Early diagnosis and treatment, before irreversible health problems or major psychosocial consequences arise, should be the goal of every family physician. Symptoms such as anxiety, depression, and insomnia may be related to alcohol use.

Inquiry into a patient's use of substances is best approached in a nonjudgmental, supportive manner. In teenagers, this can be assessed by asking whether their friends use alcohol or drugs, and if they personally have tried alcohol or illicit substances. A useful starting point for adults is the social history, looking for "red flags" such as marital or work problems, trauma, falls, blackouts, arrests, traffic tickets for driving under the influence (DUI), driving while intoxicated (DWI) or operating while intoxicated (OWI), and financial problems that may be related to purchase of drugs. It is important to elicit the substance of choice, frequency and pattern of use, and amount ingested. Patients are more likely to be deceptive about the amount they drink or how many drugs they use rather than how often they do so. The best quantitative data are obtained by asking about a specific time: "Tell me what you drank yesterday." Patients commonly use denial as a defense mechanism; it may therefore be necessary to interview family members to obtain accurate information.

When abuse is suspected, the Cut Down, Annoyed, Guilty, and Eye Opener (CAGE) Questionnaire (Box 35-2) is a useful tool. In the family practice setting, two "yes" answers have a sensitivity ranging from 70% to 85% and specificity ranging from 85% to 95%. Also useful is the Two-Item Conjoint Screen, which has nearly an 80% sensitivity and specificity. This involves asking two questions:

1. In the past year, have you ever had more to drink or used drugs more than you meant to?
2. Have you ever felt a need to cut down on your drinking or drug use?

Prior to prescribing opioids for acute or chronic pain, review the prescription drug monitoring program, obtain urine drug screening in selected individuals, and assess the risk of opioid abuse using a standardized questionnaire such as the Revised Screening and Opioid Assessment for Patients with Pain (SOAPP-R), Opioid Risk Tool (ORT), or the Current Opioid Misuse Measure (COMM). These tools have a sensitivity ranging from 77% to 83% and specificity ranging from 65% to 75%.

BOX 35-1. Alcohol and Substance-Related Symptoms

Psychosocial Complaints	Physical Complaints
Absenteeism from work	Blackouts
Antisocial behavior	Falls
Anxiety	Gastrointestinal problems
Child abuse	Gout
Depression	Headache
Domestic violence	History of trauma
Financial problems	Motor vehicle accident injuries
Interpersonal relationship problems	Muscle cramps
Irritability	Nasal congestion
Job-related problems	Nocturia
Legal problems	Palpitations or chest pains
School-related problems	Peripheral neuropathy
Suicidal ideation	Poor memory, recurrent infections, sleep disturbances, weight changes

BOX 35-2. CAGE Questions

Have you ever felt the need to *C*ut down on your drinking?
Are you *A*nnoyed by people criticizing your drinking?
Have you ever felt *G*uilty about your drinking?
Do you ever need a drink in the morning to steady your nerves or help a hangover? (*E*ye opener)

PHYSICAL EXAMINATION

The physical examination should be thorough and detailed. However, physical complications of substance abuse may not be evident early in the disease. High blood pressure may be a sign of withdrawal, chronic alcohol use, or cocaine abuse. Cirrhosis, ascites, edema, palmar erythema, testicular atrophy, rosacea, caput medusae, cardiomegaly, and peripheral neuropathy characterize end-stage alcoholism and are usually associated with heavy drinking for at least 10 years. Binge drinking can sometimes precipitate cardiac arrhythmias or the "holiday heart" syndrome. Nasal irritation, septal perforation, tachycardia, chest pain, and paranoia are associated with cocaine, whereas methamphetamine use is associated with poor dentition (meth mouth). Marijuana smoking can cause cough and dark-colored or bloody sputum. Dilated pupils are associated with stimulant abuse, whereas constricted pupils in combination with sedation and slurred speech suggest opioid use. Those going through opioid withdrawal have heighted autonomic activity and frequently have diarrhea, lacrimation, rhinorrhea, diaphoresis, abdominal cramps, nausea, vomiting, and piloerection.

DIFFERENTIAL DIAGNOSIS

The psychosocial and physical problems outlined in Boxes 35-1 and 35-3 also form the differential diagnosis for substance abuse. In evaluating patients presenting with these various complaints, consideration of underlying substance abuse is very important. Clinical and laboratory evidence of substance abuse may not be evident in early stages; hence, the diagnosis depends on a constellation of medical, social, and psychological clues. Substance abuse is often complicated by anxiety, depression, chronic pain, or marital distress, and these must be considered in evaluating the patient.

BOX 35-3. Alcohol-Related Health Problems

Cardiovascular
Hypertension
Cardiomyopathy
Arrhythmias

Endocrine
Testicular atrophy
Feminization
Amenorrhea

Gastrointestinal
Hepatitis
Cirrhosis
Esophagitis
Gastritis
Diarrhea
Pancreatitis
Gastrointestinal bleeding

Pregnancy
Low birth weight
Fetal alcohol syndrome

Hematopoietic System
Anemia
Thrombocytopenia

Neurologic System
Cognitive impairment
Dementia
Korsakoff psychosis
Wernicke encephalopathy
Peripheral neuropathy

Musculoskeletal
Cramps
Osteoporosis

Skin
Rosacea
Telangiectasia
Palmar erythema

DIAGNOSTIC EVALUATION

Although laboratory tests may not be diagnostic of substance abuse, they can be helpful. Most frequently urine drug screens and/or serum drug screens are performed in those with symptoms suspicious for substance use or withdrawal. Blood alcohol levels (BALs) confirm alcohol in the blood stream, and an elevated BAL without significant signs of intoxication suggests tolerance and chronic use. Liver enzyme abnormalities can provide objective evidence of problem drinking. Serum gamma glutamyl transferase (GGT) is the most sensitive indicator of alcohol-induced liver damage; however, it is not specific. Elevation of the liver enzyme aspartate aminotransferase (AST) to alanine aminotransferase (ALT) in a >2:1 ratio is typical of alcohol-related hepatitis. In cases of alcoholism, a CBC may reveal an elevated mean corpuscular volume (MCV) and/or anemia secondary to folate or B_{12} deficiency. Among alcohol-dependent patients, 30% exhibit signs of old rib fractures on radiographs compared to 1% of controls. Hyperlipidemia, thiamine deficiency, and elevated uric acid levels are also commonly seen.

TREATMENT

Primary interventions to quell alcohol and other substance use and their complications include greater enforcement of laws regarding substance abuse, decreased opioid prescribing, monitoring opioid use/abuse by using a prescription monitoring database, increasing the legal drinking age, hosting needle/syringe exchanges, and increasing alcohol taxes.

The goal of treatment is to reduce the consequences of the patient's substance abuse and prevent further abuse. A multifaceted team approach is usually best including participation from psychologists, psychiatrists, family medicine physicians, community health contacts, counselors, care managers, social workers, health educators, peer workers, recovery coaches, and most importantly families. For at-risk individuals or those with a short history of abusing alcohol, evidence suggests that even brief interactions may be of benefit. These may consist of short counseling sessions in which the physician educates the patient about the consequences of continued use and recommends quitting or cutting down. Setting specific goals and making a follow-up appointment to review the patient's progress are also important parts of such intervention. However, organizing a surprise intervention (Johnson intervention), as frequently seen on television, with multiple loved ones talking to the patient is not effective and is most often met with anger and resistance.

Self-help groups, such as Alcoholics Anonymous or Narcotics Anonymous, are a mainstay of treatment for patients willing to participate. Programs such as Al-Anon are also available for relatives and friends of individuals with substance abuse problems. Referral to an addiction specialist or outpatient treatment center is another treatment option. Examples include recovery coaches, recovery housing, intensive outpatient therapy, and step-down services following inpatient "residential" treatments. Counseling sessions may comprise individuals, groups, or families. Inpatient programs are usually reserved for those who fail outpatient therapy.

The treatment of alcohol withdrawal is aimed at reducing the patient's discomfort and preventing the progression of symptoms. Symptoms can range from minor manifestations such as tachycardia, elevated blood pressure, shakiness, and irritability to life-threatening problems such as seizures, delirium tremens (DTs), and coma. Normalization of vital signs and moderate sedation are two of the end points for managing withdrawal. During inpatient hospitalizations for alcohol or opioid withdrawal, patients are regularly assessed using the Clinical Institute Withdrawal Assessment for Alcohol (CIWA) and Clinical Opioid Withdrawal Scoring (COWS), respectively. Long-acting benzodiazepines (BZDs), such as diazepam or chlordiazepoxide, either given as a loading dose until the patient is sedated or using symptom-adjusted dosing, are effective for managing withdrawal. Short-acting BZDs, such as lorazepam, are preferred in patients with severe liver disease. Beta blockers, such as atenolol, can help reduce adrenergic symptoms and control blood pressure and tachycardia. Although beta blockers may reduce BZD requirements, they should not be used as monotherapy because they do not prevent seizures, hallucinations, or DTs. Clonidine, a central-acting antihypertensive medication, can also be used to help control blood pressure and withdrawal symptoms. Thiamine and magnesium deficiencies are common and associated with encephalopathy. Thiamine and magesium replacement should be given to all known alcohol-dependent patients and for those at risk for alcohol withdrawal.

Outpatient therapy is appropriate for patients with mild withdrawal symptoms and a supportive social structure. A family member should be available around the clock and always in control of medications. Inpatient care is needed for those with more severe symptoms, a history of severe withdrawal, or a poor social support network. Withdrawal from BZDs is best accomplished with a long-acting BZD or phenobarbital with scheduled dose reductions over a period of 8 to 12 weeks. Withdrawal of other sedative hypnotic drugs is usually managed using phenobarbital. Opiate overdose can be treated by nonmedical bystanders with a naloxone autoinjector, which is injected either intramuscularly or subcutaneously into the anterolateral thigh. A naloxone injector should be prescribed to patients who exceed 50 morphine milligram equivalents (MME) daily, have a history of overdose, or concomitantly use BZDs. Recently, nasal naloxone has become available as an alternative to the autoinjector. Opiate withdrawal can be treated with either propoxyphene or methadone. Clonidine and imodium are useful as adjunctive therapies. No drug is currently indicated for managing cocaine withdrawal, although tricyclic antidepressants, SSRIs, and dopamine agonists such as bromocriptine may reduce cravings.

Some patients seeking total abstinence from alcohol may request disulfiram. Disulfiram therapy sensitizes patients to alcohol and causes reactions such as flushing, palpitations, headache, nausea, and vomiting if alcohol is consumed. Naltrexone, an opioid antagonist, is also useful in alcohol abuse and can be given as a naltrexone depot intramuscular injection that is effective for 4 weeks. It appears to inhibit the pleasurable effects of alcohol and reduce cravings. Contraindications include opiate use and hepatocellular disease.

It is important to remember that alcoholics and addicts have a lifelong condition even if they are abstinent. In order to stay abstinent, many need to change jobs, create new social networks, and discover new hobbies. Approximately 15% of alcoholics relapse within 4 to 5 years. Therefore, the family physician should be cautious about prescribing narcotic- or stimulant-containing medications to these patients at any time during their medical care.

KEY POINTS

- The estimated prevalence of substance abuse disorders ranges from 10% to 20%, with an estimated 5% of the adult population using illicit substances.

- Liver enzyme abnormalities can provide objective evidence of problem drinking. Serum GGT is the most sensitive indicator of alcohol-induced liver damage; however, it is not specific.

- The goal of treatment is to reduce the consequences of the patient's substance abuse and prevent further substance abuse.

- Outpatient therapy is appropriate for patients with mild withdrawal symptoms and a supportive social structure. Inpatient care is needed for those with more severe symptoms, a history of severe withdrawal, or a poor social support network.

36 | Anemia

Anemia is defined as a hemoglobin value 2 standard deviations below the mean for gender, race, and age. In general, for adults, this is defined as hemoglobin <13.7 g/dL in males or 12.2 g/dL in females. In the United States, the most common cause of anemia in elderly individuals is anemia of chronic disease, whereas in females of reproductive age, the most common cause is iron deficiency. The most common cause of anemia worldwide is iron deficiency.

PATHOGENESIS

Anemia can result from blood loss, increased destruction of RBCs, or inadequate RBC production. Individuals with anemia may experience tissue hypoxia, which is detected by the oxygen-sensing cells in the area of the juxtaglomerular apparatus of the kidney. In response, the kidney secretes erythropoietin, the primary regulatory hormone for erythropoiesis. In chronic renal disease (GFR <60 mL/min), anemia may result from a decrease in renal production of erythropoietin. In anemia related to chronic illnesses, iron cannot be mobilized from its storage as ferritin impairing the incorporation of iron into hemoglobin, causing anemia. The three major disease categories associated with anemia of chronic disease are infection, malignancy, and inflammatory states such as connective tissue disorders. Malnutrition or drugs may also contribute to the pathogenesis of anemia of chronic disease.

For normal erythropoiesis, an adequate supply of iron is needed. Normally, the circulating RBC (erythrocyte) has a life span of $\sim$120 days, and most iron is supplied by recycling the iron from senescent red cells destroyed by the reticuloendothelial system. In a healthy, nonmenstruating adult, the daily loss of iron is minimal and only 1 to 2 mg of iron is required per day. Iron is primarily absorbed from the duodenum and transported to the bone marrow, where it is used to form hemoglobin. Excess iron is converted to ferritin and stored in the liver and bone marrow. When the stores of iron are inadequate due to blood loss or chronic dietary deficiency, normal hemoglobin synthesis is disrupted and a microcytic, hypochromic anemia results. Iron requirements differ based on age and sex. For example, a woman having periods needs more iron than a postmenopausal women and adolescents need more iron than adults over age 50.

Deficiencies in vitamin B_{12} (cobalamin) and folate impair deoxyribonucleic acid (DNA) synthesis. Although DNA synthesis is slowed, cytoplasmic development continues and there is more cytoplasm than normal, resulting in larger cells or a megaloblastic anemia. Folate deficiency generally results from inadequate dietary intake. In addition to inadequate intake, causes of B_{12} deficiency include malabsorption and lack of intrinsic factor (IF). In order for vitamin B_{12} to be absorbed, it must first bind with IF, which is secreted by the parietal cells of the stomach. Conditions such as gastric atrophy or gastrectomy can result in a vitamin B_{12} deficiency due to lack of IF. Because the cobalamin–IF complex is absorbed in the ileum, intestinal disease involving the terminal ileum, such as Crohn disease, may also lead to lack of absorption of the cobalamin–IF complex.

Genetic factors can cause abnormal hemoglobin synthesis. The normal hemoglobin molecule consists of two alpha chains and two beta chains. An abnormality in the synthesis of the alpha or beta chains can result in low hemoglobin or abnormal hemoglobin consisting of only alpha or beta chains. The abnormal hemoglobin may aggregate and form insoluble cytoplasmic inclusion bodies that damage the cells, leading to premature destruction of these cells by the spleen and liver.

CLINICAL MANIFESTATIONS

HISTORY

Anemia can lead to an inadequate supply of oxygen to the tissues, which may cause symptoms in vulnerable organ systems. For example, patients with heart disease may present with angina pectoris or decompensated CHF. However, many patients are asymptomatic until their hemoglobin level falls below 8 g/dL. General symptoms include dizziness and fatigue or weakness, either at rest or brought on by exertion.

The history should focus on potential sources of blood loss. The GI tract is the most common source of blood loss, and the presence of melena, hematochezia, or hematemesis indicates GI bleeding. Premenopausal women should be assessed for abnormal vaginal bleeding because this is a common cause of iron deficiency anemia in a young woman. In the elderly population, it is important to inquire about chronic illnesses such as hepatic, renal, inflammatory, neoplastic, and infectious diseases because these conditions are associated with anemia of chronic disease. A family history of anemia may point to an inherited cause, such as thalassemia. Alcohol consumption should be assessed because excess alcohol can suppress the bone marrow, cause chronic liver disease, and is associated with deficiencies of folate and other vitamins. If the patient reports a history of jaundice, pruritus, and a history of gallstones, hemolytic anemia should be suspected. Medications should be reviewed because chemotherapeutic drugs and other medications can suppress the bone marrow.

PHYSICAL EXAMINATION

Physical findings include pallor, tachycardia, and dyspnea. A systolic ejection murmur may be heard due to hyperdynamic circulation. Abdominal and rectal examinations can detect organomegaly and occult blood loss. Signs of iron deficiency include cheilosis (scaling at the corner of the mouth), koilonychia (spoon-shaped nails), and brittle nails.

Patients with B_{12} deficiency may have glossitis and neurologic deficits, such as abnormal reflexes, ataxia, Babinski sign, and poor position and vibration sense. These neurologic findings are not found with folate deficiency.

DIFFERENTIAL DIAGNOSIS

Anemias can be classified based on MCV into three categories: microcytic, macrocytic, or normocytic. **Microcytic anemia** is defined as an MCV below 80 fL, **macrocytic anemia** as an MCV > 100 fL, and **normocytic anemia** with MCV between 80 and 100 fL. The differential diagnosis varies by cell size. For example, the three major causes of microcytic anemia are iron deficiency, thalassemia, and anemia of chronic disease, whereas the most common causes of macrocytic anemia are B_{12} and folate deficiency.

Most iron deficiency is caused by GI or menstrual blood loss. Colon cancer is another common cause of iron deficiency anemia for adults, particularly over the age of 50 years. Iron deficiency due to nutritional deficiency is common in children, most commonly seen with excessive intake of cow milk. Anemia of chronic disease is associated with chronic infections, neoplastic diseases, renal disease, connective tissue disease, or endocrine disorders.

Macrocytic anemia from B_{12} and folate deficiency may be secondary to autoimmune disease, nutritional deficits, infections, gastrectomy, or ileal resection surgery. Since B_{12} is found only in foods of animal origin, vegetarians are at increased risk of developing B_{12} deficiency. The most common cause of B_{12} deficiency is **pernicious anemia**, an autoimmune disease in which the parietal cells that make IF are destroyed.

The most common cause of folate deficiency is decreased dietary intake. Alcoholics often present with folate deficiency. Drugs such as phenytoin, TMP/SMX, and sulfasalazine may also impair the absorption of folate.

Causes of normocytic anemia are many and include acute blood loss as well as the hemolytic anemias, which may be inherited or acquired. As many as 40% of patients with iron deficiency anemia have normocytic cells. A full review of the many causes of normocytic anemia is beyond the scope of this book.

DIAGNOSTIC EVALUATION

The classification of an anemia as microcytic, macrocytic, or normocytic helps direct the workup (see Table 36-1 and Fig. 36-1). In addition, a reticulocyte count is important to help differentiate between hemolytic anemias, blood loss, and bone marrow disorders. The reticulocyte count must be corrected for the level of anemia. (**Corrected reticulocyte count = Reticulocyte count × Patient Hematocrit (Hct)/Normal Hct.**) A corrected reticulocyte count of 2% or less suggests decreased RBC production and a hypoproliferative bone marrow. Follow-up tests should screen for renal, hepatic, and endocrine etiologies and may include examination of the bone marrow. A hypoproliferative state may also be seen in hematinic deficiencies such as low iron or B_{12}.

TABLE 36-1. Common Causes of Anemia Based on Cell Size

Microcytic (<80)

Iron deficiency
Thalassemia
Anemia of chronic disease
Sideroblastic anemia

Macrocytic (>100)

B_{12} deficiency
Folate deficiency
Excessive alcohol use
Severe hypothyroidism
Myelodysplastic syndromes

Normocytic

Anemia of chronic disease (can also be microcytic)
Aplastic anemia
Renal disease
Multiple myeloma
Myelophthisis (marrow infiltration that inhibits bone marrow function)

If the reticulocyte count is >3%, blood loss or hemolytic anemia should be suspected. A low haptoglobin, elevated lactate dehydrogenase, and an increase in unconjugated bilirubin can confirm hemolysis. A Coombs test helps distinguish between immune and nonimmune hemolysis.

The serum iron level should be checked in cases of microcytic anemia. A decreased serum iron level suggests either iron deficiency or anemia of chronic disease. In iron deficiency, the total iron-binding capacity (TIBC) is elevated and the percent saturation is low, whereas in anemia of chronic disease, the TIBC is low and the percent saturation is normal or increased. Ferritin level is also decreased in iron deficiency, but is elevated or normal in anemia of chronic disease. Typically, in anemia of chronic disease, the hemoglobin does not fall below 8 g/dL, the MCV is usually only mildly decreased, and the reticulocyte count is low and does not respond to iron therapy. Although rarely needed, bone marrow aspiration and staining for iron stores is the

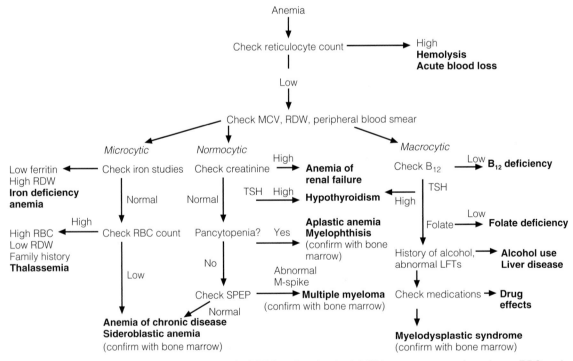

FIGURE 36-1. An approach to evaluation of anemia. LFT, liver function test; MCV, mean corpuscular volume; RBC, red blood cells; RDW, red cell distribution width; SPEP, serum protein electrophoresis; TSH, thyroid-stimulating hormone. (From Young VB, Kormos WA, Chick DA. *Blueprints: Medicine.* 6th ed. Philadelphia, PA: Wolters Kluwer; 2016.)

definitive test for iron deficiency. Other indications for a bone marrow include pancytopenia, anemias of underproduction that remain undiagnosed, macrocytic anemia of unknown etiology, and suspicion of bone marrow infiltration or malignancy. If serum iron is increased, a **sideroblastic anemia** should be suspected. Sideroblastic anemias are characterized by the presence of ringed sideroblasts that represent abnormal iron accumulation in the mitochondria. Sideroblastic anemias can be inherited, or from drugs such as isoniazid, alcohol use, pyridoxine deficiency, or lead poisoning. If the serum iron level is normal in a microcytic anemia and the cause remains uncertain, hemoglobin electrophoresis should be performed to evaluate the possibility of hemoglobinopathy, such as thalassemia, as the cause of anemia.

B_{12} and folate levels should be measured if there is macrocytic anemia. RBC folate levels are more accurate than serum folate levels. Another useful test to differentiate between B_{12} and folate deficiency is to measure the serum methylmalonic acid and homocysteine (HC) levels. Both methylmalonic acid and HC are elevated in B_{12} deficiency, whereas only HC is elevated in folate deficiency.

It is important to examine the peripheral blood smear. If sickle cells are found, a hemoglobin electrophoresis is required to rule out sickle cell anemia. Spherocytes suggest a hemolytic process causing the anemia. Basophilic stippling with microcytic anemia is seen in lead poisoning and thalassemia. In thalassemia, liver disease, and hemolysis, target cells are also found in the peripheral smear. Teardrop cells seen in myelofibrosis and abnormal types of circulating cells such as blast cells suggest a malignancy. Howell–Jolly bodies are common in post-splenectomy patients and sickle cell anemia. Hypersegmented neutrophils may indicate the presence of megaloblastic anemia.

TREATMENT

Management of anemia depends on an accurate diagnosis. Oral ferrous sulfate ($FeSO_4$) is the preferred form of iron therapy because it is soluble, inexpensive, and easily administered. The required amount of elemental iron is 150 to 200 mg/day, which can be achieved by taking 325 mg of $FeSO_4$ two to three times daily. Although foods such as milk or foods that raise the gastric pH can impair iron absorption, side effects such as nausea, constipation, and heartburn may require giving $FeSO_4$ with meals. Absorption can be increased if given with foods that lower the gastric pH, such as foods rich in vitamin C. Other iron preparations such as ferrous gluconate and ferrous fumarate may be better tolerated than $FeSO_4$ but are more expensive. Indications for parenteral iron therapy are an inability to tolerate oral therapy, malabsorption, inflammatory bowel disease, severe iron deficiency, and ongoing blood loss. Iron deficiency anemia responds to treatment within 7 to 10 days, evidenced by an elevated reticulocyte count. Hemoglobin levels should return to normal within 1 to 2 months unless there is continued blood loss, and iron supplements should be continued for 6 months or until ferritin $\geq$50 ng/L. Definitive therapy of iron deficiency anemia involves identifying and treating the underlying cause. Most men and women above 35 to 40 years of age or without a history of significant menstrual bleeding require an evaluation for GI bleeding.

Patients with renal failure or AIDS or those undergoing chemotherapy may benefit from recombinant erythropoietin. In thalassemia major, only symptomatic therapy is available, and patients may need multiple transfusions. Since this can lead to iron overdose, chelation therapy with deferoxamine may be required. Other therapies include splenectomy and bone marrow transplant.

For patients with B_{12} deficiency from IF deficiency, parenteral replacement of B_{12} or high-dose oral therapy is indicated. If folate deficiency is suspected, 1 mg/day of folate should be given, along with B_{12}. If both B_{12} and folate deficiencies are present, it is important to replace both, since folate replacement alone may improve the anemia while masking the B_{12} deficiency and allowing the neurologic symptoms of B_{12} deficiency to worsen. In normocytic anemias, the underlying process causing the anemia should be treated.

KEY POINTS

- Anemia can result from blood loss, increased destruction of RBCs, or inadequate RBC production.

- Anemia can result in an inadequate supply of oxygen to the tissues, causing symptoms in vulnerable organ systems. Most individuals do not experience symptoms unless their hemoglobin is below 8 g/dL or there is an acute drop in hemoglobin.

- The classification of anemia as microcytic, macrocytic, or normocytic helps direct the workup.

- The three major causes of microcytic anemia are iron deficiency, thalassemia, and anemia of chronic disease, whereas the most common causes of macrocytic anemia are B_{12} and folate deficiencies.

- In normocytic anemia, the reticulocyte count is the most important test because it helps to differentiate between hemolytic anemias, blood loss, and bone marrow disorders.

- Oral $FeSO_4$ is preferred for iron therapy, since it is soluble, inexpensive, and easily administered.

37 | Anxiety

Anxiety is the experience of dread, foreboding, or panic, accompanied by a variety of physical symptoms. The distress can be both physical and psychological. It is a very common complaint and accounts for $\sim$ 11% of all visits to a family physician. Anxiety disorders are a group of disorders that share anxiety as a major symptom. Box 37-1 lists brief descriptions for the different types of anxiety disorders. Anxiety may also be a symptom of other psychological diseases, intoxication or withdrawal, or a medical illness.

PATHOGENESIS

Anxiety is a normal response to many situations. Pathologic anxiety results when anxiety occurs in the absence of appropriate stimulus or is of excessive duration and intensity. Both behavioral and biologic theories exist for anxiety disorders. Biologic theories implicate the involvement of several different monoamine and neuropeptide neurotransmitters. The locus caeruleus, which is the main CNS nucleus responsible for distributing norepinephrine throughout the brain, exhibits increased activity and is implicated in the pathology of some anxiety disorders. The inhibitory neurotransmitter gamma aminobutyric acid may serve an anxiolytic function in the nervous system.

CLINICAL MANIFESTATIONS

HISTORY

The history is an essential element of the evaluation. Inquiring about stresses, fears, substance use, and precipitating factors is important. Psychological complaints include apprehension, agitation, poor concentration, feeling "on edge," difficulty sleeping,

and heightened arousal. Physical symptoms are usually related to increased autonomic activity. Typically, symptoms involve the cardiopulmonary system, GI system, urinary system, and neurologic system. Dyspnea, dizziness, palpitations, sweating, nausea, abdominal pain, diarrhea, frequent urination, sweaty palms, chronic headaches, and difficulty swallowing are common symptoms. Anxiety may also cause heightened motor tension, with trembling, twitching, muscle spasms, and easy fatigability.

PHYSICAL EXAMINATION

A physical examination helps detect medical illness that may present as anxiety. For example, an enlarged thyroid, abnormal lung examination, or irregular heart rhythm may suggest an underlying organic etiology.

DIFFERENTIAL DIAGNOSIS

In addition to anxiety disorders, similar symptoms can be seen in a wide variety of psychological and medical illnesses. Medications such as sympathomimetics (pseudoephedrine), antihistamines, bromocriptine, and bronchodilators as well as excessive caffeine may all cause anxiety-like symptoms. Neuroleptics (e.g., phenothiazines) may cause akathisia and anxiety, whereas some antidepressants (e.g., SSRIs) may cause anxiety-like reactions. Drug or alcohol withdrawal is an important differential consideration. Stimulant abuse (e.g., cocaine, amphetamines) can cause agitation, irritability, and anxiety. Other psychiatric disorders that may have anxiety as a prominent component include depression, manic-depressive disease, alcoholism, psychosis, and grief reaction. Medical illnesses may present with signs and symptoms of anxiety. Box 37-2 lists some of the conditions that may present as anxiety.

BOX 37-1. Glossary of Terms

Generalized Anxiety Disorder
Excessive or unrealistic worry about numerous issues for >6 months causing significant impairment in important areas of function. Symptoms occur more days than not and the individual is unable to control the worry. In addition to worry, symptoms include fatigue, poor concentration, irritability, increased muscle tension, and sleep disturbance
Lifetime prevalence: 5%
Typical age of onset: Early 20s but may begin anytime
Rx: SSRIs, venlafaxine, duloxetine, buspirone, BZDs, and behavioral therapy

Panic Disorder
Recurrent episodic periods of intense fear or apprehension accompanied by at least four somatic complaints: for example, diaphoresis, dyspnea, dizziness, or flushing, accompanied by behavior changes because of unrealistic and persistent worry. For a month following an attack, the patient continues to worry about future attacks that adversely affect his or her life and/or avoid similar situations.
Sudden onset, can peak within minutes and lasts from 5 to 30 minutes
Can occur with or without agoraphobia
More common in women
Lifetime prevalence: 2% to 3%, most cases begin before age 30
Rx: SSRIs, TCAs, behavioral training to desensitize patient.

Phobia
Persistent or irrational fear of a specific object, activity, or situation.
Occurs in 25% of the population at some time
More prevalent in women
Can be divided into category-specific subtype and one general type: animal type, natural environment type, blood-injection-injury type, situational type, and others
Social phobia is when an individual has an intense fear of being scrutinized in social or public situations such as public speaking.
Rx: Behavioral exposure therapy. Beta blockers or BZDs may be useful prior to exposures.

Obsessive–Compulsive Disorder
Intrusive, unwanted thoughts (obsession), and repetitive behaviors performed in a ritualistic manner to reduce the anxiety of the obsession (compulsion). The patient has insight to the behavior being excessive.
Rx: Behavioral therapy, SSRIs, clomipramine.

Acute Stress Disorder
Severe anxiety following a life-threatening event with symptoms lasting <1 month.
Rx: Depends on duration and intensity of symptoms.

Posttraumatic Stress Syndrome
Anxiety symptoms lasting at least 1 month, which develop after an individual experiences a distressing event outside the normal human response (e.g., combat, rape, natural catastrophe). There may be delayed onset and the patient may experience flashbacks.
Central etiologic factor is a traumatic event.
Rx: Group psychotherapy, SSRIs, beta blockers, and sometimes prazosin.

Adjustment Disorder with Anxious Mood
Anxious mood develops as a maladaptive response to an identifiable stressor with symptoms. This is a diagnosis of exclusion and does not meet any other psychiatric diagnosis.
Usually resolves within 6 months
Rx: Depends on severity of symptoms.

BOX 37-2. Medical Conditions That May Mimic Anxiety

Cardiopulmonary
Arrhythmias
Hypoxia
Ischemic heart disease
Mitral valve prolapse
Pulmonary edema
Pulmonary embolus
Asthma
Congestive heart failure

Neurologic Diseases
Encephalopathies
Temporal lobe epilepsy
Primary sleep disorders
Postconcussion syndrome

Endocrine
Hyperthyroidism
Pheochromocytoma
Hypoglycemia
Hypocalcemia
Hypercalcemia
Cushing disease
Carcinoid syndrome

Stimulant Toxicity
Withdrawal syndrome

Hematologic Disorders
Anemia

DIAGNOSTIC EVALUATION

The diagnostic goal is to assess the anxious patient for medical causes and psychiatric illnesses. The initial focus should be on any clinical conditions the patient may currently have and to review all his or her medications. Attention should be given to disorders such as hyperthyroidism, arrhythmia, and drug withdrawal syndromes that have anxiety as a prominent feature. Laboratory testing may not be necessary and should be directed by clinical findings. For example, pulmonary function testing may be indicated in patients with wheezing or a complete blood count in patients with pallor and dizziness. Validated screening tools can be useful in primary care offices to detect generalized anxiety disorder, panic disorders, social anxiety, and posttraumatic stress disorders (PTSDs). The GAD-7 is an example of a diagnostic and severity assessment tool for generalized anxiety disorder (Fig. 37-1). These screening tools assist in improving detection and treatment of anxiety disorders once thought to be uncommon in the primary care setting.

TREATMENT

Treatment strategies for anxiety include psychotherapeutic and pharmacologic interventions. Psychotherapy in the form of cognitive behavioral therapy can be as effective as medication for the treatment of generalized anxiety disorder. The family physician can provide supportive counseling consisting of empathetic listening, meaningful reassurance, education, guidance, and encouragement. Understanding that a patient may be unable to identify the cause of his or her anxiety coupled with an empathetic willingness to listen may help alleviate symptoms. Education begins with informing the patient of the diagnosis and discussing the underlying problems and potential treatment. Discussing the patient's fears of serious illness and of "going crazy" may have a cathartic effect.

An important element of treatment is assessing the degree of anxiety. Severely affected patients, atypical presentations, and poor response to treatment may merit referral to a psychiatrist or psychologist. Nonpharmacologic treatment that has been found beneficial includes psychotherapy, behavioral therapy, relaxation techniques, physical activity, reconditioning, and cognitive behavioral therapy. Cognitive behavioral therapy is the first line of therapy for the pediatric population with a diagnosis of anxiety. Group therapy is effective for patients with PTSD. These therapies are often augmented and enhanced by the use of anxiolytic agents. The goal of medication is to help the patient resume function and alleviate anxiety symptoms that interfere with the patient's life. Medications should generally be of limited duration and administered using a scheduled dose, rather than on an "as-needed" basis. Fixed goals should be set: for example, improved sleep or reduction in intrusive symptoms.

SSRIs are first-line therapeutic agents for anxiety disorders. They can benefit patients with panic disorder, GAD, PTSD, and obsessive-compulsive disorder (OCD). SSRIs may take a few weeks to become effective. BZDs may be prescribed concomitantly for a short term during crises and then

GAD-7

Over the <u>last 2 weeks</u>, how often have you been bothered by the following problems? *(Use "✓" to indicate your answer)*	Not at all	Several days	More than half the days	Nearly every day
1. Feeling nervous, anxious or on edge	0	1	2	3
2. Not being able to stop or control worrying	0	1	2	3
3. Worrying too much about different things	0	1	2	3
4. Trouble relaxing	0	1	2	3
5. Being so restless that it is hard to sit still	0	1	2	3
6. Becoming easily annoyed or irritable	0	1	2	3
7. Feeling afraid as if something awful might happen	0	1	2	3

For office coding: Total Score T____ = ____ + ____ + ____)

Developed by Drs. Robert L. Spitzer, Janet B.W. Williams, Kurt Kroenke and colleagues, with an educational grant from Pfizer Inc. No permission required to reproduce, translate, display or distribute.

FIGURE 37-1. GAD-7 screening tool scoring: 5-9, mild; 10 or greater, moderate to severe.

tapered as the SSRIs take effect. SSRIs should be continued for 12 months after symptoms improve before tapering to avoid relapses. Fluoxetine and sertraline are safer SSRIs for use in pregnancy and lactation. Paroxetine should be avoided in pregnancy due to risk of congenital heart defects. Buspirone and gabapentin are non-BZD medications that have mild anxiolytic effects. They are nonaddictive and have no withdrawal effects, thus making them good choices for patients at risk of abuse. Tricyclic antidepressants (TCAs) and monoamine oxidase inhibitors (MAOIs) are also effective but are not first-line treatment due to side effects. Duloxetine, venlafaxine, pregabalin, quetiapine, and antihistamines are also sometimes used as anxiolytics.

BZDs are primarily indicated for short-term relief during acute crises and are useful for treatment augmentation. Side effects include physical dependency, tolerance, sedation, respiratory depression, and suicidality. To avoid dependence especially in short-acting BZDs like alprazolam, physicians should prescribe a fixed amount and remain aware of signs of misuse, such as "lost" prescriptions. The patient should be seen regularly, and after symptoms are controlled, chronic therapy should be discontinued by tapering doses over several weeks. Abrupt cessation, especially in short-acting BZDs like alprazolam, can result in withdrawal symptoms or even seizures. Patients with increased risk for controlled substance abuse may be better served by prescribing an antihistamine such as hydroxyzine. BZDs are not appropriate for pregnancy because of risk of teratogenicity and neonatal withdrawal symptoms.

Beta blockers, such as propranolol, can blunt adrenergic symptoms such as palpitations, tremors, and tachycardia. They can help patients who suffer from anxiety-related cardiovascular symptoms, patients with panic attacks, and are useful for treating stage fright/phobias on an as-needed basis.

KEY POINTS

- Anxiety is the experience of dread, foreboding, or panic accompanied by a variety of body symptoms.

- Pathologic anxiety results when anxiety occurs in the absence of an appropriate stimulus or is of excessive duration and intensity that affects daily activities.

- Medications such as sympathomimetics (pseudoephedrine), levothyroxine, antihistamines, bromocriptine, and bronchodilators as well as excessive caffeine may cause anxiety-like symptoms.

- Treatment strategies for anxiety include psychotherapeutic and pharmacologic interventions.

- SSRIs are the first-line medications for multiple anxiety disorders.

38 | Asthma

Asthma is a chronic inflammatory disease of the airways triggered by exposure to airborne allergens, irritants, cold air, or exercise.

EPIDEMIOLOGY

Asthma affects 7% to 8% of the US population and is increasing in prevalence. Over 6 million children have asthma, which makes it the most common chronic disease of childhood. The greatest prevalence and mortality is among inner-city residents with death rates for asthma highest among African American youth between the ages of 15 and 24 years. Risk factors for mortality include a previous history of intubation, admission to an intensive care unit, two or more hospitalizations, or more than two emergency room visits in a single year. Other risk factors include the use of two canisters of short-acting beta$_2$ agonists in a single month, inability to perceive airway obstruction, and the use of systemic steroids.

Recognition of the importance of the underlying inflammatory process of asthma has made anti-inflammatory therapeutic agents the cornerstone of asthma management. Effective outpatient treatment of asthma can prevent exacerbations and reduce emergency room visits and hospitalizations.

PATHOGENESIS

The initial inflammatory event involves the degranulation of presensitized mast cells as a result of re-exposure to triggering agents and the release of inflammatory mediators (histamine, cytokines, leukotrienes, platelet activating factor, etc.), resulting in increased bronchiolar vascular permeability and edema, increased glandular and mucous secretions, and induction of bronchospasm. All this narrows the airway diameter and increases airway resistance, making it difficult to "breathe in" air and even more difficult to "breathe out" air. These events result in the **early-phase asthmatic response**, producing classic symptoms of wheezing, cough, and dyspnea. Degranulation of mast cells also stimulates alveolar macrophages, T-helper lymphocytes (Th2 cells), and bronchial epithelial cells to release chemotactic factors for the recruitment and activation of additional mediator-releasing leukocytes (eosinophils and neutrophils). The migration and activation of eosinophils and neutrophils occur 6 to 12 hours after the mast cell degranulation phase (acute-phase reaction) and constitute the **late-phase asthmatic response**, which if untreated can last up to 48 hours. During this phase, the release of mediators from eosinophils causes epithelial damage, hypersecretion of mucus, and hyperresponsiveness of bronchial smooth muscles, as well as further airway edema, bronchiolar constriction, and mast cell degranulation. Therefore, the recruited eosinophils amplify and sustain the initial inflammatory response without additional exposure to the triggering agent.

Over time, chronic inflammation can change the morphology of the bronchioles, resulting in an increase in the number of mucus-producing goblet cells at the epithelial surface, hypertrophy of submucosal mucous glands (more mucus production), thickening of the basement membrane (thus decreasing airway compliance), edema and inflammatory infiltrates in the bronchial walls with prominence of eosinophils, and hypertrophy of bronchial wall muscle. These changes in bronchiole morphology are referred to as **airway remodeling** and are signs of chronic, longstanding airway inflammation.

CLINICAL MANIFESTATIONS

HISTORY

Patients with asthma present with symptoms of wheezing, dyspnea, cough, and sputum production. In the classification of a patient's asthma, the asthma is described as being either intermittent or persistent. As outlined in Table 38-1, persistent asthma is further classified as mild, moderate, or severe. These classifications are important to determine therapy recommendations.

The frequency of symptoms and the presence of nocturnal symptoms are important elements of the history. In addition, identification of the triggers of the patient's asthma, his or her current symptoms, and previous attempts at treatment should be determined. Triggers include cold air, exercise, inhaled irritants (e.g., smoke), stress, NSAIDS, beta blockers, and inhaled allergens. The past medical history should cover the onset of the disease, prescribed and OTC medications, use of alternative medical therapies, history of allergies, past hospitalizations, and the use of steroids. A history of intubation for the treatment of asthma is a significant predictor of its severity and the need for aggressive therapy. The family history may be significant for atopy or asthma. Assessment of the home environment—including exposure to smoke, pets, and other irritants or potential triggers—is important to determine the proper treatment.

PHYSICAL EXAMINATION

Vital signs may reveal tachypnea and tachycardia during acute episodes. Fever suggests an underlying viral or bacterial illness as a trigger. The physical examination focuses on the lung examination and listening for the wheezing, rhonchi, and prolonged expiration characteristic of asthma. With severe exacerbations and limited air movement, the lung fields may be deceptively quiet. In severe cases, one can appreciate the difficulty with airway movement with physical examination findings such as nasal flaring, tracheal tugging, intercostal retractions and use of accessory muscles, and abdominal breathing.

DIFFERENTIAL DIAGNOSIS

In children, conditions that can also present with wheezing, cough, and increased sputum production include bronchiolitis, cystic fibrosis, croup,

TABLE 38-1. Asthma Classifications

Classification	Symptoms	Nighttime Symptoms	Lung Function
Intermittent	Symptoms ≤2 times per week	≤2 times per month	FEV_1 or PEF ≥ 80% predicted
	Brief exacerbations		PEF variability <20%
	Asymptomatic between attacks		
Persistent–mild	Symptoms >2 times per week but <1 time a day	>3–4 times per month	FEV_1 or PEF ≥80% predicted
	Attacks may affect activity		PEF variability 20%–30%
Persistent–moderate	Daily symptoms	>1 time a week but not nightly	FEV_1 or PEF 60%–80% predicted
	Daily use of beta$_2$ agonists		
	Attacks affect activity		PEF variability >30%
	Exacerbations may last for days		
Persistent–severe	Continual symptoms with use of beta$_2$ agonist multiple times in 1 day	Frequent; at times almost each night	FEV_1 or PEF ≤ 60% predicted
	Limited physical activity		
	Frequent attacks		PEF variability >30%

FEV_1, Forced expiratory volume in 1 second; PEF, peak expiratory flow.

epiglottitis, bronchitis, and foreign body aspiration. Bronchiolitis has many similarities to asthma but presents as an acute illness and is not a chronic disease. Cystic fibrosis is a chronic disease that initially may be confused with asthma, but patients also develop GI symptoms, growth disturbances, recurrent sinus infections, and pneumonia. Croup, epiglottitis, bronchitis, and foreign body aspiration are episodic and not chronic diseases. In adults, the primary diseases confused with asthma are COPD and CHF. In cases with chronic cough, GERD can be commonly confused for asthma as well. These diseases usually have their onset in adulthood. A CXR, ECG, spirometry, and other testing can help distinguish between CHF and pulmonary disease.

DIAGNOSTIC EVALUATION

The history and physical examination suggest the diagnosis. Reversal of the signs and symptoms by bronchodilators is also suggestive of asthma. In cases where the diagnosis is still uncertain, complete pulmonary function testing can also be obtained in individuals older than 5 years of age. A CXR is recommended during the initial evaluation of the wheezing patient if there is no improvement with a bronchodilator. It can detect pneumonia, a foreign body, CHF, or other nonasthmatic causes of wheezing. The CXR in the asthmatic patient may be normal or show hyperinflation due to air trapping. Peak flow testing helps to monitor patients with asthma. Airway obstruction exists when the peak flow is

<80% of the predicted value based on the patient's age, height, and gender. In patients with suspected allergic triggers, allergy testing may be helpful. For patients with suspected cystic fibrosis, sweat chloride testing is a useful screen.

TREATMENT

For appropriate management, asthma can be divided into four categories (see Table 38-1). The goals of asthma therapy are to prevent symptoms, maintain normal pulmonary function and activity level, prevent emergency room visits and hospitalizations, and minimize the adverse effects of medications.

Effective asthma treatment has four components:

1. Objectively assessing and monitoring lung function using a peak expiratory flow (PEF) meter: PEF monitoring is advocated for patients with moderate and severe persistent asthma. Patients first establish their personal best and are then asked to respond to PEF measurement on the basis of a "color zone" system. The green zone, defined as >80% of personal best PEF, indicates good control. The yellow zone, between 50% and 79% of personal best, indicates the need for prompt inhaled short-acting $beta_2$ agonists and contact with a physician about adjustments in current medication. The red zone, <50% of personal best, indicates immediate need for inhaled $beta_2$ agonists and emergency assessment by a physician (Fig. 38-1).

Green Zone	Yellow Zone	Red zone
No asthma symptoms. Able to do usual activities and sleep without coughing, wheezing, or breathing difficulty.	There may be coughing, wheezing, and mild shortness of breath. Sleep and usual activities may be disturbed. May be more tired than usual.	Symptoms may include frequent, severe cough, severe shortness of breath, wheezing, trouble talking while walking, and rapid breathing.
Action: Keep controlling/preventing your asthma symptoms. Continue to take your asthma medicine exactly as prescribed by your healthcare specialists, even if you have no symptoms and feel fine.	**Action:** Keep controlling your asthma symptoms and add your prescribed quick-relief medicine. Call to discuss the situation with your doctor or healthcare specialist.	**Action:** Go to an emergency room. **Peak flow:** <50% predicted
Peak flow: ≥80% predicted	**Peak flow:** 50%–79% predicted	

FIGURE 38-1. Patient instructions related to peak flow results. (From Anatomical Chart Company. *Understanding Asthma Anatomical Chart.* Alphen aan den Rijn, The Netherlands: Wolters Kluwer; 2005.)

2. Environmental control of asthma triggers to limit exacerbations: It is imperative that patients be made aware not only of the basic facts of their disease but also advised of triggers for their asthma (e.g., "respiratory infections," pollen, change of weather, tobacco smoke, animal dander, mold, dust), so that they can take appropriate environmental control measures to limit their exposures. Patients also require the influenza vaccine yearly.

3. Treatment for long-term management (Table 38-2).

4. Thorough and detailed patient education: This includes education about asthma, medications, proper use of inhalers and spacers, establishing a plan of action for episodes of exacerbation, and recognizing signs of airway obstruction.

Asthma medications are classified into **long-term control medications** (anti-inflammatories) **to prevent** exacerbations and symptoms and **quick-relief medications** (bronchodilators) **to treat** symptoms and exacerbations. All patients with persistent asthma need both types of medication.

Inhaled short-acting bronchodilators are useful for treating acute symptoms and are the only therapy needed by those with intermittent disease. Albuterol is the most commonly used beta$_2$ agonist and is generally administered as two puffs every 4 to 6 hours, as needed, to control acute symptoms. Side effects may include flushing, tremors, and tachycardia.

Inhaled corticosteroids are the most potent and effective anti-inflammatory agents used for the long-term treatment of persistent asthma. They prevent irreversible airway injury, improve lung function, and reduce asthma deaths. Most patients can be adequately maintained on twice-daily doses. Patients should be advised to gargle and rinse their mouths with water after using inhaled steroids in order to prevent oral candidiasis. As the severity of asthma increases, so must the strength of the inhaled corticosteroid. High-dose inhaled steroids used for severe asthma may interfere with the normal vertical growth of children. For this reason, oral leukotriene inhibitors, which have an additive effect when given in conjunction with inhaled steroids, can be added to low- or moderate-dose inhaled corticosteroids to reduce the need for high-dose steroids.

Cromolyn sodium is a mast cell stabilizer; it prevents mast cell degranulation in addition to inhibiting bronchoconstriction. It has a mild-to-moderate anti-inflammatory effect and is relatively safe to use in children and pregnant women with persistent, mild asthma. It is also effective against exercise-induced asthma in a single inhaled dose taken 15 to 30 minutes before exercise.

TABLE 38-2. Stepwise Approach to Asthma Management		
	Long-Term Control	**Quick Relief Medication**
Step 1		Short-acting inhaled beta$_2$ agonist
Step 2	**Preferred:** Low-dose inhaled corticosteroid **Alternative:** Cromolyn or nedocromil, leukotriene modifiers or theophylline	Short-acting inhaled beta$_2$ agonist
Step 3	**Preferred:** Low-dose inhaled corticosteroid plus long-acting beta$_2$ agonist OR medium-dose inhaled corticosteroid **Alternative:** Low-dose inhaled corticosteroid, plus leukotriene receptor agonist, theophylline, or zileuton	Short-acting inhaled beta$_2$ agonist
Step 4	**Preferred:** Medium-dose inhaled corticosteroid, plus long-acting inhaled beta$_2$ agonist **Alternative:** Medium-dose inhaled corticosteroid, plus leukotriene receptor agonist, theophylline, or zileuton	Short-acting inhaled beta$_2$ agonist
Step 5	**Preferred:** High-dose inhaled corticosteroid, plus long-acting beta$_2$ agonist AND consider omalizumab for patients with allergies	Short-acting inhaled beta$_2$ agonist
Step 6	**Preferred:** High-dose inhaled corticosteroid, plus long-acting beta$_2$ agonist, plus oral corticosteroid, AND consider omalizumab for patients with allergies	Short-acting inhaled beta$_2$ agonist

Salmeterol, a long-acting beta$_2$ agonist (LABA), is useful in the management of chronic nocturnal symptoms and exercise-induced asthma. It is more effective than cromolyn in the treatment of exercise-induced asthma because of its longer duration of action. Salmeterol used alone has been shown to increase risk of asthma-related death and increase risk of adolescent asthma-related hospitalization. Therefore, salmeterol should be used only in uncontrolled moderate persistent asthma in conjunction with inhaled corticosteroids. If there is a risk of nonadherence of the inhaled steroid, then a combined LABA with corticosteroid inhaler can be given. Studies have shown that salmeterol combined with low-dose steroids is more efficacious in improving symptoms and reducing the use of rescue medication than simply doubling the dose of inhaled steroids.

Oral (systemic) corticosteroids are recommended and effective as "burst" therapy for gaining initial control of asthma when therapy is being initiated or during an acute exacerbation. One method of administering burst therapy is to give prednisone (adults, 40 to 60 mg/day, children 1 to 2 mg/kg/day) for 3 to 10 days or until the PEF improves to 80% of personal best. Long-term use of oral steroids should be considered only for patients who are refractory to all other therapies because of their potential for causing side effects and growth retardation.

Anticholinergics for asthma include inhaled ipratropium (Atrovent), which inhibits vagally mediated bronchoconstriction and mucus production. It is effective when used in conjunction with a short-acting beta$_2$ agonist for the treatment of severe asthma exacerbations.

A monoclonal antibody (omalizumab) is available for treatment in cases of severe allergy. Its use is limited by its cost and safety concerns. It is generally prescribed in consultation with a specialist experienced in its use.

Nonadherence and poor asthma control are usually related to inadequate understanding of the disease and its treatment, improper use of inhaled medication, lack of environmental control of asthma triggers (e.g., outdoor allergens, tobacco smoke, animal dander, dust, cockroaches, molds), or poor continuity of care. Patient education remains the cornerstone of a successful asthma management strategy: increasing patient involvement, and fostering a strong partnership between patients, their families, and the physician. This relationship is imperative to help ensure not only the patient's adherence to the treatment regimen but also the continuous follow-up with his or her family physician.

KEY POINTS

- Asthma is a chronic inflammatory respiratory condition (type I hypersensitivity reaction).

- The symptoms of asthma include cough, wheezing, and dyspnea.

- The pathophysiology of asthma includes airway edema, increased mucus production, and bronchospasm.

- Asthma can be classified into intermittent, mild-persistent, moderate-persistent, and severe-persistent types.

- Short-term control includes short-acting inhaled bronchodilators (beta$_2$ agonists); long-term control includes inhaled corticosteroids.

- Intermittent asthma does not require daily medication; persistent asthma is controlled by inhaled corticosteroids as well as short-acting inhaled bronchodilators.

- Table 38-2 outlines a stepwise approach to the management of asthma. Patients should be reassessed after 2 to 6 weeks of step-up or step-down if any further changes are needed.

39 | Atopic Dermatitis

"Atopic dermatitis" (AD) is a clinical term describing one of the most common skin diseases and the most common form of eczematous dermatitis. The term "atopy" describes a genetic condition involving a personal or family history of hay fever, asthma, dry skin (xerosis), or eczema. AD is itchy, recurrent, symmetric, and commonly involves the skin in the flexural creases (e.g., popliteal and antecubital regions) in older children and extensor surfaces in children <2 years old. It begins early in life, followed by periods of remission and exacerbation, and usually resolves by age 30. The highest incidence is among children, with 65% of cases presenting within the first 12 months of life.

PATHOGENESIS

The precise pathogenesis of AD is unclear. Genetic factors, altered immune function, and abnormalities within the epidermis are thought to play a role in the development of AD. About 30% have mutations in the gene for filaggrin that plays a role in keeping the skin moisturized and provides some antimicrobial benefit. Individuals with AD appear to inherit cellular changes that lead to mast cell and basophil hyperactivity in association with IgE-mediated cross-linking and activation of these cells. With activation, histamine, leukotrienes, and other factors are released, leading to vascular leakage, which manifests as erythema, edema, and pruritus. During the late phase response and with chronic disease, inflammatory cells are present in the skin. These abnormalities in mast cell and basophil reactivity are not specific to the skin, and patients with AD frequently have other manifestations of atopic disease, such as asthma or allergic rhinitis.

CLINICAL MANIFESTATIONS

HISTORY

AD may present in slightly different patterns at different ages. The age of the patient and any history of skin disease help narrow the differential diagnosis. In addition, it is important to ask about family history of atopic disease and to get detailed information about potential triggers for the patient's AD. Infants may present around 3 months of age with inflammation occurring initially on the cheeks and later involving the forehead and extensor surfaces of arms and legs while sparing the diaper area (Fig. 39-1). AD will resolve in ∼ 50% of infants by 18 months of age and the rest will progress into childhood with this condition.

During childhood, there may be lichenification and inflammation of flexural areas, including the antecubital and popliteal fossae, neck, wrists, and

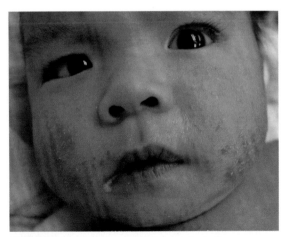

FIGURE 39-1. Atopic dermatitis in an infant. (From Dr. Barankin Dermatology Collection.)

ankles. Exudative lesions, which are more typical of the infant phase, are less common. Other areas—such as the hands, eyelids, and anogenital regions—are more commonly involved in adolescents and adults (Fig. 39-2).

AD tends to be cyclic, with remissions and exacerbations. Factors that cause dryness of the skin or increase the desire to scratch worsen and often trigger AD. These include excessive washing (especially with hot water), decreased humidity, occlusive clothing, sweating, contact with irritating substances (wool, cosmetics, some soaps, fabric softeners, household chemicals, etc.), contact allergy, and aeroallergens (dust mites, pollen, animal dander, molds, etc.). Stress and foods such as eggs, milk, seafood, nuts, wheat, or soy can also provoke exacerbations of AD.

PHYSICAL EXAMINATION

The location and nature of any skin lesion should be noted. During an acute eruption of AD, the skin may have papules and vesicles, with eventual crusting of the vesicles. Chronic skin lesions suggesting possible AD include scaling plaques and lichenification of the skin, particularly in the flexural creases. Dry skin and keratosis pilaris are other commonly associated skin findings. Signs of secondary bacterial infection should be noted, as the skin of patients with AD is more susceptible to infections with staphylococcal or streptococcal bacteria. The examination should also include a search for other manifestations of atopic disease, such as asthma, allergic rhinitis, and allergic conjunctivitis.

DIFFERENTIAL DIAGNOSIS

Eczema can also include diseases other than AD, such as dyshidrotic eczema and lichen simplex chronicus. Lesions in uncommon locations such as the axillary, gluteal and groin area should prompt consideration of a secondary cause such as psoriasis. The differential diagnosis for eczema includes other skin and systemic diseases, as outlined in Box 39-1.

DIAGNOSTIC EVALUATION

Atopic dermatitis can be clinically diagnosed by the presence of three essential criteria: personal or family history (first-degree relative) of atopy, pruritus, and the specific patterns of eruption, for example, on flexural surfaces in older children and cheeks, forehead and extensor surfaces in younger children.

AD is an itch that will erupt when scratched, leading to the phrase "the itch that rashes." The skin lesions generally do not appear before rubbing or scratching traumatizes the skin. Patients with AD often have abnormally dry skin and a lowered threshold for itching. The finding of papules, vesicles, and plaques located in the flexural creases supports the diagnosis of eczema. In addition, lichenification and dry, scaly skin should raise suspicion for eczema even in the absence of active lesions. Allergy testing should be considered in order to identify triggers of the patient's eczema, particularly in those who are refractory to therapy and with no triggers identified by history.

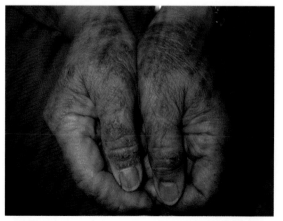

FIGURE 39-2. Atopic dermatitis affecting the hands in an adult. (From Dr. Barankin Dermatology Collection.)

BOX 39-1. Differential Diagnosis of Atopic Dermatitis

Hand dermatitis

Dyshidrotic eczema

Lichen simplex chronicus

Stasis dermatitis

Seborrheic dermatitis

Contact dermatitis

Psoriasis

Scabies

Fungal infections

Immunodeficiency diseases

TREATMENT

The goal of the therapy is to decrease inflammation, promptly treat secondary infections, and preserve and restore the stratum corneum barrier. In general, steroids are used to suppress the inflammation of acute flare-ups. Antibiotics are used to treat any secondary infection of the atopic lesions. The most common pathogen is *Staphylococcus aureus*. Trigger avoidance, emollients, and antihistamines are used in efforts to maintain the integrity of the skin.

During an acute exacerbation, weeping and vesiculated lesions may be dried with aluminum subacetate (Domeboro) compresses. Baths with an oatmeal-based emollient like Aveeno may help relieve itching. Antihistamines help control the pruritus. Sedating antihistamines are useful at night for those patients with sleep disturbances secondary to the pruritus.

Topical steroid ointments or creams are first-line agents for treating skin lesions. Emollients need to be used at least twice a day to help maintain skin hydration. Emollients work by sealing in moisture and are most effective when used after a shower or bath when the skin is well hydrated. Many physicians prefer ointments rather than creams in patients with AD because of their added moisturizing effects. Topical steroid treatment has been shown to be effective and safe for use in acute flare-ups for up

to 4 weeks, although in many cases the AD flare-up can be adequately treated in a shorter time. Important side effects of long-term daily use of topical steroids include skin atrophy, striae, telangiectasia, and worsening of acne conditions and all patients must be educated on these adverse reactions prior to implementing topical steroid treatment.

Chronically, trigger avoidance and keeping the skin moist are important aspects of treatment. Chemical irritants should be avoided. The hands should be protected from prolonged water exposure. Cotton clothing should be worn and non-soap cleansers that are labeled gentle or sensitive, such as Dove Sensitive or Basis Sensitive, are recommended. Bathing should be in warm but not hot water and daily moisturizers, ointments, oils, or petroleum jelly should be applied daily after bathing. After a shower, the skin should be dried by patting instead of rubbing. Scratching should be kept to a minimum through use of antihistamines and topical steroids. Other medications that have been used for treating AD include tars, oral steroids, and ultraviolet (UV) light. Patients do not usually tolerate topical tar medications because of their inconvenience and the staining associated with their use. Patients not controlled with topical steroids, antihistamines, use of emollients, and trigger avoidance merit referral to a dermatologist or allergist. The treatment of eczema is summarized in Table 39-1.

TABLE 39-1. Treatment of Atopic Dermatitis	
Topical	Topical steroids
	Topical immunomodulators as second-line treatment
	Tar preparations
	Moisturizers should be applied after showers and hand washing
	Lipid-free lotion cleansers
Antibiotics	Erythromycin (250 mg q.i.d.)
(suppress *Staphylococcus aureus*)	Dicloxacillin (250 mg q.i.d.)
	Cephalexin (250 mg q.i.d.) or
	Cefadroxil (500 mg bid)
Antihistamines	Hydroxyzine, Diphenhydramine
(sedation and controlling pruritus)	Topical doxepin is second line if other antihistamines fail due to risk of allergic contact dermatitis after application.
Severe cases	Oral prednisone
	Intramuscular triamcinolone
	Psoralen plus Type A ultraviolet light
	Tar plus Type B ultraviolet light
	High potency topical steroids

Nonsteroidal immunomodulators like tacrolimus (Protopic) and pimecrolimus (Elidel) are second-line treatment options for moderate-to-severe and mild-to-moderate eczema or in cases refractory to standard treatment. Tacrolimus is available in 0.1% and 0.03% ointments for adults and 0.03% ointments for children 2 years of age and above; pimecrolimus is available in 0.1% ointment for adults and children 2 years of age and above. Side effects include temporary stinging and burning on initial application, which eventually abate as the skin heals, and adverse effects in the sun with UV exposure. Of note, there has been controversy over whether or not these agents induce local or distant malignancy. The FDA mandated label revisions that include that it is a second-line treatment, along with patient and enhanced warnings. These ointments are used for short treatment periods and are contraindicated in children <2 years of age, in breastfeeding women, and women who plan to become pregnant.

People with AD, regardless of severity, should not receive the smallpox vaccination or be exposed to those who have newly received the smallpox vaccination as the live virus can cause severe and even life-threatening reactions in those with eczema. Exposure includes touching the inoculation site before it has healed and transmission of the live virus through towels, clothing, or bandages worn by the person vaccinated. The transmission period may last from 3 weeks to 1 month.

KEY POINTS

- The highest incidence of AD is among children, with 60% of cases presenting within the first 12 months of life.

- Lichenification and inflammation of flexural areas (antecubital/popliteal fossae, neck, wrists, and ankles) are common findings in AD.

- The mainstays of therapy are steroids, trigger avoidance, emollients, and antihistamines.

40 | Chronic Obstructive Pulmonary Disease

Obstructive lung diseases include asthma, cystic fibrosis, bronchiectasis, and COPD. "COPD" is a collective term used to describe emphysema, chronic bronchitis, or both and is characterized by an airflow limitation that is not fully reversible. Chronic bronchitis is defined as a productive cough that occurs for at least 3 months a year for >2 consecutive years. Emphysema is defined as an abnormal dilatation of the terminal airspaces with destruction of alveolar septa. Thus, chronic bronchitis is defined clinically whereas emphysema is defined pathologically. It is estimated that 16 million Americans are diagnosed with COPD and an equal number have the disease but are yet undiagnosed. Deaths from COPD are on the rise and it is now the third leading cause of death in the United States. Cigarette smoking is the most common cause of COPD, accounting for up to 90% of these cases. Occupational exposures and air pollution also contribute to the burden of disease.

PATHOGENESIS

The pathogenesis of COPD is not completely understood, but it is thought to result from chronic inflammation. Smoking and other inhaled irritants may promote an inflammatory response in the airways, resulting in mucosal edema, increased mucus production, and reactive airways characteristic of chronic bronchitis. Bronchospasm causes airway narrowing, which—along with impaired ciliary function—results in difficulty clearing secretions, air trapping, and alterations in gas exchange. Host susceptibility also plays a role and explains why only 20 to 30% of smokers develop COPD.

Similar changes may occur in patients with emphysema; however, the inflammatory response predominantly affects the smaller airways, leading to tissue destruction and loss of the normal elastic recoil of the lung. This results in increased dead space and air trapping creating functionless areas of lung tissue where there is minimal to no air exchange.

There is considerable overlap between these two categories of COPD and although in some individuals one presentation predominates, patients usually have features of both chronic bronchitis and emphysema. In addition to cough and increased mucus production, changes that occur because of COPD include decreased blood oxygen and decreased clearance of carbon dioxide from the blood. This results in lower oxygen delivery to the various organs and can lead to compromised organ function. For example, decreased oxygen delivery to the lung tissue increases pulmonary artery blood pressure, which can lead to right-sided heart failure or cor pulmonale.

CLINICAL MANIFESTATIONS

HISTORY

Early in the course of the disease, COPD patients will have minimal or no symptoms. Often a productive chronic cough is the first symptom, followed by shortness of breath with exertion as the disease progresses. Ultimately, the cough may become disabling and patients may develop dyspnea in the recumbent position, requiring them to sleep in the upright position.

Other important historic factors include smoking history, defined in pack-years (packs per day times number of years smoking), personal or family history of respiratory disorders, and exposure to secondhand smoke or environmental irritants. An assessment of the patient's limitations in activities may help assess the severity of his or her disease prior to pulmonary function testing.

PHYSICAL EXAMINATION

The patient with COPD may appear overweight and cyanotic, as typified by the "blue bloater" associated with chronic bronchitis. Alternatively, he or she may appear thin and barrel-chested, typical of the "pink puffer" associated with emphysema. The use of accessory muscles of respiration should be noted. On percussion, hyperresonance associated with air trapping may be present and auscultation may reveal diminished peripheral breath sounds due to limited air movement. Many patients with chronic bronchitis or those with an acute exacerbation of chronic bronchitis have rhonchi or wheezing. Skin examination can reveal the presence of cyanosis as well as clubbing of digits (Fig. 40-1). Heart sounds may be more distant due to the altered chest configuration and increased air between the chest wall and the heart. In addition, the presence of rhonchi and wheezing may obscure the heart sounds. With cor pulmonale and right-sided heart failure, other symptoms and signs such as peripheral edema, jugular venous distention, and hepatojugular reflux may be present.

DIFFERENTIAL DIAGNOSIS

Respiratory symptoms and cough may have several different etiologies. In addition to COPD, other diseases such as upper respiratory infections, bronchitis, or pneumonia may cause shortness of breath and cough. Allergies, asthma, and cystic fibrosis are chronic conditions that typically present in childhood and may include increased cough, mucus production, shortness of breath, and wheezing. Patients with decompensated CHF commonly have shortness of breath and on examination may have wheezing, rales, and peripheral edema.

Alpha$_1$ antitrypsin deficiency should be considered in patients below 45 years of age presenting with features of COPD, particularly in the absence of smoking. Up to 10% of these patients will also have serious liver disease and may have findings consistent with hepatitis or cirrhosis.

DIAGNOSTIC EVALUATION

Evaluation of a patient suspected of having COPD should include a detailed history and physical examination, which will provide the diagnosis in most cases. Other tests that may be performed to confirm the diagnosis and exclude other diseases include pulmonary function testing and a CXR. In patients with a diagnosis of COPD, arterial blood gases, pulse oximetry, and an ECG may be helpful to assess disease severity and detect cor pulmonale.

Chest radiographs are not diagnostic of COPD, and findings in patients with COPD may vary depending on the predominant component (bronchitis or emphysema). The classic findings in patients with chronic bronchitis are increased lung markings, termed a "dirty-chest" appearance. In patients with predominant emphysema, there are decreased lung markings, hyperlucency of the lung fields, and flattening of the diaphragms, all consistent with the hyperinflation of the lungs found in emphysema. In advanced COPD, the ECG may show evidence of right atrial enlargement, right ventricular hypertrophy, and right axis deviation.

Pulmonary function testing measures air exchange and lung volumes. With COPD, there is difficulty and delay in the movement of air out of the lungs, resulting in prolonged expiration on both physical examination and pulmonary function testing. In addition, because of the air trapping that occurs from incomplete emptying of the lungs, residual volumes are increased. The forced expiratory volume in 1 second (FEV_1) is a measure of the volume of air exhaled in 1 second following maximal inhalation. The FEV_1 is the most accurate and reproducible measure of outflow obstruction. It is significantly decreased in patients with COPD and is the primary measure used to assess disease severity. The FEV_1 relative to the forced vital capacity (FVC) is a ratio that defines obstructive lung disease. An $FEV_1/FVC < 0.7$ establishes airflow obstruction and a post bronchodilator response of $<12\%$ that is considered irreversible establishes

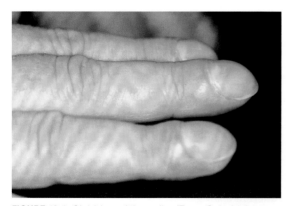

FIGURE 40-1. Clubbing of the nails. (From Schalock PC, Hsu JTS, Arndt KA. *Lippincott's Primary Care Dermatology*. Philadelphia, PA: Wolters Kluwer; 2010.)

the diagnosis of COPD. The FEV_1 correlates with patient symptoms and disease severity and is the best predictor of survival. Patients with mild disease will have minimal limitations in activities and an FEV_1 80% or more of their predicted FEV_1 (based on age, gender, height, and weight). Patients with moderate disease are limited in their activities because of the COPD; they have FEV_1 measures of 50% to 80% of their predicted FEV_1. Patients with severe disease are increasingly limited in activity; their FEV_1 is between 30% and 50% of their predicted level. Patients with very severe disease often have symptoms at rest and have an $FEV_1 < 30\%$ of predicted level. In patients with severe and very severe disease, arterial blood gases, pulse oximetry, or ECGs may help in management of the disease and are important to identify patients who might benefit from supplemental oxygen.

TREATMENT

Preventing disease progression through early identification and aggressive smoking cessation programs should be the primary goal in treating patients with COPD. Pulmonary function testing can follow decreases in lung function and the accelerated decline in lung function associated with smoking helps motivate patients to stop smoking. With smoking cessation, lung function will show a modest improvement initially and then follows the normal age-related decline, as with nonsmokers.

For patients with established COPD, goals of therapy are improvement in lung function, avoiding or reducing hospitalizations, early treatment or prevention of acute exacerbations, and minimizing disability to improve quality of life. Smoking cessation and oxygen therapy for hypoxic individuals (e.g., <88% saturation or <55 mmHg) are the only therapies that improve survival. Other long-term benefits of oxygen supplementation include decreases in polycythemia, pulmonary artery pressure, dyspnea, hypoxemia during sleep, and nocturnal arrhythmia events. For effective long-term oxygen therapy, patients should use oxygen for at least 15 hours/day with maximum effect seen at 20 or more hours of use. Pulmonary rehabilitation does not actually improve pulmonary function testing but may enhance physical endurance and thus overall function. Preventive medicine is extremely important and patients should receive the pneumococcal vaccines and annual influenza vaccinations.

Other mainstay treatments include bronchodilators, steroids, and antibiotics. Figure 40-2 outlines steps used in the treatment. Bronchodilators, in the form of anticholinergics (e.g., ipratropium), which cause bronchodilation through inhibition of vagal stimulation, or $beta_2$ agonists (e.g., albuterol) are used to treat acute exacerbations of COPD and can be used in patients who have daily symptoms. When used together, anticholinergics and $beta_2$ agonists have a synergistic effect. For patients with daily symptoms, a long-acting $beta_2$ agonist, such as salmeterol, is available for twice-daily use. Short-acting bronchodilators can then be used for breakthrough symptoms. Theophylline also has a bronchodilatory effect and may improve diaphragmatic function. Serum levels must be monitored, since nausea, palpitations, and seizures can result from toxic levels.

Oral steroids are used to treat acute exacerbations of COPD in a 2-week tapering dose. Long-term use of oral steroids has the potential for significant side effects and their use is not well defined. Inhaled corticosteroids may be helpful in limiting inflammation, improving airway reactivity, and reducing the frequency of COPD exacerbations. However, like oral steroids, they have not been shown to affect survival and their role in COPD is not clearly defined. Still, inhaled corticosteroids are a treatment option but should be used in conjunction with long-acting $beta_2$ agonists.

Antibiotics are useful for treating acute exacerbations of COPD, particularly in those patients with an increase in dyspnea, cough, and mucus production. Antibiotics commonly used include tetracyclines, sulfonamides, penicillins (e.g., amoxicillin with or without clavulanic acid), fluoroquinolones, macrolides, and cephalosporins. Antibiotics should provide coverage for the most common organisms associated with COPD exacerbations, namely *Streptococcus pneumoniae, Haemophilus influenzae*, and *Moraxella catarrhalis*. Patients with severe disease often need supplemental oxygen. Candidates for oxygen supplementation are those with a PO_2 of <55, pulse oximetry <88%, or with cor pulmonale and signs of heart failure. The use of continuous positive airway pressure (CPAP), either daily or at night, can improve functional status, oxygenation, and arterial blood gases. The use of CPAP is generally reserved for those patients with COPD who are hypercapneic. For patients with cor pulmonale and right-sided heart failure, treatment of the heart failure and the use of diuretics may be beneficial.

CHRONIC OBSTRUCTIVE PULMONARY DISEASE (COPD), DIAGNOSIS AND TREATMENT

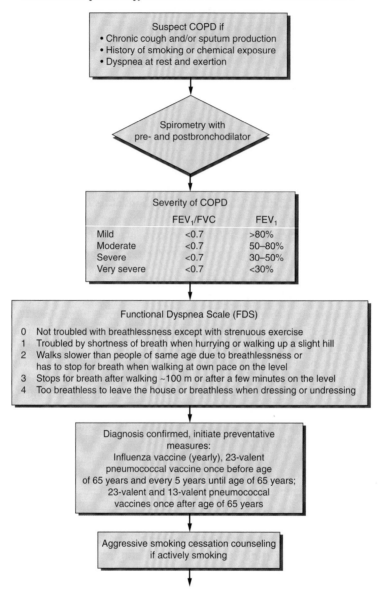

FIGURE 40-2. Diagnosis and treatment algorithm for chronic obstructive pulmonary disease. (From Domino FJ, Baldor RA, Golding J, et al. *5-Minute Clinical Consult 2018*. 26th ed. Alphen aan den Rijn, The Netherlands: Wolters Kluwer; 2017.)

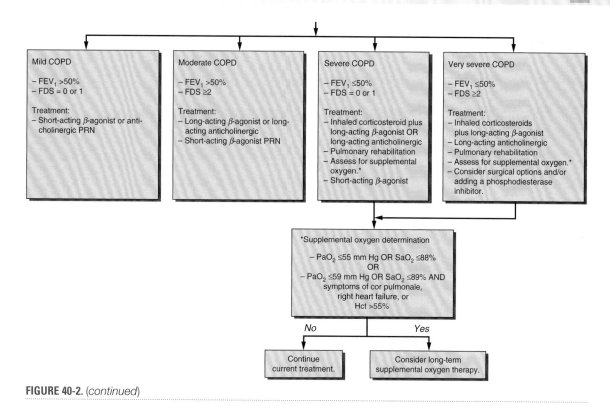

FIGURE 40-2. (continued)

KEY POINTS

- COPD is related to smoking in over 90% of cases.
- Pulmonary function testing (FEV_1) can help assess disease severity.
- Smoking cessation is an important aspect of therapy for COPD.
- Bronchodilators, steroids, antibiotics, and oxygen are the mainstays of therapy.

41 | Congestive Heart Failure

CHF affects an estimated 5 million Americans and is the most frequent cause of hospitalization in the elderly. One percent of adults aged 50 to 60 years and 10% of those in their 80's are affected by it. The overall 5-year mortality is 60% for men and 45% for women. The three major risk factors for heart failure are hypertension, CAD, and valvular heart disease.

PATHOGENESIS

Heart failure occurs if the heart is unable to perfuse body tissues adequately. Cardiac output depends on three factors: preload, contractility, and afterload. **Preload** (also referred to as the left ventricular end diastolic pressure) is the pressure required to distend the ventricle at a given volume. The relationship of pressure and volume defines compliance. **Contractility** describes the functional state of the myocardial muscle. Normally, as preload increases, the cardiac output and the amount of blood pumped by the heart muscle increase. **Afterload** is the resistance against which the heart contracts and is clinically reflected by the systolic blood pressure.

Heart failure begins with symptoms that occur only during periods of stress, as during illness or exercise; but as the disease progresses, symptoms may occur with rest. Heart failure may be due to either systolic or diastolic dysfunction. Systolic dysfunction is characterized by decreased contractility of the left ventricle, resulting in a reduced ejection fraction. A decreased ejection fraction leads to a compensatory increase in preload to maintain cardiac output. Eventually, there is a limit to which increases in preload can compensate and pulmonary congestion occurs, resulting in signs and symptoms such as orthopnea, paroxysmal nocturnal dyspnea (PND), rales, jugular venous distention (JVD), and edema. Systolic congestive heart failure is present when the ejection fraction is <40%.

Decreases in cardiac output trigger a host of compensatory mechanisms, including activation of the renin-angiotensin-aldosterone system, increased levels of catecholamines, and the secretion of atrial natriuretic hormone. These compensatory mechanisms result in systemic vasoconstriction, fluid retention, and increased afterload, which further inhibits cardiac output, thus creating a vicious feedback cycle. Late changes effected by these compensatory mechanisms include myocardial and vascular remodeling and fibrosis.

About 40% of patients have diastolic dysfunction. Diastolic dysfunction results from an inability of the ventricle to relax properly, which leads to a higher filling pressure, pulmonary congestion, and decreased cardiac return. Changes that occur with aging predispose elderly individuals to developing diastolic dysfunction. Other causes include ischemia, hypertension, ventricular hypertrophy, volume overload, and pericardial disease. It is also common for patients with systolic dysfunction to have some element of diastolic dysfunction.

CLINICAL MANIFESTATIONS

HISTORY

Symptoms of CHF include dyspnea, orthopnea, PND, nocturia, edema, weight gain, fatigue, chest pain, abdominal pain, anorexia, and mental status changes (Box 41-1). While taking the patient's history, it is useful to determine what activities make the patient short of breath, since classification of severity of disease is based on whether the patient is asymptomatic, has dyspnea with exertion, or has dyspnea at rest. The need to sleep on more than one pillow suggests orthopnea. Chest pain, palpitations,

BOX 41-1. Initial Assessment Questions to Determine Severity of CHF

Dyspnea, orthopnea, PND
Recent weight increase, edema, ascites
Chest pain or palpitations
Causes of anemia (blood loss, etc.)
Recent signs and/or symptoms of recent illness
Exercise tolerance
Claudication
Fatigue
Dietary changes (increased salt intake, eating a balanced diet)
Social history: Smoking history, alcohol and/or illicit drug abuse

and excessive salt intake are additional important historic factors associated with heart failure. Previous and current medical conditions and risk factors for CAD should be thoroughly reviewed.

PHYSICAL EXAMINATION

Checking general appearance and vital signs is important in order to determine whether the patient has an arrhythmia, is hypertensive or hypotensive, or is in respiratory distress (Box 41-2). Examination of the neck may reveal JVD, a sign of elevated filling pressures. The point of maximal impulse (PMI) of the left ventricle is often displaced laterally and downward in individuals with cardiomegaly. Auscultation

BOX 41-2. Physical Examination Findings

Vital signs: Increase of weight from documented baseline
General: Diaphoresis
Skin: Skin changes (pallor, cyanosis, jaundice)
Neck: Elevated jugular venous pressure, hepatojugular reflex
Cardiovascular: Tachycardia, bradycardia, arrhythmias, S_3, S_4 heart sounds, murmur, lateral displacement of PMI, diminished peripheral pulses
Respiratory: Labored breathing with use of assessory muscles, rales above the lower 25% of the lung that do not clear after cough
Abdomen: Hepatomegaly, tender liver, or ascites
Extremities: Edema in lower extremities without evidence of venous insufficiency

of the lungs may reveal bibasilar rales. When rales are present, measurement of the lung field level at which they are heard (e.g., a quarter of the way up from the base bilaterally) is a useful way of following treatment. Cardiac auscultation may reveal third and fourth heart sounds, which are often present in patients who are fluid-overloaded and/or who have a stiff ventricle. Murmurs may indicate valvular pathology as the cause of heart failure. Abdominal examination often reveals hepatomegaly, which is a sign of right-sided heart failure and indicates moderate-to-severe venous congestion. Lower extremity edema is a common finding; if this is of long duration, it is often accompanied by stasis dermatitis. Quantifying the degree of edema is useful for following the treatment.

DIFFERENTIAL DIAGNOSIS

The differential diagnosis depends on the presenting symptom. For patients complaining of dyspnea, the major differential is pulmonary diseases such as COPD, interstitial lung disease, pulmonary infections, and pulmonary embolus. Dyspnea may also be a sign of anemia.

For patients with fluid retention and edema, the differential diagnosis includes hypoalbuminemic states, cirrhosis, nephrotic syndrome, and chronic venous stasis. In the elderly, some common signs of heart failure may be misleading. For example, many patients have edema from chronic venous insufficiency and may not have heart failure. In these patients, the examination and constellation of symptoms combined with diagnostic testing are needed to establish the presence or absence of heart failure.

DIAGNOSTIC EVALUATION

The goals of the diagnostic evaluation are to determine the underlying reason for heart failure and to search for causes of acute decompensation. Box 41-3 lists some causes of heart failure.

The CXR remains an excellent, readily available test for identifying heart failure. Characteristic findings include cardiomegaly, redistribution of vascular markings, prominent interstitial markings, Kerley B lines, and perihilar haziness. In more advanced cases, pleural effusions may be identified. The CXR may also identify pulmonary disease, which may be causing or contributing to symptoms. An ECG is useful for

BOX 41-3. Causes of Heart Failure

Myocardial Damage
Ischemia/Infarction
Infections: Bacterial, viral, and parasites
Hypertensive cardiomyopathy
Valvular heart disease
Dilated cardiomyopathy
Toxins (e.g., alcohol, adriamycin, cocaine, radiation)

Diastolic Dysfunction
Infiltrative heart disease (e.g., amyloid, sarcoid)
Ischemia
Hypertensive cardiomyopathy
Congenital heart disease, including metabolic disorders (e.g., glycogen storage disease)
Constrictive pericarditis

Extracardiac
Anemia
Renal failure
Thyroid disease
Connective tissue disease

BOX 41-4. Causes of Cardiac Decompensation

Myocardial ischemia	Myocardial infarction
Arrhythmia	Anemia
Acute valvular disease	Superimposed medical illness
Pneumonia	Pulmonary embolus
Uncontrolled hypertension	Dietary indiscretion
Fever	Emotional stress
Excess exertion	

detecting an arrhythmia or for providing evidence of ischemic disease, left ventricular hypertrophy (LVH), or left atrial enlargement.

Virtually all patients with heart failure should have an echocardiogram. It can determine whether the mechanism of heart failure is primarily systolic or diastolic dysfunction. In patients with systolic dysfunction, the ejection fraction is reduced (<40%), whereas in diastolic dysfunction the ejection fraction is preserved or even high. Doppler US techniques help confirm diastolic dysfunction by identifying abnormal flow across the mitral valve. Echocardiogram can also detect LVH, valvular disease, pericardial disease, and wall motion abnormalities suggestive of ischemia.

Blood work should include a CBC, UA, electrolytes including liver function tests (LFTs), BUN, creatinine, albumin, PT/INR, and TSH. In patients with acute symptoms, cardiac markers are useful for detecting acute myocardial damage. Brain natriuretic peptide (BNP) helps distinguish between pulmonary disease and heart failure as the cause for dyspnea. A normal value virtually eliminates CHF as the cause. The BNP is elevated in CHF and can be used along with clinical assessment to monitor disease status. Elevated BNP values can also be caused by noncardiac disease, such as renal insufficiency.

Depending on the patient's initial clinical evaluation, other tests may be useful. For example, an exercise or pharmacologic stress echocardiogram test helps detect ischemic heart disease.

Common causes of cardiac decompensation are listed in Box 41-4 and should be considered in patients with previously stable heart failure. CAD, atrial fibrillation, valvular disease, alcohol abuse, thyroid disease, and hypertension are examples of potentially treatable causes of heart failure.

TREATMENT

The goals of management are to reduce symptoms, prevent complications, slow or reverse deterioration in myocardial function, and improve survival. All patients should follow a no-added-sodium diet (<2 to 3 g of sodium daily), stop smoking, limit alcohol, monitor their daily weight, and stay as active as possible. Box 41-5 outlines the goals of heart failure therapy. **Diuretics** are a mainstay of therapy for systolic dysfunction and for acute pulmonary congestion in patients with diastolic dysfunction. Diuretic therapy helps control symptoms but does not extend life. Loop diuretics are introduced first for fluid control in patients with overt CHF with the goal of reducing symptoms such as dyspnea and edema. Single larger doses of loop diuretics are more effective than smaller divided doses. Symptom improvement can be seen in hours to days, whereas other agents may show benefits weeks to months after initiation. Hypokalemia is a common side effect and requires treatment if the potassium level is below 4.0 meq/L. Close monitoring of BUN and creatinine as well as daily weights is important, as an increase in either may indicate the need to adjust diuretic therapy. Once symptoms are controlled, the

BOX 41-5. Treatment Principles of Heart Failure

Identify and correct reversible causes
Identify and correct causes for decompensation
Determine if heart failure is primarily systolic or
diastolic
Use vasodilators in patients with systolic
dysfunction
Initiate low sodium diet to control fluid retention
Cautious use of beta blockers in systolic
dysfunction to minimize the risk of cardiac
decompensation
Control heart rate in diastolic dysfunction
Digoxin in patients with systolic dysfunction
who remain symptomatic despite vasodilators/
diuretics

diuretic dose may be reduced or discontinued with close monitoring for evidence of fluid production.

ACE inhibitors slow the progression of heart failure, decrease the number of hospitalizations, and decrease mortality in patients with left ventricular systolic dysfunction (LVSD). ACE inhibitors are generally started prior to beta blockers because they provide rapid hemodynamic benefit. Patients should start on a low dose of an ACE inhibitor (e.g., 6.25 mg of captopril twice daily, 2.5 to 5 mg of lisinopril daily) to reduce the risk of hypotension and azotemia while reducing concurrent diuretic therapy. Common side effects include hypotension, hyperkalemia, dehydration, and cough. Patients with preexisting renal artery stenosis may experience renal impairment with an ACE inhibitor. Deterioration of renal function ($>30\%$) should result in either a dose reduction or discontinuation of the medication. If a patient cannot tolerate an ACE inhibitor, an angiotensin receptor blocker (ARB) or the combination of hydralazine and nitrates are alternative therapies.

Randomized trials demonstrate a decrease in mortality and sudden death in patients with heart failure who are treated with **beta blockers**. These should be added after ACE inhibitors and diuretics in patients with stable heart failure because they have delayed hemodynamic benefits. Beta blockers are also helpful in heart failure secondary to ischemia, diastolic dysfunction, and atrial arrhythmia. When adding beta blockers to heart failure therapy, start with a low dose (e.g., 3.25 mg/day of carvedilol or 12.5 to 25 mg/day of metoprolol) and titrate slowly upward to achieve a resting heart rate of 50 to 60 beats/minute, as some patients are more sensitive to the effects of beta blockers. Long-term benefits of left ventricular ejection fraction (LVEF) improvements and survival are dose dependent and are maximized by titrating doses base until the heart rate is <60. Patients should be monitored closely for fluid retention and clinical deterioration. Relative contraindications to beta blocker use are listed in Box 41-6. Diuretic doses may have to be adjusted upward if fluid retention occurs.

Spironolactone, a mild diuretic that blocks the effects of aldosterone, also lowers the risk of hospitalization and sudden cardiac death from heart failure. Spironolactone is indicated for patients with symptoms at rest who are already being treated with ACE inhibitors, beta blockers, and loop diuretics. Important side effects include renal and electrolyte abnormalities, especially hyperkalemia. The risk of hyperkalemia is especially high in patients on an ACE inhibitor and spironolactone; however, spironolactone and other aldosterone antagonists may be used to assist in managing diuretic-induced hypokalemia in those patients classified as having mild-to-moderate CHF.

Digoxin is useful in individuals with systolic dysfunction and moderate-to-severe heart failure whose symptoms, such as fatigue, dyspnea, and exercise intolerance, are uncontrolled with an ACE inhibitor and diuretics. Digoxin therapy reduces hospitalizations but not mortality from CHF. Digoxin is not useful in patients with diastolic dysfunction or those with acutely decompensated heart failure.

Exercise training is another ancillary approach to improve symptoms and clinical status in patients with reduced LVEF and CHF. Exercise training, also known as cardiac rehabilitation, has been shown to improve symptoms, increase exercise capacity, reduce hospitalizations, and improve quality of life along with survival in those with CHF. Exercise training should be used in conjunction with medications

BOX 41-6. Relative Contraindications for Beta Blocker Use in CHF

Heart rate <60 beats/minute
Symptomatic hypotension
Signs of peripheral hypoperfusion
PR interval >0.24 seconds
Second- or third-degree AV block
History of asthma or lung disease
Peripheral artery disease with resting limb ischemia

and is indicated in patients with mild-to-moderate CHF. There is no reported data to recommend this adjuvant therapy in those with advanced heart failure.

Treatment goals for diastolic dysfunction are prevention of LVH and control of symptoms by reducing end-diastolic pressure without reducing cardiac output. Rate control and the maintenance of sinus rhythm are essential. Slowing of the heart rate allows more time for ventricular filling during diastole. Diuretics are indicated for volume overload and for correcting precipitating factors such as hypertension. If calcium channel blockers are used for diastolic failure, they should be in the nondihydropyridine class, such as verapamil and diltiazem. The dihydropyridine (e.g., nifedipine) class causes a reflex tachycardia that decreases filling time.

KEY POINTS

- One percent of adults aged 50 to 60 years and 10% of those in their 80s are affected by CHF.

- Systolic dysfunction is characterized by decreased contractility of the left ventricle, resulting in a reduced ejection fraction.

- About 40% of patients with CHF have diastolic dysfunction. Diastolic dysfunction results from the ventricle's inability to relax properly, which leads to a higher filling pressure, pulmonary congestion, and decreased cardiac return.

- Characteristic CXR findings in CHF include cardiomegaly, redistribution of vascular markings, prominent interstitial markings, Kerley B lines, and perihilar haziness.

- The goals of management are reduction of symptoms, prevention of complications, and improvement of survival.

- ACE inhibitors slow the progression of heart failure, decrease the number of hospitalizations, and decrease mortality in patients with LVSD; they are recommended in patients with LVSD.

- Randomized trials demonstrate a decrease in mortality and sudden death in patients with heart failure who are treated with beta blockers.

42 | Depression

Feeling blue or sad is an appropriate response to a difficult situation. Clinical depression occurs if the reaction is more severe or prolonged than expected. Major depression is a mood disorder characterized by at least 2 weeks of depressed mood, a loss of interest or pleasure in usual activities, and a feeling of hopelessness associated with other findings such as sleep disturbances and loss of energy. It is a chronic debilitating disease with an overall prevalence of 4.7% in men and 8.5% in women and a lifetime incidence of 16%. It often accompanies chronic medical illnesses and substance abuse and is a major risk factor for stroke and death from coronary artery disease.

A less severe form of depression is dysthymia or persistent depressive disorder. It lasts at least 2 years and is described by some as a depressive type of personality. Symptoms of dysthymia are not as severe and there are fewer neurovegetative symptoms compared to major depression. Symptoms persist too long to be considered an adjustment reaction. Most patients with depression seek help from a family physician rather than a psychiatrist, making it important that the family physician feels comfortable managing this illness. Dysthymia and major depression can coexist when a major depressive episode occurs in a dysthymic individual. Despite the prevalence of depression, the diagnosis is missed in up to 50% of family practice patients and even when diagnosed is often undertreated. Table 42-1 lists the indications for screening for depression in adults, children, and adolescents.

TABLE 42-1. Depression: Indications for Screening

Adults	Children and Adolescents
First-degree biologic relative with history of depression	Antisocial behavior
Two or more chronic diseases	Diminished school performance
Obesity	Withdrawal from friends or social activities
Chronic pain (e.g., backache, headache)	Excessive weight gain or loss
Impoverished home environment	Substance abuse, such as alcohol or illicit drugs
Financial strain	Aggression
Experiencing major life changes	Agitation or irritability
Pregnant or postpartum	
Socially isolated	
Multiple vague or somatic symptoms (e.g., gastrointestinal, cardiovascular, neurologic)	
Fatigue or sleep disturbance	
Substance abuse, such as alcohol or street drugs	
Loss of interest in sexual activity	
Old age	

Source: Adapted with permission from Sharp LK, Lipsky MS. Screening for depression across the lifespan: a review of measures for use in primary care settings. *Am Fam Physician*. 2002;66(6):1001–1008. Copyright © 2002 American Academy of Family Physicians. All Rights Reserved.

PATHOGENESIS

Most theories explaining depression emphasize a biologic model. Depression is thought to be related to dysregulation of the brain's neurotransmitters. Although an imbalance in neurotransmitters provides an explanation for symptoms, it is still unclear why the imbalance develops. Research suggests that genetic factors and/or early childhood experiences play a role and that some individuals appear to be predisposed to developing depression in response to stressors. Potential stressors include medical illness, stressful life events, unresolved losses, poor support systems, and changes affecting lifestyle, such as divorce or financial loss. The process by which environmental factors interact with biologic factors to cause depression is still poorly understood.

CLINICAL MANIFESTATIONS

HISTORY

Depression can cause a wide range of psychological and somatic complaints. Box 42-1 lists a summary of the criteria used for diagnosing depression. The average age of onset of depression is from 20 to 40 years, although it can first present at any age. Identifiable stressors often play a role in the first episode of depression but may play a limited role or have no role in subsequent episodes. Concern expressed by a family member or friend about tearfulness, withdrawn behavior, or depressed mood should prompt the physician to ask questions about depression. The patient's past medical history should be reviewed because illnesses such as stroke, epilepsy, cardiovascular disease, chronic fatigue syndrome, dementia, diabetes, cancer, rheumatoid arthritis, and HIV are frequently associated with depression. A family history of depression significantly increases the risk of depression. A careful review of medications is indicated because some medications can precipitate depression. Box 42-2 lists medications associated with depressive symptoms as a side effect.

Many patients with depression first seek treatment for physical symptoms, and depression should be considered in patients with somatic complaints such as headache, backache, fatigue, chronic abdominal or pelvic pain, sleep disorders, sexual dysfunction, and a generalized positive review of systems. A good rule of thumb is consider a psychogenic cause whenever several somatic complaints are present.

Eliciting the patient's social history, particularly regarding alcohol and other substance use, is important. Some individuals presenting with depression have a coexisting mood disorder, so it is important to ask about episodes of mania. The severity of depression may be assessed by asking about suicidal thoughts and psychotic symptoms. Risk factors for suicide include social isolation (e.g., divorced, widowed, living alone), substance use, elderly male, persons with terminal or chronic illnesses, and those who have developed a specific plan. Although women attempt suicide more often, men succeed more often.

PHYSICAL EXAMINATION

A physical examination helps screen for medical disorders. Assessing mental status and appearance, mood, affect, speech, thought content, perceptual disturbances, and cognition is important. Psychomotor retardation, poor eye contact, tearfulness, poor grooming, somber affect, and impaired memory are characteristics of depression.

BOX 42-1. Diagnostic Criteria for Major Depression

The diagnosis requires 2 weeks of a depressed mood and/or disinterest/loss of pleasure with an impairment of function accompanied by four of the following:
Weight changes
Sleep disturbance
Loss of energy
Feelings of worthlessness or guilt
Poor concentration
Psychomotor retardation or agitation
Thoughts of death
Recurrent suicidal ideations

BOX 42-2. Common Medications Associated with Depression

Alpha methyldopa
Amphetamine withdrawal
Beta blockers
Digitalis
Cimetidine
Clonidine
Indomethacin
Isotretinoin
Levodopa
Oral contraceptives
Phenothiazines
Reserpine
Steroids

DIFFERENTIAL DIAGNOSIS

Several conditions besides depression can cause a depressed mood. An adjustment disorder with a depressed mood occurs when an identifiable stressor causes more symptoms than expected but does not last >6 months. Grief reactions may also present with symptoms mimicking depression; however, in grief reactions symptoms begin to improve after a few months. An anxiety disorder can mimic depression but is not usually accompanied by depressive symptoms such as changes in weight and fatigue. Anxiety disorder is dominated by feelings of apprehension, whereas depression is dominated by sadness and hopelessness. Bipolar disorder or substance abuse may also present with symptoms similar to those of depression. In addition to psychological diseases, certain medications (see Box 42-2) and medical illnesses such as chronic infections (e.g., HIV, TB), endocrine disorders (e.g., hypothyroidism, hyperthyroidism, Cushing disease, and Addison disease), connective tissue diseases, neurologic disorders, and cancers are associated with depression.

DIAGNOSTIC EVALUATION

The clinical interview is the most effective means of diagnosing depression. Techniques for screening include a two-question approach asking about anhedonia: "Over the last 2 weeks have you felt little interest or pleasure in doing things?" Or about a depressed mood, "Over the last 2 weeks, have you felt down, depressed, or hopeless?" Laboratory testing such as a CBC, basic chemistries, UA, STI panel, HIV testing, and vitamins B_{12} and D levels may be helpful in ruling out a medical disorder. A baseline ECG should be performed in patients with a history of cardiac disease or those who are over age 40 if tricyclic antidepressants are going to be prescribed. Neuroimaging and an electroencephalogram (EEG) should be considered for patients with new onset psychotic depression.

TREATMENT

Common treatments include **supportive counseling** and **pharmacotherapy**. Examples of supportive counseling include providing education, empathizing with the patient, challenging a patient's exaggerated negative or self-critical thoughts and encouraging him or her to be more active and schedule enjoyable activities. Sometimes encouraging patients to break their problems down into smaller components is helpful. Often a willingness to explore issues is therapeutic, although the physician should not be expected to address and solve all problems. Patients with family or marital issues may benefit from therapy. Patients with persistent symptoms or major depression should be treated pharmacologically.

The different classes of antidepressant medications are equally effective although responses from individual patients differ. SSRIs are a common first choice in medication due to their effectiveness and safety profile. However, choice of medication will depend on the patient's symptoms, current medications, and side-effect profile. If the patient has insomnia, a more sedating medication such as amitriptyline, trazodone, or mirtazapine is a good choice. If somnolence or a lack of energy is a problem, a more energizing antidepressant such as desvenlafaxine (Pristiq), duloxetine (Cymbalta), or bupropion (Wellbutrin) might be helpful.

Although some of the SSRIs may be energizing, about 15% of patients experience sedation as a side effect. Although TCAs have been available for years, they have many unpleasant side effects. Their anticholinergic properties can precipitate an attack of acute angle glaucoma or bladder outlet obstruction. They can also cause constipation, dry mouth, orthostatic hypotension, tachycardia, cardiac arrhythmias, tremor, and weight gain. SSRIs appear to be safe in patients with cardiac disease and cause less orthostatic hypotension in elderly patients. Common side effects include GI disturbances, headache, agitation, insomnia, sexual dysfunction, tremor, and somnolence. Trazodone has minimal anticholinergic side effects, but is very sedating, and on rare occasion causes priapism in males. Venlafaxine (Effexor) combines SSRI properties with noradrenergic effects. It is often used for refractory depression, but its side-effect profile limits its use as a first-line agent. MAOIs are effective but less commonly used because of their potential for drug and food interactions.

About 60% of patients will respond to a given antidepressant, and 80% will respond to a second alternative or added antidepressant medication. Patients should be assessed for therapeutic response and adverse effects of their medication within the first 2 weeks; however, therapy should be continued for 6 to 8 weeks before evaluating for effectiveness or changing the medication. The greatest risk of increased suicidal thoughts and behaviors is in the first to second month of treatment, and close follow-up is recommended to identify these risks early.

For severe cases of major depression, some patients may require multiple medications to achieve a therapeutic response to treatment, though consulting a psychiatrist is generally recommended for those patients requiring this level of treatment.

For a first episode of depression, antidepressants should be continued for 4 to 9 months after symptoms improve. Following a major depressive episode, about 50% of the patients relapse; the highest risk for recurrence is within the first few months of tapering an antidepressant. Patients suffering relapses should promptly be restarted on medications. The risk of relapse increases with each progressive episode, and patients who relapse should be considered for long-term therapy. Patients who fail to respond to therapy, abuse substances, are suicidal, have accompanying psychosis, or show symptoms of mania should be referred to a psychiatrist.

KEY POINTS

- Major depression is a mood disorder characterized by at least 2 weeks of depressed mood, a loss of interest or pleasure in usual activities, and a feeling of hopelessness associated with other findings such as sleep disturbances and loss of energy.

- Major depression is a chronic debilitating disease with a lifetime prevalence of 4.7% in men and 8.5% in women.

- Despite the prevalence of depression, the diagnosis is missed in up to 50% of patients in the primary care setting and, even when diagnosed, is often undertreated.

- Conditions such as stroke, myocardial infarction, pregnancy, chronic fatigue syndrome, dementia, diabetes, cancer, rheumatoid arthritis, and HIV are frequently associated with depression.

- The different classes of antidepressant medications are equally effective. The choice of medication depends on the patient's symptoms, current medications, and side-effect profile.

43 | Diabetes Mellitus Type 2

Diabetes mellitus is the most common endocrine problem encountered in family medicine. Diabetes is a group of heterogeneous metabolic disorders characterized by the abnormal metabolism of glucose with defects in insulin secretion, insulin action, or both. Diabetes is divided into type 1 diabetes (T1DM), characterized by little or no insulin production, and type 2 diabetes (T2DM) caused by insulin resistance and over time a progressive insulin secretory defect.

EPIDEMIOLOGY

Diabetes mellitus affects about 9% of the population. T2DM accounts for approximately 90% to 95% of individuals with diabetes. Of the approximately 29 million patients with T2DM, many have few symptoms and about 8.1 million remain undiagnosed. Previously, T2DM was primarily a disease of the middle aged and elderly; however, there is an increased incidence in young adults and children because of the obesity epidemic seen in the United States (Fig. 43-1).

PATHOGENESIS

T1DM is believed to be an autoimmune disorder with the production of autoimmune antibodies that destroy pancreatic islet cells. The disease typically develops during childhood, possibly triggered by a viral infection. Type 1 patients are vulnerable to ketoacidosis and always require exogenous insulin. In T2DM, the pancreas produces insulin but cells are resistant to its action. However, since insulin is produced, T2DM patients do not generally develop ketoacidosis.

Early in T2DM, insulin levels may be elevated as the pancreas attempts to compensate for insulin resistance. Eventually the beta cell can no longer compensate for the insulin resistance and hyperglycemia occurs. Insulin resistance is usually caused by obesity or increased percentage of body fat. T2DM also affects lipid metabolism and patients with T2DM frequently have low levels of high-density lipoprotein (HDL), moderately elevated total cholesterol levels, and high triglycerides. T2DM occurs more commonly in African Americans, Hispanics, and American Indians. Other risk factors include having a first-degree relative with diabetes mellitus, obesity—especially central obesity—and a sedentary lifestyle.

Gestational diabetes mellitus (GDM) affects 1% to 2% of pregnancies, usually during the third trimester. Blood sugars typically return to normal after delivery, but over time as many as 30% of women with GDM develop diabetes mellitus.

Acute complications of diabetes include ketoacidosis, hyperglycemic hyperosmolar state (HHS), and hypoglycemic reactions related to treatment. HHS is a syndrome characterized by severe fluid deficits induced by hyperglycemic diuresis.

Most of the morbidity and mortality associated with diabetes mellitus results from its long-term complications. These can be divided into microvascular and macrovascular complications. Microvascular complications include retinopathy, neuropathy, and nephropathy. Macrovascular complications are related to premature atherosclerosis, which affects the cardiovascular, cerebrovascular, and peripheral vascular systems. MI is the primary cause of the excess morbidity seen in diabetic individuals. Foot problems including ulcers, deformities, and infections can also manifest from neurologic and microvascular complications.

CLINICAL MANIFESTATIONS

HISTORY

Patients with T1DM usually present abruptly, often with ketoacidosis caused by an acute stress such as an infection. Other common initial symptoms

Obesity (BMI 30 kg/m^2)

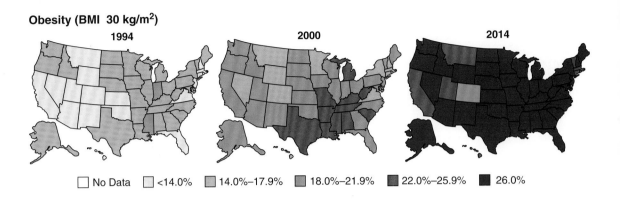

☐ No Data   ☐ <14.0%   ◼ 14.0%–17.9%   ◼ 18.0%–21.9%   ◼ 22.0%–25.9%   ◼ 26.0%

Diabetes

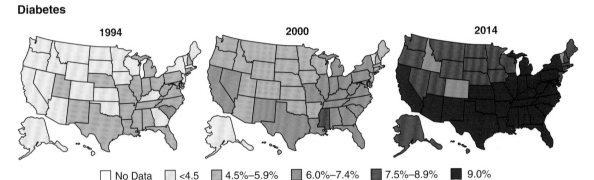

☐ No Data   ☐ <4.5   ◼ 4.5%–5.9%   ◼ 6.0%–7.4%   ◼ 7.5%–8.9%   ◼ 9.0%

FIGURE 43-1. Age-adjusted prevalence of obesity and diagnosed diabetes among US adults. BMI, body mass index. (From CDC: Division of Diabetes Translation. United States Surveillance System available at https://www.cdc.gov/diabetes/statistics/slides/maps_diabetesobesity_trends.pdf).

are nausea, abdominal pain, polyuria, polydipsia, polyphagia, and weight loss.

T2DM presents more gradually. Classic symptoms include polyuria, polydipsia, and polyphagia. However, patients more commonly present with fatigue, blurred vision, recurrent infections, or with symptoms related to complications such as a burning sensation in the feet due to a painful neuropathy. Many patients are asymptomatic and are first diagnosed by elevated blood glucose. The history should also identify risk factors for cardiovascular disease and inquiring about symptoms such as chest pain or claudication, which may indicate macrovascular disease. A medication history is indicated since drug-induced diabetes may occur with high doses of thiazide diuretics, corticosteroids, niacin, phenytoin, and atypical antipsychotics.

PHYSICAL EXAMINATION

The physical examination should include a review of vital signs and an assessment of height, weight, and body mass index (BMI). Obesity (BMI > 30 kg/m^2)

and hypertension are common in T2DM. Skin findings associated with T2DM include acanthosis nigricans and skin tags. A funduscopic eye examination may show evidence of diabetic retinopathy, such as exudates, hemorrhages, and microaneurysms. Cardiovascular and peripheral vascular examinations listening for carotid bruit and assessing peripheral pulses, respectively, are important. A foot examination looking for ulceration, deformities, and skin infection should be performed. Neurologic examination can detect signs of neuropathy such as sensory loss.

DIFFERENTIAL DIAGNOSIS

Transient hyperglycemia may result from stresses such as an infection or a heart attack that subsequently resolves when the inciting event is under control. Elevated blood sugars may also be related to pancreatic disease from pancreatitis, pancreatic cancer, pancreatic resection, and hemochromatosis (from iron overload damaging the pancreas), which is often referred to as "bronze diabetes." Excess secretion of counter regulatory hormones seen in endocrinopathies such as Cushing disease, pheochromocytoma, and acromegaly may also cause hyperglycemia.

DIAGNOSTIC EVALUATION

The American Diabetes Association (ADA) recommends that all patients over age 45 be screened with a fasting blood sugar every 3 years; those with risk factors should be screened earlier (see Box 43-1 for risk factors). The diagnosis of diabetes mellitus can be established by one of four criteria: (1) HbA_{1C} or glycosylated hemoglobin level $\geq$6.5%; (2) fasting blood glucose $>$ 126 mg/dL; (3) random blood glucose $>$ 200 mg/dL with polyuria, polydipsia, and polyphagia; and (4) a 2-hour postprandial glucose $>$ 200 mg/dL. Normally about 4% to 6% of hemoglobin is glycosylated. The percentage of glycosylated hemoglobin rises with the average level of blood glucose. Because the average lifespan of a red blood cell is 120 days, the HbA_{1C} reflects the average glucose levels over the past 2 to 3 months (Box 43-2). HbA_{1C} testing may not be accurate if the patient is pregnant, anemic, has a hemoglobinopathy, has had recent blood loss or transfusion, or is on erythropoietin therapy.

BOX 43-1. Risk Factors for Diabetes Mellitus Type 2

Family history of type 2 diabetes mellitus
Age
BMI $>$ 25 kg/m^2
Low HDL cholesterol ($<$35 mg/dL) and/or high triglycerides ($>$250 mg/dL)
Blood pressure $>$ 140/90 mmHg
History of gestational diabetes or birth of macrosomic baby (birth weight $>$ 9 lb)
Previous impaired fasting glucose with fasting plasma glucose 110–125 mg/dL
Previous impaired glucose tolerance with oral glucose tolerance test 2-hour glucose value 140–199 mg/dL
Clinical condition associated with insulin resistance such as polycystic ovarian syndrome (PCOS) or acanthosis nigricans
Habit of physical inactivity
Vascular disease
Ethnic groups at increased risk of T2DM: African Americans, Native Americans, Hispanic Americans, Asian Americans, and Pacific Islanders

BOX 43-2. Correlation Between Average Glucose Values and Hemoglobin A1c

Hemoglobin A1c	Average Glucose Reading (approx., mg/dL)
6%	120
7%	150
8%	180
9%	210
10%	240

In addition to establishing the diagnosis of diabetes, the initial evaluation should aim at evaluating risk factors and detecting diabetic complications. Routine laboratory testing should include a fasting lipid profile, glycosylated hemoglobin, electrolytes, BUN, and creatinine. Screening for coronary artery disease in asymptomatic patients with T2DM is not recommended because it has not been shown to improve clinical outcomes if cardiovascular disease risk factors are treated. For patients over 30 years of age or those with diabetes mellitus of $>$5 years' duration, urine screening for microalbuminuria should be performed annually.

TREATMENT

This section focuses on T2DM, which is far more common in the family practice setting. Treatment goals include alleviating symptoms, restoring glycemic control, preventing or minimizing long-term complications, and improving quality of life. Although treatment targets should be individualized, the generally recommended target in adults is to achieve a hemoglobin A1c (HbA_{1c}) below 7%. Less stringent goals may be appropriate for older patients, cognitively impaired individuals, those with limited life expectancy or with multiple chronic illnesses, and those at risk for hypoglycemia.

Diet and exercise are the cornerstones of treatment; 80% to 90% of individuals with T2DM are overweight or obese. Even a modest weight loss of 10 to 20 lbs may be sufficient to significantly improve glycemic control. Reducing fat intake is also important, because diabetic patients are at risk for developing hyperlipidemia and vascular disease. As the risk of atherosclerosis is high, statin therapy is recommended for LDL cholesterol levels over 70 mg/dL. Exercise is important for controlling weight and may also improve insulin resistance. The ADA recommends physical activity for ≥150 minutes/week.

If lifestyle modifications fail to control blood sugar, then pharmacologic therapy is the next step. In addition to insulin, there are several pharmacologic treatment options, including biguanides, sulfonylureas, thiazolidinediones, meglitinides, alpha glucosidase inhibitors, sodium glucose cotransporter 2 (SGL2) inhibitors, glucagon-like peptide-1 receptor (GLP-4) agonists, and dipeptidyl peptidase-4 inhibitors (DPP-4 inhibitors) (Figs. 43-2 and 43-3).

Metformin is the only biguanide available in the United States and, in the absence of contra-indications, it is the drug of choice for T2DM because of its low cost, proven effectiveness, and potential cardiovascular benefit. It works by inhibiting hepatic gluconeogenesis and increasing glucose uptake in the peripheral tissues. When used alone, metformin does not cause hypoglycemia, but can potentiate hypoglycemia when used in conjunction with insulin or sulfonylureas. The most common side effects are nausea, diarrhea, and dyspepsia. A rare but potentially fatal complication is lactic acidosis. The risk of lactic acidosis can be reduced by avoiding the use of metformin in patients with renal dysfunction (estimated GFR <30 mL/minute), CHF, acute or chronic acidosis, or hepatic dysfunction.

Sulfonylureas (e.g., glipizide, glyburide) stimulate insulin release from pancreatic beta cells. Contraindications include allergy, pregnancy, and significant renal dysfunction. The most common serious side effects of these medications are weight gain and hypoglycemia. Hypoglycemic reactions occur in about 4% of patients per year but most are mild. Sulfonylureas generally improve fasting

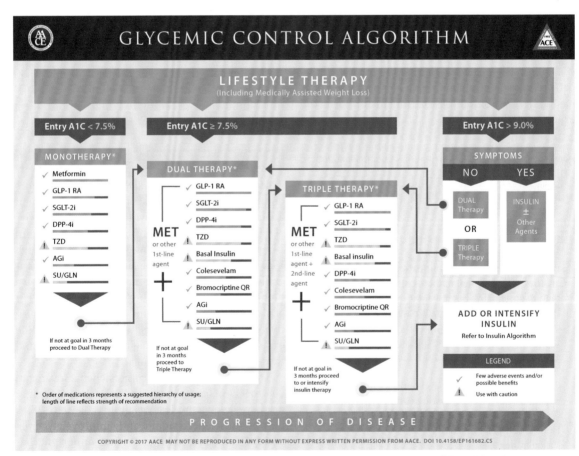

FIGURE 43-2. Glycemic control algorithm. AGI, alpha glucosidase inhibitor; Bromocriptine QR, quick-release bromocriptine; DPP-4i, dipeptidyl peptidase 4 inhibitors; GLN, glinides; GLP-4, glucagon-like peptide-1 receptor; SGL2, sodium glucose cotransporter 2; SU, sulfonylureas; TZD, thiazolidinediones. (Reprinted with permission from American Association of Clinical Endocrinologists, copyright © 2017 AACE. Garber AJ, Abrahamson MJ, Barzilay JI, et al. AACE/ACE comprehensive type 2 diabetes management algorithm 2017. *Endocr Pract.* 2017;23[2]:207–238.)

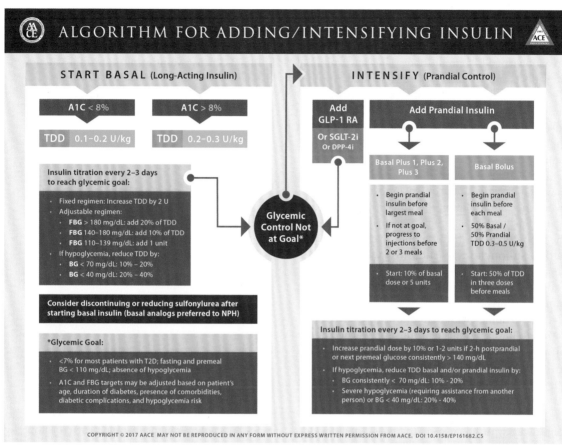

FIGURE 43-3. Algorithm for adding/intensifying insulin. BG, blood glucose; DPP-4i, dipeptidyl peptidase 4 inhibitors; FBG, fasting blood glucose; GLP-4, glucagon-like peptide-1 receptor; NPH, neutral protein hagedorn insulin; SGLT2 inhibitors, sodium-glucose cotransporter 2 inhibitors; TDD, total daily dose. (Reprinted with permission from American Association of Clinical Endocrinologists, copyright © 2017 AACE. Garber AJ, Abrahamson MJ, Barzilay JI, et al. AACE/ACE comprehensive type 2 diabetes management algorithm—2017. *Endocr Pract.* 2017;23[2]:207–238.)

blood sugars by 30 to 60 mg/dL and HbA_{1C} by 1.5% to 2.0%. About 50% to 70% of patients can initially be controlled solely with a sulfonylurea but as beta cell function worsens, 5% to 10% of patients per year previously controlled with a sulfonylurea will lose glycemic control.

The **meglitinides** (Prandin, Starlix) stimulate insulin release in the presence of glucose by increasing calcium and decreasing potassium in pancreatic beta cells. The two FDA-approved medications include repaglinide and nateglinide; both are taken 1 to 30 minutes before meals to maximize the release of insulin and can help control postprandial glucose excursions. Adverse effects associated with meglitinides include weight gain up to 3 kg and hypoglycemia.

Thiazolidinediones (rosiglitazone, pioglitazone) work by decreasing insulin resistance in skeletal muscle and the liver. They can cause hepatotoxicity and require monitoring of liver enzymes. Recently, there have been new FDA warnings regarding use of thiazolidinediones and an increased risk of CHF and MI in patients with cardiac conditions. Therefore, although these medications are still used to achieve adequate glucose control, they are used with caution in patients with cardiac conditions.

Alpha glucosidase inhibitors (acarbose, miglitol) inhibit an enzyme found in the intestinal brush border that hydrolyzes disaccharides, thus limiting the rate of carbohydrate absorption and reducing postprandial elevation of glucose. The major side effects are flatulence, diarrhea, and abdominal pain. These are less used than other agents because of their side effects and limited effectiveness.

Two additional classes of related medications are the **GLP-1 analogues** and **DPP-4 inhibitors**. The GLP-1 receptor agonists (exenatide, liraglutide, albiglutide) are administered as subcutaneous injections and provide modest HbA_{1c} reductions with the added benefit of weight loss. Side effects include nausea and diarrhea. DPP-4 inhibitors (sitagliptin, saxagliptin, and linagliptin) work by preventing the breakdown of GLP-1 in the body. They have minimal side effects and are generally well tolerated. Another class of medication is the **SGLT2 inhibitors**. This class of drugs works in the kidneys to block the reabsorption of glucose. As a result, glucose is released in the urine, which can lead to side effects such as urinary tract and yeast infections.

T2DM is a progressive disease, and a single agent may be ineffective at the outset or lose effectiveness over time. Combination therapy with two or more agents that work by different mechanisms may reduce the blood sugar to an acceptable level. A biguanide with a sulfonylurea is the most widely studied combination. The effect of the two medications is additive; switching from one to another does not improve control.

All individuals with diabetes who receive medication to lower blood sugar must be warned about the possibility of a hypoglycemic reaction manifested by confusion, loss of consciousness, tachycardia, shakiness, headache, or diaphoresis. Patients at risk for hypoglycemia should be instructed about the symptoms of a reaction and should carry either a hard candy or glucose gel to take if they develop hypoglycemic symptoms.

Monitoring, preventing, and treating complications are important elements in managing patients with diabetes mellitus (Box 43-3).

If dual therapy with metformin and a sulfonylurea fails, one approach is to change the sulfonylurea to long-acting insulin. Given in sufficient doses, insulin can usually control even the most refractory hyperglycemia. Characteristics of insulin preparations vary in terms of onset and duration of action. Patients on insulin usually require self-monitoring at home using a glucometer. An alternative approach to insulin is to add a third agent, such as a DPP-4 inhibitor, GLP-1 receptor agonist, or SGLT2 inhibitor.

The ADA also recommends prophylactic aspirin use in male patients age 50 years or above and female patients over the age of 60 years.

The ADA recommends monitoring the HbA_{1C} every 3 to 6 months, with a target goal of below 7% to prevent microvascular complications. Levels above 8% usually suggest the need to reexamine treatment, either by reemphasizing adherence to current therapy or by changing management. With the elderly population, glucose control may be complicated by hypoglycemic episodes. Adjusting glycemic targets for those at risk for hypoglycemia

BOX 43-3. Targets of Optimal Diabetes Type 2 Management

Blood Glucose Monitoring on Insulin Therapy:
Monitor glucose two to four times each day.
Premeal: 70–140 mg/dL
Postmeal: <160 mg/dL (2 hours after start of meal)
Bedtime: 100–160 mg/dL
More than 50% of glucose readings within target range with no severe hypoglycemic episodes

HbA_{1C}:
<7%
Test every 3 months and use to verify home glucose monitoring readings.

Blood Pressure:
Goal <130/80 mmHg

Lipids: Statin therapy for LDL >70 mg/dL

to avoid complications of hypoglycemic episodes may be appropriate.

Currently, the ADA recommends annual dilated eye examinations and screening for microalbuminuria in patients with diabetes. Patients with retinopathy need monitoring by an ophthalmologist. Microalbuminuria is defined as the excretion of 30 to 300 mg of urinary protein over 24 hours. The presence of microalbuminuria should prompt a careful retinal evaluation, because retinopathy usually precedes nephropathy. Reducing blood pressure to 130/80 mmHg and using an ACE inhibitor are strategies that may slow the progression of nephropathy. For patients who cannot tolerate an ACE inhibitor, an ARB agent is an alternative. Neuropathy is one of the most common diabetic complications. In addition to sensory loss, diabetic neuropathy can cause bladder and bowel problems, impotence, and orthostatic hypotension. Patients with sensory neuropathies frequently also have peripheral vascular disease and are especially prone to develop foot problems. Painful neuropathies may respond to tricyclic antidepressants, carbamazepine, or gabapentin.

Another important intervention to reduce complications in diabetic patients includes tobacco cessation using support groups and counseling. Annual influenza vaccines and pneumococcal vaccinations are also recommended to prevent severe infection. Dental examinations every 6 months are also recommended to maintain proper oral hygiene, again to deter serious infections that can be complicated with T2DM.

KEY POINTS

- There are two main types of diabetes mellitus: type 1, characterized by little or no insulin production, and type 2, in which the initial defect is insulin resistance.

- Many individuals with T2DM are asymptomatic and are identified by blood testing.

- Glycemic control reduces the risk of developing complications and slows the progression of diabetes in those who already have established complications.

- The cornerstones of treatment in T2DM are diet and exercise, with pharmacologic treatment reserved for those who do not reach treatment goals with diet and exercise alone.

44 | Diverticulitis

Diverticuli are herniations in the colonic mucosa; they are present in 20% of individuals over the age of 40 and in up to 70% of people over age 85. Approximately 95% of patients with diverticuli have sigmoid diverticuli. Most patients with diverticuli are asymptomatic; however, up to 15% will develop complications such as diverticulitis, GI obstruction, or bleeding. Risk factors for the development of diverticulitis include older age, a low-fiber diet, a previous history of diverticulitis, constipating conditions, obesity, opiates, NSAID and aspirin use, smoking, and the presence of a large number of diverticuli in the colon.

PATHOGENESIS

Diverticuli are outpouchings, or herniations, of the colonic mucosa through the muscularis layer. These occur in areas of mucosal weakness where an artery penetrates the muscularis to reach the submucosa and the mucosa. The weakened colonic muscle wall resistance is related to increased elastin deposits, age-related collagen changes, and disordered motility. The sigmoid colon is more commonly involved because the luminal size is smaller and the pressures generated are greater than in other areas of the colon. Normally, diverticuli are asymptomatic; however, they may become obstructed with fecal material, which can cause inflammation and microabscess formation within and around the diverticulum. This inflammatory process is called diverticulitis. The inflammation may progress to involve a larger segment of colon and cause a narrowing or stricture. Larger abscesses may form and encroach on neighboring structures, leading to development of fistulas. Diverticular bleeding is usually not associated with pain and occurs when fecal matter traumatizes one of the perforating arteries at the site of a diverticulum.

CLINICAL MANIFESTATIONS

HISTORY

The clinical manifestations of diverticular disease vary from asymptomatic disease to abdominal pain or bleeding. Only 10% to 25% of people with diverticulosis develop symptoms. Patients with diverticulitis usually present with complaints of colicky left lower quadrant abdominal pain that may be aggravated by eating and relieved by a bowel movement. On occasion, the abdominal pain may occur in other locations, such as the right lower quadrant. These patients also experience fever, chills, nausea, vomiting, and decreased appetite; they are often constipated. Patients may present with massive GI bleeding but without other symptoms or pain. Colon cancer should be suspected in elderly patients with weight loss, abdominal pain, and changes in bowel habits.

PHYSICAL EXAMINATION

General symptoms such as fever may or may not be present. The physical examination may reveal peritoneal signs such as rigidity, rebound tenderness, and guarding. The abdomen may be distended and tympanic. Often a mass or fullness is palpated in the left lower quadrant. Bowel sounds are either decreased or normal early in presentation; however, they may be increased with obstruction. The physical examination should include a rectal examination to exclude the presence of a mass or bleeding. In cases of severe bleeding, patients may have signs of hypovolemia and anemia.

DIFFERENTIAL DIAGNOSIS

Box 44-1 lists some causes of lower abdominal pain. The differential diagnosis for rectal bleeding includes polyps, colon cancer, angiodysplasia, and

BOX 44-1. Causes for Lower Abdominal Pain

Inflammatory bowel disease (Crohn disease, ulcerative colitis)
Irritable bowel syndrome
Large bowel obstruction or ileus
Carcinoma of the colon
Ischemic colitis
Nephrolithiasis
Appendicitis
Mesenteric ischemia
Colon spasm
Incarcerated hernia
Urinary tract infections
Gynecologic disorders (ovarian pathology, ectopic pregnancy, endometriosis)

diverticular disease. Patients with left lower quadrant abdominal pain may have infectious, inflammatory, or ischemic colitis, IBS, or colon cancer. With right-sided abdominal pain, appendicitis should be considered. Nephrolithiasis may cause abdominal pain but is usually not associated with tenderness or fever. In women, gynecologic complaints such as an ovarian mass, ruptured ovarian cyst, torsion, and endometriosis are part of the differential diagnosis.

DIAGNOSTIC EVALUATION

Diverticulitis is initially a clinical diagnosis, especially in patients with previous diverticulitis. Diagnosis may be supported by laboratory and diagnostic testing. An elevated WBC count along with a left shift suggests an inflammatory process. Hemoglobin testing is useful for evaluating GI bleeding and UA is useful in ruling out urinary tract disorders such as stones or infection. Plain abdominal films do not demonstrate specific findings with diverticulitis but may show an ileus pattern. CT of the abdomen with contrast is the imaging test of choice for patients with suspected diverticulitis and provides diagnostic evidence of diverticulitis in >90% of cases (sensitivity 90% to 100% and specificity 95% to 100%). CT findings may include pericolic fat infiltration (considered diagnostic finding), thickened fascia, muscular hypertrophy, and "arrowhead sign" that shows localized colonic wall thickening with arrowhead-shaped lumen pointing to inflamed diverticuli. A CT scan can also help detect other causes for a patient's abdominal

pain. Barium enema can reveal diverticulitis but is often not advisable during an acute episode for fear of causing perforation and spillage of barium into the abdomen. In patients with diverticulitis and no recent colonoscopy, follow-up testing should include a colonoscopy 6 to 8 weeks after resolution of symptoms in order to detect an underlying malignancy. Delaying colonoscopy is important to avoid colonic perforation.

TREATMENT

Patients with diverticulosis should be encouraged to eat high-fiber diets and to engage in daily exercise. Traditionally, patients were counseled to avoid foods with small seeds and nuts, but recent research findings reveal no correlation between diverticulitis and these foods; still, some providers may counsel patients to avoid these foods if the patient reports abdominal upset with their ingestion. Fiber supplements such as psyllium are helpful. In addition to dietary maneuvers, anticholinergic or antispasmodic drugs may be helpful for the relief of crampy abdominal pain. Stool softeners may benefit those with firm stools or constipation. Patients with diverticulitis may be treated as outpatients or inpatients depending on the severity of illness and their reliability in adhering to therapy and follow-up. Patients with mild symptoms and stable vital signs who are not vomiting may be placed on a clear liquid diet with follow-up in 2 to 3 days. If the patient is improving, the diet may be advanced. Antibiotics were once routinely part of therapy; however, they are now used selectively based upon severity of symptoms and presence of complications. When used, antibiotics should be continued for 7 to 10 days. The patient should undergo colonoscopy in 6 to 8 weeks to evaluate the possibility of colon carcinoma. Patients with more severe pain, vomiting, or unstable vital signs will require hospitalization. Patients should be placed on bowel rest and started on intravenous fluids, broad spectrum antibiotics, and opiates for pain if needed. As the pain subsides, oral intake can be resumed and the patient switched to oral antibiotics. Follow-up colonoscopy is recommended in 6 to 8 weeks. Both inpatients and outpatients with diverticulitis are monitored for complications that may require surgical intervention. These include abscess formation, stricture formation with obstruction, fistulas, and peritonitis. Recurrent episodes may prompt surgical intervention.

Antibiotic selection for patients with diverticulitis should provide coverage for gram-negative and anaerobic bacteria. Common oral outpatient choices are amoxicillin/clavulanate, trimethoprim/sulfamethoxazole, or ciprofloxacin plus metronidazole with duration of treatment from 7 to 10 days. Common inpatient treatment includes metronidazole or clindamycin, plus an aminoglycoside, aztreonam, or third-generation cephalosporin (ceftriaxone, ceftazidime, cefotaxime). Ampicillin/sulbactam or piperacillin/tazobactam may also be used. Improvement should be expected within 48 to 72 hours of initiation of treatment.

Diverticular bleeding is managed with supportive care and evaluation of the source of the bleeding. The bleeding will usually resolve spontaneously but may recur in up to 25% of cases.

KEY POINTS

- Diverticular disease is common in the elderly.
- Risk factors for diverticulitis include age over 40 years, low-fiber diet, history of diverticulitis, and the number of diverticuli in the colon.
- The clinical manifestations of diverticular disease vary from totally asymptomatic disease to severe pain, bleeding, or diverticulitis.
- Patients with diverticulitis will often have left lower quadrant pain along with fever and chills.
- Elderly patients with weight loss, abdominal pain, and changes in bowel habits should be suspected of having colon cancer.
- In acute cases of diverticulitis, CT scan with contrast is the test of choice.

45 Human Immunodeficiency Virus

Over 1 million people are infected with the HIV virus. Tremendous advancements in therapy have allowed HIV to become a chronic disease and no longer a terminal illness. With proper and reliable care, HIV patients can have a near-normal life expectancy. Since HIV infection is often a disease of families, involving spouse and children, the family physician has an important role in the diagnosis, treatment, and prevention of AIDS.

PATHOGENESIS

HIV-1 is a retrovirus that by infecting lymphocytes bearing the CD4 marker causes HIV infection and if untreated over time AIDS. CD4 lymphocytes are T cells involved in cell-mediated immunity. The depletion of CD4 lymphocytes also impairs B cell activation against foreign antigens and limits antibody production. Together, these effects contribute to the immunocompromised state termed AIDS.

HIV is transmitted from person to person through blood and body fluids. HIV transmission is linked to sexual contact (90%), intravenous drug use (10%), and blood transfusions before 1980. HIV may also be transmitted to healthcare workers from needlestick injuries or from mother to infant in utero, during labor, or through breastfeeding. With sexual activity, the transmission rate from a male to a female is 0.5 to 1.5 per 1000 episodes, whereas the transmission rate from female to male is 0.3 to 0.9 per 1000 episodes. Viral load is the most powerful predictor of risk of heterosexual transmission. There is a 1.5 times greater risk of transmission during menstruation. Healthcare workers suffering from an infected needlestick have a risk of seroconversion of approximately 3.2 per 1000 with hollow-bore needles and a lower rate with a suture needle. Blood splashed on intact skin poses a very low risk of transmission.

CLINICAL MANIFESTATIONS

HISTORY

Manifestations of acute HIV infection are fever, fatigue, rash, headache, lymphadenopathy, pharyngitis, myalgia, GI upset (i.e., diarrhea, vomiting), night sweats, aseptic meningitis, and oral or genital ulcers. Symptoms of acute HIV infection usually develop within days to weeks after exposure and usually last <14 days. During the acute infection, HIV disseminates widely and spreads into lymphoid tissue. Seroconversion, or the development of antibodies to the virus, takes 3 to 4 weeks. A prolonged asymptomatic period of clinical latency (up to 12 years) may ensue, with measurable HIV-1 ribonucleic acid (RNA) and antibody levels as the only evidence of infection. Untreated, ultimately AIDS develops, characterized by immune deficiency, high-level viremia, opportunistic infections, and death.

A complete history should include risks for transmission, preexisting comorbid conditions, social history, and previous antiretroviral treatments. The patient's spouse or partner(s) and children should be evaluated for HIV infection. Patients should be questioned about symptoms associated with opportunistic infections, such as dyspnea, dysphagia, and skin lesions. Past and current history of genital symptoms or lesions should be obtained. Even though HIV patients may have a near-normal lifespan with use of antiretroviral therapy (ART), many still view HIV infection as untreatable and may become depressed or even suicidal as a result. Learning about patients' previous psychiatric illnesses and family support can help them to cope with the disease and adhere to treatments. Inquiring about prior medications used by the patient, duration of use, response, intolerance, and toxicities helps clinicians choose appropriate medications and antiviral therapy.

PHYSICAL EXAMINATION

The physical examination should focus on weight change, the presence of fever, skin lesions, signs of opportunistic infections, presence of sexually transmitted diseases (STDs), neurologic function, and emotional state. A weight loss of >10% requires aggressive evaluation and treatment. *Pneumocystis carinii* pneumonia is the most common cause of fever, and patients may have a normal lung examination despite active infection. Sinusitis is also common in early stage disease, and the presence of sinus tenderness should be noted. Other opportunistic infections that may be apparent on physical examination include oral thrush (candidiasis), CMV retinitis (with a ketchup-and-cottage cheese fundus), toxoplasmosis (an intracranial lesion manifesting as deficits in extraocular movements), and cryptococcal meningitis (headache, fever, mental status change). Common skin lesions are Kaposi sarcoma, an exacerbation of psoriasis, seborrheic dermatitis, drug-related eruptions, dry skin, molluscum contagiosum, and herpes zoster. HIV infection increases the risk of pelvic inflammatory disease and cervical carcinoma in women, making a gynecologic examination including Pap smear and STD evaluation (including syphilis) necessary. Mild confusion and memory loss may occur early in HIV disease and suggest AIDS dementia complex. Myopathies, sensory and motor neuropathies, and central lesions (CNS lymphoma) may also be found in HIV disease.

DIFFERENTIAL DIAGNOSIS

Box 45-1 lists the differential diagnosis. Early HIV infection can be confused with acute viral infections or other immunocompromised states. Family physicians should be alert to the possibility of HIV in patients presenting with fever, fatigue, and STDs.

DIAGNOSTIC EVALUATION

HIV infection initially results in a low-level viremia with progressively increasing viral levels over the first 2 weeks of the illness. After approximately 10 days, virus, and a few days later, antigen (p24 antigen) become detectable. However, IgM antibodies that form can bind to the p24 antigen and make p24 assay detection challenging. Most individuals develop measurable IgG antibodies (seroconvert) within 3 to 12 weeks of the initial infection. Current assays for detecting HIV infection combine antigen/antibody assays, evaluating IgG antibodies, and p24

BOX 45-1. Differential Diagnosis for Acute HIV Infection

Infectious Diseases
Infectious mononucleosis, influenza, primary cytomegalovirus infection, streptococcal pharyngitis, viral hepatitis, secondary syphilis, primary herpes simplex virus infection, toxoplasmosis, malaria

Immunocompromised State
Primary immunodeficiency disease in both B/T cells (i.e., immunoglobulin A deficiency, most commonly found in adults >21 years old), lymphoma

Others
Drug reactions

antigen. An algorithm for testing is presented in Figure 45-1. Nucleic acid detection methods (e.g., PCR testing for HIV RNA or DNA) can help detect acute infection in those with indeterminate results. Plasma viral load (PVL) testing, usually reported as copies/mL, is based on how much HIV RNA is in the blood and can detect HIV infection as early as 11 days. Laboratory evaluation is performed to determine the stage of HIV disease, preferably using the CD4 count and PVL. Other suggested screenings for related cancers, STDs, and HIV-related infections are listed in Box 45-2.

TREATMENT

The primary goals of initiating treatment with ART include improving quality of life, reducing HIV-related mortality and prolonging survival, restoring and preserving immunologic functions, maximizing and maintaining suppression of viral load, and preventing vertical transmission of HIV. Before initiating treatment, the patient should be counseled and educated about the potential risks and benefits; this includes long-term and short-term adverse drug effects and the need for long-term commitment and adherence to ART. The current recommendation is to offer ART to all HIV-infected patients. Early treatment and a commitment to daily therapy are critical for ART effectiveness in restoring immune function, suppressing viral loads, and minimizing risk of transmission. Lack of adherence can limit the effectiveness and put the patient at risk for future drug resistance.

CD4, PVL, and assessment for drug resistance are obtained at baseline. The effectiveness of treatments

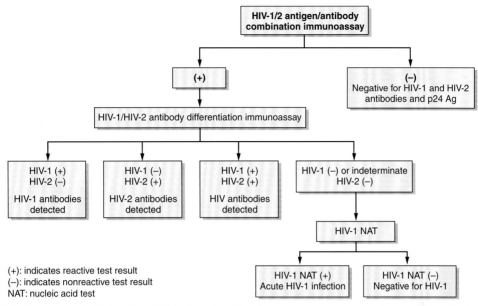

FIGURE 45-1. Recommended laboratory HIV testing algorithm for serum or plasma specimens. (From Centers for Disease Control and Prevention and Association of Public Health Laboratories. Laboratory testing for the diagnosis of HIV infection: updated recommendations. http://dx.doi.org/10.15620/cdc.23447. Published June 27, 2014. Accessed November 2, 2017.)

BOX 45-2. Initial Laboratory Evaluation of an HIV-Positive Patient

(1) CD4 cell counts, PVL, CBC for HIV-related anemia or thrombocytopenia
(2) Pap smear, gonococcal (GC)/chlamydial infection, syphilis (VDRL test)
(3) Hepatitis C, hepatitis B panel, tuberculin skin test, toxoplasma titer, cytomegalovirus titer
(4) Basic metabolic profile: BUN, creatinine, electrolytes, liver function tests, total protein, serum albumin

is measured against baseline PVL, with follow-up laboratory tests done 4 to 8 weeks after the start of therapy until the viral load is <200 copies/mL, at which time PVL is assessed every 3 to 6 months. The viral load should become undetectable after 16 to 24 weeks of therapy. CD4 counts are assessed at baseline and prophylaxis for opportunistic infections is started as outlined in Table 45-1. CD4 counts are evaluated every 3 months for the first 2 years and if stable over 300 cells/mL, then yearly or with changes in clinical condition. The treatment regimens for HIV infection should include a combination of antiretroviral medications that include at least three drugs from

TABLE 45-1. Primary Prophylaxis Against Opportunistic Infections

Infection	Indications	Primary Treatment	Secondary Treatment
PCP[a]	CD4 cells <200/mm^3	Bactrim	Dapsone
Toxoplasmosis	CD4 cells <100/mm^3	Bactrim	Dapsone
MAC	CD4 cells <50/mm^3	Azithromycin or Clarithromycin	Rifabutin
TB	PPD > 5 mm	INH w/pyridoxine	Rifampin
VZV	Exposure	VZIG	Acyclovir

[a]In neonates, PCP prophylaxis treatment (Bactrim or dapsone) begins when zidovudine therapy is stopped or the child reaches age 6 weeks, and is continued until the child is found to be HIV-free or for at least 1 year.
MAC, *Mycobacterium avium* complex; PCP, *Pneumocystic carinii* pneumonia; PPD, purified protein derivative; TB, tuberculosis; VZIG, varicella zoster immunoglobulin; INH, Isoniazid; VZV, varicella zoster virus.

two classes to avoid resistance. Therapy should be continued indefinitely. Four different categories of antiviral agents are available: the nucleoside reverse transcriptase inhibitors (NRTIs), the nonnucleoside reverse transcriptase inhibitors (NNRTIs), protease inhibitors (PIs), and integrase inhibitors. Either an integrase inhibitor or a protease inhibitor plus two NRTIs are recommended for initial therapy in treatment-naive patients. Resistance to ART can develop, and a change of medications as well as resistance testing may be necessary in case of therapeutic failure. Treatment can be difficult because the regimens may involve taking multiple pills at different times throughout the day. Side effects can include nausea, vomiting, diarrhea, osteoporosis, lipid abnormalities, and blood sugar elevations. A full discussion of medication dosing and side effects is beyond the scope of this chapter.

Studies in obstetric HIV patients have shown that ART and selective use of cesarean section along with concurrent ART decrease the vertical transmission rate dramatically. Because maternal immunoglobulins against HIV cross the placenta, all neonates born to an HIV-positive mother will have a positive test for HIV in the first 6 months. Current recommendations for children born to HIV-positive mothers state that infants should receive ART for at least the first 4 to 6 weeks of life. Repeat testing following treatment is indicated to determine the status of the infant. The mother should be counseled about avoiding breastfeeding.

Postexposure prophylaxis using an ART regimen for 4 weeks along with diagnostic testing is recommended following occupational or other known exposures to limit risks of HIV transmission (https://stacks.cdc.gov/view/cdc/20711). Pre-exposure prophylaxis is also recommended for patients with ongoing risk, such as HIV-discordant couples. Daily medication use (e.g., tenofovir DF plus emtricitabine) can limit the risk of transmission in these cases by up to 90% or more (https://www.cdc.gov/hiv/pdf/prepprovidersupplement2014.pdf).

KEY POINTS

- Symptoms of acute HIV infection usually develop within days to weeks after exposure and usually last <14 days. The development of antibodies (seroconversion) takes place 3 to 4 weeks after the exposure.

- HIV infection is detected by assays for both HIV antibody and antigen, with nucleic acid identification methods in patients with indeterminate results.

- Treatment regimens for HIV infection should include a combination of antiretroviral medications continued indefinitely.

- Postexposure prophylaxis using an ART regimen for 4 weeks along with diagnostic testing is recommended following occupational or other known exposures to limit risks of HIV transmission.

46 | Hypertension

Hypertension (HTN) is defined in the 2017 guidelines endorsed by the American Heart Association (AHA) and American College of Cardiology (ACC) as a systolic blood pressure (BP) ≥130 mmHg or diastolic pressure ≥80 mmHg.

EPIDEMIOLOGY

In older guidelines, HTN affects about 75 million Americans (about 30% of the adult population). In lowering the definition of hypertension from 140/90 mmHg, almost half of the US adult population will have hypertension. Hypertension remains a major risk factor for cardiovascular and cerebrovascular disease. Prevalence increases with age, such that by the age of 60, HTN is present in approximately 71% of African Americans, 61% of Mexican Americans, and 60% of non-Hispanic whites. Primary HTN accounts for 90% to 95% of all cases of HTN; secondary HTN causes about 5% to 10% of all adult HTN. Nearly another 1 in 3 has elevated BP where their BP numbers are higher than normal but not yet in the hypertensive range. Although HTN is defined at 130/80 mmHg, the mortality risk from stroke and heart disease doubles for each 20 mmHg increase in systolic pressure or 10 mmHg in diastolic pressure increase over 115/75 mmHg.

PATHOGENESIS

HTN can be either **primary (essential)** or **secondary**. Primary HTN does not have a known cause and is a complex process that results from a variety of physiologic and environmental factors. Secondary HTN has an identifiable underlying cause such as exogenous substances (e.g., stimulants, alcohol, NSAIDs), renal failure, sleep apnea, renovascular disease, primary aldosteronism, pheochromocytoma, and Cushing syndrome.

Insulin resistance is also associated with increased arterial BP. Hyperinsulinemia can increase vascular tone by any of the following four mechanisms: (1) promoting $Na+$ retention; (2) promoting hypertrophy or hyperplasia of vascular smooth muscles through its mitogenic properties; (3) modifying ion transport, leading to an increase in intracellular calcium; and (4) sympathetic activation.

Poorly controlled HTN leads to complications or damage in several target organs. The risk of cardiovascular complications correlates with the degree of BP elevation.

CLINICAL MANIFESTATIONS

HISTORY

HTN is referred to as the "**silent killer**" because it is generally asymptomatic until there is end organ damage and as a result is usually diagnosed during a routine office visit screening. Target organs include the heart, peripheral vasculature, eyes, and kidneys. Clinical manifestations include ischemic heart disease, stroke, peripheral vascular disease, renal insufficiency, retinopathy characterized by exudates or hemorrhages, and, in severe HTN, papilledema.

The history for hypertensive individuals should focus on symptoms of end organ damage, additional risk factors for cardiovascular disease, clues to suggest a secondary cause of HTN, and calculation of cardiac risk (http://www.cvriskcalculator.com/). It is essential to ask about cardiovascular symptoms, such as chest pain, shortness of breath, prior TIAs or strokes, and renal disease. It is important to inquire about a family history of heart disease, HTN, hyperlipidemia, diabetes, and renal disease. Additional behavioral risk factors such as tobacco and alcohol use, exercise, and dietary habits should be assessed. Inquiring about medications is important, because drugs such as NSAIDs, decongestants, estrogen, progesterone, appetite suppressants, and MAOIs may elevate BP. Features of the history that suggest a secondary cause include the following:

1. Early or late onset of HTN (younger than 20 and older than 50 years of age).
2. An associated history of tachycardia, sweating, and headache.
3. A personal or family history of renal disease.
4. Treatment resistant HTN in a compliant patient.
5. Symptoms consistent with sleep apnea.
6. History of amphetamine, cocaine, or alcohol abuse.
7. Use of oral contraceptives, estrogens, corticosteroids, NSAIDs.
8. History of hirsutism or easy bruising.
9. Accelerated onset of high BP.

PHYSICAL EXAMINATION

The diagnosis of HTN requires an increased BP (SBP ≥ 130 or DBP ≥ 80 mmHg) on at least two consecutive visits 2 weeks apart. The exception is one SBP ≥ 210, one DBP ≥ 120, or the presence of significant end organ damage at the time of the first reading. Because several factors—such as pain, fear, anxiety, physical activity, and exogenous substances or medication—can influence BP readings, a standard approach must be followed to ensure accurate BP readings and avoid incorrectly labeling a patient as hypertensive (Box 46-1).

BOX 46-1. Essentials of Blood Pressure Measurement

1. Seated at rest for 5 minutes
2. No caffeine or cigarettes in preceding 30 minutes
3. Bladder of blood pressure cuff encircles 80% of arm
4. Arm supported at heart level
5. Inflate cuff and determine systolic range by palpably checking for obliteration of radial pulse
6. Auscultate over brachial artery after inflating cuff 10–20 mmHg above palpable systolic pressure
7. Systolic pressure = onset of Korotkoff sounds
8. Diastolic pressure = muffling or cessation of Korotkoff sounds

Additional elements of the physical examination include the skin examination, looking for signs of Cushing syndrome or neurofibromatosis; funduscopic examination, looking for target organ damage such as retinal hemorrhages, increased vascular tortuosity, and "arteriovenous (AV) nicking"; checking the thyroid for enlargement or nodularity; auscultating the carotids for bruits; listening to the lungs for signs of heart failure; palpating the chest for displacement of the PMI (suggestive of cardiomegaly); listening to the heart for murmurs and S_3 or S_4 heart sounds; examining the abdomen for bruits or masses; conducting a neurologic examination for focal deficits; and checking the extremities for pulses and the presence of edema.

DIFFERENTIAL DIAGNOSIS

The differential diagnosis generally involves distinguishing between primary and secondary HTN. Additional considerations in evaluating elevated BP readings are transient factors, such as stress or an acute illness causing the elevated reading, as well as "white coat" HTN and "pseudohypertension."

Primary HTN tends to run in families; the physical examination and laboratory screening do not identify a specific etiology for the increased BP. Although secondary HTN accounts for only 5% of hypertensive individuals, it is important to identify these cases because they are potentially curable.

White coat HTN and pseudohypertension are conditions where the patient does not truly have HTN, but the BP is elevated under the conditions or time it is being measured. For example, with white coat HTN, the patient's BP is elevated in the physician's office but not at other times. In pseudohypertension, the patient is generally elderly; has calcified, rigid blood vessels; and the intra-arterial BP is actually lower than what can be measured with the BP cuff.

DIAGNOSTIC EVALUATION

Once the diagnosis of HTN has been made, four main questions must be addressed:

1. Is this HTN primary (essential) or secondary?
2. What other cardiovascular risk factors are present?
3. Is there evidence of target organ damage?
4. Are there any comorbid conditions that would affect the choice of therapy?

Laboratory and diagnostic studies are indicated to assess end organ damage, identify additional cardiovascular risk factors, exclude secondary causes, and assist in the choice of medications. A CBC is recommended as a baseline for future evaluation in the event of medication-induced neutropenia or agranulocytosis. A fasting serum glucose, K+, serum creatinine, UA, and lipid profile are recommended for newly diagnosed hypertensive patients. A high fasting serum glucose can indicate diabetes mellitus, unprovoked hypokalemia (<3.5 meq/L) suggests hyperaldosteronism, an elevated creatinine may indicate renal insufficiency, and proteinuria or microalbuminuria suggests renal end organ damage. Two other recommended tests are serum calcium (with albumin) and uric acid, because hypercalcemia or hyperuricemia may preclude the use of thiazide diuretics and hypercalcemia can identify hyperparathyroidism.

An ECG helps assess for prior MI, heart block, or left ventricular hypertrophy. A plain CXR can detect cardiomegaly, CHF, and coarctation of the aorta. In patients with suspected white coat HTN, ambulatory BP monitoring may help determine whether HTN is an appropriate diagnosis. A serum TSH can help diagnose thyroid disease, which can elevate BP. Individuals with symptoms suggesting sleep apnea are candidates for a sleep study.

A common clinical dilemma is when to test for renovascular hypertension due to renal artery stenosis (RAS). Current ACC/AHA guidelines recommend screening only those patients in whom a corrective procedure would be considered. Clinical clues suggesting the presence of RAS include onset of hypertension before age 30 or onset of severe hypertension after age 55, sudden worsening of previously controlled blood pressure, resistant hypertension, malignant hypertension, worsening renal function after starting an ACEi or ARB, size discrepancy of >1.5 cm between the kidneys, and unexplained renal failure. While several procedures exist to screen for RAS, the ACC/AHA guidelines recommend ultrasound because of its safety, good sensitivity and specificity, low cost, and ability to be repeated with little risk or discomfort to the patient.

TREATMENT

Once the diagnosis of HTN has been established, treatment should be initiated. The Joint National Committee (JNC) on Detection, Evaluation and Treatment of High Blood Pressure classified HTN into three stages (Table 46-1) to help guide therapy.

The first step in treatment for patients is lifestyle modification (Box 46-2). About 60% of hypertensive

BOX 46-2. Treatment Overview

Treat patients with an estimated 10 year CV risk >10% to BP <130/80
Treat all patients to BP <140/90
Most patients require two medications for optimal control.
Encourage lifestyle modifications:
- Weight loss
- Dietary approaches to stop hypertension (DASH) diet
- Sodium restriction
- Aerobic physical activity for at least 30–40 minutes per day
- Moderate alcohol consumption
- Smoking cessation

Initial drug treatment:
- Stage 1 hypertension and CV risk >10% (130–139/80–89 mmHg): thiazide-type diuretics; may consider ACEI, ARB, CCB, or combination
- Stage 2 hypertension (>140/90 mmHg): two-drug combination using thiazide-type diuretic plus ACEI, ARB, or CCB
- Consider BB in patients with cardiovascular disease

TABLE 46-1. Stages of Hypertension			
Stage	**Systolic Pressure**	**Diastolic Pressure**	**Treatment**
	Range (mmHg)	Range (mmHg)	
Normal	<120	<80	No treatment
Elevated BP	120–129	<80	• Lifestyle modification
Stage 1	130–139	80–89	• Lifestyle modification • If not at target in 3 months, consider medication • Initiate medication if CV risk >10%
Stage 2	>140	>90	• Lifestyle modification • Consider initiating two medications

patients are salt sensitive and may benefit from sodium restriction (<2.4 g/day) by avoiding added salt and salty or processed food. Other lifestyle changes include weight reduction, regular aerobic exercise (30- to 60-minute sessions three to four times a week), smoking cessation, and limiting alcohol intake (<24 oz beer per day, <8 oz of wine per day, <2 oz of whisky per day). Lifestyle modification alone effectively controls BP in about 10% of patients.

If an individual remains hypertensive after 3 to 6 months of lifestyle modification, it is appropriate to start antihypertensive medication. Patients with stage 2 HTN warrant earlier initiation of pharmacologic therapy in addition to lifestyle recommendations. Isolated systolic HTN (SBP ≥ 140 mmHg) is common in the elderly. The Systolic HTN in the Elderly Program (SHEP) demonstrated that the treatment of patients more than age 60 with isolated systolic HTN by using low-dose diuretics and beta blockers (BBs) significantly reduces the incidence of strokes and MIs. Despite the proven benefits of treating hypertension, only about 40% of adults in the United States with high BP have their condition under good control.

The classes of medications most commonly used as **first-line agents** are **diuretics, calcium channel blockers,** and **ACE inhibitors.** Other agents, such as beta blockers, centrally acting agents, alpha blockers, and direct vasodilators have less evidence for improving clinical outcomes and are reserved for those who have separate indications for these drugs or who fail first-line therapy. Most patients will require two or more antihypertensive medications to achieve adequate control. For patients with BP >20/10 mmHg above goal BP, consideration should be given to initiating therapy with two agents.

DIURETICS

Thiazides were the first major drugs introduced for the treatment of HTN and are still the most widely used. They inhibit Na+ reabsorption from the renal tubules and thus reduce total blood volume. In addition, they blunt the effect of endogenous vasoconstrictors on the vascular smooth muscles, causing a decrease in peripheral vascular resistance. Thiazides are useful in patients without renal impairment ([GFR] >25 or creatinine levels <2 and <1.5 in the elderly). Although thiazides may cause adverse metabolic side effects—such as hypokalemia, hyperuricemia, carbohydrate intolerance, and hyperlipidemia—these effects can be minimized with doses kept below the equivalent of 25 mg/day of hydrochlorothiazide (HCTZ). Most patients can be successfully treated with 12.5 to 25 mg of HCTZ. Side effects include sexual dysfunction, dyslipidemia, hyperglycemia, and elevations in uric acid levels.

For patients with renal impairment (creatinine >2 to 2.5), loop diuretics (i.e., furosemide) are more effective. They tend to produce more diuresis and hypokalemia than thiazides. Concomitant use of NSAIDs interferes with the delivery of loop diuretics to their site of action. Loop diuretics tend to lower serum calcium, whereas thiazides tend to cause hypercalcemia.

Before diuretics are administered, the serum K+ level should be checked and then monitored periodically after diuretic therapy is initiated.

ACE INHIBITORS AND ANGIOTENSIN RECEPTOR BLOCKERS

ACEIs act through the renin–angiotensin system by inhibiting the enzyme that converts angiotensin I to angiotensin II. ACEIs are particularly beneficial to patients with CHF and provide renal protection for those with diabetes. Patients epidemiologically associated with "low-renin" states, such as the elderly and African American populations, may be less likely to respond to the antihypertensive effects of these medications. ACEIs are generally well tolerated; the most common side effect is cough. Other less common but serious reactions include angioedema and neutropenia. In those with RAS, ACEIs may cause an acute reversible renal failure. ARBs act by blocking the receptor site. They appear to be equipotent for lowering BP but may not be as effective as ACEIs in treating CHF and diabetic nephropathy. Unlike ACEIs, they do not cause a cough and only rarely cause skin rashes, making these agents useful for patients who cannot tolerate ACEIs because of these side effects.

CALCIUM CHANNEL BLOCKERS

The CCBs recommended for first-line HTN treatment are the long-acting dihydropyridine agents, such as amlodipine. Diltiazem, verapamil, and short-acting dihydropyridines may lower BP but are less effective, have more side effects, and are not recommended as first-line agents. CCBs lower BP through a peripheral vasodilatory action. Diltiazem and verapamil also depress the AV node and myocardial contractility. The dihydropyridines have a purer vasodilatory action and can cause reflex tachycardia, but they have less effect on cardiac contractility. The use of short-acting dihydropyridines to lower BP may precipitate ischemic events in individuals with coronary artery disease because of reflex tachycardia. No such association has been found with use of long-acting dihydropyridines. Other side effects of CCBs include dizziness, edema, constipation, headache, and flushing. Diltiazem and verapamil should be avoided or used cautiously in patients with second- or third-degree heart block, CHF, and those already taking BBs.

BETA BLOCKERS

Beta blockers are no longer considered first-line antihypertensive agents except in those with underlying cardiovascular disease. Beta-adrenergic receptor blockers work by decreasing heart rate and cardiac contractility. In addition, they modulate the output of the central and peripheral sympathetic nervous systems and decrease release of renin from the juxtaglomerular apparatus. Their renin-mediated mechanism of action may account for the decreased responsiveness in "low-renin" patients (elderly, African Americans).

Within the BB class of medications, there are nonselective and selective beta receptor blockers. Nonselective agents block both $beta_1$ and $beta_2$ receptors, whereas selective agents block only $beta_1$ receptors. The use of a selective agent is indicated in patients with a history of reactive airway disease, where the selectivity may lessen the likelihood of medication-induced bronchospasm. In addition to selective and nonselective subcategories, there are BBs with intrinsic sympathomimetic activity (ISA). BBs with ISA are thought to be less likely to elevate triglycerides or lower HDL cholesterol, and they cause less of a decrease in heart rate.

Side effects of BBs include bradycardia, fatigue, depression, insomnia, sexual dysfunction, and adverse effects on the lipid profile. BBs should be avoided or used cautiously in patients with asthma, COPD, second- or third-degree heart block, peripheral vascular disease, and insulin-dependent diabetes mellitus. Sudden withdrawal of these medications should be avoided, as it can cause tachyarrhythmias and rebound HTN due to the upregulation of beta receptors associated with chronic therapy.

OTHER HYPERTENSIVE MEDICATIONS

Less commonly used but still important classes of antihypertensives include the centrally acting agents and alpha-adrenergic blockers. The centrally acting sympatholytic inhibitors include agents such as clonidine, methyldopa, guanfacine, and reserpine, one of the first available antihypertensives. They lower BP by stimulating alpha-adrenergic receptors in the CNS, which in turn reduces peripheral sympathetic outflow. These agents are usually second-line medications because of the high frequency of side effects, including sedation, fatigue, dry mouth, sexual dysfunction, and postural hypotension. Rebound HTN has been reported with their abrupt withdrawal. Alpha blockers block the alpha-adrenergic receptors, thereby relaxing smooth muscle and decreasing peripheral resistance. These agents include prazosin, terazosin, and doxazosin. Tachyphylaxis, headache, and postural hypotension are relatively common. The hypotension includes a marked first-dose phenomenon. Therefore, the first dose should be small and given at bedtime. The alpha blockers also relax smooth muscle in the prostate and are good choices for men with HTN and BPH.

KEY POINTS

- As defined by the 2017 guidelines about half of adult Americans have HTN and it is a major risk factor for the development of cardiovascular disease and cerebrovascular disease.
- Primary HTN accounts for 90% to 95% of all cases of HTN.
- The history, physical examination, and laboratory evaluation of hypertensive individuals involve assessment for end organ damage, additional risk factors for cardiovascular disease, and secondary causes of HTN.
- The first step in therapy generally involves lifestyle modifications; if patients still remain hypertensive after 3 to 6 months, antihypertensive medications should be started.

47 | Hyperthyroidism

Family physicians must be aware of the varied clinical manifestations of thyroid disease as well as their different causes and treatment options. Thyroid hormone affects virtually every cell in the human body.

PATHOGENESIS

The thyroid gland is derived from the pharyngeal epithelium that descends into the neck during embryogenesis to its location anterior to the larynx, with the thyroglossal duct indicating its path of descent. TSH secretion is stimulated by the pituitary gland by hypothalamic thyrotropin-releasing hormone (TRH). TSH causes increased trapping of iodine by the thyroid gland, elevated production and release of triiodothyronine (T3) and thyroxine (T4), and stimulates growth of the gland itself. Thus, elevated levels of TSH may lead to diffuse or nodular enlargement of the thyroid gland (i.e., goiter). Rising levels of thyroid hormone cause the pituitary gland to be less sensitive to TRH, creating an effective feedback loop to maintain a euthyroid state.

T4 and T3 are the active thyroid hormones and are 99% protein bound by thyroxine-binding globulin (TBG) and other serum proteins. In the peripheral tissues, T4 is converted into free T3, which has a 40 times greater affinity for cellular receptors than T4. Thus, at the cellular level, T3 is the metabolically active thyroid hormone and is primarily responsible for the metabolic effects of the thyroid hormone. However, because of extremely low concentrations of serum T3, free T4 is more easily measured.

Many things can alter TBG levels, thus affecting measured thyroid hormone levels. Conditions that increase TBG include pregnancy, acute liver disease, the newborn state, and medications such as oral contraceptive pills (OCPs) and tamoxifen. Elevated levels of androgens, chronic liver disease, glucocorticoid excess, severe illness, and nephrotic syndrome all lower TBG levels.

In **Graves disease**, circulating antibodies mimic the activity of TSH, causing thyroid gland enlargement and abnormally elevated levels of circulating thyroid hormone. Thyroid nodules occasionally release T3 and T4 independent of TSH. These autonomously functioning nodules often produce excessive levels of thyroid hormone, resulting in systemic abnormalities and atrophy of the remaining normal thyroid tissue. Postpartum and autoimmune thyroiditis (Hashimoto thyroiditis) are inflammatory conditions of the thyroid that can result in hyperthyroidism early in the process as a result of excess release of preformed thyroid hormone associated with thyroid cellular injury. Eventually these patients can become hypothyroid.

CLINICAL MANIFESTATIONS

HISTORY

Patients with symptomatic hyperthyroidism (also known as thyrotoxicosis) complain of weight loss despite normal or high caloric intake, nervousness, heat intolerance, fatigue, increased perspiration, more frequent bowel movements, and inability to sleep. Older patients may complain of angina, palpitations, and shortness of breath. Premenopausal women often experience irregular vaginal bleeding. Those with Graves disease may describe a doughy, swollen appearance of their pretibial area (i.e., myxedema). Individuals with Graves disease may also present with visual changes secondary to exophthalmos. In patients with a thyroid nodule, it is important to obtain a history of head and neck radiation because radiation exposure increases the risk of thyroid carcinoma.

The history should also explore the possibility of excess exogenous hormone. The most obvious case is iatrogenic over replacement but some patients may be taking thyroxine surreptitiously for weight loss. Others may take an over the counter thyroid supplement.

PHYSICAL EXAMINATION

Individuals suffering from hyperthyroidism often appear restless and fidgety. Their skin may be moist and velvety, and palmar erythema is often detectable. Patients often have a fine resting tremor and a "frightened" facial appearance secondary to ocular abnormalities that include widened palpebral fissures, infrequent blinking, and lid lag (Fig. 47-1). The cardiovascular examination may reveal atrial fibrillation, sinus tachycardia, widened pulse pressure, and heart failure. Examination of the neck may demonstrate the presence of a goiter or nodule. Patients with thyroiditis may have thyroid tenderness in addition to enlargement of the gland. If a goiter is present, auscultation may reveal a bruit or venous hum. Deep tendon reflexes are typically brisk and symmetric.

DIFFERENTIAL DIAGNOSIS

The most common causes of hyperthyroidism are Graves disease, toxic multinodular goiter, and thyroiditis. Other potential causes are thyroid adenomas (a variant of toxic multinodular goiter) and, rarely, pituitary disorders. Graves disease is the primary cause in those between 20 and 50 years of age, whereas multinodular goiter is more common in the elderly. In areas of the world where there is insufficient iodine, ingestion of iodine or amiodarone may stimulate the thyroid and lead to hyperthyroidism as well.

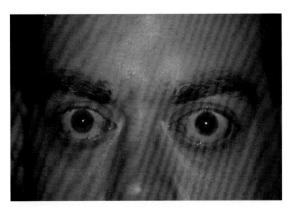

FIGURE 47-1. Thyroid ophthalmopathy. (From Shields JA, Shields CL. *Eyelid, Conjunctival, and Orbital Tumors: An Atlas and Textbook*. 3rd ed. Alphen aan den Rijn, The Netherlands: Wolters Kluwer; 2016.)

DIAGNOSTIC EVALUATION

The diagnosis of hyperthyroidism is established by a raised serum total or free T4 and/or T3 hormone levels, reduced TSH level, and increased radioiodine uptake in the thyroid gland with features of hyperthyroidism. The TSH is often the initial test ordered in evaluating for thyroid disease. TSH is very sensitive for detecting both hyper- and hypothyroidism. Follow-up testing of abnormal TSH results formerly involved measurement of total serum T4, T3 resin uptake, and free T4 index. Although these tests are still available, free T4 and T3 have largely supplanted their use, because the free levels of these hormones define disease activity in hyperthyroidism. TSH is decreased in patients with Graves disease, toxic multinodular goiter, toxic nodule, and occasionally with thyroiditis. Patients with these conditions have primary hyperthyroidism and will have elevated levels of thyroid hormone (free T4 and T3). A thyroid radioactive iodine uptake scan is useful in the setting of hyperthyroidism to differentiate between a diffuse process (e.g., Graves disease or thyroiditis) and a nodular disorder. The thyroid scan will show diffusely increased uptake in Graves disease and multifocal uptake in toxic multinodular goiter. There will be decreased radioactive iodine uptake in thyroiditis. In patients with a palpable nodule, the thyroid scan also helps to differentiate between hot (hyperfunctioning) and cold (hypofunctioning) nodules. Thyroid scanning, ultrasound, and fine-needle aspiration are often used to monitor thyroid nodules. Ultrasound can determine whether the nodule is solid or cystic. Thyroid antibodies are commonly found in patients with thyroiditis (Hashimoto) and Graves disease. Graves disease is positive for TSH-receptor stimulating antibodies, which include thyroid stimulating immunoglobulin (TSI) or thyroid binding inhibitor immunoglobulin. In hyperthyroid patients with abnormally high levels of TSH, MRI is useful in further evaluating for pituitary pathology. Table 47-1 shows different causes of hyperthyroidism and their diagnostic features.

TREATMENT

Initial therapy for hyperthyroidism is targeted toward controlling thyroid hormone production with medications. Definitive treatment depends on the underlying disease process, patient's age, comorbidities, and patient's preferences. There are three distinct treatments for hyperthyroidism: antithyroid medications, thyroidectomy, and radioactive iodine.

TABLE 47-1. Causes of Hyperthyroidism

Disorder	Characteristics	Diagnostic Features
Graves disease	Diffuse thyromegaly	Diffuse increased RAIU
Subacute granulomatous thyroiditis (de Quervain thyroiditis)	Tender thyromegaly	Decreased RAIU
Toxic Adenoma	Solitary nodule with decreased TSH (hyperfunctioning/hot nodule)	Localized increased RAIU
Toxic multinodular goiter	Diffuse hyperplasia of thyroid follicular cells	Multifocal increased RAIU
Factitious hyperthyroidism	Exogenous source	Decreased RAIU

RAIU, radioactive iodine uptake; TSH, thyroid-stimulating hormone.

Antithyroid medications as definitive therapy are most commonly used in patients below 40 years of age; they include propylthiouracil (PTU) and methimazole. These medications are relatively safe and inhibit iodine processing during the production of thyroid hormone; they also inhibit the peripheral conversion of T4 to T3. Agranulocytosis is a rare but serious side effect of these medications; thus, CBCs should be monitored during treatment. Other side effects include nausea, arthropathy, skin rashes, allergic reactions, and elevations of liver enzymes. Both medications are typically introduced in a loading dose for about 4 to 6 weeks, and then as the patient's condition improves the dose can usually be reduced. Treatment typically lasts for 1 year, followed by a gradual taper. Approximately 50% of those with Graves disease will have no further episodes. For those in whom hyperthyroidism returns, options include retreatment, radioactive iodine, and surgery. Radioactive iodine (iodine 131 or ^{131}I) is an effective treatment for thyrotoxicosis, but is contraindicated in young children and pregnant women. The primary disadvantage is resultant hypothyroidism, for which lifelong treatment with thyroid replacement is necessary. Maximum treatment effects are noted after 3 to 4 months and treatment may need to be repeated after 6 months if hyperthyroidism returns. Pretreatment with antithyroid medications is often initiated to avoid excess release of thyroid hormone resulting from radiation-induced damage to the thyroid tissue.

Symptomatic treatment of thyrotoxicosis is another important consideration. Beta blockers like propranolol are titrated up until the symptoms of anxiety, restlessness, and tachycardia are adequately controlled. Definitive treatment of other forms of hyperthyroidism is typically achieved by radioactive iodine treatment, antithyroid medications, or surgery.

Surgery is a useful treatment and offers a quick and definitive cure. It is most often performed in younger patients and those with a hyperfunctioning nodule. Postsurgical hypothyroidism may occur, but is less common than in those undergoing radioactive iodine treatments. The main risks include those associated with neck surgery, such as recurrent laryngeal nerve damage, damage to the parathyroid gland, infection, bleeding, and hypothyroidism.

Thyroid storm is a rare, life-threatening syndrome of severe thyrotoxicosis that usually occurs in an individual with unknown or inadequately treated hyperthyroidism. Symptoms include nausea, fever, heart failure, tachycardia, and diaphoresis. Treatment is similar to that used to treat hyperthyroidism but more aggressive; it includes high-dose antithyroid medications, intravenous iodine, intravenous beta blockers, and high-dose steroids.

Patients with Graves disease and exophthalmos are at risk for corneal ulcers and permanent visual deficits secondary to optic nerve compression and extraocular muscle involvement. To prevent corneal ulcers, eye patches, protective glasses, and artificial tears are often employed. Steroids tapered over several weeks are also commonly used to prevent permanent ocular damage. In severe cases, radiation of the extraocular muscles or orbital decompression is indicated. Treatment of the pretibial myxedema usually consists of a topical steroid.

Patients with thyroid nodules must be evaluated over time to detect malignancies. Those with hyperfunctioning solitary nodules may be treated surgically or with thyroid suppression, using exogenous thyroid hormone. Because approximately 1 out of 20 nodules (functioning and nonfunctioning) is malignant, all thyroid nodules must be evaluated using ultrasound and biopsy.

KEY POINTS

- Patients with symptomatic hyperthyroidism (also known as thyrotoxicosis) often complain of weight loss despite normal or high caloric intake, nervousness, heat intolerance, fatigue, increased perspiration, more frequent bowel movements, and insomnia.

- The most common causes of hyperthyroidism are Graves disease, toxic multinodular goiter, and thyroiditis.

- The TSH is often the initial test ordered in evaluating for thyroid disease. If abnormal, it is followed by serum free T4 and T3 to define disease activity in hyperthyroidism.

- A thyroid radioactive iodine uptake scan is useful in hyperthyroidism to differentiate between a diffuse process (e.g., Graves disease or thyroiditis) and a nodular disorder.

- Definitive treatment of hyperthyroidism is typically achieved by radioactive iodine treatment, antithyroid medications, or surgery.

48 | Hypothyroidism

Hypothyroidism has an overall prevalence of 1% to 2% in the United States, increasing to about 10% in individuals over 65. The incidence is 6 to 10 times greater in women than in men. Other risk factors include a history of head and neck radiation, family or personal history of autoimmune disease, and Turner or Down syndromes. Clinical symptoms of hypothyroidism are often nonspecific and range from mild fatigue to coma.

PATHOGENESIS

Thyroid hormone regulates cellular metabolism. Causes of hypothyroidism include agenesis or other congenital abnormalities of the thyroid, inadequate production of thyroid hormone by the thyroid gland, or inadequate stimulation from either the hypothalamus or pituitary glands. Iodine is necessary to produce thyroid hormone, and geographic areas that lack sufficient iodine have an increased rate of endemic hypothyroidism and goiter (enlarged thyroid gland). As a result, many nations provide iodine as a dietary supplement, usually in salt. Because untreated congenital hypothyroidism results in physical and intellectual disabilities, all newborns in the United States are screened for congenital hypothyroidism. Mandatory screening and early treatment virtually eliminate mental retardation related to congenital hypothyroidism.

Autoimmune destruction of the thyroid gland is the most common noniatrogenic cause of hypothyroidism in the United States. Hashimoto thyroiditis is the most common autoimmune disease affecting the thyroid and is characterized by elevated levels of antibodies to thyroid peroxidase (TPO). TPO is involved in thyroid hormone synthesis. These antibodies cause inflammation of the thyroid and lead to diminished production of thyroid hormone.

Hashimoto thyroiditis is more common in women, has a genetic predisposition, and is often associated with other autoimmune disorders.

Iatrogenic hypothyroidism may occur as a result of neck irradiation, radioactive iodine therapy, or thyroid surgery. Medications such as lithium, amiodarone, and interferon may also cause hypothyroidism. Any disorder causing dysfunction of the hypothalamus or pituitary glands, such as pituitary adenoma or postpartum pituitary necrosis, may lower levels of TRH and TSH. This then results in diminished production of thyroid hormone. Other disorders associated with hypothyroidism include postpartum thyroiditis, acute suppurative thyroiditis, subacute (de Quervain) thyroiditis, and silent thyroiditis. Table 48.1 lists some causes of hypothyroidism.

CLINICAL MANIFESTATIONS

HISTORY

Symptoms of hypothyroidism include weakness, fatigue, weight gain, cold intolerance, constipation, dry skin, depression, and thinning hair. However, early hypothyroid symptoms may be subtle and overlooked by the patient. Women may complain of altered menstruation and infertility, and older patients may present with memory loss. Patients with long-standing hypothyroidism often experience a delay in thought, hoarse voice, muscle cramps, and a diminished acuity of taste, smell, or hearing.

Congenital hypothyroidism has a subtle presentation that may include feeding problems, a hoarse cry, jaundice, and constipation. Later findings include developmental delay, failure to thrive, short stature, and delayed dentition. Newborn screening for this condition has greatly reduced the sequelae of this condition in the United States.

TABLE 48-1. Causes of Hypothyroidism

Primary

Agenesis

Gland destruction

- Surgical removal
- Irradiation (therapeutic radioiodine, external irradiation)
- Autoimmune disease (Hashimoto thyroiditis)
- Idiopathic atrophy
- Infiltrative process

Inhibition of thyroid hormone synthesis and release

- Iodine deficiency
- Excess iodide in susceptible persons
- Drugs (e.g., Interferon alpha, lithium, amiodarone)

Transient

- Postsurgery or therapeutic radioiodine
- Postpartum thyroiditis

Secondary

Hypothalamic disease

Pituitary disease

- Infiltrative disorders
- Postpartum necrosis (Sheehan syndrome)
- Surgery or irradiation
- Trauma
- Adenomas

PHYSICAL EXAMINATION

Physical examination findings vary according to the degree of hypothyroidism. The general appearance can reveal coarse, dry hair, brittle nails, thinning of the outer halves of eyebrows, peripheral edema, and facial puffiness. Vital signs may show hypothermia, bradycardia, and normal-to-low BP. The neck should be evaluated for the presence of goiter, which may or may not be tender. Cardiovascular examination may reveal evidence of a pericardial effusion or cardiac enlargement. Deep tendon reflexes are usually prolonged, with a slow return phase. Rarely, a patient may present with myxedema coma, a life-threatening condition that includes mental status change, hypothermia, respiratory depression, and hypotension that is often precipitated by physiologic stress including infection, hypothermia, or surgery.

DIAGNOSTIC EVALUATION

TSH, which is synthesized and secreted by the pituitary gland, is the most sensitive indicator of hypothyroidism caused by thyroid dysfunction. It is elevated in patients with hypothyroidism except in the rare cases of central hypothyroidism, where the pituitary fails to secrete TSH. Both TSH and free T4 are low in cases of hypothalamic or pituitary dysfunction. In subclinical hypothyroidism, TSH is elevated, whereas free T4 is normal. High titers of thyroid antibodies are seen most commonly in those with Hashimoto thyroiditis, but they may be present in other conditions as well, such as subacute lymphocytic thyroiditis. Pituitary failure can be confirmed by the failure of TSH to respond to TRH stimulation. Patients with low TSH and low free T4 should have MRI to evaluate for abnormalities of the pituitary or hypothalamus.

Hypothyroid patients may have elevations of cholesterol, CPK, and liver enzymes. Anemia is present in 20% to 60% of patients with hypothyroidism. Anemia of chronic disease is the most common etiology, but one may see microcytic, macrocytic, or normocytic anemias in this population. Serum electrolytes occasionally show hyponatremia. The ECG and CXR may reveal findings consistent with a pericardial effusion.

TREATMENT

Hypothyroidism is gratifying to treat because of the ease and completeness with which it responds to treatment. Levothyroxine is nearly always the treatment of choice. Widely available and inexpensive, it is converted to T3 in the peripheral tissues at a rate similar to that seen in euthyroid individuals. Most patients require a daily dose between 75 and 150 µg. Older patients and those with cardiovascular disease are often very sensitive to thyroid replacement. In order to avoid precipitating an anginal attack or palpitations, these patients should be started on lower doses of levothyroxine, such as 25 µg, with incremental increases to therapeutic levels over 4 to 6 months. Thyroid levels in the hypothyroid newborn must be corrected quickly and maintained in order to avoid permanent damage. Dosages in this population are based on weight and age. Repeat TSH testing is recommended in 6 to 8 weeks and after a dosage change. After serum TSH normalizes with therapy, an annual TSH is recommended. Hypothyroidism in pregnancy is a special consideration. Typically, women with hypothyroidism who become pregnant require a 50% increase in their daily dose of levothyroxine continued until after delivery.

Patients with subclinical hypothyroidism have an elevated TSH and normal free T4 levels. These patients are at higher risk for subsequently developing hypothyroidism, especially if they have elevated anti-TPO antibodies. Therapy is initiated if the patient becomes symptomatic, if the TSH levels rise above 10 mIU/L, or if free T4 levels fall below normal. Treating patients with TSH levels between 5 and 10 mIU/L remains controversial. Treatment should be individualized on the basis of patient preference, symptoms, age, and associated medical conditions. Factors favoring treatment include younger age, symptoms consistent with hypothyroidism, abnormal lipids, a persistent and gradual increase in TSH, presence of antithyroid antibodies, and/or an enlarged thyroid.

Myxedema coma is a medical emergency associated with a high rate of mortality. Intravenous levothyroxine and steroids, and treatment of the underlying cause along with respiratory and hemodynamic support in an intensive care unit are the mainstays of treatment.

KEY POINTS

- Hypothyroidism occurs in about 1% to 3% of the population and affects people of all ages, including newborns and the elderly.

- Symptoms of hypothyroidism include weakness, fatigue, cold intolerance, constipation, dry skin, depression, weight gain, and thinning hair.

- Physical examination findings often reveal coarse, dry hair, brittle nails, thinning of the outer halves of eyebrows, peripheral edema, and facial puffiness.

- The two most common causes are thyroid gland failure caused by Hashimoto thyroiditis and hypothyroidism secondary to surgery or radiation therapy.

- TSH, which is synthesized and secreted by the pituitary gland, is the most sensitive indicator of hypothyroidism due to thyroid dysfunction.

49 | Obesity

Obesity is characterized by the presence of excessively large amounts of adipose tissue. The preferred method to assess obesity is to use a measure known as the body mass index (BMI). BMI is calculated by dividing the weight in kilograms by the height in meters squared. The BMI has the advantage of being independent of gender and frame size and serves as a surrogate measure of body fat. Using BMI, **overweight** in adults is defined as **BMI of 25 to 29.9 kg/m²**, and **obesity** as a **BMI >30 kg/m²**. **Morbid or extreme obesity is defined as a BMI >40 kg/m².** In the United States, approximately 35% of men and 40% of women meet the criteria for obesity. Unfortunately, the percentage of obese Americans is increasing (Fig. 49-1), particularly among children and adolescents.

Several studies suggest that central obesity may be associated with more adverse health conditions than lower body obesity. Central obesity can be determined by calculating a waist-to-hip ratio. Central obesity is present if the waist-to-hip ratio is >0.85 in women and 1.0 in men. Because of its impact on health, obesity is a leading cause of preventable death, with minority groups disproportionately affected.

PATHOGENESIS

People gain weight when the caloric intake exceeds the body's energy expenditure. The reason why an individual's caloric intake exceeds demand is complex and represents a heterogeneous disorder

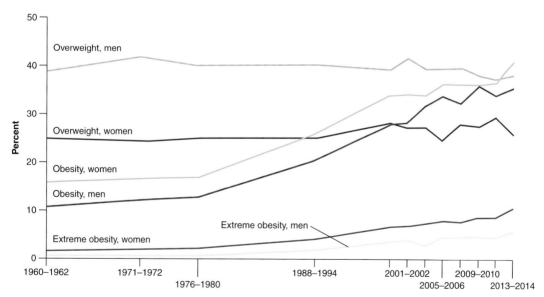

FIGURE 49-1. Trends in adult overweight, obesity, and extreme obesity for men and women aged 20 to 74: United States, 1960 to 2014. (From Frayer C, Carroll M. Ogden C. Prevalence of overweight, obesity, and extreme obesity among adults aged 20 and over. 2016. https://www.cdc.gov/nchs/data/hestat/obesity_adult_13_14/obesity_adult_13_14.htm.)

reflecting genetic, socioeconomic, and environmental influences. Clinically, physicians should view obesity as a chronic metabolic disease with serious health consequences rather than solely as a cosmetic or behavioral problem.

The current American social environment has contributed to the increased incidence of obesity. Many individuals have sedentary jobs and lifestyles that reduce or eliminate calorie-burning activities. More people can afford to eat at restaurants, where large portions of high-calorie foods contribute to added weight. In addition to environmental and social influences, some individuals overeat in response to emotional stress or have become conditioned to eat not for sustenance but for the pleasure associated with various activities (e.g., watching television and movies and attending parties).

Studies of identical twins indicate that energy expenditure and fat distribution appear to be influenced by heredity. Leptin is an appetite-controlling hormone that is also thought to play a role in obesity. It is secreted by fat cells and may signal the hypothalamus with a measure of the level of stored fat. There have been cases of obese individuals having mutations of the leptin gene or decreased sensitivity to leptin levels. Ghrelin is another hormone that influences appetite. Produced by the stomach, it modulates appetite control and is secreted when the stomach is empty. In a few cases, genetic syndromes such as Prader–Willi syndrome cause obesity. These syndromes are usually identified in childhood.

Research has suggested that the intestinal microbiome may influence weight. Gut flora appears to differ between lean and obese individuals and may affect metabolism. The clinical relevance of these findings remains uncertain.

There is evidence that the body regulates its weight around a certain weight or set point. The body defends the set point by adjusting the metabolic rate, and one theory proposes that obese patients regulate their weight around a higher set point. Some experts believe that physical activity and the amount of dietary fat may help modify this set point. Despite advances in understanding the pathophysiology of obesity, it is unlikely that these advances will lead to significant improvements in treatment in the near future.

CLINICAL MANIFESTATIONS

HISTORY

Obese patients generally have symptoms related to decreased exercise tolerance or to illnesses associated

BOX 49-1. Conditions Associated with Obesity

Cancer of the uterus, breast, prostate, and colon	Coronary disease
Degenerative arthritis	Diabetes
Fatty liver	Gallbladder disease
Gout	Hyperlipidemia
Hypertension	Increased operative risk
Low back pain	Reflux esophagitis
Sleep apnea	Low self-esteem
Thromboembolic disease	Intertrigo

with obesity. Box 49-1 lists some health conditions associated with obesity. In addition, obese individuals may suffer from psychological impairments, such as poor self-image or social isolation.

The history should also include information about current diet, previous diets attempted and their outcome, motivation to lose weight, and knowledge about health and diet. It is also important to ask about mood disorders and psychiatric history, including binge eating, night eating syndrome, bulimia, and depression.

PHYSICAL EXAMINATION

The physical examination should include the patient's BP, height, weight, and BMI. Although anthropomorphic measures are important, visual assessment of the patient is generally accurate—that is, if the patient *looks* overweight, then he or she is overweight. In addition, signs of obesity-influenced conditions should be sought and an assessment made of the patient's mobility.

DIFFERENTIAL DIAGNOSIS

Obesity can be either primary or secondary. Secondary causes of obesity account for <1% of cases. Medicines associated with weight gain include tricyclic antidepressants, beta blockers, phenothiazines, glucocorticoids, oral contraceptives, sulfonylureas, and insulin.

Neuroendocrine problems such as hypothyroidism, Cushing syndrome, and hypothalamic disease can also cause obesity. Genetic disorders causing obesity are extremely rare and are usually clinically evident in childhood.

DIAGNOSTIC EVALUATION

Few tests are routinely indicated in the obese patient. Laboratory evaluation depends on the individual and his or her age, but should usually include a fasting blood glucose and lipid profile. Liver enzymes can be evaluated to screen for nonalcoholic steatohepatitis (fatty liver disease). A TSH is helpful in cases of suspected hypothyroidism.

TREATMENT

Individuals must be motivated to lose weight and to make lifestyle changes in diet and exercise. Poorly motivated patients are unlikely to adhere to a weight loss program.

Treatment options include diet, exercise, drugs, and surgery. The degree of obesity and the presence of associated illness should influence management strategies. Conservative therapy relying on diet and exercise forms the basis of most weight loss programs. High-cost programs or hazardous procedures such as surgery should be reserved for morbidly obese patients and those at greatest risk from obesity who have failed more conservative treatment.

Most obese people would like to achieve an "ideal body weight." Unfortunately, short of surgery, most diet, exercise, or drug programs result in about a 10% weight loss. For many individuals, the goal might be to achieve a healthful weight rather than an ideal weight. Even modest weight reduction (5% to 10%) can be clinically significant, especially in obese individuals with diabetes or hypertension. Emphasizing realistic goals and then reinforcing them can help prevent failure, which would only contribute further to poor self-esteem. Sometimes preventing further weight gain may be the most appropriate goal for an individual who is unwilling or unable to lose weight.

Ideally, the patient and the physician should work together to create a nutritionally sound diet that incorporates the patient's food preferences. A dietitian can also be helpful in planning a diet.

Avoiding behaviors associated with obesity such as the consumption of restaurant and fast food, large portion sizes, and sugar-added beverages is standard advice. Conversely, behaviors associated with weight loss such as an increased intake of fruits, vegetables, and eating a healthy breakfast should be recommended. Weight is a product of energy balance, and the loss of 1 lb of fat requires a 3500-calorie deficit. Therefore, a calorie deficit of 500 to 1000 calories per day will result in a weight loss of 1 to 2 lb/week, which is appropriate for most patients. Gradual dietary changes tend to produce better, longer-lasting results. Simple suggestions include eating three meals a day, eating only at mealtimes, and limiting portions to one serving. Reducing dietary fat to 20% to 30% of total calories also enhances weight loss and is consistent with recommendations to reduce the risk of cardiac disease. Low-carbohydrate diets are more acceptable to many patients because of the increased satiety associated with them. Low-carbohydrate diets have achieved better short-term weight loss, but long-term results are comparable to those with traditional low-fat calorie-restricted diets. Very low-calorie, medically supervised diets have a limited role in management and are usually reserved for the morbidly obese or individuals at very high risk, such as those with sleep apnea. A minimum of 800 calories per day is recommended. Risks for very low-calorie diets include cardiac arrhythmias and gallstones. Exercise alone, without calorie restriction, is not an efficient weight loss strategy. However, exercise enhances overall health, improves waist-to-hip ratio, and helps to keep an individual's metabolic rate from resetting during periods of caloric restriction. Studies show that people who exercise regularly with an expenditure of 2000 kcal/week are more likely to maintain weight loss.

Exercise is most likely to be sustained if it is something that the patient enjoys and can fit into his or her lifestyle. Opportunities should be explored to integrate exercise into daily activities whenever possible, such as climbing stairs instead of taking the elevator. Even if exercise produces only minimal weight loss, it still improves cardiovascular risk factors, and obese patients with good fitness levels have been shown to have a reduced mortality risk from cardiovascular disease compared to lean but unfit individuals.

Drug therapy should be considered for morbidly obese individuals or those with significant obesity-related comorbidities. It should be provided only as an adjunct to diet and exercise. Medications include appetite suppressants such as phentermine. Side effects include insomnia, hypertension, tachycardia, nausea, diarrhea, and anxiety. Amphetamines and amphetamine-like products are rarely used because of their side effects and addictive potential.

Orlistat is a GI lipase inhibitor that interferes with fat absorption. It appears to be modestly effective, with a mean difference in weight loss of 2.9 kg. Side effects are triggered by dietary indiscretions and primarily affect the GI tract; they include oily stools, diarrhea, and leakage of stool. Symptoms usually improve with time and adherence to a low-fat diet.

Lorcaserin is a 5-HT$_{2C}$ receptor agonist. It works on the receptors in the brain and provides satiety, which leads to weight loss.

Surgery for obesity, such as gastric stapling, should be reserved for patients with morbid refractory obesity. Although it is the most effective treatment, its cost and risks of serious complication, including fat embolus, hemorrhage, and even death, limits its use to patients with a BMI >40 kg/m^2 or those with a BMI between 30 and 39 kg/m^2 and significant comorbidities. In these individuals, bariatric surgery is associated with reduced mortality, better long-term weight loss, reduction in comorbidities, and improved fertility in women. Liposuction can remove localized deposits of fat by the use of a suction probe.

Childhood obesity is increasing, and children who are overweight by age 6 are at much greater risk for being obese as adults than are other children. Involvement of the parents in managing the diet and activity of younger children is essential. Often, slowing weight gain is the goal, so that the child can grow out of the obesity. In adolescents, the degree of parental involvement should be individualized. Schools may also represent an important opportunity for preventing childhood obesity. Programs aimed at decreasing television and video viewing time, increased physical activity, healthy eating, and eliminating sugar-sweetened beverage intake have shown some success in decreasing the prevalence of obesity.

KEY POINTS

- BMI is the weight in kilograms divided by the height in meters squared. BMI is independent of gender and frame size.
- Obesity is defined as a BMI >30 kg/m^2. Morbid or extreme obesity is defined as a BMI >40 kg/m^2.
- Obesity is a heterogeneous disorder reflecting genetic, socioeconomic, behavioral, and environmental influences.
- The loss of 1 lb of fat requires a 3500-calorie deficit.

50 | Oral Health

Oral health contributes to an individual's overall health, and its importance is often underappreciated by physicians. Poor access to dental care contributes to oral health disparities and The Health Resources and Services Administration (HRSA) recommends expanding clinical competency in oral health to primary care clinicians, who should be able to appropriately manage, educate, prevent, and refer basic conditions. This chapter provides an overview of some common outpatient oral health issues.

XEROSTOMIA

Xerostomia or "dry mouth" is a common and troubling problem. Xerostomia is not a disease; instead, it is a symptom of an underlying process. Prevalence varies depending on the population examined but is estimated at between 12% and 20% and may be as high as 50% in patients over age 65.

PATHOPHYSIOLOGY

Saliva lubricates the oral mucosa and is important for eating, swallowing, speaking, digestion, taste, and maintaining good dentition. Although composed primarily of water, saliva contains electrolytes that help support the enamel and IgA, which fights infection. Decreased saliva flow rates increase the risk of both tooth decay and respiratory infection.

Salivary glands secrete less saliva with age, and as people age they are also at greater risk for diseases or for taking medications that adversely affect salivary gland function. Dryness is subjective and the complaint of dry mouth is not always associated with decreased salivary flow. Pseudoxerostomia occurs when patients subjectively complain of dryness despite objective measures of normal saliva flow. Sjogren syndrome is an autoimmune disorder that damages the salivary glands accompanied by a systemic autoimmune disorder such as rheumatoid arthritis.

HISTORY

In addition to dryness, patients may complain of difficulty eating, speaking, swallowing, or discomfort wearing dentures. Dry mouth and dry eyes characterize Sjogren syndrome, and patients complain of itchy or gritty eyes. Several medications affect salivation, making it important to take a detailed medication history. Radiation therapy damages salivary glands and can cause severe xerostomia; most patients undergoing chemotherapy also suffer from some degree of xerostomia.

PHYSICAL EXAMINATION

The mucous membranes may appear dry and the lips fissured. Sjogren syndrome may cause salivary gland enlargement, and patients can have findings related to an associated connective tissue disease. Physical findings include the consequences of xerostomia, including poor dentition, halitosis, and fungal infections.

DIFFERENTIAL DIAGNOSIS

Dry mouth is most commonly related to medications and far less often to a connective tissue disorder. Drugs with anticholinergic activity (e.g., diphenhydramine, oxybutynin) are notorious for causing dry mouth. Dry mouth is also associated with vitamin deficiencies (especially B complex), Parkinson disease, diabetes, and hypercalcemia. Individuals with depression or an anxiety disorder frequently experience dry mouth. Local factors that can cause xerostomia include damage to the salivary glands from radiation therapy and, less commonly, sialoadenitis, sialolithiasis, oral neoplasms, and acute infections. Smoking and alcohol inhibit saliva secretion.

TREATMENT

Discontinuing or adjusting the dose of medications suspected of contributing to dry mouth may improve symptoms. Table 50.1 lists medications commonly associated with xerostomia. Education about proper oral hygiene to avoid dental complications and counseling that smoking and alcohol contribute to dryness are important. Patient education also includes advice to avoid dry foods such as crackers and to chew gum and/or to suck on lozenges (e.g., lemon drops) to stimulate saliva production. Maintaining good hydration, taking frequent sips of water, and sucking on ice cubes can also be of benefit. In persistent and more severe cases, lubricating agents such as Biotene or other saliva substitutes help some patients. Several cholinergic sialagogues are available by prescription, but many patients do not tolerate these drugs because of troublesome side effects.

TEMPOROMANDIBULAR JOINT DYSFUNCTION

Temporomandibular joint dysfunction (TJD) affects 20% to 30% of the adult population, with a peak incidence from age 20 to 40. Symptoms are twice as common in women as in men. After toothache, TJD is the second most common cause of orofacial pain. Although not life threatening, TJD can significantly impact a patient's quality of life.

PATHOPHYSIOLOGY

The temporomandibular joint (TMJ) is a synovial joint connecting the mandible to the temporal bone of the skull. It allows both hinge and sliding movements that enable individuals to chew, swallow, and speak. Pain may occur with arthritic disorders, such as degenerative joint disease, or from trauma, which damage the joint or its supporting structures. In most cases, the source of TJD pain and underlying etiology remain uncertain but are probably caused by

TABLE 50.1. Medications Associated with Dry Mouth

| Diuretics |
| Phenothiazines |
| Opioids |
| Antihistamines |
| Anticholinergics |
| Antidepressants |
| Benzodiazepines |

complex interactions involving the muscles, nerves, myofascial tissue, and joint. Abnormal occlusion, teeth clenching, grinding, and stress can contribute to joint and myofascial inflammation and painful muscle spasm. Other factors associated with TJD include fibromyalgia, sleep apnea, depression, and anxiety.

HISTORY

The most important feature of the history is an ache in the muscles of mastication aggravated by chewing and other joint motion. Many patients complain of jaw clicking or popping and, occasionally, limited motion. In some instances, the pain radiates to the neck or shoulder. Inquiring about trauma such as a whiplash injury, nighttime teeth grinding, jaw clenching, or excessive chewing is important because these can contribute to TJD.

PHYSICAL EXAMINATION

Examination includes palpation of the TMJ and surrounding structures. Patients may exhibit limited range of motion and tenderness when palpating the jaw muscles. Some patients have distinct joint clicking and popping that can be felt or heard when opening their jaw. However, clicking does not always correlate with the degree of pain and functional limitation. Up to 50% of asymptomatic individuals make clicking, popping, or grating sounds with jaw movement.

Other structures near the TMJ can cause pain and mimic TJD. An ear examination, palpating for temporal artery tenderness, and checking for dental problems such as diseased wisdom teeth are parts of a thorough evaluation.

DIFFERENTIAL DIAGNOSIS

The differential diagnosis of TJD includes joint disease, temporal arteritis, ear infections, dental disease, salivary gland disorders, partial dislocation, and malocclusion. The clinical evaluation is typically sufficient for excluding other diagnoses. Usually only severe or chronic symptoms merit diagnostic imaging or other testing.

TREATMENT

For most patients, TJD improves over time with or without treatment. As many as 50% improve within 1 year and 85% are symptom free within 3 years. As a result, noninvasive treatments are the mainstay of treatment and need sufficient time to work. Invasive or permanent treatments are considered a last resort.

Reassurance and education are important first steps for patients with new or intermittent symptoms.

Avoiding gum chewing, cutting smaller bite sizes when eating, and consuming softer foods such as cooked rather than raw carrots often improve symptoms. Some patients benefit from occlusive devices such as a splint or mouth guards worn at night. Physical modalities such as heat or cold frequently improve symptoms, and some individuals benefit from relaxation techniques to help reduce muscle spasm. Pharmacologic treatment with NSAIDs or acetaminophen may provide relief to those who fail to respond to nonpharmacologic therapy. Muscle relaxants, benzodiazepines, and tricyclic antidepressants may help if more conservative treatments fail. Alternative medicine modalities such as acupuncture and biofeedback benefit some patients.

Severe and persistent cases that fail to respond to conservative management frequently benefit from referral to a dentist or other provider specializing in TJD.

PERIODONTITIS

Periodontal disease is a common problem affecting 10% to 15% of the adult population. In addition to being the most common cause of tooth loss, periodontitis is associated with systemic conditions such as atherosclerosis and diabetes. Individuals with periodontitis may not seek regular dental care but might see a primary care physician for a medical complaint, providing an opportunity to educate patients about prevention and to identify patients needing referral.

PATHOPHYSIOLOGY

Periodontitis is an inflammatory disease caused by a chronic microbial infection characterized by irreversible damage to the bone, ligaments, and soft tissue supporting the teeth. Inflammation of the supporting tissues without permanent damage to the attached ligament or bone differentiates gingivitis from periodontitis. Whereas gingivitis does not always progress to periodontitis, it usually precedes periodontitis. The microbial infection of periodontal disease triggers an inflammatory cascade that increases inflammatory markers systemically, which may explain the association of periodontal disease and systemic diseases such as atherosclerosis.

HISTORY

Bleeding gums, bad breath, and painful chewing are symptoms of periodontal disease. Assessing contributing factors such as smoking, diabetes, and infrequent or absent dental care are important.

PHYSICAL EXAMINATION

Common findings include inflamed, receding, swollen, or bleeding gums and loose or absent teeth.

DIFFERENTIAL DIAGNOSIS

Patients need dental referral to confirm the diagnosis and to assess disease severity by probing the depths of the pocket between the tooth and the gum. Radiographs to assess bone loss may augment clinical examination.

TREATMENT

Family physicians need to recognize the important role of periodontal disease in overall health and to provide prevention education and referral. Good dental hygiene disrupts the biofilm that contributes to polymicrobial infection and consists of brushing for 2 minutes twice a day, daily flossing, and the use of an antiplaque mouthwash. Routine dental checkups to prevent, diagnose, and treat periodontitis are important. Family physicians contribute to treatment by counseling about smoking cessation, improving glycemic control, and avoiding drugs that inhibit salivary flow.

ODONTOGENIC (DENTAL) PAIN

Patients with dental pain may present to their family physician, and it is important to be able to provide appropriate care and referral. The most common cause is a toothache from pain arising from the teeth and/or their support structures. The primary physician needs to be able to assess severity, to make an appropriate and timely referral, and to rule out nondental causes for the pain.

PATHOPHYSIOLOGY

Odontogenic pain is pain arising from teeth or their supportive structures. Teeth are calcified structures covered by enamel and dentin with an inner core structure (the pulp) that contains blood vessels and nerves. The pain usually results from tooth decay, infection, or injury that irritates the nerve in the tooth root.

Tooth enamel lacks innervation. In its initial stages, tooth decay affects the surface enamel and tends to be painless. However, if decay deepens into the dentin, hot, cold, or sweet substances can cause pain. In early stages, the pain may be poorly localized and is one reason why a patient might seek medical rather than dental care. Unchecked decay results in pulpitis, an inflammation and infection of the pulp. If the pulp is completely damaged, the pain may subside until the infection extends beyond the tooth into the adjacent soft tissues, causing edema, redness, and pain. Spread through the soft tissues can cause a severe cervical or facial cellulitis.

Since dentin responds to stimuli, some patients with gingival recession and exposed dentin experience dentin hypersensitivity triggered by cold, sweet, or spicy foods, and brushing. Unlike pulpitis, the pain of dentin sensitivity tends to be shorter and less severe.

HISTORY

Tooth sensitivity to heat, cold pressure, and pain with chewing suggests a dental cause of pain. Inquiring about recent trauma or dental work is important. A nondental pain source often involves multiple teeth and pain centered either above or below the jaw. Asking about sinus symptoms, cardiac disease, and TJD helps rule out a nondental cause. Sharp, severe, intermittent pain along the trigeminal nerve suggests trigeminal neuralgia. Recurrent, self-healing painful ulcerations suggest aphthous stomatitis.

PHYSICAL EXAMINATION

The clinical examination usually identifies whether orofacial pain is dental or nondental. The examination includes palpating the TMJ and careful examination of the ears, sinuses, and salivary glands. The oral cavity should be inspected for poor dentition, fractured or missing teeth, stomatitis, and gum ulcerations. Facial swelling, fever, tenderness, redness, and fluctuance along the gumline suggest an abscess or cellulitis.

The presence of multiple painful oral vesicles and fever suggests a primary viral stomatitis. Primary herpes stomatitis is the most common viral stomatitis affecting mainly children and is characterized by painful ulcers on the buccal mucosa and gums. Herpangina, caused by Coxsackie A virus, also causes painful ulcerations but usually to the soft palate and anterior pillar of the mouth and not the oral mucosa. A secondary herpes infection or cold sore most commonly forms at the vermillion border. Aphthous ulcers, also known as canker sores, are recurrent, benign, and noncontagious ulcerations that appear on oral mucosal surfaces but spare the hard palate and gums.

DIFFERENTIAL DIAGNOSIS

The key role for the physician is to determine whether the pain is odontogenic or from a nondental cause. The most common nondental causes are TJD or maxillary sinusitis. Less common causes include salivary gland disorders, neuralgias, aphthous ulcers, viral stomatitis, cluster headaches, and, rarely, neoplasms. A careful history and physical examination usually point to these conditions. Radiographs help identify mandibular disorders such as an osteomyelitis, bone cyst, or bone infarction. Dental disorders include caries, pulpitis, dentin hypersensitivity, and alveolar osteitis. Alveolar osteitis is a complication following tooth extraction (usually a wisdom tooth), in which a blood clot either does not form or dislodges from the socket, exposing the bone below. The pain is moderate to severe, throbbing, and localized to the socket.

Ludwig angina is a rare but potentially life-threatening bacterial facial space infection that usually stems from an infected back molar. It typically presents with a sore throat, and, as it spreads, painful neck swelling can progress and cause dysphagia, drooling, severe pain and lead to airway obstruction.

TREATMENT

Treatment depends on the underlying cause and if dental related, needs referral for definitive treatment such as tooth restoration, a root canal, extraction, or abscess drainage. Prescribing an NSAID provides pain management while arranging for definitive treatment. Dental pain alone is not an indication for antibiotic therapy, and antibiotics should be reserved for those with adjacent soft-tissue swelling or fluctuance. Penicillin or, if allergic to penicillin, clindamycin provides adequate microbial coverage. Patients who appear toxic with facial swelling, trismus, fever, and drooling merit hospitalization, intravenous antibiotics, and consultation with an oral surgeon. Dry sockets respond to warm gargles and antibiotic mouthwashes and usually resolve in 2 to 6 weeks.

Most patients with aphthous stomatitis have minor symptoms and do not require specific therapy other than to avoid spicy foods and acidic beverages that trigger discomfort. Topical Orabase, a paste that adheres to the oral mucosa to form a protective barrier, is available in combination with benzocaine to reduce the pain. In more severe cases, combining Orabase with a topical steroid adds benefit.

Treatment for viral stomatitis consists of maintaining good fluid intake, good oral hygiene, and pain management with an NSAID or acetaminophen. Some physicians recommend a soothing mouthwash preparation, such as an antacid combined with diphenhydramine, lidocaine, and hydrocortisone. Sucking on popsicles can reduce pain and help maintain adequate fluid intake. In healthy individuals, the lesions heal spontaneously in 1 to 2 weeks, but severe cases may require parenteral fluids.

KEY POINTS

- Oral health contributes to an individual's overall health, and its importance is often underappreciated by physicians.

- Xerostomia is a symptom of an underlying process. Prevalence varies depending on the population examined but is estimated between 12% and 20% and may be as high as 50% in patients over age 65.

- Dry mouth is most commonly related to medications especially drugs with anticholinergic activity (e.g., diphenhydramine, oxybutynin).

- TJD affects 20% to 30% of the adult population, with a peak incidence from age 20 to 40.

- For most patients, TJD improves over time with or without treatment. As many as 50% improve within 1 year and 85% are symptom free within 3 years. Invasive treatments should be avoided.

- Periodontitis affects 10% to 15% of adults and is an inflammatory disease caused by a chronic microbial infection. It is characterized by irreversible damage to the bone, ligaments, and soft tissue supporting.

- Odontogenic pain is a pain arising from teeth or their supportive structures.

51 | Osteoporosis

Osteoporosis is a reduction in bone mass per unit of volume with microarchitectural deterioration of bone tissue that compromises bone strength and increases susceptibility to fracture. It is seen primarily in elderly individuals.

EPIDEMIOLOGY

As the population in the United States has aged, the number of individuals with osteoporosis has grown to over 10 million, with an additional 34 million individuals at high risk for developing this condition. Most of these are women (80%); one in two women will have an osteoporosis-related fracture over her lifetime; and by age 75, one out of three white women will suffer an osteoporotic hip fracture. Although the incidence among men is lower, one in four men over age 50 will have an osteoporosis-related fracture over his lifetime. Osteoporosis is responsible for 1.5 million fractures each year, with an annual cost of over $17 billion. Approximately 10% to 20% of patients who suffer a hip fracture die of a medical complication within 6 months of the fracture, and those who survive are often unable to live independently.

PATHOGENESIS

The resorption and formation of bone is a continuous process. Under steady state, these processes are equal and linked. At around age 35, bone mass peaks, and both genders begin to lose bone mass after age 40. Estrogen receptors are present on osteoblasts, the cells that form bone, which may explain why estrogen-deficient states result in bone loss. There also appears to be an uncoupling of osteoblasts from the action of osteoclasts, the cells that resorb bone. Several different chemical modulators may mediate this uncoupling, but the precise mechanisms for developing osteoporosis have not yet been determined.

Osteoporosis can be either primary or secondary to an underlying disease, such as hyperparathyroidism. Primary osteoporosis is an age-related bone disorder that results from aging and changes in sex hormones. It consists of two types: Type I osteoporosis, or postmenopausal osteoporosis, is associated with declines in estrogen and typically develops between the ages of 50 and 70. It primarily affects trabecular bone and is due to increased osteoclast activity. Trabecular bone is present in the hip, vertebrae, distal radius, and heel. Type II osteoporosis, or senile osteoporosis, involves loss of both cortical and trabecular bones and primarily affects individuals over age 70. Type II changes appear to correlate with age-related decreases in calcium absorption and decreases in vitamin D absorption and synthesis. The effects of types I and II osteoporosis are additive and most individuals with osteoporosis have elements of both types. Secondary osteoporosis can be caused by many medical conditions and a variety of medicines, particularly glucocorticoids.

CLINICAL MANIFESTATIONS

HISTORY

Patients with osteoporosis are generally asymptomatic. However, chronic pain and tenderness over the affected area may occur, particularly in association with osteoporotic fractures. The bones most commonly affected by osteoporotic fractures are the spine, hip, and distal radius. It is important to elicit other symptoms that may occur as complications of osteoporosis. For example, a vertebral fracture may result in spinal cord compression and neurologic findings. Osteoporosis of facet joints may also contribute to back pain.

History is useful to identify those patients with risk factors for osteoporosis. These risk factors can be grouped into several different categories: (1) genetic: Caucasian or Asian ethnicity, small stature, and a family history of osteoporosis; (2) lifestyle: tobacco, alcohol, and caffeine consumption, lack of physical activity; (3) nutritional: low calcium and vitamin D intake; and (4) other risk factors such as older age and postmenopausal state.

PHYSICAL EXAMINATION

On physical examination, height reduction >1.5 inches, dorsal kyphosis (dowager or widow hump) (Fig. 51-1), exaggerated cervical lordosis, gait deficits, and low body weight are common findings associated with osteoporosis. Dorsal kyphosis is due to wedge-shaped deformity in the middorsal vertebrae. Because of the risk of spinal cord compression, it is important to perform a complete neurologic examination to rule out neurologic involvement from an osteoporotic fracture.

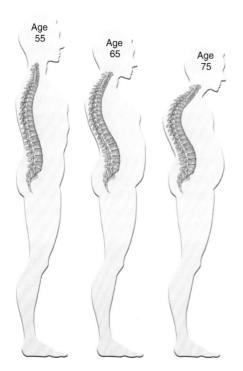

Progressive Spinal Deformity in Osteoporosis
Osteoporosis weakens the bones, which can lead to fractures of the vertebrae. The vertebral fractures lead to loss of height and to kyphosis (humpback). Although vertebral fractures may be painful, the majority occur without any symptoms. Individuals may be aware only of deformity and progressive loss of height.

FIGURE 51-1. Osteoporotic kyphoscoliosis. (From Anatomical Chart Company. *Understand Osteoporosis Anatomical Chart*. Alphen aan den Rijn, The Netherlands: Wolters Kluwer; 2002.)

DIFFERENTIAL DIAGNOSIS

Although osteoporosis is commonly age related, other diseases or conditions may secondarily cause osteoporosis. These can be divided into five different categories (Box 51-1). Identification and treatment of these underlying diseases can limit bone loss. Glucocorticoid-induced disease is the most common cause of secondary osteoporosis. When the disease or condition is not modifiable, as in patients requiring chronic corticosteroids, the use of preventive medicines such as a bisphosphonate (e.g., alendronate) may help prevent bone loss.

BOX 51-1. Secondary Causes of Osteoporosis

Endocrine
Acromegaly
Diabetes mellitus
Cushing disease
Hyperparathyroidism
Hypogonadism
Hyperthyroidism

Nutritional
Malabsorption
Malnutrition
Anorexia nervosa
Liver disease
Vitamin D deficiency
Alcoholism

Collagen Vascular
Rheumatoid arthritis
Ehlers–Danlos syndrome
Marfan syndrome
Osteoporosis imperfecta

Cancer
Multiple myeloma
Bone metastases
Breast cancer
Lymphoma
Leukemia

Medications
Glucosteroid
Phenobarbital
Phenytoin
Heparin
Methotrexate
Excess thyroid hormone replacement

DIAGNOSTIC EVALUATION

Patients at risk for developing osteoporosis are candidates for screening. These include (1) postmenopausal women below 65 years of age with one or more risk factors besides menopause; (2) all postmenopausal women over age 65; (3) postmenopausal women with a history of fractures; (4) those who are on long-term corticosteroid treatment; and (5) some but not all groups recommend screening for men over age 70. In addition, those who are considering treatments or preventive measures for osteoporosis may benefit from information gained through screening. For patients with normal results, the frequency of repeat screening is uncertain but screening at 4-year intervals is recommended by some experts. Patients being treated for osteoporosis require repeat testing to assess therapy though the frequency of repeat testing is uncertain. Measurement of bone mineral density (BMD) is the standard method for screening and establishing the diagnosis of osteoporosis. Dual energy x-ray absorptiometry (DEXA) is the preferred method for confirming the diagnosis and monitoring therapy because it represents the best combination of sensitivity, technical simplicity, reproducibility, and cost while also minimizing radiation exposure. When using DEXA to determine the effects of therapy, the same machine should be used, if possible, in order to limit variations in measurements between different DEXA scanners. BMD determinations of both the spine and hip provide the best assessments, since the degree of osteoporosis can differ between sites.

The BMD report provides a T score and Z score. The T score compares the patient's BMD with that of a normal adult 25 to 30 years of age and of the same gender. The Z score compares the patient's BMD with that of the same age group and gender. Osteoporosis is defined as a T score of >2.5 standard deviations below the mean (-2.5 SD). Osteopenia, or low bone mass, is defined as a T score between -1.0 and -2.5. Z scores of -1.5 suggest a secondary cause of osteoporosis. The risk for an osteoporotic fracture increases two- to fourfold for every standard deviation in reduced BMD.

In addition to a DEXA scan, blood tests are useful for identifying and managing secondary cases of osteoporosis. Initial tests consist of a CBC, ESR, 25-hydroxy vitamin D; chemistry panel including serum calcium, phosphorus, and alkaline phosphatase, and renal function. Calcium and phosphate measurements help detect hyperparathyroidism and vitamin D deficiencies. In patients with anemia and an elevated ESR, multiple myeloma should be considered. Electrolyte abnormalities can identify patients with chronic acidosis or renal tubular acidosis. Serum alkaline phosphatase is a marker of osteoblastic activity and is elevated in malignancy, hyperparathyroidism, and other high-turnover states. More selective tests such as a 24-hour urine calcium test or parathyroid hormone (PTH) levels should be selectively ordered based on history, physical examination, and preliminary laboratory findings.

TREATMENT

The first line of prevention for osteoporosis is lifestyle changes, whereas pharmaceutical agents are the first line of treatment for osteoporosis. Smoking cessation, avoiding excess alcohol, weightbearing exercise, and improved dietary habits help preserve bone mass. It is recommended that calcium intake exceed 1000 mg/day for premenopausal women and 1500 mg/day for postmenopausal women. Vitamin D supplementation increases bone density in patients with an established deficiency. Vitamin D deficiency has also been associated with cardiovascular disease, diabetes, autoimmune disease, and some types of cancer. In vitamin D deficient individuals stores should be normalized with supplementation over a period of 2 to 3 months with repeat testing to assure adequate levels. As patients age, the risk of falls increases and fall prevention is another priority for reducing the number of osteoporotic fractures. Improving vision, adjusting sedative medications, and incorporating balance exercises are beneficial. Environmental adjustments such as minimizing clutter, anchoring rugs, adding handrails, and better lighting in dark hallways help prevent falls.

Pharmaceutical therapy for osteoporosis should be considered for individuals with a BMD T score below -2.5 without risk factors or T score below -1.5 with multiple risk factors, women above age 70 with multiple risk factors, and patients undergoing long-term corticosteroid treatment. Preventive therapy for osteopenia should be provided to those with T score values below -1.0. Bisphosphonates are the preferred first line of therapy and Table 51-1 also lists other medications available for treatment. The bisphosphonates must be taken on an empty stomach with a large glass of water, with the patient remaining upright without eating for at least 30 minutes. More convenient formulations that

TABLE 51-1. General Guidelines for Pharmacologic Agents

Agent	Benefits	Contraindications
Hormone replacement therapy (HRT)	Inhibits bone reabsorption in estrogen-deficient patients	Breast cancer
		Estrogen-dependent neoplasm
	Control vasomotor symptoms	Undiagnosed vaginal bleeding
		History of thromboembolic disorder
		History of migraine
		Low HDL
Bisphosphonates	Inhibits bone resorption	Gastric ulcer (oral formulations)
		Abnormal esophageal motility (oral formulations)
		Unable to sit upright for 30 min (oral formulations)
Calcitonins	Most effective in spine	Allergy to salmon protein
	Analgesic effect in back pain	Unable to tolerate nasal spray
SERM (Selective estrogen receptor modulators, e.g., raloxifene, tamoxifen)	Patients with contraindications to HRT use	Vasomotor symptoms not relieved
	Decreased total and LDL cholesterol	
	Not affecting HDL	History of thromboembolic disorder
Human monoclonal antibody	Effective for preventing vertebral and nonvertebral fractures	Twice a year subcutaneous injections; most expensive
Human recombinant PTH	Effective for preventing both vertebral and nonvertebral fractures	Daily subcutaneous injection; can cause hypercalcemia or hyperuricemia

HDL, high density lipoprotein; HRT, hormone replacement therapy; LDL, low density lipoprotein; PTH, parathyroid hormone; SERM, selective estrogen receptor modulator.

allow these medicines to be administered orally, intravenously or SQ in single weekly, monthly, quarterly, or annual doses make therapy easier. Common side effects include stomach pain, nausea, and musculoskeletal pain. Osteonecrosis of the jaw or atypical femoral fractures are very rare but serious side effects. These side effects occur primarily in patients with metastatic cancer or multiple myeloma on high-dose therapy for longer durations. Thus, cessation of bisphosphonate therapy after 5 years should be considered in those without a history of fractures.

KEY POINTS

- Osteoporosis is a reduction in bone mass per unit of volume that is seen primarily in older individuals.
- Approximately 20% of patients who suffer a hip fracture die within a year of the fracture.
- Osteoporosis can be either primary or secondary. Secondary causes include medications, cancers, endocrine disorders, collagen vascular disease, or nutritional problems.
- DEXA is the preferred method for detecting osteoporosis and is reported as a T score that compares the patient's BMD with peak bone mass and a Z score that compares the patient's BMD with age- and gender-matched controls.

52 | Prostate Disease

Prostate problems are most common in men after age 50 but may occur earlier. Prostate pathology includes enlargement (commonly known as benign prostatic hypertrophy or BPH), inflammation (prostatitis), and cancer. BPH is a noncancerous enlargement of the prostate gland, with or without the cellular changes of true hyperplasia, which affects up to 90% of men by age 80. Prostatitis is an inflammation of the prostate gland, with a prevalence of around 8%. Prostatitis may be acute, chronic, asymptomatic, and bacterial or nonbacterial in origin. Prostate cancer is the most common noncutaneous cancer in men and the second leading cause of cancer death. Despite being a leading cause of death, over 50% of diagnosed prostate cancers remain asymptomatic giving credence to the adage that many men die with prostate cancer rather than from it.

TABLE 52-1. NIH Classification of Prostatitis
Acute bacterial prostatitis: Acute infection of the prostate gland
Chronic bacterial prostatitis: Recurrent infection of the prostate gland
CPPS • Inflammatory: WBCs in prostate secretions or postprostatic massage urine • Noninflammatory: No WBCs in prostate secretions or post-prostatic massage urine
Asymptomatic inflammatory prostatitis: Incidental finding for workup of elevated PSA or abnormal semen analysis

CPPS, Chronic pelvic pain syndrome; NIH, National Institutes of Health; PSA, prostate-specific antigen; WBC, White blood corpuscles.

PATHOGENESIS

The prostate remains small from birth until puberty when testosterone levels increase and stimulate growth in the androgen-sensitive cells of the prostate. After adolescence, a second growth phase begins in most men after around age 50. As the prostate gland enlarges, it can block the urethra, which may cause problems urinating. As a result, the prevalence of symptomatic BPH increases with age, from about 8% of men under 40 to 80% of men older than 80. Although testosterone stimulates prostate cell growth, exactly how it influences BPH remains uncertain.

Prostatitis, one of the most common urologic problems in men under age 50, is classified by the National Institutes of Health (NIH) based on etiology and duration into acute bacterial, chronic bacterial, asymptomatic inflammatory disease, and chronic pelvic pain syndrome (Table 52-1). Bacterial prostatitis may develop through the introduction of bacteria into the prostate in association with sexual activity or as part of a more generalized urinary tract infection (UTI). Chronic prostatitis or chronic pelvic pain syndrome (CPPS) is a poorly understood process, which may either be inflammatory or noninflammatory. Although the cause of CPPS remains uncertain, researchers speculate there may be a connection to physical trauma, infection, nerve damage, or an immune response to a previous UTI. CPPS has also been linked to other disorders such as chronic fatigue and irritable bowel syndrome. Asymptomatic prostatitis is an incidental finding where the prostate is inflamed but asymptomatic and is found when evaluating other conditions. Some evidence links prostatic inflammation to infertility and treatment may improve male reproductive function.

Prostate cancer is an adenocarcinoma that develops when normal cells, most often in the peripheral zone, mutate into cancerous cells. Risk factors for prostate cancer include older age, African American race, and family history. The greater prevalence of prostate cancer in the western world and analysis of migrant population data also implicates lifestyle and environmental factors.

An enlarged prostate from either a benign or a cancerous process can obstruct urinary flow at the neck of the bladder. Early in the process, the detrusor muscle hypertrophies, but still contracts effectively allowing the bladder to empty. However, a hypertrophied detrusor muscle may contract involuntarily, leading to symptoms of urgency, frequency, and nocturia. As the obstructive process progresses, bladder emptying is incomplete and muscle contractility may become less effective leading to symptoms of incomplete emptying, hesitancy, and a weak urinary stream. More severe obstruction requires abdominal straining in order to establish urinary flow, and ultimately, urinary dribbling and overflow incontinence may occur.

CLINICAL MANIFESTATIONS

HISTORY

Symptoms of prostatic disease include difficulty voiding, a sensation of incomplete bladder emptying, dysuria, urinary frequency, urgency, decreased force of stream, dribbling, and nocturia. In addition, patients may complain of vague symptoms such as discomfort in the genital region, perineum, or rectum. Pain with ejaculation may also be present. Signs of prostatic enlargement and the degree of obstruction are indicated by positive responses to the questions about symptoms presented in Table 52-2. Other important historic factors include personal or family history of prostate disease.

TABLE 52-2. Questions to Elicit Symptoms of Prostate Disease
1. Do you have the sensation of not emptying your bladder completely after you have finished voiding?
2. Do you have to urinate again <2 hours after you finished urinating before?
3. Does your urinary stream stop and start again several times during urination?
4. Do you find it difficult to postpone urination?
5. Have you noticed a weak urinary stream?
6. Do you have to push or strain to initiate urination?
7. Do you awaken to urinate more than one time per night?

Acute prostatitis is associated with a more acute onset and more severe symptoms including fever, chills, dysuria, and frequency. In contrast, the main symptom of CPPS is pain or discomfort lasting >3 months in the lower pelvis, abdomen, lower back, or genitals. Pain during or after ejaculation, dysuria, and urgency are other common symptoms.

PHYSICAL EXAMINATION

Physical examination should assess the abdomen, genitals, and prostate. Abdominal examination can detect bladder distention, indicating urinary retention. The penis and testicles should be examined for tenderness, signs of inflammation, or STIs. A prostate examination should be performed with either the patient standing and bent over the examination table with his elbows resting on the table or lying on side with upper leg flexed. The normal prostate is a rounded, heart-shaped structure with a median groove or sulcus, and ~2.5 cm in length. A midline groove should be identifiable. Enlargement is indicated by both an increase in size and loss of the midline groove. Tenderness or a boggy texture on palpation suggests an inflammatory process. A palpable nodule raises the possibility of cancer but many cancers present with increased firmness of the prostate without a discrete mass. A prostate examination is not indicated when evaluating urinary or prostate-related symptoms in an ill-appearing febrile patient in whom acute bacterial prostatitis is suspected. In these instances, bacteremia may occur with a prostate examination; treatment should be initiated and the examination deferred until the patient is stabilized.

DIFFERENTIAL DIAGNOSIS

Lower urinary tract symptoms of urinary frequency, hesitancy, urgency, dysuria, and nocturia may result from conditions involving the bladder, prostate, urethra, or neurologic systems. Urethral strictures should be suspected in those with a history of urethral catheterization, instrumentation, or urethritis. Bladder lesions such as cancer or cystitis may cause symptoms suggestive of prostatic disease. Neurologic diseases such as MS and spinal cord injury may cause voiding dysfunction, with symptoms overlapping those seen with prostatic disease. Peripheral neuropathies associated with diabetes mellitus or alcoholism may affect the autonomic fibers to the bladder, leading to obstructive urinary tract symptoms. Pharmacologic agents with anticholinergic or alpha-adrenergic agonist properties may precipitate urinary retention. Finally, paruresis or "shy bladder syndrome" is defined as trouble urinating when other people are present.

DIAGNOSTIC EVALUATION

Evaluation begins with a focused history and physical examination. Inquiring about medications, neurologic disease, and prior urologic disease may suggest the underlying cause for the patient's symptoms. Evaluation of the patient begins with a UA and culture to assess for hematuria, signs of inflammation, and infection. In patients with suspected obstruction, BUN and creatinine values should be obtained, along with U/S of the renal system looking for signs of obstruction. The evaluation for individuals with hematuria is found in Chapter 18. Glycosuria should prompt consideration of diabetes with or without neuropathy as a cause of urinary symptoms. BPH is usually diagnosed by history combined with an enlarged prostate found on examination.

Several tests can help differentiate the types of prostatitis. These include urine Gram stain and culture, along with microscopic examination of prostatic secretions using either the 2-glass preprostatic and postprostatic massage or Meares-Stamey 4-Glass Test (see Table 52-3). WBCs present after prostate massage indicate bacterial or nonbacterial prostatitis, with a culture distinguishing between the two. The absence of WBCs in the urine or in prostatic secretions after prostatic massage suggests noninflammatory CPPS as the underlying cause. Patients with a history of urethral disorders, infections, or instrumentation may be evaluated for stricture by cystoscopy or by performing a urethrogram. Patients with urinary tract symptoms and fever should have their urine and blood cultured and treated with an antibiotic. Individuals with suspected acute bacterial prostatitis and who appear ill or septic should be hospitalized.

Screening tests for prostate cancer include both a prostate-specific antigen (PSA) test and a digital rectal examination (DRE). Although this was the standard of care for several decades, the USPSTF now recommends against routine PSA screening for prostate cancer because evidence indicates with a moderate to high degree of certainty that the harms of testing outweigh the benefits. PSA testing lacks specificity and may be elevated in the setting of BPH or prostatitis and many patients with prostate cancer will have normal PSA levels. According to the USPSTF, "There is convincing evidence that PSA-based screening programs result in the detection of many cases of asymptomatic prostate cancer. There is also convincing evidence that a substantial percentage of men who have asymptomatic cancer detected by PSA screening have a tumor that either will not progress or will progress so slowly that it would have remained asymptomatic for the man's lifetime". The terms "over diagnosis" or "pseudodisease" are used to describe both situations. As a result, many nonharmful cancers are discovered and treated, which can result in significant morbidities including urinary incontinence and erectile dysfunction. The AAFP also recommends against routine DRE for prostate cancer screening for the same reasons. Instead of universal screening for prostate cancer, the AAFP recommends that physicians engage their patients in a conversation about the benefits and harms of screening and to participate in shared decision making. Patients at higher risk of prostate cancer include American and Caribbean men of African descent and those with a positive family history.

TREATMENT

Acute bacterial prostatitis generally requires 6 weeks of antibiotic therapy with agents such as TMP/SMX or a fluoroquinolone active against gram-negative bacteria. Patients requiring hospitalization are given intravenous treatment with a broad-spectrum penicillin combined with a beta-lactamase inhibitor, third-generation cephalosporin or fluoroquinolone, possibly combined with an aminoglycoside. Patients with chronic prostatitis who have positive cultures should have therapy based on antibiotic sensitivities. Empiric therapy for those with negative cultures can be provided with TMP/SMX or a fluoroquinolone. Patients may require therapy for 4 to 12 weeks or more.

TABLE 52-3. Localization of Inflammation with Urinary and Prostatic Infections

Meares-Stamey 4-Glass Test

1. Initial = urethral

2. Midstream = bladder/kidney

3. Prostate secretions from massage = prostate

4. Postprostatic massage urine = prostate

2-Glass Test

1. Midstream = bladder/kidney

2. Postprostatic massage urine = prostate

Patients with CPPS may be treated with antibiotics initially. In patients failing to respond to antibiotics, alpha blockers, NSAIDs, or tricyclic antidepressants may help. Nonpharmacologic management includes biofeedback, cognitive behavioral therapy, or other treatments. Unfortunately, none of these therapies consistently shows benefit for patients with CPPS. Since management of CPPS is complex, referral to urology may help.

Treatment for benign prostatic enlargement is directed at attempting to decrease the size of the prostate or to relax the muscle at the bladder outlet. Finasteride inhibits the conversion of testosterone to dihydrotestosterone, the active metabolite of testosterone. This blocks the effects of testosterone on the prostate, and over 6 to 12 months can decrease prostatic size by about 20% and may improve obstructive symptoms. Finasteride causes about a 50% decline in PSA values, a factor that must be considered when ordering a PSA in this patient population. A rise in PSA for patients on finasteride merits an evaluation for prostate cancer. Although finasteride reduces the risk of prostate cancer, those who get prostate cancer while taking the drug tend to have a more aggressive form.

Alpha-adrenergic blockers such as terazosin, doxazosin, and tamsulosin block action at the alpha-adrenergic receptors on the smooth muscle in the bladder neck, allowing for relaxation and enhanced bladder emptying. These agents have an advantage over finasteride in their higher efficacy and prompt onset of action in relieving symptoms. The alpha blockers—doxazosin, terazosin and prazosin—also lower blood pressure and may be of value in patients with concomitant hypertension. Tamsulosin and alfuzosin are more selective agents for treating BPH and have little effect on blood pressure and less associated dizziness. Orthostatic hypotension is increased when these agents are combined with phosphodiesterase inhibitors such as sildenafil (Viagra) used to treat erectile dysfunction and should either be avoided or separated by several hours. Alpha blockers may also be used in combination with finasteride. Patients refractory to medical therapy require referral to a urologist for consideration of surgical procedures such as transurethral resection of the prostate (TURP), transurethral incision, ablation, or resection of the prostate in order to provide symptom relief.

Patients with suspected cancer of the prostate should be referred to a urologist for a transrectal US-guided biopsy of the prostate gland. Biopsy is done in the outpatient setting and usually well tolerated, although some patients experience discomfort and bleeding. A microscopic evaluation of the biopsy results in a Gleason score that correlates with chances of metastasis. Staging of prostate cancer may include a PSA, a bone scan, laboratory testing, and CT or MRI. Treatment depends on patient preference, Gleason score, and the stage of disease. Watchful waiting (also known as active surveillance), surgery, radiation, hormone therapy, and chemotherapy are all potential options. PSA levels should be monitored after prostate cancer surgery and are generally not detectable following curative prostatectomy. Elevation of the PSA level after surgery suggests recurrent or residual disease. For patients with metastases, hormonal suppression through orchiectomy or the administration of luteinizing hormone-releasing hormone (LH-RH) agonists (e.g., Lupron) or antiandrogens may slow disease progression. Radiation therapy is often used to shrink bone metastases.

KEY POINTS

- Prostate disease will affect over 90% of men during their lifetimes.
- Prostate cancer affects 1 in 6 men.

- Urologic consultation should be obtained for patients with prostate disease refractory to medical therapy or those suspected of having prostate cancer.

53 | Sexually Transmitted Diseases

STDs are common infections; >8 to 12 million STDs are diagnosed annually in the United States. Although HIV is considered an STD, it is discussed in more detail separately in Chapter 45.

PATHOGENESIS

Sexually transmitted organisms enter through the mucosa or skin to cause disease. On mucosal surfaces, the organisms attach to the surface and cause an inflammatory reaction that enables the organism to penetrate. Organisms that produce skin ulcers usually gain access by small abrasions in the upper layers of the epidermis. These abrasions occur secondary to microtrauma associated with sexual intercourse, accounting for the fact that the most common locations for STD lesions are the penis, vagina, labia, and rectal surfaces.

Younger women are at a greater risk for STDs than older women because they have a more exposed transformation zone (squamous-columnar junction). Exposed columnar cells have a higher affinity for *Chlamydia trachomatis* and *Neisseria gonorrhoeae* than squamous cells and are also more vulnerable to infection by HPV. In addition, progesterone deficiency, commonly seen in younger women, results in a thinner protective mucous layer on the cervix, which facilitates the migration of pathogens to the upper genital tract.

CLINICAL MANIFESTATIONS

HISTORY

Most individuals with STDs seek care because of genitourinary symptoms or because they notice a genital lesion. The most commonly encountered symptoms in men are related to urethritis and epididymitis. In women, urethral symptoms and vaginal discharge are the most common presenting complaints. Both men and women can develop genital lesions such as ulcers and genital warts.

Some patients are asymptomatic but seek care because of exposure to a partner with an STD or because of a high-risk sexual contact. A sexual history inquiring about numbers of partners, sexual practices, history of STDs, and any high-risk sexual contacts identifies individuals at risk. Table 53-1 outlines the five Ps of sexual history: Partners, practices, prevention of pregnancy, protection from STDs, and past history of STDs.

PHYSICAL EXAMINATION

Careful examination of the genitalia is critically important for evaluating a patient with a suspected STD. The examination should focus on detecting skin lesions, rashes, lymphadenopathy, ulcers, and mucosal lesions. Specific clinical syndromes are listed below and summarized in Table 53-2.

Urethritis

In men, the most common symptom of a gonococcal infection is a urethral discharge. Typically, the discharge from gonococcal urethritis is more purulent than that from a nongonococcal urethritis (NGU). NGU is usually caused by a chlamydial infection but may also occur due to *Ureaplasma* or *Mycoplasma* infections.

Hepatitis B

Sexual transmission accounts for 30% to 60% of hepatitis B cases. Common signs and symptoms of hepatitis B infections include jaundice, nausea, vomiting, arthralgias, fever, and abdominal pain.

Hepatitis A

Hepatitis A infection is usually transmitted by the fecal-oral route. However, the most frequent source of hepatitis A infection is household or sexual contact with an infected person.

TABLE 53-1. The Five Ps: Partners, Practices, Prevention of Pregnancy, Past History

1. Partners

"Do you have sex with men, women, or both?"

"In the past 2 months, how many partners have you had sex with?"

"In the past 12 months, how many partners have you had sex with?"

"Is it possible that any of your sex partners in the past 12 months had sex with someone else while they were still in a sexual relationship with you?"

2. Practices

"To understand your risks for STDs, I need to understand the kind of sex you have had recently."

"Have you had vaginal sex, meaning 'penis in vagina sex'?" If yes, "Do you use condoms: never, sometimes, or always?"

"Have you had anal sex, meaning 'penis in rectum/anus sex'?" If yes, "Do you use condoms: never, sometimes, or always?"

"Have you had oral sex, meaning 'mouth on penis/vagina'?"

For condom answers:

If "never": "Why don't you use condoms?"

If "sometimes": "In what situations (or with whom) do you use condoms?"

3. Prevention of pregnancy

"What are you doing to prevent pregnancy?"

4. Protection from STDs

"What do you do to protect yourself from STDs and HIV?"

5. Past history of STDs

"Have you ever had an STD?"

"Have any of your partners had an STD?"

Additional questions to identify HIV and viral hepatitis risk include the following:

"Have you or any of your partners ever injected drugs?"

"Have your or any of your partners exchanged money or drugs for sex?"

"Is there anything else about your sexual practices that I need to know?

HIV, human immunodeficiency virus; STD, sexually transmitted diseases.

TABLE 53-2. Clinical Characteristics of Sexually Transmitted Diseases

Disease	Characteristics
Urethritis	Urethral discharge, dysuria, periurethral irritation
Hepatitis B	Flulike prodrome, nausea, vomiting, arthralgias, rash, jaundice
Hepatitis A	Nausea, vomiting, diarrhea, jaundice
Human papillomavirus	Genital warts, abnormal pap smear
Herpes simplex	Painful genital vesicles and ulcers, dysuria, fever (primary infection), recurrences
Chancroid	Painful ulcer and inguinal lymphadenopathy
Syphilis	Primary: nontender, painless ulcers; secondary: rash, flulike illness; tertiary: aortic insufficiency, aortic aneurysm, peripheral neuropathy, meningitis, psychiatric disease
Cervicitis	Vaginal discharge, dysuria
Bacterial vaginosis	Malodorous vaginal discharge, pruritus
Epididymitis	Testicular pain and swelling, urethral discharge

Genital Warts

The HPV causes anogenital warts (condylomata acuminata) (Fig. 53-1). The lesions are typically cauliflower-like but can be smooth and either flesh colored or pigmented. The lesions are usually asymptomatic and discovered by the patient or physician upon examination. About 95% of anal cancers are caused by HPV: most are connected to type 16. The HPV strains most closely associated with cervical cancer are types 16 and 18, accounting for about 70% of cervical cancer cases. These are discussed in Chapter 58.

Genital Ulcers

Herpes simplex virus (HSV) and chancroid cause painful ulcers, whereas the ulcers of syphilis are painless. HSV is the most common cause of genital ulceration. Primary genital herpes usually presents 2 days to 2 weeks after exposure, with widespread vesicles and ulcers on the genitalia. Symptoms such as dysuria and fever are common and can be mistaken for that of a UTI. The initial infection is usually more severe than recurrences, presumably because of the body's immune response. Reactivation triggers include sunlight, skin trauma, cold or heat, stress, concurrent infection, and menstruation.

Chancroid is caused by *Haemophilus ducreyi* and is associated with inguinal lymphadenopathy and painful genital ulcers. Chancroid ulcers are deep and tender, with irregular borders and a purulent base.

Syphilitic chancres are caused by the spirochete *Treponema pallidum* and are painless, nontender, indurated ulcers with a clean base (Fig. 53-2). The chancre develops about 3 weeks after exposure. Even without treatment, the primary lesion usually resolves within 4 to 6 weeks. The secondary stage of syphilis typically presents with a generalized maculopapular rash, often involving the palms and soles. Other symptoms include general malaise, fever, rhinorrhea, sore throat, myalgias, headaches, and generalized lymphadenopathy. Secondary syphilis may evolve into a latent asymptomatic stage with no symptoms but with positive serology testing. One-third of these patients eventually develop tertiary syphilis, which can cause significant morbidity and a shortened life span due to the associated cardiovascular and neurologic complications.

Cervicitis and Pelvic Inflammatory Disease

Either *C. trachomatis* or *N. gonorrhoeae* most commonly causes cervicitis. Many women with cervicitis are asymptomatic, whereas others may experience a vaginal discharge, dysuria, or vaginal spotting. Pharyngeal and anorectal gonorrheal infections can develop in patients who engage in oral or rectal sex. Pelvic inflammatory disease (PID), often marked by the development of abdominal pain and

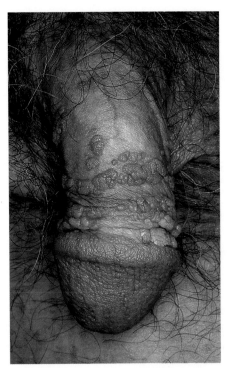

FIGURE 53-1. Penile warts. (From Edwards L, Lynch P. *Genital Dermatology Atlas*. 2nd ed. Philadelphia, PA: Lippincott Williams & Wilkins; 2011.)

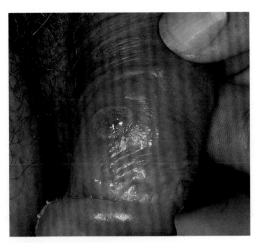

FIGURE 53-2. Genital syphilis with chancre. (From Edwards L, Lynch P. *Genital Dermatology Atlas*. 3rd ed. Philadelphia, PA: Wolters Kluwer; 2017.)

TABLE 53-3.	Criteria for the Diagnosis of Pelvic Inflammatory Disease
Minimal criteria	Lower abdominal pain, adnexal tenderness, cervical motion tenderness
Additional criteria	Oral temp >101°F (38.3°C), abnormal cervical or vaginal discharge, elevated ESR, C-reactive protein, documented *N. gonorrhoeae* or *C. trachomatis* infection
Definitive criteria	Histopathologic evidence of endometritis on endometrial biopsy, transvaginal ultrasound, or other imaging modes showing thickened fluid-filled tubes with or without free pelvic fluid or tubo-ovarian complex, laparoscopic abnormalities consistent with PID

ESR, erythrocyte sedimentation rate; PID, pelvic inflammatory disease.

fever, can occur if the upper female genital tract is involved. Physical examination may reveal pain with cervical motion, adnexal tenderness, and rebound tenderness. Table 53-3 lists the diagnostic criteria for PID. Although PID is most commonly caused by *N. gonorrhoeae* and *C. trachomatis*, other pathogens including anaerobes, gram-negative facultative bacteria (e.g., *Bacteroides fragilis*), and streptococci may play a role. Perihepatitis, also known as Fitzhugh-Curtis syndrome, is a rare complication of PID. Long-term complications of PID include tubal scarring, which can cause infertility, chronic pain, and an increased risk of ectopic pregnancy.

Approximately 1% to 2% of patients with gonorrheal infections develop bacteremia. These individuals can develop septic arthritis and petechial or pustular skin lesions, which are found primarily on the dorsal aspect of the distal extremities, ankle, or wrist joints.

Bacterial Vaginosis

Although bacterial vaginosis (BV) is associated with multiple sexual partners, it is still uncertain whether BV is transmitted sexually. BV is discussed in Chapter 63.

Vaginitis

Trichomonas is usually asymptomatic in men who may transmit it to women. *Candida* may be harbored under the foreskin in men and can be found in asymptomatic women. Candidal infections are not generally considered STDs. Vaginitis is discussed more fully in Chapter 63.

Epididymitis

Epididymitis is most common in young, sexually active men and is usually caused by gonorrhea or chlamydial infection. On examination, the epididymis, which is located on the posterior aspect of the testis, is tender and swollen. Infection with gram-negative bacilli can also cause epididymitis and this infection is generally associated with lower risk, older patients.

DIFFERENTIAL DIAGNOSIS

Lesions that can mimic condyloma acuminatum (HPV infection) are seborrheic keratosis, nevi, molluscum contagiosum, pearly penile papules, and condyloma latum (syphilitic lesions). Urethral symptoms such as dysuria can be present in UTIs, prostatitis, and vaginitis. The differential diagnosis for PID includes appendicitis, ectopic pregnancy, ovarian torsion, ruptured ovarian cyst, endometriosis, IBS, and somatization disorder.

DIAGNOSTIC EVALUATION

Evaluation of STDs begins with a clinical assessment. In male patients with urethritis, a Gram stain of the discharge looking for neutrophils and the presence of organisms is helpful. A urethral swab can also be sent for culture, DNA analysis, and either culture or immunofluorescence testing for *Chlamydia*. Finding intracellular gram-negative diplococci on the Gram stain is diagnostic for gonorrhea. More recently, many providers use urine testing which relies on DNA amplification techniques to detect gonorrhea and chlamydia instead of a urethral or cervical culture. Urine testing offers the advantage for women of not having to have a pelvic exam and for men avoiding the discomfort of a urethral swab. In women with urethral symptoms, it is important to rule out a UTI or vaginitis. Vaginal discharge can also be a sign of cervicitis or PID, and swabs of the discharge should be sent for culture, DNA analysis, or immunofluorescent testing. Gram stains are less valuable in women. A wet mount, KOH test, pH determination, and whiff test are useful in characterizing a vaginal discharge.

Painful genital ulcers suggest HSV or chancroid. Painless ulcers suggest syphilis. The presence of multinucleated giant cells on a smear or a positive viral culture can diagnose HSV, whereas *H. ducreyi* can be isolated by cultures. Spirochetes seen on a dark-field examination from a scraping of an ulcer or direct immunofluorescent microscopy can confirm the diagnosis of syphilis.

The common serologic screening tests for syphilis—an RPR or a venereal disease research laboratory (VDRL) test—turn positive as early as 4 to 7 days after a chancre appears. The VDRL or RPR titer can be used to determine disease activity following treatment. False-positive tests for syphilis may occur in conditions such as antiphospholipid syndrome, advancing age, narcotic use, chronic liver disease, HIV, tuberculosis, and acute herpetic infection. Generally higher titers ($>$1:8) are more likely to represent true disease. A fluorescent treponemal antibody absorption (FTA-Abs) test should be used to confirm a positive RPR or VDRL result. The FTA-Abs will remain positive indefinitely and therefore cannot be used to determine disease activity.

HPV is commonly diagnosed by its appearance, but if necessary the diagnosis can be confirmed by tissue biopsy. Pap smears can detect cervical changes associated with HPV infection.

TREATMENT

Treatment guidelines for STDs are presented in Table 53-4. Primary prevention, by encouraging condom use and avoiding high-risk sexual activity, is an important part of STD management. Vaccination for hepatitis B remains the most effective measure to prevent this disease. Hepatitis B immune globulin can be used in conjunction with the vaccine series in unimmunized individuals who have been exposed to the virus. There are three licensed HPV vaccines in the United States that protect against HPV infections. Safe sex practices also reduce the risk of infection.

The treatment for genital warts depends on the number, size, morphology, and anatomic sites of the warts. Treatments include patient-applied therapies such as podofilox and imiquimod and provider-applied therapies such as cryotherapy, trichloroacetic acid, bichloroacetic acid, and surgical removal. Podofilox is not recommended for perianal, vaginal, or urethral warts and should not be used during pregnancy. Imiquimod directly eradicates HPV but is not recommended in pregnant women. Cryotherapy with liquid nitrogen eradicates warts by thermally induced cytolysis. Generally, two to three sessions are required for treating the warts.

Acyclovir (Zovirax), valacyclovir (Valtrex), and famciclovir (Famvir) are used to treat HSV. Treatment shortens the course of the infection and reduces the length of time that the virus is shed. Suppressive therapy is indicated for patients with frequent recurrences.

Uncomplicated chlamydial infections can be treated with doxycycline for 7 days or with a single 1 g dose of azithromycin. Uncomplicated gonorrhea can be treated with intramuscular (IM) ceftriaxone or spectinomycin or a single oral dose of cefixime. Fluoroquinolone resistance is as high as 15% in some areas, and therefore, preferred therapies for gonorrhea are cefixime or IM ceftriaxone. Treatment for gonorrhea should generally be followed by a regimen effective against *Chlamydia.* Erythromycin, ceftriaxone, or azithromycin are each active against chancroid.

Regimens of outpatient antibiotics are recommended for mild PID and include single dose cephalosporin (ceftriaxone IM, cefoxitin IM, or oral cefixime) plus 2 weeks of oral doxycycline. The indications for hospitalizing patients with PID include pregnancy, failed outpatient therapy, the inability to follow or tolerate an outpatient oral regimen, severe illness, high fever, a tubo-ovarian abscess, immunodeficiency, or in cases where the diagnosis is uncertain. Inpatient therapy can include cefoxitin intravenously every 6 hours along with intravenous doxycycline or clindamycin and gentamycin. Following a clinical response, each of these regimens is generally followed by 2 weeks of oral doxycycline. Recommended regimens for women with BV include oral metronidazole and topical metronidazole or clindamycin. Penicillin is the treatment of choice for syphilis. For individuals with penicillin allergy, doxycycline or tetracycline can be used.

Sexually Transmitted Diseases: Summary of 2015 CDC Treatment Guidelines

These summary guidelines reflect the 2015 CDC Guidelines for the Treatment of Sexually Transmitted Diseases. They are intended as a source of clinical guidance. An important component of STD treatment is partner management. Providers can arrange for the evaluation and treatment of sex partners either directly or with assistance from state and local health departments. Complete guidelines can be ordered online at www.cdc.gov/std/treatment or by calling 1 (800) CDC-INFO (1-800-232-4636).

Disease	Recommended Rx		Dose/Route	Alternatives	
Bacterial Vaginosis	metronidazole oral[1]	OR	500 mg orally 2x/day for 7 days	tinidazole 2 g orally 1x/day for 2 days	OR
	metronidazole gel 0.75%[1]	OR	One 5 g applicator intravaginally 1x/day for 5 days	tinidazole 1 g orally 1x/day for 5 days	OR
	clindamycin cream 2%[1,2]		One 5 g applicator intravaginally at bedtime for 7 days	clindamycin 300 mg orally 2x/day for 7 days	OR
	★ Treatment is recommended for all symptomatic pregnant women.			clindamycin ovules 100 mg intravaginally at bedtime for 3 days	
Cervicitis	azithromycin	OR	1 g orally in a single dose	Consider concurrent treatment for gonococcal infection if at risk of gonorrhea or lives in a community where the prevalence of gonorrhea is high. Presumptive treatment with antimicrobials for *C. trachomatis* and *N. gonorrhoeae* should be provided for women at increased risk (e.g., those aged <25 years and those with a new sex partner, a sex partner with concurrent partners, or a sex partner who has a sexually transmitted infection), especially if follow-up cannot be ensured or if NAAT testing is not possible.	
	doxycycline[3]		100 mg orally 2x/day for 7 days		
Chlamydial Infections Adults and adolescents	azithromycin	OR	1 g orally in a single dose	erythromycin base[4] 500 mg orally 4x/day for 7 days	OR
	doxycycline[3]		100 mg orally 2x/day for 7 days	erythromycin ethylsuccinate[5] 800 mg orally 4x/day for 7 days	OR
				levofloxacin[6] 500 mg 1x/day orally for 7 days	OR
				ofloxacin[6] 300 mg orally 2x/day for 7 days	
Pregnancy[3]	azithromycin[7]		1 g orally in a single dose	★ amoxicillin 500 mg orally 3x/day for 7 days	OR
				erythromycin base[4,8] 500 mg orally 4x/day for 7 days	OR
				erythromycin base 250 mg orally 4x/day for 14 days	OR
				erythromycin ethylsuccinate 800 mg orally 4x/day for 7 days	OR
				erythromycin ethylsuccinate 400 mg orally 4x/day for 14 days	OR
Infants and Children (<45 kg): urogenital, rectal	erythromycin base[9] ethylsuccinate	OR	50 mg/kg/day orally (4 divided doses) daily for 14 days	★ Data are limited on the effectiveness and optimal dose of azithromycin for chlamydial infection in infants and children <45 kg	
Neonates: opthalmia neonatorum, pneumonia	erythromycin base[9] ethylsuccinate	OR	50 mg/kg/day orally (4 divided doses) daily for 14 days	★ azithromycin 20 mg/kg/day orally, 1 dose daily for 3 days	

(continued)

TABLE 53-4. Summary of STI Treatment Guidelines (from: https://www.cdc.gov/std/tg2015/2015-wall-chart.pdf) (*continued*)

Disease	Recommended Rx		Dose/Route	Alternatives
Epididymitis[10,11]				
For acute epididymitis most likely caused by sexually transmitted CT and GC	ceftriaxone	PLUS	250 mg IM in a single dose	
	doxycycline		100 mg orally 2x/day for 10 days	
★ For acute epididymitis most likely caused by sexually-transmitted chlamydia and gonorrhea and enteric organisms (men who practice insertive anal sex)	ceftriaxone	PLUS	250 mg IM in a single dose	
	levofloxacin	OR	500 mg orally 1x/day for 10 days	
	ofloxacin		300 mg orally 2x/day for 10 days	
For acute epididymitis most likely caused by enteric organisms	levofloxacin	OR	500 mg orally 1x/day for 10 days	
	ofloxacin		300 mg orally 2x/day for 10 days	
Genital Herpes Simplex				
First clinical episode of genital herpes	acyclovir	OR	400 mg orally 3x/day for 7-10 days[13]	
	acyclovir	OR	200 mg orally 5x/day for 7-10 days[13]	
	valacyclovir[12]	OR	1 g orally 2x/day for 7-10 days[13]	
	famciclovir[12]		250 mg orally 3x/day for 7-10 days[13]	
Episodic therapy for recurrent genital herpes	acyclovir OR		400 mg orally 3x/day for 5 days	
	acyclovir OR		800 mg orally 2x/day for 5 days	
	acyclovir OR		800 mg orally 3x/day for 2 days	
	valacyclovir[12]	OR	500 mg orally 2x/day for 3 days	
	valacyclovir[12]	OR	1 g orally 1x/day for 5 days	
	famciclovir[12]	OR	125 mg orally 2x/day for 5 days	
	famciclovir[12]	OR	1000 mg orally 2x/day for 1 day[13]	
	famciclovir[12]		500 mg orally once, followed by 250 mg 2x/day for 2 day	
Suppressive therapy[14] for recurrent genital herpes	acyclovir	OR	400 mg orally 2x/day	
	valacyclovir[12]	OR	500 mg orally 1x/day	
	valacyclovir[12]	OR	1 g orally once a day	
	famciclovir[12]		250 mg orally 2x/day	
Recommended regimens for episodic infection in persons with HIV infection	acyclovir	OR	400 mg orally 3x/day for 5-10 days	
	valacyclovir[12]	OR	1 g orally 2x/day for 5-10 days	
	famciclovir[12]		500 mg orally 2x/day for 5-10 days	
Recommended regimens for daily suppressive therapy in persons with HIV infection	acyclovir	OR	400-800 mg orally 2-3x/day	
	valacyclovir[12]	OR	500 mg orally 2x/day	
	famciclovir[12]		500 mg orally 2x/day	

Genital Warts[15] (Human Papillomavirus) External genital and perianal warts	**Patient Applied** ★ imiquimod 3.75% or 5%[12] cream OR podofilox 0.5%[15] solution or gel OR sinecatechins 15% ointment[2,12] OR **Provider Administered** Cryotherapy OR trichloroacetic acid or bichloroacetic acid 80%–90% OR surgical removal	See complete CDC guidelines. Apply small amount, dry, apply weekly if necessary	★ podophyllin resin 10%–25% in compound tincture of benzoin may be considered for provider-administered treatment if strict adherence to the recommendations for application. intralesional interferon OR photodynamic therapy OR topical cidofovir OR	
Gonococcal Infections[16] Adults, adolescents, and children >45 kg: uncomplicated gonococcal infections of the cervix, urethra, and rectum	ceftriaxone PLUS azithromycin[7]	250 mg IM in a single dose 1 g orally in a single dose	If ceftriaxone is not available: cefixime[17] 400 mg orally in a single dose azithromycin[7] 1 g orally in a single dose ★ If cephalosporin allergy: gemifloxacin 320 mg orally in a single dose azithromycin 2 g orally in a single dose ★ gentamicin 240 mg IM single dose azithromycin 2 g orally in a single dose	
Pharyngeal[18]	ceftriaxone PLUS azithromycin[7]	250 mg IM in a single dose 1 g orally in a single dose		
Pregnancy	See complete CDC guidelines.			
Adults and adolescents: conjunctivitis	ceftriaxone PLUS azithromycin[7]	1 g IM in a single dose 1 g orally in a single dose		
Children (≤45 kg): urogenital, rectal, pharyngeal	ceftriaxone[19]	25-50 mg/kg IV or IM, not to exceed 125 mg IM in a single dose		
Lymphogranuloma venereum	doxycycline[3]	100 mg orally 2x/day for 21 days	erythromycin base 500 mg orally 4x/day for 21 days	
Nongonococcal Urethritis (NGU) ★ Persistent and recurrent NGU[3,20,21]	azithromycin[7] OR doxycycline[3] Men initially treated with doxycycline: azithromycin Men who fail a regimen of azithromycin: moxifloxacin Heterosexual men who live in areas where *T. vaginalis* is highly prevalent: metronidazole[22] OR tinidazole	1 g orally in a single dose 100 mg orally 2x/day for 7 days 1 g orally in a single dose 400 mg orally 1x/day for 7 days 2 g orally in a single dose 2 g orally in a single dose	erythromycin base[4] 500 mg orally 4x/day for 7 days OR erythromycin ethylsuccinate[5] 800 mg orally 4x/day for 7 days OR levofloxacin 500 mg orally 1x/day for 7 days OR ofloxacin 300 mg orally 2x/day for 7 days	

(*continued*)

Disease	Recommended Rx		Dose/Route	Alternatives	
Pediculosis Pubis	permethrin 1% cream rinse	OR	Apply to affected area, wash off after 10 minutes	malathion 0.5% lotion, applied 8–12 hrs then washed off	OR
	pyrethrins with piperonyl butoxide		Apply to affected area, wash off after 10 minutes	ivermectin 250 µg/kg, orally repeated in 2 weeks	
Pelvic Inflammatory Disease[10]	Parenteral Regimens			Parenteral Regimen	
	Cefotetan	PLUS	2 g IV every 12 hours	Ampicillin/Sulbactam 3 g IV every 6 hours	
	Doxycycline	OR	100 mg orally or IV every 12 hours	Doxycycline 100 mg orally or IV every 12 hours	
	Cefoxitin	PLUS	2 g IV every 6 hours	The complete list of recommended regimens can be found in CDC's 2015	
	Doxycycline		100 mg orally or IV every 12 hours	STD Treatment Guidelines.	
	Recommended Intramuscular/Oral Regimens		250 mg IM in a single dose		
	Ceftriaxone	PLUS	100 mg orally twice a day for 14 days		
	Doxycycline	WITH or	500 mg orally twice a day for 14 days		
	Metronidazole	WITHOUT	2 g IM in a single dose		
		OR	1 g orally administered concurrently in a single dose		
	Cefoxitin	PLUS	100 mg orally twice a day for 14 days		
	Probenecid,	PLUS	500 mg orally twice a day for 14 days		
	Doxycycline	WITH or			
	Metronidazole	WITHOUT			
Scabies	permethrin 5% cream	OR	Apply to all areas of body from neck down, wash off after 8–14 hours 200 µg/kg orally, repeated in 2 weeks	lindane 1%[23,24] 1 oz. of lotion or 30 g of cream, applied thinly to all areas of the body from the neck down, wash off after 8 hours	
	ivermectin				
Syphilis	benzathine penicillin G		2.4 million units IM in a single dose	doxycycline[3,25] 100 mg 2x/day for 14 days	OR
Primary, secondary, or early latent <1 year	benzathine penicillin G		2.4 million units IM in 3 doses each at 1 week intervals (7.2 million units total)	tetracycline[3,25] 500 mg orally 4x/day for 14 days	
Latent >1 year, latent of unknown duration	See complete CDC guidelines. aqueous crystalline penicillin G		18–24 million units per day, administered as 3–4 million units IV every 4 hours or continuous infusion, for 10–14 days	doxycycline[3,25] 100 mg 2x/day for 28 days	OR
Pregnancy	See complete CDC guidelines.			tetracycline[3,25] 500 mg orally 4x/day for 28 days	
Neurosyphilis	benzathine penicillin G		50,000 units/kg IM in a single dose (maximum 2.4 million units)	procaine penicillin G 2.4 MU IM 1x daily	PLUS
★ Congenital syphilis	benzathine penicillin G		50,000 units/kg IM for 3 doses at 1 week intervals (maximum total 7.2 million units)	probenecid 500 mg orally 4x/day, both for 10–14 days.	
Children: Primary, secondary, or early latent <1 year				See CDC STD Treatment guidelines for discussion of alternative therapy in patients with penicillin allergy.	
Children: Latent >1 year, latent of unknown duration					

Trichomoniasis			metronidazole[22] 500 mg 2x/day for 7 days
Persistent or recurrent trichomoniasis	metronidazole[22]	OR	
	tinidazole[26]		
	metronidazole		
	If this regimen fails:		
	metronidazole	OR	
	tinidazole		
	If this regimen fails, susceptibility testing is recommended.		
	2 g orally in a single dose		
	2 g orally in a single dose		
	500mg orally 2x/day for 7 days		
	2g orally for 7 days		
	2g orally for 7 days		

1. The recommended regimens are equally efficacious.
2. These creams are oil-based and may weaken latex condoms and diaphragms. Refer to product labeling for further information.
3. Should not be administered during pregnancy, lactation, or to children <8 years of age.
4. If patient cannot tolerate high-dose erythromycin base schedules, change to 250 mg 4x/day for 14 days.
5. If patient cannot tolerate high-dose erythromycin ethylsuccinate schedules, change to 400 mg orally 4 times a day for 14 days.
6. Contraindicated for pregnant or lactating women.
7. Clinical experience and published studies suggest that azithromycin is safe and effective.
8. Erythromycin estolate is contraindicated during pregnancy.
9. Effectiveness of erythromycin treatment is approximately 80%; a second course of therapy may be required.
10. Patients who do not respond to therapy (within 72 hours) should be re-evaluated.
11. For patients with suspected sexually transmitted epididymitis, close follow-up is essential.
12. No definitive information available on prenatal exposure.
13. Treatment may be extended if healing is incomplete after 10 days of therapy.
14. Consider discontinuation of treatment after one year to assess frequency of recurrence.
15. Vaginal, cervical, urethral meatal, and anal warts may require referral to an appropriate specialist.
16. CDC recommends that treatment for uncomplicated gonococcal infections of the cervix, urethra, and/or rectum should include dual therapy, i.e., both a cephalosporin (e.g., ceftriaxone) plus azithromycin.
17. CDC recommends that cefixime in combination with azithromycin or doxycycline be used as an alternative when ceftriaxone is not available.
18. Only ceftriaxone is recommended for the treatment of pharyngeal infection. Providers should inquire about oral sexual exposure.
19. Use with caution in hyperbilirubinemic infants, especially those born prematurely.
20. MSM are unlikely to benefit from the addition of nitroimidazoles.
21. Moxifloxacin 400mg orally 1x/day for 7 days is effective against *Mycoplasma genitalium*.
22. Pregnant patients can be treated with 2 g single dose.
23. Contraindicated for pregnant or lactating women, or children <2 years of age.
24. Do not use after a bath; should not be used by persons who have extensive dermatitis.
25. Pregnant patients allergic to penicillin should be treated with penicillin after desensitization.
26. Randomized controlled trials comparing single 2 g doses of metronidazole and tinidazole suggest that tinidazole is equivalent to, or superior to, metronidazole in achieving parasitologic cure and resolution of symptoms.
★ Indicates update from the 2010 CDC Guidelines for the Treatment of Sexually Transmitted Diseases.

KEY POINTS

- Both hepatitis A and B are considered STDs because sexual transmission accounts for the majority of reported incidences.

- HSV and chancroid cause painful ulcers, whereas the ulcers of syphilis are painless.

- Either *C. trachomatis* or *N. gonorrhoeae* most commonly causes cervicitis. PID, often marked by the development of abdominal pain and fever, can occur if the upper tracts are involved.

- The differential diagnosis for PID includes appendicitis, ectopic pregnancy, ovarian torsion, ruptured ovarian cyst, endometriosis, IBS, and somatization disorder.

- The treatment for genital warts depends on the number, size, morphology, and anatomic sites of the warts. Treatments include patient-applied therapies such as podofilox and imiquimod and provider-applied therapies such as cryotherapy, trichloroacetic acid, bichloroacetic acid, and surgical removal.

- Uncomplicated chlamydial infections can be treated with doxycycline or a single 1 g oral dose of azithromycin. Uncomplicated gonorrhea can be treated with intramuscular ceftriaxone or single oral doses of cefixime, or spectinomycin.

54 | Skin Infections

Skin serves as a barrier to fluid loss and protects internal organs against mechanical injury, infections, temperature changes, noxious agents, and trauma. When the skin's defenses are altered or destroyed, bacteria, viruses, fungi, and parasitic organisms can infect or infest it.

PATHOGENESIS

Clinical infection results from breaks in the skin (i.e., abrasions, needle punctures, pressure ulcers, fungal infections, and catheters), loss of local immunity, and changes in the skin flora. Although more than 100 bacteria are known to cause cellulitis, two gram-positive cocci, *Staphylococcus aureus* and group A beta hemolytic streptococcus, account for most skin and soft-tissue infections. *S. aureus* can cause folliculitis, cellulitis, and furuncles (abscess/boil). Toxins elaborated by *S. aureus* can result in bullous impetigo and staphylococcal scalded skin syndrome. Streptococci are usually secondary invaders of traumatic skin lesions and can cause impetigo, erysipelas, cellulitis, and lymphangitis.

Viruses damage host cells by entering the cell and replicating at the host's expense. HSV infections can occur anywhere on the skin and are caused by two types of the virus: HSV-1 and HSV-2. HSV-1 is usually seen in oral infections, whereas HSV-2 is associated with genital infections. HSV infections have two phases: a primary phase representing infection transmitted by direct contact with an active lesion or infected secretions; and a secondary phase representing a reactivation of latent virus which may occur from months to years later.

The varicella virus, which causes chicken pox, is a highly contagious viral infection transmitted by airborne droplets or vesicular fluid. Patients are contagious from 2 days before onset of the rash until all lesions have crusted. Varicella can lay dormant in the dorsal root ganglion for many years. It reactivates and presents as herpes zoster (shingles) typically involving a painful vesicular rash in the distribution of a single or multiple dermatomes. Warts are benign skin tumors confined to the epidermis resulting from HPV, which is transferred by touch and commonly occurs at sites of trauma. Molluscum contagiosum is caused by a poxvirus and produces an umbilicated skin lesion that is spread by autoinoculation, scratching, or touching a lesion.

The dermatophytes, or ringworm fungi, infect and survive only on dead keratin, namely, the top layer of the skin (stratum corneum), the hair, and the nails. Dermatophyte infections are clinically classified by body region with varying disease responses. "Tinea" means "fungus infection"; so the term "tinea capitis" refers to a fungal infection of the scalp.

The fungus *Candida albicans* and other *Candida* species live normally in the mouth, vagina, and gut. They may become pathogenic and produce budding spores, pseudohyphae (elongated cells), or true hyphae. In individuals with altered defenses against yeast (e.g., due to pregnancy, oral contraceptives, antibiotics, diabetes, skin maceration, topical steroid therapy, and some endocrinopathies), *Candida* can infect the stratum corneum of mucous membranes (mouth, anogenital tract) and warm, moist intertriginous skin areas (axillae, groin, breast folds, digit spaces).

Scabies infestation begins when a fertilized female mite burrows through the stratum corneum to begin a 30-day life cycle of egg laying and deposition of fecal matter (scybala). After the eggs have hatched, the mites can migrate to other areas such as the finger webs, wrists, extensor surfaces of the elbows and knees, axillae, breasts, waist, sides of hands and feet, ankles, penis, buttocks, scrotum, and palms and soles of infants, causing symptoms to intensify. The disease is transmitted by direct skin contact with an infected patient.

Three kinds of lice infest humans: *Pediculus humanus capitis* (head louse), *Pediculus humanus corporis* (body louse), and *Phthirus pubis* (pubic or crab louse). Pediculosis capitis is most common in children. Live nits fluoresce and can be detected by Wood's light. Pediculosis corporis is a disease of poor hygiene, where the lice live and lay their nits in the seams of clothing and return to the skin surface only to feed. Pediculosis pubis is an extremely contagious STD and may involve not only the groin but also other hairy areas of the body. Eyelash infestation in a child may be a sign of sexual abuse by an infested adult.

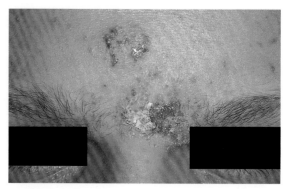

FIGURE 54-1. Impetigo. (From Frankel DH. *Field Guide to Clinical Dermatology*. 2nd ed. Philadelphia, PA: Lippincott Williams & Wilkins; 2006.)

CLINICAL MANIFESTATIONS

HISTORY

The onset of the skin lesions and associated symptoms—such as fever, warmth, or pruritus—should be part of the history. Tenderness, pain, mild paresthesias, or burning may occur at the site of inoculation with herpes virus infections. A prodrome of localized pain, tender lymphadenopathy, headache, generalized aching, and fever may occur. Shingles may also present with a prodrome of itching, pain, and burning in the affected dermatome before the rash develops. Associated underlying skin conditions or trauma should be noted. Local trauma or systemic changes such as menses, fatigue, or fever may trigger a recurrence of herpes simplex infections. Known contact with cases of scabies, lice, viral, or fungal infection may suggest that transmission has occurred.

Medications and medication allergies may be important in identifying other potential causes for the rash and in determining therapy. An attack of chicken pox usually confers lifelong immunity to chicken pox, but a previous varicella infection can reactivate and cause shingles. Unlike chicken pox, an episode of shingles does not confer lifelong immunity.

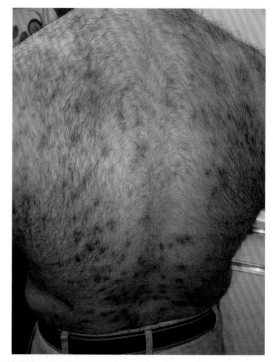

FIGURE 54-2. Folliculitis. (From Dr. Barankin Dermatology Collection.)

PHYSICAL EXAMINATION

The lesions of impetigo are superficial and are characterized by honey-colored crusts (Fig. 54-1). Erythema, warmth, edema, pain, and sometimes fever characterize cellulitis. Folliculitis is characterized by a pustule in association with a hair follicle (Fig. 54-2). Furuncles are larger fluctuant erythematous lesions that also occur in association with hairy regions (Fig. 54-3). Nikolsky sign aids in the diagnosis of staphylococcal

scalded skin syndrome and is elicited when local skin separation occurs after minor pressure.

Herpes simplex appears as grouped vesicles on an erythematous base which are uniform in size, unlike the vesicles seen in herpes zoster or chicken pox. The chicken pox rash has a centripetal distribution, starting at the trunk and spreading to the face and extremities. Lesions appear as "dewdrops on a rose petal," with a thin-walled vesicle filled with clear fluid on a red base; they appear

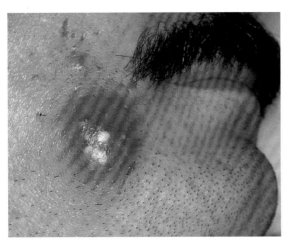

FIGURE 54-3. Furuncles. (From Frankel DH. *Field Guide to Clinical Dermatology*. 2nd ed. Philadelphia, PA: Lippincott Williams & Wilkins; 2006.)

as constellations of lesions in different stages at the same time. Warts are small tumors of the skin that obscure normal skin lines, have a mosaic surface pattern, and may have thrombosed vessels appearing as black dots on the surface. The lesions of molluscum contagiosum are discrete 2 to 5 mm, slightly umbilicated, flesh-colored, dome-shaped papules occurring on the face, trunk, axillae, and extremities in children and in the pubic and genital areas in adults (Fig. 54-4).

Fungal infections are characterized by erythematous as well as hypopigmented or hyperpigmented lesions associated with scaling. They occur on various parts of the body. The classic ringworm lesion has a central clear area and a raised edge.

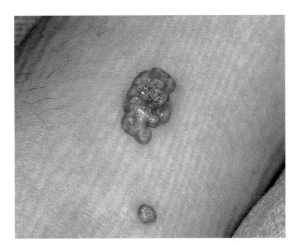

FIGURE 54-4. Molluscum contagiosum. (From Frankel DH. *Field Guide to Clinical Dermatology*. 2nd ed. Philadelphia, PA: Lippincott Williams & Wilkins; 2006.)

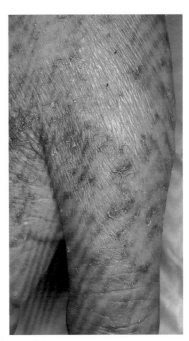

FIGURE 54-5. Scabies. (From Frankel DH. *Field Guide to Clinical Dermatology*. 2nd ed. Philadelphia, PA: Lippincott Williams & Wilkins; 2006.)

Lice are suspected when a patient itches without an apparent rash. Lice and nits may be identified on close visual examination. Scabies are associated with linear burrows on the distal extremities and occur as scattered pruritic papules on the rest of the body (Fig. 54-5).

DIFFERENTIAL DIAGNOSIS

The differential diagnosis for bacterial infections includes other forms of dermatitis, such as eczema and contact or stasis dermatitis. Herpes virus infections—including shingles, chicken pox, and herpes simplex—may be confused with eczema, impetigo, or contact dermatitis. The lesions of molluscum contagiosum may mimic warts or herpes simplex. Both warts and molluscum may be confused with skin tags, dermatofibromas, or nevi. The differential diagnosis for fungal infections includes pityriasis alba, pityriasis rosea, eczema, or in some instances psoriasis or seborrheic dermatitis. Scabies lesions may form vesicles, leading to the consideration of diagnoses such as herpes and contact dermatitis.

DIAGNOSTIC EVALUATION

Skin infections are usually diagnosed clinically. Additional diagnostic measures obtained to assist with diagnosis include blood cultures, wound cultures,

TABLE 54-1. Diagnostic Testing and Treatment of Common Skin Infection

Infection	Diagnostic Test	Treatment
Impetigo	Clinical examination	Topical mupirocin, oral dicloxacillin, cephalexin
Cellulitis	Clinical examination, blood or wound cultures	Oral or intravenous dicloxacillin, cefazolin, cephalexin; trimethoprim-sulfamethoxazole, clindamycin
Furuncles	Clinical examination, culture of drainage	Incision and drainage, antibiotics
Herpes simplex	Clinical examination, Tzanck smear, culture	Antivirals: acyclovir, famciclovir, valacyclovir
Chicken pox, herpes zoster	Clinical examination, culture, serology	Antivirals as for herpes simplex
Warts	Clinical examination, biopsy	Electrocautery, cryotherapy, topical salicylic acid, imiquimod, or squaric acid, immunotherapy
Molluscum contagiosum	Clinical examination, biopsy	Curettage, cryotherapy, tretinoin, salicylic acid

viral cultures of suspicious lesions, and microscopic examination of skin scrapings or suspected organisms (Table 54-1). Blood cultures are usually negative, but bacteremia can occur with extensive cellulitis. Wound cultures are in general not helpful, though some advocate obtaining "leading edge" cultures by injecting and aspirating from the edge of the infection. More helpful is a culture obtained from a purulent infection such as an abscess or furuncle. Viral culture is the most definitive method for diagnosing herpes infections. The diagnosis of fungal infections is made by KOH wet-mount preparations, which allow direct visualization under the microscope of the branching hyphae of dermatophytes in keratinized material. Culture is necessary for scalp, hair, and nail fungal infections to identify the true source of infection and determine proper treatment. Mycosel agar, dermatophyte test medium, and Sabouraud dextrose agar are the most common fungal culture media.

TREATMENT

Treatment generally involves use of a topical or oral medication directed at the offending organism. More extensive bacterial infections may require hospitalization and intravenous antibiotics. Furuncles are self-limited and usually respond to frequent moist, warm compresses followed by incision, drainage, and packing. Antibiotics are often prescribed but may not be necessary for furuncles that have been properly drained. For patients with recurrent impetigo or furuncles, nasal cultures for *S. aureus* and treating those with positive cultures by applying mupirocin ointment intranasally helps to eradicate carriage of this bacterium and prevent recurrence. In addition, good hygiene and cleansing with an antibacterial soap may aid with eradication and prevention.

Although there is an increasing concern about antibiotic resistance in community-acquired cellulitis, in most cases of nonpurulent and uncomplicated cellulitis coverage for methicillin-resistant *S. aureus* (MRSA) and gram-negative infections adds little benefit. In these cases, a first-generation cephalosporin (e.g., cephalexin), an antistaphylococcal penicillin (e.g., dicloxicillin), or amoxicillin clavulanate are acceptable outpatient choices. If there is a true penicillin allergy, clindamycin is an acceptable alternative. If there is a purulent cellulitis caused by suspected (i.e., the patient has risk factors for MRSA) or known MRSA, adding trimethoprim-sulfamethoxazole or doxycycline is appropriate. Risk factors for MRSA include recent hospitalization, residing in a long-term care facility, participating in contact sports, recent antibiotic treatment, living in crowded or unsanitary conditions, men having sex with men, intravenous drug use, and individuals with previous MRSA exposure. Duration of therapy is based on the clinical response but, in general, outpatient treatment ranges from 5 to 10 days.

Treatment for herpes simplex and varicella infections consists of measures to relieve discomfort, promote healing, and prevent recurrence. Antiviral agents decrease the duration of viral excretion, new lesion formation, and vesicles. Antipruritic lotions, antihistamines, and antibiotics for if a secondary bacterial infection develops are also recommended. Antiviral agents started within the first 48 to 72 hours may shorten the course of illness and, in the case of herpes zoster, may decrease the likelihood of developing postherpetic neuralgia. Acyclovir and varicella zoster immune globulin (VZIG) are also indicated in immunocompromised patients.

Wart treatment depends on the site and severity of the wart; options include electrocautery, blunt dissection, topical salicylic acid or imiquimod, liquid nitrogen, or tape occlusion. For warts refractory to other therapies, topical immunotherapy with contact allergens such as squaric acid or dinitrochlorobenzene has been successful for many patients. In addition to topical or systemic antifungal agents, treatment of candidal infections should include keeping the infected skin area clean and dry. Permethrin is the first line of treatment for scabies, which involves application of the lotion to the entire body for 12 hours before rinsing. Reapplication and treatment 1 week later may improve treatment success. Second-line scabies treatment with gamma benzene hexachloride (Lindane) must be used exactly as directed to avoid potential neurotoxicity. Persistent itching may be treated with oral antihistamines or, if inflammation is present, topical steroids. Permethrin shampoo is the first line of therapy for lice and malathion is the second line of therapy and also very effective. To eradicate head lice, nit removal is an important component of treatment, because the nits may hatch and reinfect the patient. A nit comb is effective following the use of the shampoo. Treatment is then repeated 1 week later to increase success in treatment (see Table 54-1).

KEY POINTS

- Clinical infection results from breaks in the skin (i.e., abrasions, needle punctures, and catheters), loss of local immunity, and changes in the skin flora.

- Although more than 100 bacteria have been identified as causing cellulitis, two gram-positive cocci, *S. aureus*, and group A beta hemolytic streptococcus account for most skin and soft-tissue infections.

- HSV-1 is usually seen in oral infections, whereas HSV-2 is associated with genital infections.

- Wart treatment depends on the site and severity of the wart; options include electrocautery, blunt dissection, topical agents, liquid nitrogen, and tape occlusion.

- Oral antibiotics are usually effective for treating most cases of cellulitis. Unless MRSA is suspected, penicillinase-resistant antibiotics (cloxacillin or dicloxacillin), or cephalosporins (e.g., cephalexin) are good empiric choices.

55 | Tobacco Abuse

Tobacco abuse is the leading preventable cause of death and disability in the United States. Each year in the United States, about 1 in 5 deaths are attributable to tobacco use. Both changes in public health policy such as not allowing smoking in public places and increased pricing have contributed to a decline in the overall percentage of smokers in the United States to about 15%. The incidence of adolescent smoking has also fallen continuously since its peak in the 1970s (Fig. 55-1). However, despite these positive trends, millions of Americans continue to smoke. Multiple studies indicate that advising patients to stop smoking and offering smoking cessation therapies can help.

PATHOGENESIS

Smoking is a complex behavior that is still not completely understood. Pharmacologic and psychological models have been proposed. The psychological and behavioral models propose that smoking is a learned behavior that continues because the individual receives gratification from it. Smoking also becomes a habit, triggered by situations such as stress or alcohol. There also appears to be a link between depression and smoking.

The pharmacologic model emphasizes physical addiction to smoking. There is abundant evidence that nicotine is an addictive drug capable of creating tolerance and physical dependence, as well as causing

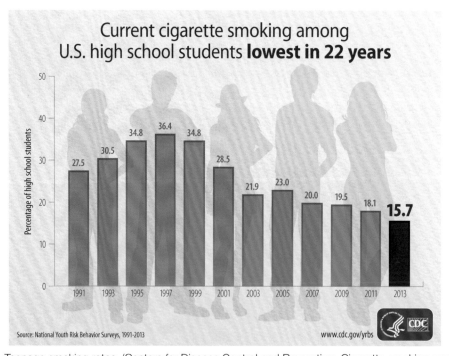

FIGURE 55-1. Teenage smoking rates. (Centers for Disease Control and Prevention. Cigarette smoking among U.S. high school students at lowest level in 22 years. https://www.cdc.gov/media/releases/2014/images/p0612-YRBS.pdf, accessed January, 2018.)

withdrawal symptoms. According to this model, smokers use tobacco to maintain their nicotine levels and avoid withdrawal. Withdrawal symptoms include craving for cigarettes, restlessness, irritability, poor concentration, headache, and nausea. Withdrawal varies greatly among smokers. Clinically, those who need to smoke shortly after rising, smoke at least one pack a day, or have difficulty abstaining for even a few hours, are at greatest risk for withdrawal symptoms. Although withdrawal symptoms explain why many smokers fail to quit during the first week, they do not explain why many smokers have trouble abstaining for long periods of time.

Epidemiologic data clearly identify multiple benefits for smoking cessation. Box 55-1 lists some health consequences of smoking. Even older individuals benefit from stopping tobacco use after years of smoking or from quitting after a smoking-related illness. Lung cancer risk drops significantly 10 years after a smoker quits.

Cigarette smoking increases cardiovascular morbidity and mortality and affects all phases of atherosclerosis from endothelial dysfunction to acute clinical events. The exact mechanisms involved in tobacco-related cardiovascular dysfunction are largely unknown, but smoking is linked to increases in inflammation, thrombosis, and oxidation of low-density lipoprotein cholesterol. Coronary risk reduction occurs much more rapidly; the excess risk of a second MI is cut in half within 1 to 2 years of quitting.

CLINICAL MANIFESTATIONS

HISTORY

Smokers may present with symptoms of one of the smoking-related illnesses listed in Box 55-1. More commonly, smokers complain of cough, sore throat, shortness of breath, and frequent infections. The history should focus on when and why the patient began to smoke. Smoking can be quantified in pack-years, obtained by multiplying the average number of packs smoked per day by the number of years of smoking. Asking whether the patient has thought about quitting, tried to quit, or intends to quit helps assess readiness and motivation to quit. By understanding and accepting the patient's past failures or fears about quitting, the physician can help address barriers to smoking cessation.

PHYSICAL EXAMINATION

The physical examination may show signs of underlying smoking-related disease. The mouth and

BOX 55-1. Health Consequences Associated with Smoking

Cancers
Lung cancer
Oral cancers
Laryngeal cancers
Pharyngeal cancers
Esophageal cancers
Genitourinary cancers: kidney, bladder, cervical
Gastrointestinal cancers: pancreas, stomach

Cardiovascular
Myocardial infarction
Cerebrovascular disease
Peripheral vascular disease

Pulmonary
Chronic obstructive pulmonary disease
Recurring respiratory infections

Secondhand smoke–related problems
High incidence of respiratory tract infections
Asthma in children of smokers
Higher risk of lung cancer in household members of smokers

Pregnancy
Lower birth weight babies
Higher incidence of sudden infant death syndrome

Others
Osteoporosis
Peptic ulcer disease
Skin wrinkling
Discolored skin and teeth
Halitosis

oral cavity should be examined for lesions that appear cancerous. The tongue in smokers often has a brownish discoloration because of exposure to the tar in smoke. Wheezing and diminished breath sounds may indicate COPD. Peripheral pulses may be diminished, suggesting vascular disease.

DIFFERENTIAL DIAGNOSIS

In general, laboratory tests are not helpful for the diagnosis, but may be indicated to evaluate the consequences of smoking. Pulmonary function tests may help quantify pulmonary damage and provide evidence of the importance of smoking cessation.

If the tests are normal, it is important to stress the importance of stopping smoking immediately to prevent future damage.

CLINICAL EVALUATION

By providing all smokers seen in the office with even brief advice, the physician can help increase the proportion of smokers who quit. The National Cancer Institute lists the five A's for office-based intervention:

1. **Ask**—about smoking at every opportunity. Ask those who smoke whether they are interested in stopping.
2. **Advise**—every smoker with a clear, unambiguous, direct message. Tailor the advice to the patient's individual situation.
3. **Assess**—a patient's willingness to quit.
4. **Assist**—patients in their efforts to stop. If a smoker is ready to quit, ask him or her to set a quit date. Provide self-help material and offer pharmacologic therapy, such as nicotine replacement. Consider a referral to a formal smoking cessation program. If the individual is not ready to quit, discuss the benefits of and barriers to smoking cessation. Make the information as relevant to the individual as possible. Advise the smoker to avoid exposing family members to secondhand smoke. Indicate a willingness to help in the future, when the smoker is ready, and continue to ask about quitting in follow-up visits.
5. **Arrange**—a follow-up appointment, generally within 1 to 2 weeks after the quit date. Make sure you congratulate those who have quit and reinforce the benefits of giving up smoking. Discuss high-risk situations for relapse, and review coping mechanisms. For those who fail to quit, provide positive reinforcement for taking the first steps toward quitting. Ask what obstacles the patient encountered, and discuss strategies to overcome these problems in the future. Encourage the smoker to set another quit date.

TREATMENT

The most effective approaches address nicotine addiction and behavioral dependence. Nicotine replacement mitigates some of the symptoms of withdrawal by continuing nicotine exposure, although at reduced and tapered doses. Nicotine delivery can be achieved with transdermal patches, nicotine-containing chewing gum, lozenges, or nicotine inhalers. All are ideally used for 2 to 3 months and then discontinued. They may be utilized for more extended periods of time if needed to ensure continued abstinence from smoking.

Nicotine replacement is not a panacea, but does improve the quit rate by about 50% to 70%. They should be offered to smokers willing to set a quit date, who will not smoke while on nicotine replacement therapy (NRT), and who ideally will follow a behavioral program, either individually or in a group setting. The side effects of the nicotine patch are mild, generally limited to skin irritation. Nicotine gum was the original form of nicotine replacement. Side effects of the gum are mostly related to vigorous chewing and the release of excess nicotine. These symptoms include sore jaw, mouth irritation, hiccups, nausea, dizziness, and headache. Data suggest that combined use of patches to provide a continuous release of nicotine and adding rapid-release forms of nicotine (inhalers, gum, lozenges) to address periods of increased desire for nicotine is an effective strategy.

Bupropion, originally marketed as an antidepressant, also enhances quit rates. Its use is contraindicated in individuals with a history of seizures. It is useful for people who do not want to, or have been unable to quit with nicotine replacement. It is generally started 1 week before the target quit date. Bupropion has been used in conjunction with nicotine replacement, and some evidence suggests that the combination of the two is more effective than either one alone. Varenicline is a nicotinic receptor agonist, and has been shown to be an effective oral therapy. It decreases the urge to smoke and reduces withdrawal symptoms and it can be prescribed with nicotine replacement therapy. Varenicline is taken for 1 week while the patient may still be smoking, and during the second week the dose is increased and the patient stops smoking. Nausea is the most common adverse effect, and there have been reports of neuropsychiatric side effects including suicidal ideation.

The behavioral model has also stimulated a host of strategies to help manipulate the environment. The physician can work with the patients to develop strategies like spending time in places where smoking is not permitted, or rewarding themselves with the money saved by not smoking. Organized group programs such as those sponsored by the American Cancer Society or the American Lung Association may also be of benefit. These societies sponsor telephone services that provide education, encouragement, advice, and referral. Giving up smoking is associated with weight gain, and patients should be encouraged to increase their activity and watch their diets. The health benefits from smoking cessation are far greater than the risk from the weight gain associated with giving up smoking.

KEY POINTS

- Tobacco abuse is the leading preventable cause of death and disability in the United States.

- There are benefits even for older individuals who stop smoking after many years or quit after a smoking-related illness.

- By providing all smokers seen in the office with even brief advice, the physician can help increase the proportion of smokers who quit.

- Bupropion, varenicline, and nicotine replacement are medication options.

56 | Urinary Tract Infection

Urinary tract infections (UTIs) affect women more often than men. Bacteriuria is present in 1% of infants of both genders, 1% to 2% of school-age girls, and 3% to 4% of women of childbearing age, whereas males have a prevalence of bacteriuria of 0.3% after infancy; 8% of girls and 2% of boys have UTIs by age 7. With advancing age, the occurrence of bacteriuria increases for both genders to about 15% of the geriatric population.

Symptomatic UTI is much less common in men than in women. Most UTIs in males occur in infants or the elderly, usually associated with urologic abnormalities like bladder outlet obstruction and prostatic hyperplasia. In contrast, up to 10% of women experience an infection in a given year, and about 50% of women have at least one infection over their lifetime.

PATHOGENESIS

Normal urine is sterile because of the antibacterial properties of the bladder mucosa and urine and the removal of bacteria through voiding. In most UTIs, bacteria gain access to the bladder via the urethra. Women are more vulnerable to UTIs because bacteria can access the bladder through the shorter female urethra. Further, bacterial ascent from the bladder is the mechanism responsible for most renal parenchymal infections. Among sexually active women, risk factors for infection include frequency of sexual intercourse, spermicide use, and a history of UTI.

UTIs can be divided into lower tract infections (urethritis, cystitis, and prostatitis) and upper tract infections (acute pyelonephritis and intrarenal and perinephric abscesses), which may occur together or independently. Infections of the urethra and bladder are usually superficial, whereas prostatitis, pyelonephritis, and renal suppuration signify tissue invasion.

Gram-negative bacilli are the most common cause of infection. *Escherichia coli* is the most common pathogen and accounts for 70% to 80% of cases of UTI. Other gram-negative rods—such as *Proteus, Klebsiella, Enterobacter, Serratia*, and *Pseudomonas*—account for a smaller proportion of infections and are associated with urologic manipulation, calculi, obstruction, and catheter-associated infections. *Proteus* species, by virtue of urease production, and *Klebsiella* species, through the production of extracellular slime and polysaccharides, predispose individuals to formation of stones.

Although gram-positive cocci are less common, *Staphylococcus saprophyticus* accounts for 10% to 15% of acute symptomatic UTIs in young sexually active women. Enterococci frequently cause infection in geriatric patients, and enterococci and *Staphylococcus aureus* infections are more common in patients with renal stones or previous instrumentation. Isolation of *S. aureus* from the urine should arouse suspicion for a bacteremia seeding to the kidneys.

Sexual intercourse increases the likelihood of cystitis. In addition, the use of a diaphragm and/or a spermicide is associated with increased vaginal colonization with *E. coli* and the risk of urinary infection. Any impediment to the free flow of urine—such as tumor, stricture, stone, neurologic disease, or prostatic hypertrophy—is associated with an increased frequency of UTI. Urinary infections are detected in 2% to 8% of pregnant women, and 20% to 30% of pregnant women with asymptomatic bacteriuria subsequently develop pyelonephritis. This predisposition to upper tract infection during pregnancy results from decreased ureteral tone and peristalsis and temporary incompetence of the vesicoureteral valves.

Vesicoureteral reflux occurs during voiding or with elevation of pressure in the bladder, and predisposes individuals to upper tract infections. Vesicoureteral reflux is common among children with a family history of vesicoureteral reflux and those with anatomic abnormalities of the urinary tract. Over time, reflux with infection can cause renal scarring and lead to hypertension.

CLINICAL MANIFESTATIONS

HISTORY

Patients with cystitis usually experience dysuria, frequency, urgency, and suprapubic pain, and may have hematuria. The urine becomes grossly cloudy, malodorous, and bloody in about 30% of cases. Symptoms of acute pyelonephritis include fever (>101°F or 38.3°C), shaking chills, nausea, vomiting, diarrhea, and flank pain. Symptoms of cystitis may or may not precede an upper tract infection. Patients should be asked about previous UTIs, renal disease, kidney stones, and recent surgical procedures or antibiotic use, sexual activity, and contraceptive use. Inquiring about other medical problems, such as diabetes, is important because an underlying condition may affect management.

Older children experience UTI symptoms similar to those found in adults. In infants and younger children, irritability, fever, nausea, vomiting, bed-wetting, and diarrhea may be presenting symptoms of a UTI. Elderly patients may also present with nonspecific symptoms, such as change in mental status, malaise, incontinence, and poor appetite.

PHYSICAL EXAMINATION

The physical examination should include temperature, an abdominal examination, and checking for CVA tenderness. For individuals unable to distinguish between the "internal" dysuria associated with urethritis or cystitis and "external" dysuria that may occur with vaginitis, a genital examination can be helpful. Suprapubic tenderness is consistent with cystitis, whereas a fever (>101°F), ill appearance, and CVA tenderness suggest pyelonephritis.

DIFFERENTIAL DIAGNOSIS

The differential diagnosis of dysuria includes UTI, vaginitis, and urethritis. Approximately 30% of patients with acute dysuria, frequency, and pyuria have midstream urine cultures with either no growth or insignificant bacterial growth. Clinically, these patients cannot be readily distinguished from those with cystitis. In this situation, sexually transmitted pathogens—such as *Chlamydia trachomatis*, *Neisseria gonorrhoeae*, and HSV—or a low-count *E. coli* or staphylococcal UTI may account for the symptoms. Chlamydial or gonococcal infection should be suspected when there is a gradual onset of illness, no hematuria, no suprapubic pain, and more than 7 days of symptoms. A new sex partner or exposure to chlamydial or gonococcal urethritis should heighten suspicion for a sexually transmitted infection. Infection with *C. trachomatis*, *N. gonorrhoeae*, *Trichomonas*, *Candida*, and herpes simplex virus (HSV) should be considered in patients with vaginal discharge, mucopurulent cervicitis, genital lesions, urethritis, but negative urine cultures.

Noninfectious causes, such as urethral or bladder irritation from conditions such as trauma or exposure to chemical irritants (e.g., coffee, spicy foods, citrus), can cause dysuria. A negative culture and a normal UA characterize interstitial cystitis, which is most common in young women. Cystoscopy may reveal inflammation and mucosal hemorrhage. Bladder tumors, instrumentation, and trauma may also cause cystitis symptoms.

Dysuria is less common in men. In younger sexually active men, urethritis rather than cystitis is the usual etiology. Older men may have irritative symptoms secondary to BPH rather than from an infection. Other considerations in men include prostatitis or epididymitis.

Patients with upper tract infection usually experience back pain. Noninfectious causes of flank pain include renal stones, renal infarction, and papillary necrosis.

DIAGNOSTIC EVALUATION

Many experts recommend treating healthy young women with characteristic symptoms of acute uncomplicated cystitis and pyuria without doing an initial urine culture. Urinalysis for evaluation of pyuria is the most valuable laboratory diagnostic test for UTI, and the most accurate method for assessing pyuria is a voided midstream urine specimen. The absence of pyuria suggests an alternative diagnosis. The leukocyte esterase "dipstick" method has a sensitivity of over 80% in identifying UTIs, and is a useful alternative when microscopy is not available. Nitrite positivity is very specific for UTIs, and the combination of leukocyte esterase and nitrite positivity is more than 90% sensitive in identifying them. Pyuria in the absence of bacteriuria (sterile pyuria) may indicate infection with organisms, such as *C. trachomatis, Ureaplasma urealyticum, Mycobacterium tuberculosis,* and fungi or noninfectious urologic conditions such as calculi, anatomic abnormality, nephrocalcinosis, or polycystic disease. WBC casts suggest upper tract involvement.

A urine culture is indicated if the diagnosis is uncertain, in males, in patients with suspected upper tract infections, and in those with complicating factors such as pregnancy or diabetes.

Given the increasing prevalence of antimicrobial resistance, obtaining a urine culture before initiating therapy is necessary if symptoms persist or recur within 3 months following previous antimicrobial therapy, or when antimicrobial resistant or complicated infection is suspected.

Growth of more than 100,000 organisms/mL from a properly collected midstream clean catch urine sample indicates infection. In urine specimens obtained by suprapubic aspiration or catheterization, colony counts of 100 to 10,000/mL generally indicate infection. In some circumstances (antibiotic treatment, high urea concentration, high osmolarity, low pH), relatively low bacterial colony counts may still indicate infection. Dilute urine or recent voiding also reduces bacterial counts in urine.

TREATMENT

Table 56-1 outlines treatment for UTIs in adults. The following principles underlie the treatment of UTIs:

1. In straightforward cases of uncomplicated cystitis, diagnosis and treatment may be based on symptoms and a UA without culture. However, in complicated or questionable cases, a UA, Gram stain, or culture is indicated to confirm infection before starting treatment. When available, antimicrobial sensitivity testing should direct or modify therapy. All cases of suspected pyelonephritis require testing.
2. If possible, identify and correct factors predisposing the patient to infection, such as obstruction and calculi.
3. In general, uncomplicated infections and lower tract infections respond to shorter courses of therapy, whereas upper tract infections require longer treatment. Early recurrences usually mean relapse. Recurrences more than 2 weeks after completing therapy usually represent reinfection with a new strain.
4. Community-acquired infections, especially initial infections, are usually due to antibiotic-sensitive strains.
5. In patients with repeated infections, instrumentation, or recent hospitalization, the presence of antibiotic-resistant strains should be suspected.

Cystitis usually responds to shorter courses of antibiotics. Single doses of fosfomycin (Monurol) and short courses (3 days) of TMP/SMX are effective in areas where resistance to *E. coli* is <20%. Nitrofurantoin (100 mg orally twice daily for 5 to 7 days) can be used for uncomplicated cystitis, but should be avoided in cases of suspected pyelonephritis. Although effective, the CDC no longer recommends fluoroquinolones as first-line therapy for uncomplicated cystitis because of concerns about increasing resistance and side effects. However, they are still first-line agents for the empiric treatment of pyelonephritis. Males with UTI often have urologic abnormalities or prostatic involvement, and should receive an antibiotic course for 7 to 14 days.

With upper tract infections, most cases respond to 10 to 14 days of therapy. In some cases, longer courses of treatment (2 to 6 weeks) aimed at eradicating a persistent focus of infection may be necessary. *E. coli* causes most cases of acute uncomplicated pyelonephritis in healthy women without underlying urologic disease. Most uncomplicated cases respond to a 14-day course of a fluoroquinolone or a third-generation cephalosporin. Ampicillin, amoxicillin, or TMP/SMX should not be used as initial therapy because 20% to 30% of strains of *E. coli* are now resistant to these drugs.

First-line agents for acute cystitis in pregnancy include amoxicillin, nitrofurantoin, or a cephalosporin. Screening for infection and treating asymptomatic bacteriuria is indicated for all pregnant women because of the risk of developing pyelonephritis. Acute pyelonephritis in pregnancy usually requires hospitalization and parenteral antibiotic therapy, generally with a cephalosporin or extended-spectrum penicillin. After treatment, a culture to document clearing of the infection is indicated, and should be repeated monthly until delivery. Continuous low-dose prophylaxis with nitrofurantoin is indicated for pregnant women with recurrent infections.

Goals of UTI treatment in infants and children are to eliminate infection, to relieve acute symptoms, including fever, dysuria, frequency, and to prevent

TABLE 56-1. Urinary Tract Infections in Adults

Category	Diagnostic Criteria	Principal Pathogens	First-Line Therapy	Comments
Acute uncomplicated cystitis	Urinalysis for pyuria and hematuria (culture not required)	• *Escherichia coli* • *Staphylococcus saprophyticus* • *Proteus mirabilis* • *Klebsiella pneumoniae*	• Fosfomycin • Nitrofurantoin • TMP/SMX DS (Bactrim, Septra) • Trimethoprim (Priloprim) • Ciprofloxacin (Cipro)	• Quinolones, fosfomycin, and nitrofurantoin are first-line agents in areas of TMP/SMX resistance or in patients who cannot tolerate TMP/SMX
Recurrent cystitis in young women	Symptoms and a urine culture with a bacterial count of >100,000 CFU/mL of urine	• Same as for acute uncomplicated cystitis	• If the patient has more than three cystitis episodes per year, treat prophylactically with postcoital or continuous daily therapy (see text)	• Repeat therapy for 7–10 days based on culture results and then use prophylactic therapy[a]
Acute cystitis in young men	Urine culture with a bacterial count of 1000–10,000 CFU/mL of urine	• Same as for acute uncomplicated cystitis	• Same as for acute uncomplicated cystitis, except nitrofurantoin is not a preferred agent	• Treat for 7–10 days
Acute uncomplicated pyelonephritis	Urine culture with a bacterial count of 100,000 CFU/mL of urine	• Same as for acute uncomplicated cystitis	• If gram-negative organism, oral fluoroquinolone • If gram-positive organism, amoxicillin • If parenteral administration is required, ceftriaxone (Rocephin) or a fluoroquinolone • If *Enterococcus* species, add oral or IV amoxicillin	• Switch from IV to oral administration when the patient is able to take medication by mouth; complete a 14-day course
Complicated urinary tract infection	Urine culture with a bacterial count of >10,000 CFU/mL of urine	• *E. coli* • *K. pneumoniae* • *P. mirabilis* • *Enterococcus* species • *Pseudomonas aeruginosa*	• If gram-negative organism, oral fluoroquinolone • If *Enterococcus* species, ampicillin or amoxicillin with or without gentamicin (Garamycin)	• Treat for 10–14 days
Asymptomatic bacteriuria in pregnancy	Urine culture with a bacterial colony count of >100,000 CFU/mL of urine	• Same as for acute uncomplicated cystitis	• Amoxicillin • Nitrofurantoin (Macrodantin) • Cephalexin (Keflex)	• Avoid tetracyclines and fluoroquinolones • Treat for 3–7 days
Catheter-associated urinary tract infection	Symptoms and a urine culture with a bacterial count of >100 CFU/mL of urine	• Depends on duration of catheterization	• If gram-negative organism, a fluoroquinolone • If gram-positive organism, ampicillin or amoxicillin plus gentamicin	• Remove catheter if possible, and treat for 7–10 days • For patients with long-term catheters and symptoms, treat for 5–7 days

[a]Patient is given a prescription for an antibiotic to take if symptoms develop.
CFU, colony-forming unit; IV, intravenous; TMP/SMX, trimethoprim–sulfamethoxazole.
Source: Data from Stamm WE, Hooton TM. Management of urinary tract infections in adults. *N Engl J Med*. 1993;329:1328–1334.

TABLE 56-2. Treatment Regimens for Uncomplicated Acute Bacterial Cystitis

Antimicrobial Agent	Dose	Adverse Events and Comments
Trimethoprim–sulfamethoxazole	One tablet (160 mg trimethoprim–800 mg sulfamethoxazole) twice daily for 3 days	Fever, rash, photosensitivity, neutropenia, thrombocytopenia, GI upset, pruritus, urticaria, and Stevens–Johnson syndrome. Avoid empiric use if community resistance >20%.
Ciprofloxacin	250 mg twice daily for 3 days	Rash, confusion, seizures, restlessness, headache, severe hypersensitivity, hypoglycemia, hyperglycemia, and Achilles tendon rupture (in patients older than 60 years). Considered a second-line agent for cystitis.
Levofloxacin	250 mg once daily for 3 days	Same as for ciprofloxacin
Nitrofurantoin monohydrated macrocrystals	100 mg twice daily for 5–7 days	Nausea, vomiting, hypersensitivity, headache, peripheral neuropathy, hepatitis, hemolytic anemia, and pulmonary reactions
Fosfomycin tromethamine	3 g dose (powder), single dose	Diarrhea, nausea, vomiting, rash, and hypersensitivity. Avoid if suspected pyelonephritis.
Beta-lactams (e.g., amoxicillin, amoxicillin clavulanate, cephalosporin)	Use for 3–7 days	Second-line agents because of resistance, considered safe during pregnancy. Common side effects include GU symptoms and allergic reactions.

GI, gastrointestinal; GU, genitourinary.
Source: From https://www.guideline.gov/summaries/summary/12628, accessed on July, 2017.

recurrence and long-term complications such as hypertension, renal scarring, and impaired renal growth and function.

E. coli remains the most common bacteria causing UTI in infants and young children. Other organisms causing UTI in the pediatric population include *Klebsiella*, *Proteus*, *Enterobacter*, and *Citrobacter*. Aminoglycosides (gentamicin and amikacin) and third-generation cephalosporins (cefpodoxime, cefixime, cefdinir, ceftibuten, cefotaxime, and ceftriaxone) are first-line agents for UTI in children. A child or infant, who is toxic, dehydrated, or unable to tolerate oral intake, requires parenteral antimicrobial therapy and hospitalization. Children who fail to improve after 2 days of antibiotic therapy need reevaluation and repeat urine testing. Imaging (US or CT) and cystoscopy are indicated in women with relapsing infection, a history of childhood infections, stones, painless hematuria, or recurrent pyelonephritis. Most males with a single UTI require investigation. Men or women presenting with acute infection and signs or symptoms suggestive of an obstruction or stones should undergo US or CT scan. Children with pyelonephritis need imaging with dimercaptosuccinic acid (DMSA) nuclear scans to assess for renal function and scarring. Girls with recurrent UTI, boys with a single UTI, and children with pyelonephritis should undergo evaluation including renal US and voiding cystourethrogram (VCUG). The VCUG is generally performed after completing a course of antibiotics and sterilizing the urine, because infection itself may cause reflux. A proposed algorithm for imaging in children is presented in Figure 56-1.

Patients with frequent symptomatic infections may benefit from long-term administration of low-dose antibiotics to prevent recurrences. Daily or thrice-weekly administration of a single dose of TMP/SMX (80/400 mg), TMP (100 mg), or nitrofurantoin (50 mg) can reduce infections. Prophylactic antibiotics and voiding after sexual intercourse reduce recurrences in women whose infections are temporally related to intercourse. Other patients for whom prophylaxis appears beneficial include men with chronic prostatitis; patients undergoing prostatectomy, both during the operation and in the postoperative period; and pregnant women with asymptomatic bacteriuria. Asymptomatic bacteriuria in older women is common and does not require therapy.

In addition to antibiotics, oral phenazopyridine is a urinary analgesic that may help alleviate dysuria and frequency until antimicrobial therapy begins to resolve the infection. Patients should be advised that phenazopyridine may turn their urine orange-red.

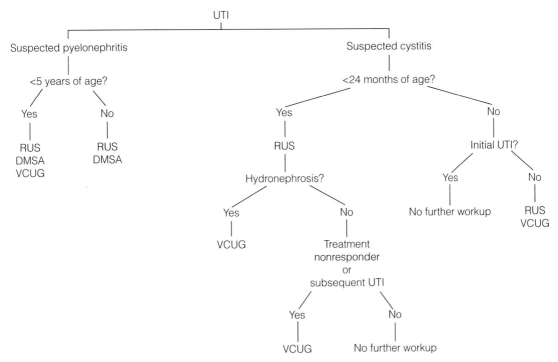

FIGURE 56-1. Algorithm for imaging with urinary tract infections in children. DMSA, dimercaptosuccinic acid; RUS, renal ultrasound; UTI, urinary tract infection; VCUG, voiding cystourethrogram. (From https://www.guideline .gov/summaries/summary/12628, accessed on July, 2017.)

KEY POINTS

- UTIs affect women more often than men.
- Gram-negative bacilli are the most common cause of infection. *E. coli* is the most common pathogen, and accounts for 70% to 80% of cases of UTI.
- The differential diagnosis of dysuria includes UTI, vaginitis, and urethritis.
- Pyuria is present in almost all urinary infections; its absence suggests an alternative diagnosis.
- In general, uncomplicated infections and lower tract infections respond to shorter courses of therapy, whereas upper tract infections require longer treatment.
- Uncomplicated cystitis in women can be treated with nitrofurantoin, TMP/SMX, or fosfomycin.
- Uncomplicated cystitis in men can be treated with TMP/SMX. Fluoroquinolones can be used for more complicated infections. Nitrofurantoin should not be used in men with cystitis.
- Patients with uncomplicated pyelonephritis can be treated as outpatients with ciprofloxacin (500 mg orally twice daily) or levofloxacin (750 mg oral once daily for 5 to 7 days).

57 | Urticaria

Urticaria, also known as hives or wheals, is a pruritic, immune-mediated skin eruption consisting of well-circumscribed papules and plaques on an erythematous base. It can affect any part of the body. Angioedema is a related condition that affects deeper layers of the skin, and often involves the face, tongue, extremities, or genitalia. Urticaria and angioedema can occur together. Urticaria affects 10% to 20% of the population, and is classified as acute (<6 weeks' duration) or chronic (>6 weeks). It can be a manifestation of many conditions, and determining the underlying cause can be challenging.

PATHOGENESIS

A number of stimuli, such as medications or foods, may serve as antigens that bind to IgE receptors on mast cells, causing them to degranulate. In other cases, physical or chemical stimuli may directly cause mast cell degranulation. Hypersensitivity to acetylcholine triggers mast cell degranulation in the physical urticarias. Autoimmune diseases associated with immune complex formation are additional causes of urticaria. These various stimuli trigger release of chemical mediators that increase blood flow and capillary permeability, causing leakage of protein-rich plasma from the local postcapillary venules and resulting in hive formation. Angioedema occurs with massive transudation of fluid into the dermis and subcutaneous tissues. Pruritus is usually present, but to a milder degree in angioedema, because there are fewer mast cells and sensory nerve endings in the deeper tissues.

CLINICAL MANIFESTATIONS

HISTORY

It is important that urticaria be differentiated from anaphylaxis, which requires much more rapid and aggressive treatment. Urticaria accompanied by symptoms of organ systems other than skin (such as wheezing, vomiting, diarrhea, or changes in level of consciousness) should be treated as anaphylaxis. The emergent management of anaphylaxis is not covered in this chapter.

The history is a critical element in trying to establish the cause of urticaria. Having the patient keep a log of activities may help identify triggers in chronic cases. All medications taken within 2 weeks of onset should be considered as a potential cause of urticaria or angioedema. Foods and food dyes may also cause urticaria. Occasionally, a patient may have urticaria or angioedema with a seasonal pattern because of a seasonal allergen that is inhaled, ingested, or contacted. Such patients may have other manifestations of atopy, such as allergic rhinitis or asthma, in reaction to the same allergens.

Viral infections, such as hepatitis B, hepatitis C, EBV, and herpes simplex, and parasitic infections may also cause urticaria; so, inquiring about recent infections and completing a thorough review of symptoms is essential. The physical urticarias result from environmental factors, such as a change in temperature or by direct stimulation of the skin from pressure, stroking, vibration, or light. In exercise-induced urticaria, pruritus, urticaria, angioedema, wheezing, and hypotension occur because of exercise.

There is an increased incidence of urticaria in association with thyroid disease (hyperthyroidism and hypothyroidism), which may resolve with the control of the thyroid disease. Urticaria with carcinoma of the colon, rectum, or lung and with lymphoid malignancies such as Hodgkin disease and B-cell lymphomas has been reported. Inquiring about systemic symptoms (weight loss, fever, chills, and night sweats) is important. Some etiologies of urticaria are outlined in Table 57-1.

TABLE 57-1. Differential Diagnosis of Urticaria
Idiopathic
Food and food additives
Medications
Infections (e.g., sinusitis, vaginitis, hepatitis, infectious mononucleosis)
Environmental allergens
Insect stings
Physical urticarias (heat, cold, pressure, exercise, vibration, sunshine)
Connective tissue disease
Malignancy
Hereditary C1 inhibitor deficiency
Thyroid disorders

PHYSICAL EXAMINATION

At the time of the office visit, the patient may be free of lesions. Skin lesions that are present should be examined; their characteristics and distribution may help identify possible causes. For example, typical urticarial lesions are erythematous plaques that blanch with pressure. Nonblanching purpuric lesions raise the possibility of an underlying vasculitis. Swelling that involves the face, lips, and periorbital region suggests angioedema.

A thorough examination looking for other associated or underlying diseases is warranted. Review the vital signs for any evidence of anaphylaxis (tachycardia or hypotension). The examination should include the ears, pharynx, sinuses, teeth, and lungs for signs of underlying infection. Examination of the abdomen should note the presence of hepatosplenomegaly or tenderness. Lymphadenopathy and joint swelling, effusion, or warmth should be documented.

DIFFERENTIAL DIAGNOSIS

Systemic vasculitides (e.g., Sjogren syndrome, rheumatoid arthritis, hepatitis, and SLE either with or without cryoglobulinemia) are associated with lesions that are visually indistinguishable from urticaria. In addition to idiopathic urticaria, the differential diagnosis includes underlying urticaria because of systemic diseases such as connective tissue diseases, infections, neoplasm, and thyroid disease. Underlying thyroid disease was found in

12% of one study population and sinus disease in 17% in another study. In up to 90% of cases of chronic urticaria (CU), no cause is identified. Studies examining the frequency of the different forms of urticaria and underlying causes vary depending on the study population. Food and medications are thought to account for a significant percentage of cases, with physical and contact urticarias occurring less often. Dermatologic conditions that can mimic urticaria include erythema multiforme, mast cell disorders, urticarial vasculitis, and bullous pemphigoid.

DIAGNOSTIC EVALUATION

For patients with acute urticaria, the history and physical examination will direct any further evaluation. In patients with CU, diagnostic testing may include a CBC with differential, liver function tests, ESR and/or CRP, and thyroid function. Further workup is directed by clinical history and physical examination, keeping in mind the differential diagnosis listed in Table 57-1. In patients with CU and no apparent cause, referral to an allergist for allergy testing (skin testing and immunoassay) is warranted. Despite evaluation, many patients remain undiagnosed.

TREATMENT

Underlying diseases such as connective tissue diseases, thyroid disease, and infections should be treated, and any identified triggers avoided. Medications that may be causing urticaria should be discontinued. For those patients with acute symptoms, the severity of the symptoms dictates treatment measures. Those with mild symptoms are treated with H_1 receptor blockers. These medications include the classic antihistamines, such as diphenhydramine, and the newer nonsedating antihistamines, such as loratadine. Those with severe symptoms should receive H_1 blockers, H_2 blockers, and a tapering course of corticosteroids (see Table 57-2).

Therapy for CU is often empiric because only a fraction of cases has an identifiable cause. Therapy includes nonpharmacologic and pharmacologic treatment. Avoiding NSAID medications, heat, and tight-fitting clothing may help. Pharmacologic treatment of CU is similar to that of acute urticaria. In refractory cases, stepwise additions of therapy may be necessary. If H_1 blockers do not provide

TABLE 57-2. Medications for Acute Urticaria

	Medication Class	Examples	Advantages	Disadvantages
Mild	Second generation H1 blockers	Loratadine Desloratadine Fexofenadine Cetirizine	Less sedating Once-daily dosing	No IV form available Slower acting
	First generation H1 blockers	Diphenhydramine Hydroxyzine	Parenteral forms available Rapid acting	Side effects include drowsiness, decreased reaction time, confusion, dizziness, impaired concentration, and decreased psychomotor performance. Use with caution in older patients.
	H2 blockers	Famotidine Ranitidine	May provide modest benefit when used in addition to H1 blockers	
Severe	Glucocorticoids	Prednisone for 3–7 days course.		Must be tapered if using >5 days course. Side effects including insomnia, gastrointestinal upset and tremor/anxiety.

adequate control, the following agents may be added: H_2 blockers, doxepin (a tricyclic antidepressant with strong antihistaminic effects), and leukotriene antagonists, such as montelukast. Corticosteroids in 7- to 14-day tapering courses are sometimes used for acute control of exacerbations. Cyclosporine or sulfasalazine may be useful as steroid-sparing agents to suppress CU. Other medications that have been studied and found beneficial to varying degrees for CU include dapsone, hydroxychloroquine, colchicine, tacrolimus, mycophenolate, and the new antiallergic, monoclonal antibody, omalizumab. Most cases of CU or angioedema resolve within 1 year, and only 10% to 20% of patients will have long-term symptoms.

KEY POINTS

- Urticaria is extremely common, affecting up to 10% to 20% of the population.

- In addition to allergens as triggers of urticaria, the differential diagnosis includes systemic disease, most notably connective tissue diseases, infections, neoplasm, and thyroid disease.

- Despite evaluation, many patients remain undiagnosed.

- For those patients with an acute urticaria, treatment includes avoidance of triggers, H_1 blockers, H_2 blockers, and/or corticosteroids. Therapy for chronic urticaria is often empiric because only a fraction of cases has any identifiable cause.

CLINICAL VIGNETTES

VIGNETTE 1

A 67-year-old male presents with dyspnea, 1+ pitting leg edema, regular rhythm that is sinus on his EKG, rales on lung examination, and pulmonary edema with a slightly enlarged cardiac silhouette on CXR.

1. Which of the following diagnostic tests will provide the most information to help guide future treatment?
   a. EKG
   b. BNP
   c. Chest CT scan
   d. Echocardiogram

2. The patient's EKG shows normal sinus rhythm (NSR) without acute changes; his cardiac markers are negative, and the echocardiogram shows normal valvular function with an ejection fraction (EF) of 35%. These findings are consistent with which of the following?
   a. Diastolic congestive heart failure
   b. Systolic congestive heart failure
   c. Normal cardiac function
   d. Pericarditis

VIGNETTE 2

A 35-year-old male presents with palpitations, temperature intolerance, and a slight tremor. Examination reveals warm and moist skin, minimal tremor upon action, brisk reflexes, and a smooth normal-size thyroid.

1. You are concerned about a thyroid disorder, and order diagnostic testing: which of the following tests would be most helpful in this patient?
   a. Thyroid ultrasound
   b. Nuclear medicine scan
   c. TSH
   d. Thyroid receptor antibodies
   e. Thyroglobulin

2. Following radioactive iodine ablation, the patient was no longer symptomatic and was started on levothyroxine as replacement for his hypothyroidism. He presents now for follow-up and his TSH is noted to be elevated at 10.5. Which of the following is correct management of this patient?
   a. Lower the levothyroxine dose
   b. Increase the levothyroxine dose
   c. No change in therapy
   d. Add liothyronine (T3) to his levothyroxine

VIGNETTE 3

A moderately overweight (BMI = 28.7) 42-year-old female with irregular menses and elevated glucose values has an HbA_{1C} of 6.7%. Her renal and liver function tests are within normal limits. She has comorbid hypertension and takes lisinopril.

1. In addition to dietary counseling and exercise, what additional therapy should you now recommend?
   a. Glargine insulin
   b. Glipizide
   c. Acarbose
   d. Metformin
   e. Pioglitazone

2. Her cholesterol is 230 with an LDL-cholesterol of 100. Her calculated cardiac risk in the next 10 years is 6%. Which of the following would you now recommend for this patient?
   a. Lovastatin 20 mg daily
   b. Pravastatin 20 mg daily
   c. Simvastatin 10 mg daily
   d. Atorvastatin 20 mg daily
   e. Rosuvastatin 40 mg daily

VIGNETTE 4

A 70-year-old female with a prior history of diabetes mellitus and a myocardial infarction 2 weeks ago presents with a depressed affect and anhedonia. She has a remote history of depression, but does not recall her medication used in prior treatment.

1. Which of the following medications would be most appropriate in treating this patient's depression?
   a. Amitriptyline
   b. Risperidone
   c. Buspirone
   d. Sertraline
   e. Methylphenidate

VIGNETTE 5

An 84-year-old male with lung cancer and brain metastases presents with extreme depression, including symptoms of anhedonia, depressed affect, and social withdrawal. The lung cancer causes shortness of breath, headaches, and recently some seizure activity related to the metastatic spread to his brain. He is currently receiving hospice/palliative care, and his physical symptoms are under control. He currently takes dexamethasone and levetiracetam.

1. Which of the following would most benefit this patient?
   a. Amitriptyline
   b. Sertraline
   c. Electroconvulsive therapy (ECT)
   d. Methylphenidate
   e. Bupropion

VIGNETTE 6

A 23-year-old female presents with recurring episodes of palpitations and dyspnea, for which she is evaluated in the emergency department. She has a normal physical examination, and laboratory tests including a D-dimer, TSH, cardiac enzymes, CBC, and metabolic panel. Her EKG is interpreted as normal with a rate of 100 and a sinus rhythm.

1. Which of the following is most consistent with this patient's presentation and workup?
   a. Pulmonary embolus
   b. Panic disorder
   c. Myocardial infarction
   d. Cushing disease
   e. Hyperthyroidism

2. Which of the following can cause symptoms that mimic an anxiety disorder or reaction?
   a. Hypothyroidism
   b. Diabetes mellitus
   c. Phenothiazines
   d. Propranolol
   e. Buspirone

VIGNETTE 7

A 34-year-old male presents to the office to seek help with the onset of withdrawal symptoms, he is experiencing because of stopping his alcohol intake abruptly 48 hours ago. He admits to drinking eight beers or more per day for years. He has never had a seizure, but gets irritable if he does not drink every day. In the office, he has a normal examination, except he appears anxious and has a slight tremor.

1. Which category of medications will be most helpful in managing this patient's symptoms?
   a. Antihistamines
   b. Benzodiazepines
   c. Antipsychotics
   d. SSRIs
   e. Anticholinergic muscle relaxant

2. When present, which of the following may play a role in the etiology of alcohol or substance abuse?
   a. An alcoholic parent
   b. Teetotaler parents
   c. Onset of drinking after age 20 years
   d. Clonidine use

VIGNETTE 8

A 32-year-old obese male is a new patient, who visits the office to establish care. He reports no significant past medical problems, takes no medications, and has no allergies. Upon review of systems, he reports stable weight, fatigue, nighttime heartburn, and snoring, but denies edema, chest pain, or shortness of breath. He complains of a nonproductive cough for the past several months that worsens at night. The cough is not associated with fever, wheezing, or shortness of breath. He does not smoke, drinks minimally, and denies illicit drug use. His vital signs and physical examination are normal, other than his BMI of 35.

1. Initial management of this patient would include which of the following?
   a. CXR
   b. EKG and exercise stress test
   c. Pulmonary function testing
   d. Empiric therapy with a PPI

2. Upon follow-up, the patient's heartburn and cough resolved with PPI therapy, but he continues to complain of excessive fatigue and now also daytime somnolence. His wife reports his snoring keeps her up at night. While continuing his current treatment, what additional testing is indicated to evaluate this patient's symptoms?
   a. EEG
   b. PSQ-9 testing
   c. Sleep study
   d. ESR

3. Since under treatment for his prior medical problems, the patient has been feeling much better, but he continues to gain weight despite lifestyle counseling and now has a BMI of 42. Physical and laboratory evaluation reveal a BP of 150/98, HbA$_{1C}$ of 6.3%. He wants the best long-term option for weight loss to avoid lifelong treatment for diabetes mellitus and hypertension. Which of the following has the best long-term weight loss results?
   a. Methylphenidate
   b. Bupropion
   c. Orlistat
   d. Bariatric surgery
   e. Phentermine

ANSWERS

VIGNETTE 1 Question 1

1. Answer D:
This patient is experiencing an exacerbation of congestive heart failure as evidenced by his dyspnea, edema, rales, and CXR findings. Although an EKG would be warranted to assess for MI or ischemia, and could impact immediate therapy, an echocardiogram will provide more long-term diagnostic and therapeutic utility. Treatment initially will include diuresis to get the patient out of pulmonary edema. However, long-term treatment decisions will benefit most from knowing if he has valvular disease, reduced EF, and whether there is systolic or diastolic dysfunction. An elevated BNP may confirm the diagnosis of CHF, but, with these physical findings, will likely add little to the clinical care. A chest CT would be of benefit for suspected PE, which may present with shortness of breath (SOB), tachycardia, peripheral edema, a normal CXR, cardiac markers, and EKG.

VIGNETTE 1 Question 2

2. Answer B:
An EF of <40% indicates systolic dysfunction and the patient will likely benefit from diuretics (furosemide, spironolactone), ACE inhibitors, and beta blockers. In diastolic dysfunction, the EF is typically within the normal range, but accompanied by impaired filling because of ventricular stiffness or poor relaxation. The role of specific agents for diastolic dysfunction is not clear, but treatment for this form of CHF centers less on volume status and more on increasing ventricular

filling. Beta blockers that slow the heart rate and allow more time for the ventricles to fill properly and ACE inhibitors to prevent ventricular muscle remodeling play a more prominent role. Some studies suggest that calcium channel blockers may reduce ventricular stiffness in some cases.

VIGNETTE 2 Question 1

1. Answer C:

The patient has signs and symptoms consistent with hyperthyroidism and a TSH can screen for hyperthyroidism. The TSH is suppressed in Graves disease, toxic goiter, factitious hyperthyroidism, and in the hyperthyroid phase of thyroiditis. Further testing may include T4, T3, nuclear scans, and antibody testing to determine the specific underlying cause because treatment will depend upon the cause. In primary hypothyroidism, the TSH is increased.

VIGNETTE 2 Question 2

2. Answer B:

Patients who undergo definitive therapy for hyperthyroidism with radioactive iodine ablation or thyroidectomy will require replacement therapy with thyroid hormone, most commonly levothyroxine. When adjusting the dose to achieve the right amount of levothyroxine, the TSH is measured. An elevated TSH signals that too little levothyroxine is being given because the hypothalamus/pituitary glands are trying to get the thyroid to increase its production with more TSH. So, in this patient, the dose should be increased. Patients receiving too much thyroid replacement will have a low TSH level with the central feedback suppressing TSH production in an attempt to tell the thyroid gland to cease production. With a suppressed TSH, the thyroid dose should be reduced. If the TSH is in the normal range, no changes would be necessary.

VIGNETTE 3 Question 1

1. Answer D:

Metformin is first-line therapy for most patients with diabetes or prediabetes. It is also useful adjunctive therapy for patients with polycystic ovaries, who may be obese and have comorbid diabetes or prediabetes. Metformin improves glucose metabolism by acting on both on the hepatic and peripheral glucose uptake. Metformin when used alone is neutral with regard to weight gain, whereas insulin and sulfonylureas increase insulin levels and are associated with weight gain. Acarbose and pioglitazone are generally not first-line agents, but can be beneficial as add-on therapy.

VIGNETTE 3 Question 2

2. Answer D:

Cholesterol therapy is indicated for diabetic patients with an LDL value between 70 and 190 mg/dL. Calculation of the 10-year cardiac risk through use of a risk calculator helps determine whether to use moderate- or high-intensity statin therapy. For those with a risk >7.5%, high-intensity statin therapy is warranted, whereas moderate intensity therapy is recommended for those with <7.5% risk. An example of a risk calculator is available at http://www.cvriskcalculator.com/.

VIGNETTE 4 Question 1

1. Answer D:

SSRIs are often recommended as first line of pharmacologic therapy for depression because of their combined efficacy and safety profile. Risperidone is not indicated as monotherapy for depression, but, while more commonly used to treat psychosis, does carry an indication for bipolar disease with mania. Buspirone is indicated for treatment of anxiety disorders, but not depression. On occasion, methylphenidate can be used to treat depression but is not a first-line agent, and should be used with caution post-MI due to its stimulant properties. Amitriptyline is contraindicated during recovery from MI, and should be used with caution in diabetics and those with heart disease because of its anticholinergic properties and the potential for orthostatic hypotension.

VIGNETTE 5 Question 1

1. Answer D:

Methylphenidate has the most rapid onset of action of the medications listed and will help the patient to remain alert. This is an important consideration for a patient with a limited lifespan and a terminal illness. Sertraline and amitriptyline may take 4 to 6 weeks for assessment of their effect and need repeated dosage titrations. Amitriptyline may also cause sedation as a side effect. ECT has no absolute contraindications, but can affect mentation, including causing amnesia. It can also cause prolonged seizures or status epilepticus in a patient who already has a lowered seizure threshold. Bupropion is contraindicated in patients who have experienced seizures.

VIGNETTE 6 Question 1

1. Answer B:

Patients with panic disorder frequently will undergo extensive medical workups to eliminate medical causes before recognizing that these episodes represent a psychiatric diagnosis of panic disorder. DSM-V criteria state the symptoms must include 4 of 13 symptoms, including palpitations, sweating, tremor, SOB, chest pain, choking sensation, dizziness, nausea, numbness, tingling, fear of dying, loss of control, chills, or hot flashes. The symptoms must be present for over 1 month and not be caused by substance abuse or underlying medical disease. The medical conditions listed were considered, and a normal D-dimer and cardiac enzymes eliminate PE and MI as considerations. A normal TSH, physical examination, and electrolytes make these endocrine diseases unlikely.

VIGNETTE 6 Question 2

2. Answer C:

Phenothiazines can cause a reaction known as akathisia, which is an agitated, restless state that can mimic anxiety, and will remit with cessation of the medication. Hypothyroidism and diabetes typically do not have associated symptoms that mimic anxiety, and propranolol and buspirone may have calming effects that can diminish symptoms of anxiety.

VIGNETTE 7 Question 1

1. Answer B:

Benzodiazepines are the mainstay of treatment for alcohol withdrawal and can control symptoms of anxiety and tremor, and help prevent development of delirium and seizures. The other medications listed would have no direct role in treating the symptoms or limiting the severity of withdrawal. Following successful withdrawal, long-term therapy and lifestyle changes are necessary to prevent relapse. Many patients are referred to a 12-step program—Alcoholics Anonymous—for ongoing support and mentoring.

VIGNETTE 7 Question 2

2. Answer A:

Factors associated with alcohol use or abuse include relatives who suffer from alcoholism, particularly first-degree relatives and parents. Age at onset of drinking also plays a significant role with early drinking (before age 15) correlating with increased risk. Patients with mental illness also frequently have comorbid substance abuse because many turn to alcohol and other drugs to self-medicate. Clonidine has been used to help manage the symptoms of withdrawal, along with benzodiazepines.

VIGNETTE 8 Question 1

1. Answer D:

The patient's symptoms suggest gastroesophageal reflux triggering his heartburn and associated nocturnal cough. An empiric trial of a PPI along with lifestyle modifications, such as dietary changes and not eating within 2 hours of bedtime, is warranted. Obesity is also a risk factor for reflux, and he should be counseled about weight loss. His age, nonsmoking status, and absence of systemic symptoms do not warrant a CXR at this first visit. His symptoms could represent reactive airways, but there is no wheezing or shortness of breath characteristic of reactive airway disease. However, although pulmonary function testing would not be warranted at this time, it may be of benefit if empiric treatment with a PPI does not result in improvement. Cardiac stress testing would be indicated with substernal chest pain, angina-type symptoms, or exertional shortness of breath.

VIGNETTE 8 Question 2

2. Answer C:

Extreme fatigue and daytime somnolence can be associated with obstructive sleep apnea (OSA). Other symptoms include dry mouth or sore throat upon awakening, poor concentration, irritability, high blood pressure, and morning headaches. Snoring and respiratory apneic spells during sleep are important concomitant findings, often reported by family members during the history. OSA is commonly associated with being overweight or obese and can improve with weight loss. A sleep study can not only document OSA, but can also be performed with CPAP to help determine if using a CPAP mask will alleviate the snoring and apneic spells. An EEG assists in documenting seizure activity; however, the history does not suggest any relationship of the patient's symptoms to seizures. PSQ-9 testing assesses depression, which can cause fatigue, but the diagnosis of depression requires additional symptoms such as sadness, anhedonia, change in appetite, or loss of concentration. An ESR is a nonspecific marker of inflammation that is elevated with underlying infections, malignancies, connective tissue disease, and polymyalgia rheumatica or temporal arteritis. This patient does not have the systemic symptoms or pain associated with these conditions to warrant testing at this time.

VIGNETTE 8 Question 3

3. Answer D:

Orlistat and phentermine carry indications for weight loss therapy and can be useful adjunctive measures for short-term weight loss. The most effective long-term therapy, especially for those with a BMI over 40 and with comorbid obesity-related diseases (DM, HTN), is bariatric surgery. Surgery is generally safe with the most common early complications being wound related or thromboembolic disease (DVT, PE). Late complications include nutritional deficiencies and bowel obstruction.

58 | Abnormal Pap Smear

The Papanicolaou (Pap) smear is a screening tool for cervical cancer developed in the late 1940s. Its widespread use led to a decrease in cervical cancer from an incidence of 14.2 cases per 100,000 in 1973 to 7.5 cases per 100,000 in 2013. False-negative rates for Pap smears vary between 15% and 45%. Errors occur from poor sampling and fixation technique and the cytologist's failure to recognize abnormalities. Despite these limitations, regular Pap smear screening and the natural history of cervical cellular changes leading to cancer make Pap smear testing an effective cancer prevention tool. The ThinPrep method, which collects cells in a fluid medium to minimize background and drying artifact, improved sensitivity of Pap smears to detect high-grade lesions from 88% to 93%.

PATHOGENESIS

Squamous and columnar epithelia line the cervix. As the cervix matures, squamous cells replace columnar cells in a process known as squamous metaplasia. It is the squamocolumnar junction—where squamous metaplasia is most active and cell turnover the greatest—that is most vulnerable to injury. Development of abnormal cells usually begins in this area (Fig. 58-1).

The observation that the immature squamous cell epithelium at the squamocolumnar junction is particularly sensitive to injury correlates with the epidemiologic observation of this area as the most common site of cervical cancer. Immature cells are also more common at menarche and during the postpartum period, which may explain why early sexuality and multiple pregnancies place women at higher risk for cervical cancer. The natural history of cervical cancer is a progression from mild dysplasia to carcinoma in situ to invasive carcinoma. HPV causes most abnormal Pap smear results. DNA fragments of HPV are found in over 90% of cervical cancer cells

with serotypes 16, 18, 31, 52, and 58 most closely associated with cervical cancer. Recent improvements in testing for these viral serotypes make testing for them an important adjunct to the traditional Pap smear.

CLINICAL MANIFESTATIONS

HISTORY

A good history can identify risk factors for cervical cancer and facilitate decision making about how frequently to obtain Pap smears. Risk factors include early age of initiating sexual activity, multiple sexual partners, history of STDs, smoking, HIV, current or prior history of condyloma, and previous abnormal Pap smears. As of 2012, US Preventive Services Task Force (USPSTF), American College of Obstetrics and Gynecology (ACOG), American Cancer Society (ACS), and American Academy of Family Physicians (AAFP) all recommend Pap smear screening at age 21 regardless of sexual history. From ages 21 to 29, they recommend screening every 3 years when results are normal. From ages 30 to 65, cotesting for HPV can be initiated, and

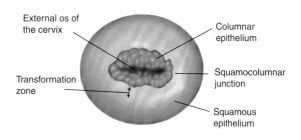

FIGURE 58-1. Normal cervix landmarks. (From *Bickley LS. Bates' Guide to Physical Examination and History Taking*. 12th ed. Alphen aan den Rijn, The Netherlands: Wolters Kluwer; 2017.)

if both are negative, to rescreen no sooner than every 5 years. If HPV testing is unavailable, then screening with a Pap smear alone every 3 years for women over 30 is acceptable. Screening can be stopped after age 65 provided the patient has had adequate prior screening (three consecutive negative cytology results or two consecutive negative HPV results within 10 years) with the most recent test occurring within 5 years.

PHYSICAL EXAMINATION

During the 24 hours before the examination, the patient should not douche, have sexual relations, or use tampons, to ensure adequate endocervical sampling. Most physicians recommend rescheduling Pap smears if a woman is menstruating because it may interfere with obtaining a satisfactory sample. To sample the cervix correctly, rotate either a spatula or brush over the cervix at the squamocolumnar junction. Obtain samples for HPV testing by rotating a cytobrush in the endocervical canal. The physical examination may be normal, but occasionally genital warts or other lesions may be visible. Bleeding and cervical friability can be a sign of cervical disease or infection. When the cervix appears abnormal, a Pap test alone may not be sufficient for evaluation. In other words, a normal Pap smear does not preclude the clinician from proceeding to colposcopy if there is a visibly suspicious lesion (Fig. 58-2).

DIFFERENTIAL DIAGNOSIS

Table 58-1 lists the descriptive changes for Pap smears. The Bethesda system is the preferred system

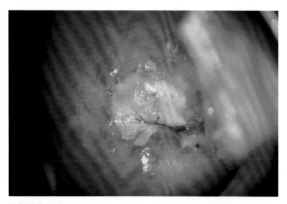

FIGURE 58-2. Lesion on cervix. Human papillomavirus (HPV)/cervical intraepithelial neoplasia II (CIN II) presents as a white lesion with surface spicules. (From Berek JS. *Berek & Novak's Gynecology.* 15th ed. Philadelphia, PA: Lippincott Williams & Wikins; 2012.)

TABLE 58-1. Bethesda System

Adequacy of Specimen

Satisfactory for evaluation

Satisfactory for evaluation but limited by (SBLB): no endocervical cell; inadequate history provided

Unsatisfactory for evaluation, specify reason

Descriptive Diagnosis

Within normal limits

Benign cellular changes:
Infection: *Trichomonas vaginalis, Candida, Coccobacilli* c/w shift in vaginal flora, *Actinomyces* species, HSV; Inflammatory changes, except cellular changes of HPV infections

Epithelial cell abnormalities

Squamous cell the lesions

ASCUS: borderline changes more reactive than definitive
LSIL: borderline changes including HPV, mild dysplasia, CIN I
HSIL: moderate dysplasia or CIN II, severe dysplasia or CIN III, and CIS, +/−HPV changes
Squamous cell carcinoma: cancer or invasive

Glandular cell

Endometrial cells, cytologically benign in a postmenopausal woman—endometrial hyperplasia or cancer
AGCUS: borderline cells between reactive changes to premalignant/malignant process
AIS: adenocarcinoma in situ
Adenocarcinoma: endocervical suggesting adenocarcinoma or ACIS, endometrium suggesting possible endometrial cancer or extrauterine that could be from vagina, ovary, tube, or metastatic

Other malignant neoplasms: small cell carcinoma, melanoma, lymphoma, sarcoma, etc.

Hormonal evaluation (vaginal smears only): hormonal pattern compatible or incompatible with age and history

Hormonal pattern incompatible with age and history: specify

Hormonal evaluation not possible due to: specify

ACIS, adenocarcinoma in situ; ASCUS, atypical squamous cells of undetermined significance; AGCUS, atypical glandular cells of undetermined significance; CIN, cervical intraepithelial neoplasia; CIS, carcinoma in situ; HPV, human papillomavirus; HSIL, high-grade squamous intraepithelial lesion; HSV, herpes simplex virus; LSIL, low-grade squamous intraepithelial lesion.

and interprets specimen adequacy as satisfactory, satisfactory but limited, or unsatisfactory. If the reading is limited, then the report should document the reason (e.g., lack of endocervical cells). Next, the smear may show findings consistent with normal cellular material, inflammatory changes, infection, dysplasia, cancer, or other. The Bethesda system also uses the term "squamous intraepithelial lesions," which includes two grades: low-grade squamous intraepithelial lesion (LSIL) and high-grade squamous intraepithelial lesion (HSIL). LSIL is consistent with mild dysplasia. HSIL includes moderate and severe dysplasia.

DIAGNOSTIC EVALUATION

The first step is to evaluate the adequacy of the Pap smear. If there are no endocervical cells present, this indicates inadequate sampling of the squamocolumnar junction. These smears usually need repeating, unless this is expected (i.e., pregnancy, menopause). In some low-risk individuals with previously normal Pap smears, a physician may exercise discretion and defer a repeat examination for 1 year. Cervical inflammation from infections such as *Chlamydia* or yeast may cause cells to appear abnormal; in such instances, repeat the Pap smear after treating the infection and documenting test of cure (usually repeated 1 month after treatment).

Atypical squamous cells fall into two categories: atypical squamous cells of undetermined significance (ASCUS) defined as changes in cells beyond the normal reactive process, but which lack the criteria for an SIL and atypical squamous cells that cannot exclude HSIL (ASC-H). Follow-up for patients with ASCUS can include either testing for HPV, repeat cytology at 6-month intervals, or colposcopy. If HPV testing is negative, then cytologic testing can be repeated in 12 months. If repeat cytologic testing is negative, then routine Pap smear screening may be resumed. Follow-up testing after colposcopy should include either HPV testing in 12 months or repeat cytologic testing every 6 months times two. A subsequent abnormal smear needs colposcopic examination. If adherence to frequent monitoring is a concern or the patient is at high risk, immediate colposcopy is indicated. Recommendations for patients with LSIL parallel those for ASCUS. Patients with HSIL need colposcopy-directed cervical biopsy and endocervical curettage (ECC). If the assessment is inadequate (i.e., the lesion cannot be fully visualized), conization or loop electroexcision procedure (LEEP) is indicated.

Occasionally, the Pap smear reports the presence of atypical glandular cells of undetermined significance (AGCUS). AGCUS merit colposcopy with ECC because of the risk of adenocarcinoma in situ (AIS) and adenocarcinoma. If the AGCUS is reported as favoring a neoplasia, then the risk of AIS or adenocarcinoma is about 20%, and cone biopsy is indicated even if colposcopy and ECC are negative. Most authorities also recommend evaluation of the upper genital tract with an endometrial biopsy for women over age 35 or those with abnormal bleeding. On occasion, endometrial cells are noted. A postmenopausal woman with this finding is at risk for endometrial carcinoma and should have an endometrial biopsy (Figs. 58-3 and 58-4).

TREATMENT

Since abnormal Pap smears are associated with HPV, a sexually transmitted virus, consider other STDs when evaluating these patients. Approximately 60% of Pap smears with ASCUS/LSIL regress spontaneously. Low-risk patients may be followed with repeat Pap smears every 6 months to 1 year until two consecutive negative smears are obtained. Patients with an abnormal smear on follow-up require colposcopy to rule out a high-grade lesion. Most experts recommend that patients with HSIL directly undergo colposcopy and directed biopsy with therapy based on the histologic readings and ECC findings. Because dysplasia can be a precursor to cervical cancer, destruction or excision of the abnormal area of the cervix is usually performed. Higher grade lesions or a positive ECC generally requires conization or a LEEP procedure. Lower grade lesions can be observed or treated with laser, cryotherapy, or LEEP depending on the size and location of the lesion. Carcinoma in situ generally requires conization and referral to a gynecologist.

Procedures such as conization or LEEP involve removing a portion of the cervix, and place patients at risk for preterm labor, incompetent cervix, or cervical stenosis in future pregnancies.

After treatment for dysplasia, women need Pap smears every 6 months for 1 year, and if negative, they may revert to the regular screening cycle. In pregnancy, ASCUS and LSIL should be followed up with colposcopy and repeated again postpartum. HSIL should undergo colposcopy performed by an experienced colposcopist during pregnancy and at 6 weeks postpartum. In either situation, ECC is always contraindicated during pregnancy.

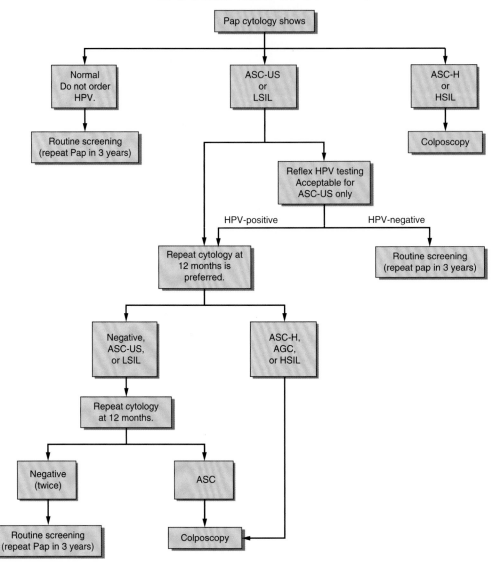

FIGURE 58-3. Algorithm for Pap results in women aged 21 to 24 years. AGC, atypical glandular cells; ASC-H, atypical squamous cells, cannot rule out high-grade SIL; ASC-US, atypical squamous cells of undetermined significance; HPV, human papillomavirus; HSIL, high-grade squamous intraepithelial lesion; LSIL, low-grade squamous intraepithelial lesion. (From Domino FJ, Baldor RA, Golding J, et al. *5-Minute Clinical Consult 2018.* 26th ed. Alphen aan den Rijn, The Netherlands: Wolters Kluwer; 2017.)

PAP, NORMAL AND ABNORMAL IN NONPREGNANT WOMEN AGES 25 YEARS AND OLDER

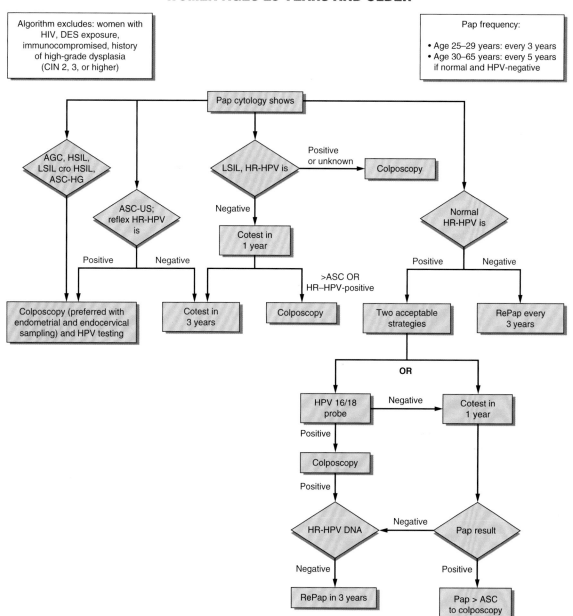

FIGURE 58-4. Algorithm for Pap results in women aged 25+ years. AGC, atypical glandular cells; ASC-US, atypical squamous cells of undetermined significance; cotest, pap cytology and HR-HPV testing; cro, cannot rule out; DES, diethylstilbestrol; HR-HPV, high-risk human papillomavirus DNA probe testing; HSIL, high-grade squamous intraepithelial lesion; LSIL, low-grade squamous intraepithelial lesion. (From Domino FJ, Baldor RA, Golding J, et al. *5-Minute Clinical Consult 2018*. 26th ed. Alphen aan den Rijn, The Netherlands: Wolters Kluwer; 2017.)

KEY POINTS

- HPV is the major cause of abnormal Pap smears. Serotypes 16, 18, 31, 52, and 58 are most closely associated with cervical cancer.

- ASCUS may be followed with repeat smears in 6 months to 1 year in a low-risk individual. High-risk individuals, HPV-positive patients, or patients whose repeat smear is abnormal should undergo colposcopy.

- Individuals with HSIL on Pap smear should undergo colposcopy, ECC, and directed cervical biopsy. Conization or LEEP may be indicated to fully evaluate and treat these higher risk patients.

- AGCUS merit colposcopy with ECC for all patients with AGCUS, because of the risk of AIS and adenocarcinoma.

59 | Abnormal Vaginal Bleeding

The normal menstrual cycle ranges from 21 to 35 days. Day 1 of the cycle is the first day of bleeding. Menstrual flow usually lasts from 2 to 7 days, with the average amount of blood loss between 30 and 45 mL: <80 mL is considered normal. Important factors to consider when assessing bleeding are the presence of anemia and interference with lifestyle manifested by disruptions in schedules, activities, and passage of blood clots or use of an excessive number of pads or tampons.

Abnormal vaginal bleeding is subdivided into the following: (1) menorrhagia—irregular cycles with excessive flow, duration, or both; (2) metrorrhagia—bleeding that occurs between cycles; (3) menometrorrhagia—excessive or prolonged bleeding at irregular intervals; (4) polymenorrhea—regular bleeding at intervals of <21 days; (5) oligomenorrhea—regular bleeding at intervals of more than 35 days; and (6) intermenstrual bleeding—uterine bleeding between regular cycles.

PATHOGENESIS

A normal menstrual cycle consists of a proliferative and a secretory phase. During the proliferative or follicular phase, follicle-stimulating hormone (FSH) released by the pituitary stimulates a primary ovarian follicle to release estrogen, which stops menses and stimulates the endometrium. At midcycle, an LH surge triggers ovulation. After ovulation, the luteal or secretory phase begins, a corpus luteum develops, and progesterone levels increase. Normal menstruation occurs if fertilization does not take place and estrogen and progesterone levels drop, resulting in the endometrium being sloughed off. Normally, this cycle recurs with a regular periodicity, with menstruation generally occurring 14 days after ovulation. Cycle length variability is primarily due to variability in the time for follicle development during the proliferative phase, which precedes the 14-day long luteal/secretory phase (Fig. 59-1).

An imbalance between estrogen and progesterone in the proliferative phase, at ovulation, or in the secretory phase can cause abnormal vaginal bleeding. Persistently low levels of estrogen are associated with a thin endometrium, and intermittent spotting with light bleeding. Excess estrogen stimulates the proliferation of endometrium; but without sufficient progesterone, the endometrium becomes abnormally thick. Eventually, the endometrium outgrows its vascular support, becomes friable, and sloughs off irregularly, resulting in estrogen breakthrough bleeding. Rapid estrogen withdrawal after ovulation may trigger self-limited vaginal bleeding (midcycle spotting).

The most common form of abnormal vaginal bleeding is dysfunctional uterine bleeding (DUB). Hormonal imbalances from a functionally abnormal hypothalamic–pituitary–ovarian axis resulting in abnormal follicle development and anovulation cause DUB. The corpus luteum does not develop and a progesterone-deficient state ensues. In DUB, the vaginal bleeding occurs irregularly (metrorrhagia), because of a progesterone-deficient luteal/secretory phase. In contrast, progesterone breakthrough bleeding can occur in patients taking oral contraceptives with a high progesterone-to-estrogen ratio or receiving IM progesterone. The endometrium in this instance becomes atrophic and ulcerated, causing metrorrhagia.

Abnormal vaginal bleeding can also be due to structural abnormalities, such as uterine fibroids, polyps, or endometrial hyperplasia. Systemic illnesses—such as coagulation disorders, platelet abnormalities, and renal or hepatic disease—may affect coagulation as well as the metabolism and excretion of estrogen and progesterone. Obesity increases peripheral estrogen production, which interferes with the hypothalamic–pituitary axis. Thyroid disease,

Ovum and Menstral Cycle

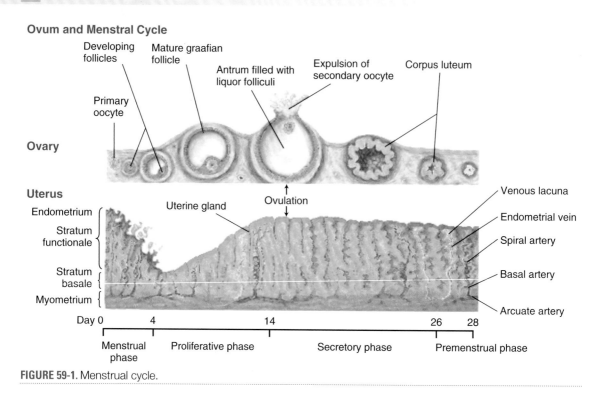

FIGURE 59-1. Menstrual cycle.

adrenal disease, and prolactin disorders alter the normal hormonal feedback mechanisms, thus again leading to alteration of menstrual flow.

CLINICAL MANIFESTATIONS

HISTORY

The menstrual history should include onset of menarche and duration of the menstrual period, as well as the frequency of menstruation, flow, and bleeding pattern. In contrast to ovulatory cycles, anovulatory cycles lack regular cycle length and a biphasic temperature curve. Women are also less likely to experience premenstrual symptoms, dysmenorrhea, breast tenderness, and a change in cervical mucus. A history of liver, renal, or thyroid disease may suggest a potential etiology for abnormal uterine bleeding. The use of anticoagulants, oral contraception, or hormone replacement therapy (HRT) are potential causes of abnormal bleeding. Review of systems—particularly regarding weight change, hirsutism, exercise, increased stress, and the presence of galactorrhea or visual changes—may help determine the cause of abnormal bleeding.

PHYSICAL EXAMINATION

The physical examination should include vital signs, including orthostatic blood pressure and pulse, signs of pregnancy, assessment for systemic disease, and a speculum and bimanual examination. Orthostatic changes indicate significant blood loss and a more acute course. Patients with polycystic ovary syndrome (PCOS) and anovulatory bleeding often have hirsutism and/or acne due to a hyperandrogenic state, in conjunction with irregular menses and obese body habitus. A cushingoid appearance may indicate an adrenal abnormality, whereas the presence of a goiter and hyporeflexia suggest thyroid disease. Characteristics of hyperprolactinemia include visual field changes and milky nipple discharge. A bleeding diathesis can present with petechiae and ecchymoses, along with menorrhagia. A speculum examination can identify vaginal or cervical lesions and directly visualize the amount of bleeding. The bimanual examination can assess cervical motion tenderness seen in PID and detect uterine and adnexal masses. The examination can usually identify if the source of bleeding is rectal, urethral, vaginal, or cervical.

DIFFERENTIAL DIAGNOSIS

Malignancy, trauma, and sexual abuse or assault are potential causes of abnormal bleeding. Table 59-1 lists some additional causes of abnormal vaginal bleeding. Establishing the pattern of bleeding as ovulatory or anovulatory helps narrow the differential diagnosis. For example, anovulatory bleeding is common in DUB, obese patients, and those suffering from infertility. Pregnancy-related bleeding can be due to an ectopic pregnancy, miscarriage, threatened abortion, trophoblastic disease, and placenta previa or abruption. Abnormal bleeding can be a side effect of oral contraception or other hormonal therapy, and of systemic disorders, particularly thyroid, adrenal, pituitary, and hypothalamic conditions. PID, coagulopathies, and anatomic lesions (e.g., cervical erosions) are other causes of premenopausal bleeding. Perimenopausal bleeding is typically irregular. The likelihood of cervical and endometrial cancer and endometrial hyperplasia is greater in those over age 35, particularly in perimenopausal and postmenopausal women. Fibroids and polyps are benign neoplasms that can cause abnormal bleeding. In postmenopausal women, vaginal bleeding is most commonly associated with endometrial carcinoma or HRT.

TABLE 59-1. Symptoms Associated with Different Patterns of Vaginal Bleeding

Type	Associations	Causes	Ovulation
Midcycle spotting	Pelvic pain (*mittelschmerz*)	Ovulatory bleed	+
Menorrhagia	von Willebrand disease, platelet disorder, structural lesion	Thrombocytopenia, uterine fibroids, adenomyosis, endometrial polyps	+
Metrorrhagia	Situational stress, weight loss, exercise training, hypothyroidism or hyperthyroidism, hyperprolactinemia, infertility, hirsutism, obesity, or amenorrhea	Hypothalamic dysfunction with progesterone-deficient state Polycystic ovarian syndrome	+ −
Menometrorrhagia	Menstrual cramps	Uterine fibroids	+
Oligomenorrhea	Frequency >35 days	Prolonged follicular phase	+
Polymenorrhea	Frequency <21 days	Inadequate luteal phase or a short follicular phase	+
Intermenstrual bleed		IUD, cervical disease	+
Postcoital bleed	Cervix ulcerations	Cervical cancer	+
	Spotting between menses	Cervical polyps, erosions, vaginal lesions	+
	Fever, pelvic pain, cervical discharge	Pelvic inflammatory diseases	+
Pregnancy	Amenorrhea, vaginal spotting, unilateral pelvic pain Painless vaginal bleeding Vaginal bleed with clots, abdominal pain	Ectopic pregnancy Placenta previa Placenta abruption	NA NA NA
Perimenopausal bleed	Metrorrhagia, vasomotor symptoms	Estrogen withdrawal	−
Postmenopausal bleed	>40 years Continuous combined estrogen with cyclic progesterone: 3 weeks on and 1 week off, estrogen	Endometrial cancer Cervical cancer Cervical or vaginal lesions Breakthrough bleed or spotting	− −

IUD, intrauterine device; NA, not applicable; +, ovulatory; −, anovulatory.

DIAGNOSTIC EVALUATION

Figure 59-2 outlines the evaluation of the patient with abnormal vaginal bleeding. The initial evaluation should include a Pap smear (unless there is a record of a recently documented normal smear), a CBC, and a pregnancy test in perimenopausal and premenopausal patients. If a genital lesion is detected, appropriate treatment or referral for evaluation and treatment should be advised. An US can confirm the finding of an enlarged uterus on examination and

the cause for the enlargement. Cervical culture may be helpful in patients at high risk for infection and those with symptoms of infection. Thyroid tests may be helpful in addition to testing for any systemic diseases suggested by the history and physical (e.g., prolactin levels in a patient with galactorrhea and abnormal bleeding).

In younger patients with menorrhagia, consider coagulation disorders when there are other signs or symptoms of a bleeding disorder. Adolescents and young women with anovulatory patterns should have

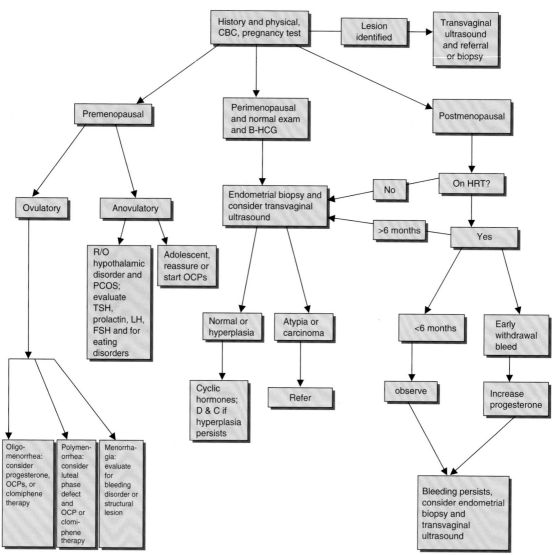

FIGURE 59-2. Algorithm for the evaluation of abnormal vaginal bleeding. B-HCG, beta-human chorionic gonadotropin; CBC, complete blood count; FSH, follicle-stimulating hormone; HRT, hormone replacement therapy; LH, luteinizing hormone; OCP, oral contraceptive pills; PCOS, polycystic ovary syndrome; TSH, thyroid-stimulating hormone.

their TSH and prolactin levels checked. Those with suspected PCOS warrant the measurement of LH, FSH, dehydroepiandrosterone sulfate (DHEA-S), and free testosterone levels on the third day of the menstrual cycle. An LH–FSH ratio greater than 2:1 is consistent with PCOS.

Women after age of 35 are more at risk for endometrial cancer, making it important to consider an US and/or endometrial biopsy for this age group. All postmenopausal women with an endometrial stripe >4 mm on US need an endometrial biopsy to rule out endometrial hyperplasia or cancer. Saline infusion sonohysteroscopy and hysteroscopy are more invasive diagnostic tests that may help if bleeding persists and remains undiagnosed. The exception to this may be in those postmenopausal women recently started on HRT. Bleeding occurs commonly in the first 6 months of HRT, and adjustment of the progesterone dosage followed by observation may be tried. Persistent abnormal bleeding merits further evaluation.

Vaginal bleeding occurring more than 12 months after menopause is considered postmenopausal bleeding. Postmenopausal bleeding is always abnormal and merits further investigation, because of increased risk of cancer in this age group.
The diagnosis of DUB is made by clinical evaluation, laboratory tests, and, in some cases, imaging to rule out an identifiable pathologic cause of abnormal bleeding. No test confirms DUB, and it is a diagnosis of exclusion. Patients with DUB are likely to be anovulatory, and it is most common during times in a woman's life such as adolescence or perimenopause when she is most likely to be anovulatory. Pathologic anovulation occurs in conditions such as hypothyroidism, hyperprolactinemia, and hyperandrogenism.

TREATMENT

Management of DUB depends on the degree of bleeding, presence of anemia, desire for fertility or contraception, and the acute versus chronic nature of the bleeding. In hemodynamically unstable patients, hospitalization, transfusion, and stabilization of the bleeding with intravenous estrogen or surgical management are necessary. For patients with DUB who are clinically stable and not anemic, observation may be sufficient, or oral contraceptives may be used to regulate the menstrual cycles and provide contraception. Iron-deficient, anemic individuals need supplemental iron. NSAIDs and tranexamic acid are other oral agents that can decrease heavy menstrual bleeding. Patients with DUB who are unresponsive to medical therapy warrant referral to gynecology.

In oligomenorrhea and PCOS, induction of menses at least every 3 months with progesterone is indicated to prevent endometrial hyperplasia and its risk for progression to cancer. Progesterone used in this manner will not prevent pregnancy; therefore, those patients with oligomenorrhea desiring contraception need oral contraceptives. Progesterone-releasing intrauterine devices (IUDs) are another option that combines lessened menstrual flow with reliable contraception. Clomiphene is useful for inducing ovulation in those desiring pregnancy.

Perimenopausal and postmenopausal women without surgical conditions can be treated with cyclic hormonal therapy or adjustment of previously prescribed doses of hormones. Lesions of the vulva and vagina should be biopsied. Patients with surgical causes or those who are not responding to medical therapy warrant referral to a gynecologist. Surgical options for DUB include endometrial ablation or hysterectomy.

KEY POINTS

- The most common cause of abnormal vaginal bleeding in a premenopausal patient is DUB secondary to anovulation; in a perimenopausal patient endometrial hyperplasia and carcinoma; and in a postmenopausal patient endometrial carcinoma and HRT.

- DUB is not associated with bleeding due to pelvic pathology, medications, systemic disease, or pregnancy.

- Because of the high likelihood of cancer in perimenopausal or postmenopausal patients, perform an endometrial biopsy and transvaginal US early in the investigation.

60 | Amenorrhea

Amenorrhea is the absence of menstrual periods in a woman of reproductive age. Physiologic amenorrhea occurs when a woman reaches menopause, becomes pregnant, or breastfeeds. The evaluation of amenorrhea depends on whether it is primary or secondary. Primary amenorrhea is defined as the absence of menarche by age 16 years with normal pubertal development or by age 14 years without the onset of puberty. Secondary amenorrhea is defined as an absence of menses for 6 months in a woman, who previously had regular menses, or an absence of menses for at least 6 cycles or 12 months in a woman with previously irregular menses. Excluding physiologic causes, secondary amenorrhea has a prevalence rate of about 4%. Primary amenorrhea is less common, with about 99% of women having menses by age 16.

PATHOGENESIS

The hypothalamus, anterior pituitary, ovary, and uterus orchestrate the menstrual cycle. The pulsatile release of gonadotropin-releasing hormone (GnRH) from the hypothalamus stimulates the anterior pituitary gland to release LH and FSH into the bloodstream. FSH stimulates the ovarian follicles, which produce estrogen and later progesterone. Estrogen stimulates the endometrial lining. An LH surge and ovulation occur midcycle, triggered by the positive feedback between FSH and the hypothalamus–pituitary axis. The dominant follicle develops into a corpus luteum and secretes progesterone. If the oocyte fails to be fertilized, the progesterone production of the degenerating corpus luteum decreases and the endometrial lining of the uterus begins to slough off. If there are no anatomic anomalies that inhibit outflow, menstruation occurs. Amenorrhea reflects an interruption of the mechanisms of normal menstruation and may result from abnormalities in the hypothalamus, anterior pituitary, ovaries, or uterus.

Stress, chronic infection, systemic illness, anorexia nervosa, and excessive exercise can suppress hypothalamic GnRH secretion through neuronal pathways in the arcuate nucleus and cause amenorrhea. Pituitary failure secondary to Kallmann syndrome, a rare genetic disorder where GnRH neurons fail to migrate from the olfactory bulb, results in delayed or absent puberty and amenorrhea. Trauma, hypotension, infiltrative or inflammatory processes, pituitary adenoma, or craniopharyngioma can impair pituitary function. Ovarian failure can result from chromosomal abnormalities, radiation, chemotherapy, and premature menopause. Hypothyroidism and hyperprolactinemia can suppress the secretion of GnRH, FSH, and LH.

CLINICAL MANIFESTATIONS

HISTORY

The history should include a menstrual history (presence of menarche, dysmenorrhea, and menstruation duration and flow), a review of development (growth and sexual development), chronic illnesses, and medications. It is also important to discuss a teenager's sexual history and substance abuse in a private setting and to assure confidentiality. Emotional stress or pronounced weight loss may be a clue to hypothalamic dysfunction. Visual changes, headache, galactorrhea (suggest pituitary adenoma), presence of goiter, fatigue, palpitations (thyroid disease), presence of abdominal pain, bloating, and normal pubertal changes (vaginal outlet obstruction) should all be noted. In female athletes, discussing nutrition, physical activity, weight changes, dieting, and body image may give clues to an underlying eating disorder.

PHYSICAL EXAMINATION

The physical examination begins with vital signs, including weight and height, followed by a careful funduscopic examination, thyroid gland palpation, breast examination with attempts to elicit galactorrhea, abdominal examination, and a bimanual pelvic examination. In patients with primary amenorrhea, evaluation of the secondary sexual characteristics and possible signs of virilization and uterine or vaginal abnormalities is important. Secondary sexual characteristics described per Tanner staging can help differentiate primary versus secondary amenorrhea (Figs. 60-1 and 60-2). A pale vaginal mucosa lacking normal rugal folds suggests estrogen deficiency. Short stature (<60 inches) in a patient with primary amenorrhea merits evaluation for Turner syndrome. Hirsutism, obesity, and acanthosis may be signs of PCOS.

DIFFERENTIAL DIAGNOSIS

Table 60-1 lists common causes of primary and secondary amenorrhea. The causes of primary amenorrhea include hormonal aberrations, congenital defects, chromosomal abnormalities, and hypothalamic or pituitary dysfunction. In patients with primary amenorrhea and normal secondary sexual characteristics, the most likely cause is an anatomic abnormality, such as the failure to develop a normal uterus or vagina. In contrast, the lack of secondary sexual characteristics suggests a hormonal problem. The most common hypothalamic etiology is Kallmann syndrome, whereas a tumor or compression from a Rathke pouch cyst may cause pituitary gland dysfunction. Ovarian function may be defective because of gonadal dysgenesis, as seen in Turner syndrome.

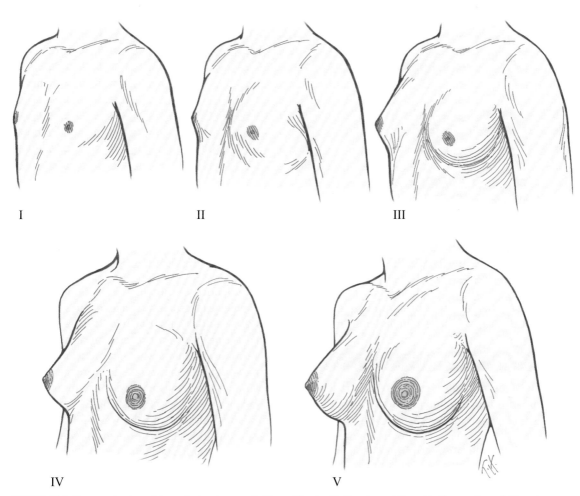

FIGURE 60-1. Tanner staging of breast development. (From Berek JS. *Berek and Novak's Gynecology*. 15th ed. Philadelphia, PA: Lippincott Williams & Wilkins; 2012.)

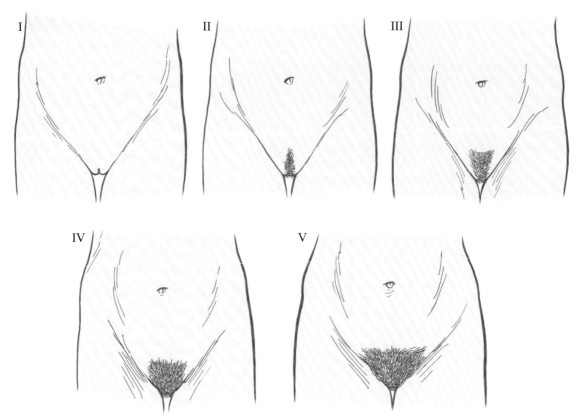

FIGURE 60-2. Tanner staging of pubic hair development. (From Berek JS. *Berek and Novak's Gynecology*. 15th ed. Philadelphia, PA: Lippincott Williams & Wilkins; 2012.)

Many of the causes of secondary amenorrhea overlap with the causes of primary amenorrhea. After pregnancy, the most common causes are hypothalamic amenorrhea due to stress or illness, hyperprolactinemia, hypothyroidism, or PCOS, which accounts for 30% of secondary amenorrhea. In a few women, Turner syndrome may present as premature ovarian failure. Abrupt and rapid onset of virilization suggests a serious underlying problem.

DIAGNOSTIC EVALUATION

The clinical examination drives the evaluation of a patient with primary amenorrhea (Fig. 60-3). If breast development and secondary sexual characteristics are present, suspect anatomic abnormalities or testicular feminization syndrome. For patients with a uterus but no breasts, gonadal dysfunction or a hypothalamic–pituitary axis problem is likely. The absence of both a uterus and breasts indicates the need for a chromosomal analysis. Consultation

with a specialist is often useful in a patient with primary amenorrhea.

The evaluation for secondary amenorrhea starts by ruling out pregnancy, even if a patient uses contraception or denies sexual activity. If the pregnancy test is negative and no obvious explanation exists for the amenorrhea, obtain a prolactin level and a TSH. Hyperprolactinemia causes about 20% of the cases of secondary amenorrhea. If these tests are normal, the next step is a progesterone challenge test to determine whether a woman produces estrogen. Medroxyprogesterone acetate (Provera) given as an oral daily dose of 10 mg for 7 days is a commonly used method for a progesterone challenge. Any bleeding, even a small amount, in the week following the progesterone indicates that the major components of the hypothalamic, pituitary, ovarian, and uterine pathways are at least minimally functional and that the patient is anovulatory. The most common cause of anovulatory periods is either PCOS or a functional abnormality in the hypothalamus. An elevated LH is

TABLE 60-1. Causes of Amenorrhea

Primary	Helpful Tests
Physiologic	
Pregnancy	B-HCG
Hypothalamic/pituitary	
Thyroid disease	TSH
Pituitary adenoma	Prolactin, MRI or CT scan
GnRH deficiency (Kallmann syndrome)	LH, FSH
Polycystic ovarian syndrome	LH, FSH, progesterone challenge
Chronic medical disease	LH, FSH, estradiol, prolactin
Stress, eating disorders	LH, FSH, estradiol, prolactin
Medications	Trial off medication
Ovarian	
Gonadal dysgenesis	LH, FSH, karyotype
Congenital adrenal hyperplasia	17-Hydroxyprogesterone
Testicular feminization	Karyotype
Outflow tract	
Imperforate hymen or transverse vaginal septum	Physical examination
Rokitansky–Küster–Hauser syndrome	Physical examination, karyotype, pelvic ultrasound
Secondary	**Helpful Tests**
Physiologic	
Pregnancy	B-HCG
Lactation	History
Menopause	History/age, FSH
Hypothalamic/pituitary	
Thyroid disease	TSH
Pituitary adenoma	Prolactin, MRI or CT scan
Polycystic ovarian syndrome	LH, FSH, progesterone challenge
Sheehan syndrome	LH, FSH
Stress, eating disorders	LH, FSH, estradiol, prolactin
Chronic medical disease	LH, FSH, estradiol, prolactin
Medications	Trial off medications
Ovarian	
Premature ovarian failure	FSH, estradiol; karyotype, age <30
Uterine	
Asherman syndrome	Hysterosalpingogram, estrogen/progesterone

B-HCG, beta-human chorionic gonadotropin; CT, computed tomography; FSH, follicle-stimulating hormone; LH, luteinizing hormone; MRI, magnetic resonance imaging; TSH, thyroid-stimulating hormone.

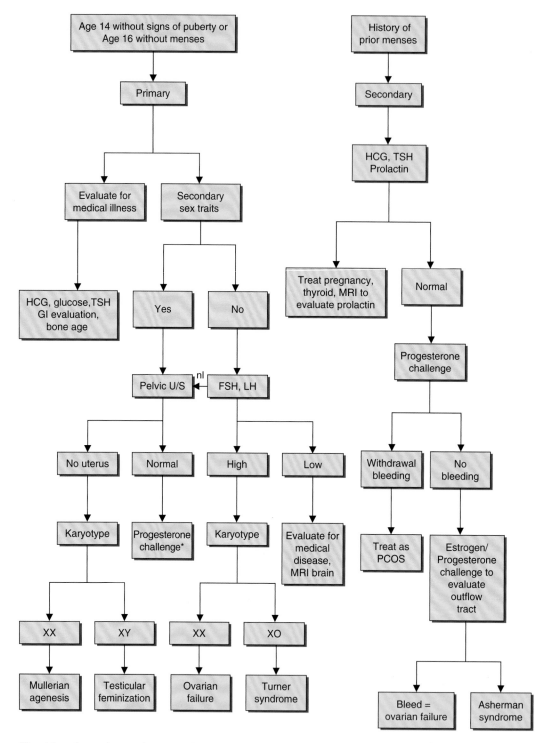

*Complete work-up as for secondary amenorrhea and if negative bleed with estrogen and progesterone, then consider imperforate hymen or transverse vaginal septum as causes since Asherman's is a result of prior uterine surgeries (i.e., D + C).

FIGURE 60-3. Algorithm for the evaluation of primary and secondary amenorrhea. D&C, dilatation and curettage; HCG, human chorionic gonadotropin; FSH, follicle-stimulating hormone; LH, luteinizing hormone; MRI, magnetic resonance imaging; PCOS, polycystic ovarian syndrome; TSH, thyroid-stimulating hormone; US, ultrasound.

highly suggestive of PCOS in a woman with clinical evidence of PCOS, such as mild hirsutism, infertility, and obesity. An LH–FSH ratio of 2.5 or greater is also consistent with PCOS.

Functional hypothalamic amenorrhea is a diagnosis of exclusion, but a history of anorexia nervosa, stress, or extreme exercise support the diagnosis. In anovulatory patients with evidence of hyperandrogenism (e.g., hirsutism), obtain testosterone and DHEA-S levels. Testosterone levels >200 mg/dL and/or DHEA-S levels >7 mg/dL require a CT scan to rule out an adrenal or ovarian tumor. In PCOS, DHEA-S is often mildly elevated. An increased ratio of testosterone to DHEA-S suggests an adrenal source and the need to check a 17-hydroxyprogesterone level to rule out late-onset congenital adrenal hyperplasia and Cushing syndrome.

The absence of withdrawal bleeding after a progesterone challenge indicates either an estrogen deficiency or an anatomic abnormality. In suspected cases of estrogen deficiency, measuring the FSH level is the next step. An elevated FSH level indicates ovarian failure. Patients below 30 years of age with ovarian failure should undergo karyotyping to evaluate for Turner syndrome. If the FSH is low or normal, an MRI scan of the hypothalamus and pituitary is indicated to rule out a CNS lesion, such as a craniopharyngioma, meningioma, pituitary adenoma, or granulomatous disease. A combined estrogen–progesterone challenge of estrogen given daily for 3 weeks and adding progesterone to the last 5 days can identify an outflow problem. Failure to bleed after a combined estrogen and progesterone challenge indicates an outflow abnormality. Imaging such as transvaginal or transabdominal ultrasound or CT of the pelvis helps identify the outflow abnormality.

TREATMENT

Management of amenorrhea depends on the underlying cause. Patients with congenital anatomic abnormalities usually require referral for surgery. Patients with primary amenorrhea with an absent uterus and no breast tissue need estrogen replacement to promote breast development and to prevent osteoporosis. Patients with breast tissue and an absent uterus do not require hormonal treatment because the amenorrhea in this case is secondary to an absent uterus and not because of hormonal deficiency.

Hypothyroid patients require replacement therapy with thyroid hormone. Those with a pituitary macroadenoma need an evaluation for possible surgery, whereas microadenomas may be managed with bromocriptine and close follow-up.

Management of patients with anovulatory periods depends on whether a patient desires pregnancy or contraception. Those patients wanting contraception may elect to take birth control pills. For patients with anovulatory periods desiring pregnancy, drugs such as clomiphene can induce ovulation. For patients failing to respond to clomiphene, adding gonadotropins may stimulate ovulation. Patients who are not sexually active or who do not want birth control pills need progesterone on a regular basis to induce withdrawal bleeding to prevent endometrial hyperplasia. Patients with premature ovarian failure need HRT to treat menopausal symptoms and atrophic vaginitis. Prescribing HRT or bisphosphonates prevents bone loss and osteoporosis. However, risks versus benefits of HRT should be weighed prior to offering and initiating treatment. Risks include increased risks for heart disease, invasive breast cancer, stroke, pulmonary embolism, and deep vein thrombosis. In addition to amenorrhea, PCOS is associated with obesity, insulin resistance, impaired glucose tolerance, hypertension, hyperlipidemia, and premature vascular disease. Medications such as metformin and thiazolidinediones can help correct the underlying metabolic defect with PCOS, and in some patients menstrual cycles may return with weight loss.

Female athletes who train intensively may experience exercise-associated amenorrhea (EAA). EAA occurs due to decreased pulse frequency of GnRH release from hypothalamus leading to decreased LH from the pituitary and ultimately a hypoestrogenic state. The mainstay of treatment for EAA is predominantly nonpharmacologic and includes education about nutrition, training regimens, as well as ruling out underlying causes such as eating disorders. Patients with prolonged EAA can face complications secondary to prolonged estrogen deficiency.

KEY POINTS

- Primary amenorrhea is the absence of menarche by 16 years of age with normal pubertal development or no pubertal development by the age of 14 years. Secondary amenorrhea is the absence of menses for 6 months or 6 previous cycles after establishing normal menses.

- Concealed pregnancy remains the most likely cause of primary or secondary amenorrhea in an otherwise normal adolescent.

- History taking should include a careful menstrual and medical history, including all medications, sexual history, a review of systems, and history of drug abuse.

- The workup for primary amenorrhea depends on the absence or presence of breast development and the absence or presence of a uterus.

- Pregnancy should be included in the differential diagnosis for amenorrhea and ruled out before more extensive testing.

- Hyperprolactinemia is a common cause of secondary amenorrhea.

- Management of amenorrhea depends on the underlying causes. The most common treatment is restoring the menstrual cycle with either a progesterone withdrawal method or combined estrogen–progesterone therapy such as OCP.

61 | Breast Masses

Discovery of a breast mass is a common occurrence. In the United States, a woman's lifetime risk of developing breast cancer is 8% to 10%, with >50% of cancers occurring in patients over age 65. Depending on the population studied, about 5% to 20% of breast masses turn out to be malignant, making it essential to rule out malignancy. Although far less common, 1% of breast cancers occur in men.

PATHOGENESIS

Breast tissue contains epithelium that forms the acini and ducts, fat, and fibrous tissue, which provides structural support (Fig. 61-1). The hormones of the menstrual cycle influence the progression and regression of the ducts, and many women experience breast tenderness around their menstrual periods. Under hormonal influence, breast tissue may be overstimulated, leading to the development of fibroadenomas, ductal dysplasia, and breast cysts. Cysts are either collections of fluid, such as colostrum, or dissolved cellular debris, from stricture and fibrosis of the small ductules.

Most breast cancers arise from malignant transformation of ductal or epithelial cells. The exact causes of breast cancer cannot be determined for the vast majority of cases. Approximately 5% of cases are thought to be attributable to inheritance of the *BRCA1* or *BRCA2* genes. Breast cancer is not considered a consequence of fibrocystic disease.

Breast cancers are usually divided into epithelial or nonepithelial (stromal) malignancies. Epithelial cancers are more common and are classified as lobular or ductal carcinomas. Lobular carcinomas are more frequent in younger patients, and ductal carcinomas more frequent in older patients. Ductal carcinomas tend to be more invasive than lobular lesions. The first site of metastases is usually the axillary lymph nodes. Less than 10% of patients with breast tumors <1 cm in diameter have metastases.

CLINICAL MANIFESTATIONS

HISTORY

The history should include questions about how long the mass has been present, how it was discovered, and whether any change has occurred. Additional helpful information includes the presence of pain or breast discharge, weight loss, or bone pain. Past personal or family history of breast cancer, menstrual history, and use of any hormonal therapies should also be obtained.

PHYSICAL EXAMINATION

The physical examination includes both inspection and palpation of the breast. One should inspect for masses, skin changes such as inflammation or edema, and skin dimpling or nipple retraction (Figs. 61-2 and 61-3). Palpation of the axillary and supraclavicular regions can be done while the patient is seated by feeling for enlarged lymph nodes. Perform careful and methodical palpation of each quadrant of the breast along with areolar pressure around the nipple to assess for breast discharge.

DIFFERENTIAL DIAGNOSIS

The most common causes of breast masses are fibrocystic changes, fibroadenomas, and breast cancer. Less common causes of breast masses include hamartomas, adenomas, abscesses, lipomas, intraductal papillomas, and fat necrosis. Mastitis and abscess formation are rare in nonlactating women.

Diffusely lumpy, tender breasts suggest fibrocystic change. Fibrocystic changes vary with the menstrual cycle and are more common in younger women.

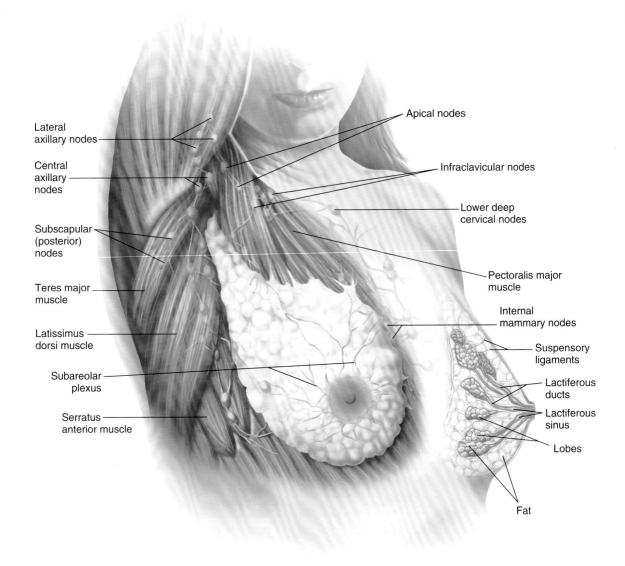

FIGURE 61-1. Breast anatomy. (From Anatomical Chart Company. *Understanding Breast Cancer Anatomical Chart.* 2nd ed. Alphen aan den Rijn, The Netherlands: Wolters Kluwer; 2006.)

Cysts that persist throughout the menstrual cycle and fail to resolve with aspiration or those with a bloody aspirate need further investigation to rule out malignancy.

Fibroadenomas are benign tumors that commonly present in younger women as discrete, mobile, painless, rubbery masses. After an initial several-month period of growth, fibroadenomas generally stabilize in size, remain mobile, and do not spread to adjacent structures or lymph nodes.

Cancer typically presents in a postmenopausal woman as an isolated, painless, hard mass usually larger than 2 cm discovered on self-examination. The mass often does not have discrete borders. Over time, cancerous masses enlarge, become fixed, and may be associated with palpable axillary lymph nodes. Other signs of breast cancer include skin dimpling, nipple inversion, nipple discharge (especially bloody discharge), and skin edema or inflammation.

DIAGNOSTIC EVALUATION

Clinical features of benign and malignant disease overlap, and most women need testing starting with a diagnostic mammogram. One exception may be a woman under age 30, in whom mammograms are

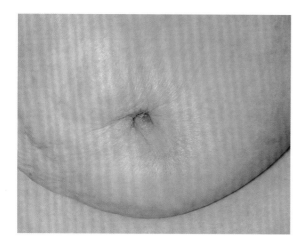

FIGURE 61-2. Skin changes with breast cancer—nipple retraction. (From Harris JR, Lippman ME, Morrow M, et al. *Diseases of the Breast*. 5th ed. Philadelphia, PA: Wolters Kluwer Health; 2014.)

more difficult to interpret because of the density of the breasts. In this case, clinical suspicion and ultrasound of the breast direct the evaluation. Easy mobility, regular borders, and a soft, squishy, or cystic feel suggest a benign mass. If the mass is accessible, fine-needle aspiration should be performed. If no mass can be palpated after aspiration and the aspirated fluid is not bloody, the patient may be followed clinically by re-examination. A persistent mass or bloody fluid mandates excisional biopsy to rule out malignancy. In addition to utilizing ultrasound to evaluate lesions and differentiate cystic from solid

masses, ultrasound helps guide needle biopsy. Solid masses with no fluid found on fine-needle aspiration generally require core-needle or excisional biopsy for evaluation.

In postmenopausal women, breast lumps should be regarded as cancer until proven otherwise. Mammography is typically the initial study. For best results, informing the radiologist about the suspicious area enables him or her to obtain special views in order to fully evaluate the abnormal area. However, a normal mammogram or a reading suggesting a benign lesion in a patient with a dominant breast mass on examination does not rule out cancer. Some 9% to 22% of palpable breast cancers are not seen on mammography. In these instances, ultrasound can characterize the mass and help to direct biopsies. Any palpable mass in a woman over the age of 40 must be biopsied to establish the diagnosis.

Mammography is still useful even if a palpable mass is present because it can help locate the mass, guide needle biopsy, or find nonclinically evident lesions in the ipsilateral or contralateral breast. In addition, an initial mammogram provides a baseline for comparison with future mammograms and aids in planning the surgical approach for lesions requiring surgery. Fine-needle aspiration biopsy of a solid breast mass provides an adequate specimen in 60% to 85% of cases; sensitivity is >80% and specificity is >99%. Thus, negative cytology does not preclude breast cancer, but a positive biopsy makes cancer very likely. Solid lesions that have negative or suspicious

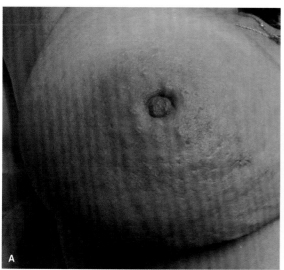
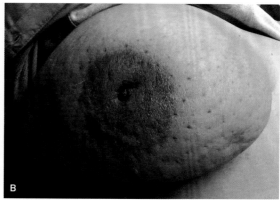

FIGURE 61-3. Classic clinical features of inflammatory breast cancer. (**A**) Erythema, edema (peau d'orange). (**B**) Enlargement of the breast. (From Harris JR, Lippman ME, Morrow M, et al. *Diseases of the Breast*. 5th ed. Philadelphia, PA: Wolters Kluwer; 2014.)

cytology, and cystic lesions with serosanguineous fluid require excisional biopsy. Some experts recommend that lesions appearing to be benign on the basis of examination, mammogram, and a negative needle biopsy can be followed with serial mammograms and clinical evaluation. Discordant results suggest the need for excisional biopsy. For cysts that are aspirated, resolve, have negative cytology, and do not return on breast examination, mammography or breast examination can be used for follow-up depending on the patient's age and risk.

Nipple discharge warrants thorough breast examination. It should be noted whether the discharge is unilateral or bilateral, bloody or milky, spontaneous or expressible, or localized to one duct. Guaiac testing and cytologic testing are helpful. Mammography is essential in evaluating these patients. If nipple discharge is unexplained, a surgeon will have to evaluate the ducts for early ductal cancer.

TREATMENT

Individuals with fibroadenomas may elect to do nothing or to undergo excision of the lesion. Women with fibrocystic change should be informed about the benign nature of the disease and that fibrocystic disease without atypical cells does not increase breast cancer risk. Treatment options include a supportive bra, vitamin E supplements, and avoiding chocolate and caffeinated beverages. More severe cases may be treated with medications such as spironolactone or short trials of cyclic progesterone, danazol, or tamoxifen.

Management of the patient with breast cancer incorporates a team approach involving the family physician along with the surgeon and oncologist.

Assessment for metastatic disease initially involves checking a CBC, liver enzymes, CXR, tumor markers (CA15-3), and in some cases a bone scan. A CT scan of the liver is indicated if liver enzymes are elevated. Surgery generally involves either a lumpectomy or modified radical mastectomy and assessment of lymph nodes, commonly with a sentinel node biopsy or axillary dissection. Postoperatively, after the patient has healed, radiation therapy and possibly chemotherapy may be provided depending on the patient's age, lymph node and estrogen-receptor status. Coordination of care requires communication and involvement between the various members of the health care team and the patient to determine the best treatment for the patient's medical and psychological well-being.

SCREENING

Different organizations have provided varying recommendations for breast cancer screening. Most recent recommendations from the USPSTF advise routine breast cancer screening biennially beginning at 50 years of age with the use of mammography. Screening is indicated earlier when there is a physical finding or clinical suspicion of cancerous lesion, personal or family history of breast cancer, or because of incidental finding with other imaging techniques (e.g., CT chest). Screening can be discontinued at age 74 because benefits of screening decrease after that age as the incidence of the onset of breast cancer decreases after 69 years of age, and the risks of treatment, either medical or surgical, may cause more harm than benefit for the patient.

 KEY POINTS

- Fibrocystic change is common in women under 50 years of age and is hormonally mediated and benign.
- Fibroadenomas are common benign solid breast masses most often found in women under age 30.
- Malignant breast tumors are diagnosed in ~20% of all dominant breast masses evaluated.
- Ultrasonography, mammography, fine-needle aspiration biopsy, and open biopsy are all methods of evaluating solid breast masses.

62 | Contraception

In 2011, CDC published statistics showing that nearly half of all pregnancies in the United States were unintentional, and about half of these pregnancies ended in abortion. Several contraceptives are available that can limit the number of unintended pregnancies. Methods of birth control include natural family planning, barrier methods, IUDs, hormonal medications, and surgical sterilization. Each birth control method has disadvantages and advantages.

The theoretical efficacy rate of a birth control method is the number of unintended pregnancies per 100 women when the method is used exactly as instructed. Actual efficacy rates reflect the rate of women actually using the method for a year. Table 62-1 lists the efficacy rates of common forms of birth control. Birth control methods that require minimal patient involvement, such as surgical sterilization, have actual rates that approach theoretical rates, whereas methods requiring more active patient involvement have actual rates much lower than theoretical rates.

NATURAL FAMILY PLANNING

Natural family planning birth control includes several different methods based on abstinence or abstinence at selected times during the menstrual cycle. With natural family planning, a woman must keep track of her normal menstrual cycle and abstain from sexual intercourse during 7 to 10 days surrounding ovulation. Measuring cycle length (calendar method), changes in cervical mucus, and changes in basal body temperature help identify the time of ovulation and when to avoid intercourse. With the calendar method, ovulation typically occurs 14 days before the onset of menses and requires that women abstain from sexual relations for several days before and after ovulation. Regular menstrual cycles make it easier to identify when ovulation will occur. In assessing cervical mucus, a woman inserts her fingers into her vagina to determine the amount and consistency of the mucus. Intercourse should be avoided when the mucus is thin and copious. The basal body temperature method requires that a woman measures her temperature first thing in the morning before getting out of bed. At ovulation, the temperature rises by 0.4°C to 0.8°C. Again, sexual intercourse should be avoided during the period surrounding ovulation. The recent availability of home hormonal assays can also play a part in natural family planning. Some couples combine barrier methods with natural planning.

Natural methods are not effective directly after childbirth because it may take several months for the resumption of normal and regular menstrual cycles, especially if the mother is breastfeeding. Natural methods are also not to be recommended for women with irregular menses. Candidates for this type of contraception must be highly motivated, because prolonged periods of abstinence are necessary, and also be willing to learn reproductive physiology. Studies reveal the failure rate for this form of contraception to be approximately 20% per year.

BARRIER METHODS

Commonly used barrier methods are diaphragms and condoms. Because both require active patient participation, patient motivation must be taken into account when choosing barrier methods.

Diaphragm use requires instruction and is more effective in older women who are familiar and comfortable with using a diaphragm. The failure rate ranges from 2.4 to 19.6 per 100 woman-years and is highly dependent on the user. In users over 25 years of age with at least 5 months' experience using a diaphragm, the failure rate was 2.4 per 100 woman-years. The diaphragm is placed into the

TABLE 62-1. Failure Rates for Various Contraceptive Methods

Method	Percent of Women Who Become Pregnant	
	Theoretical Failure Rate	Actual Failure Rate
No method	85.0	85.0
Periodic abstinence	–	20.0
Calendar	9.0	
Ovulation method	3.0	
Symptothermal	2.0	
Postovulation	1.0	
Withdrawal	4.0	18.0
Lactational amenorrhea	2.0	15.0–55.0
Condom		
Male condom	2.0	12.0
Female condom	6.0	21.0–26.0
Diaphragm with spermicide	6.0	18.0
Cervical cap	6.0	18.0
Sponge		
Parous women	9.0	28.0
Nulliparous women	6.0	18.0
Spermicide alone	3.0	21.0
IUDs		
Progestasert	2.0	2.0
Paraguard copper T	0.8	0.7
Combination pill	0.1	3.0
Progestin-only pill	0.5	3.0–6.0
Norplant	0.09	0.09
Depo-Provera	0.3	0.3
Tubal ligation	0.2	0.4
Vasectomy	0.1	0.15

IUDs, intrauterine devices.
Source: Adapted from Speroff L, Darney P. *A Clinical Guide for Contraception*. 4th ed. Philadelphia, PA: Lippincott, Williams & Wilkins; 2011:4–5.

vagina along the anterior vaginal wall and should cover the entire cervix, thus preventing passage of semen into the cervix. Diaphragms come in different sizes that need to be fitted to the patient. After an initial fitting, patients must be refitted after pregnancy, pelvic surgery, or a weight change of more than 10 lb. The diaphragm must be used together with a spermicidal lubricant containing nonoxynol-9, inserted no longer than 6 hours before coitus and left in the vagina for at least 6 hours but not longer than 24 hours after coitus. Additional spermicide should be placed intravaginally without removing the diaphragm for each episode of intercourse. Women using this form of contraception may be more prone to develop UTIs. Another disadvantage is that a diaphragm needs to be fitted by a clinician, making its initial cost greater than OTC barrier methods.

There are two general types of condoms—one for the male and one for the female. The male condom is a sleeve made of latex, polyurethane (for latex-sensitive individuals), or lambskin that prevents passage of semen into the vagina. The condom must be placed on the erect penis before penetration. When used properly, condoms can be up to 98% effective in preventing pregnancy. However, the actual use rate is about 85% to 95%. The female condom is placed in the vagina before intercourse and also prevents passage of semen into the vagina. Female condoms have a failure rate of 20% to 25%. Condoms can be used with other forms of contraception (e.g., spermicide), and latex condoms have the added benefit of preventing transmission of STDs. Condoms have few side effects outside of hypersensitivity reactions.

HORMONAL CONTRACEPTIVE MEDICATIONS

Oral contraceptives (OCs), specifically estrogen and progestin preparations, are among the most reliable form of birth control. Pregnancy rates are <0.5 per 100 woman-years with perfect use and about 3% with typical use in the general population. OCs containing estrogen (most frequently ethinyl estradiol) together with one of several different progestin components inhibit gonadotropin secretion and ovulation and induce changes in the cervical mucus and endometrial lining that inhibit sperm passage and ovum implantation.

Box 62-1 lists some noncontraceptive benefits of OCs. Women with a history of ovarian cysts or dysmenorrhea often benefit from the effects of OCs in ovarian suppression and thinning the endometrium.

OC use is contraindicated in women 35 years of age and older who smoke because of the increased risk of venous thrombosis and cardiovascular complications. Additional contraindications for OC use include a history of venous thromboembolic disease, known cardiovascular disease, undiagnosed vaginal bleeding, breast cancer, and active liver disease. Relative contraindications include depression, diabetes, gallbladder disease, lactation, and obesity.

BOX 62-1. Noncontraceptive Benefits of Oral Contraceptives

Reduce the Risk of the Following Conditions:
Ovarian cancer
Endometrial cancer
Ectopic pregnancy
Pelvic inflammatory disease
Anemia
Dysmenorrhea
Functional ovarian cysts
Benign breast disease
Osteoporosis

Abnormal bleeding and nausea are the most common side effects of OCs. Nausea is usually related to the OC's estrogen content; decreasing the dose of estrogen to 20 μg often helps relieve nausea but increases the risk of breakthrough bleeding. Other side effects include weight gain, headache, breast tenderness, acne, fluid retention, and depression. Multiphasic pills that vary the dose of progestin were developed to decrease the incidence of progestin-related side effects and breakthrough bleeding. However, there is no convincing evidence that multiphasic pills reduce side effects. Women with acne or hirsutism may benefit from a pill containing one of the less androgenic progestins (e.g., desogestrel or norgestimate). Another progestin, drospirenone, is a derivative of spironolactone and partially blocks the effects of mineralocorticoids; pills with drospirenone may cause less bloating, weight gain, breast tenderness, and swelling than other OC preparations.

Many women experience side effects of OCs during the first few months, but encouragement to continue the same regimen for at least 3 months is important because many of these annoying but benign side effects will resolve with time. Some women prefer an extended-cycle regimen, where they take 84 active pills in a row followed by 7 days of placebo pills or 7 days of low estrogen pills, respectively, to reduce menses to four times per year. Women desiring pregnancy after discontinuation of the pill should be counseled that there might be a delay of several months in the resumption of ovulation and regular menstrual cycles. Postpartum OCs can be started as early as 2 to 3 weeks in non–breast-feeding individuals; however, many providers advise waiting until 6 weeks because of the risks of venous thromboembolism. Lactation can be suppressed by OCs containing more than 50 mg of estrogen, and progestin-only pills are generally indicated for nursing mothers.

Progestin-only hormonal contraception is available orally, by injection, and as a subdermal implant. They work by thickening the cervical mucus, inhibiting sperm motility, and thinning the endometrial lining, so that it is not suitable for implantation. These agents may be used in patients who are unable to tolerate estrogenic side effects or who have a contraindication to estrogen use (e.g., cardiovascular disease, venous thromboembolic disease). The oral progestin-only contraceptive, also known as the "minipill," is slightly less effective than the combination pill. The injectable form of steroid contraception, depot medroxyprogesterone acetate, is 99% effective in preventing conception. It is given as 150 mg IM every 3 months. The subdermal hormone implant is also an effective form of reversible contraception. The major disadvantages of implants are the expense and occasional difficulty in removing the implants. Side effects of progestin-only contraception include acne, headache, weight gain, and irregular bleeding. Spotting and bleeding are the most common and troublesome side effects of these agents. Progestin-only agents do not affect lactation.

Another option among hormone contraceptive medications is the monthly injectable combination of medroxyprogesterone acetate and estradiol cypionate, which has a 1-year cumulative pregnancy rate of 0.2%. Return to fertility is rapid when injections are stopped, with ovulation usually returning during the third month posttreatment. The most frequent reasons for discontinuation are weight gain, excessive bleeding, breast pain, menorrhagia, and dysmenorrhea. Birth control patches containing both estrogen and progesterone are also available. The patches are changed weekly, and menses occurs during the "off" week. Its efficacy and side effects are similar to those of OCs.

Hormone-releasing vaginal rings provide a low-dose release of 120 µg of etonogestrel and 15 µg of ethinyl estradiol per day. The ring is "one size fits all," stays in place for 3 weeks, and is removed for the fourth week. Efficacy data show that it is comparable to other combined hormonal forms of contraception. Disadvantages include not wishing to have a foreign body in the vagina and the fear of expulsion.

INTRAUTERINE DEVICES

IUDs work by interfering with sperm mobility and fertilization. IUDs have a failure rate of two to three pregnancies per 100 women-years. This form of contraception is independent of the act of intercourse, highly effective, inexpensive, and reversible. Thus, women who use IUDs are among the most satisfied of all contraceptive users. Worldwide IUDs are one of the most widely used methods of reversible contraception.

Two main types of IUDs in use are the copper-containing T-shaped devices and the progesterone-releasing devices. Copper-containing IUDs can remain in place for 10 years, whereas progesterone-releasing devices must be changed more frequently. The copper-containing IUDs may cause irregular uterine bleeding, an effect that is less prevalent with the progesterone IUDs. The levonorgestrel intrauterine system (Mirena) releases low doses of levonorgestrel at 20 µg/day in the uterine cavity for 5 years.

The 5-year cumulative failure rate is 0.71 per 100 women, nearly equal to that of sterilization.

Both copper IUDs and hormonal IUD (Mirena) are recommended for use in patients who have had at least one vaginal pregnancy. The reason for this recommendation relates to the size of the device; the end-to-end flange length of both IUDs is ~32 mm and requires passing an insertion tube ranging from 4.1 to 4.4 mm in diameter through the cervical canal. Insertion is more difficult and painful for the nulliparous patient.

Two additional hormonal IUDs are approved by the FDA. Skyla, a levonorgestrel-based IUD known as the "mini Mirena," gives the same localized hormonal effect with fewer systemic side effects because it releases lower doses of levonorgestrel. It is smaller in size and uses a smaller insertion tube that allows nulliparous women, or women with only surgical deliveries, to use the IUD. A disadvantage is a shorter duration of contraception: A Skyla lasts for 3 years.

The FDA has also approved Kyleena, which combined the advantages of Mirena and Skyla together. Kyleena is the same size as the Skyla, but releases a larger dose of levonorgestrel, 17.5 µg/day, and lasts for 5 years. Kyleena is also approved for use in nulliparous women.

IUDs must be inserted under sterile conditions. It is recommended that an IUD should be placed within 5 days of the menstrual cycle, but it may be inserted at any time the patient is not pregnant. Contraindications to IUD insertion include pregnancy, undiagnosed vaginal bleeding, and PID. Relative contraindications include nulliparity, prior ectopic pregnancy, history of multiple sexual partners, history of a previous STD, an abnormal Pap smear that has not been fully evaluated, and uterine anomalies. The most common side effects are cramping and bleeding, which usually diminish with time. These symptoms can be helped by NSAIDs. All of the IUDs are visible on x-ray.

Complications of IUD use include pelvic inflammatory disease, ectopic pregnancy, spontaneous abortion, dysmenorrhea, metrorrhagia, and uterine perforation. The risk of PID associated with IUD use correlates most closely with the presence of contamination at the time of insertion. Many clinicians recommend against placing IUDs in women at high risk for STDs.

STERILIZATION

Approximately 1 million sterilizations are performed in the United States each year. The two most common forms of sterilization performed are vasectomy and tubal ligation. Of these two procedures, tubal ligation is performed more often than vasectomy and is the most commonly used birth control method in the world. In order to avoid postprocedure regret, it is extremely important to **stress the irreversibility** of these procedures. Risk factors for regret include depression, young age, low parity, unstable marriage, and having the procedure at the time of a cesarean section.

Tubal ligation is an invasive procedure that can be performed laparoscopically, through a minilap incision or at the time of a cesarean section. Tubal continuity is interrupted surgically, thus preventing passage of the sperm or ovum. A newer procedure, performed hysteroscopically, is the placement of Essure coils within the fallopian tubes, leading to their occlusion. Confirmation of tubal occlusion by hysterosalpingogram is recommended 3 months after placing the coils.

Vasectomies can be performed as outpatient procedures under local anesthesia, with less time away from work and a more rapid recovery than a tubal ligation. The procedure involves incising the scrotum, identifying the vas deferens, and then surgically removing a portion of each vas, thus preventing the passage of sperm. Vasectomy does not result in immediate sterility. Clearing stored sperm occurs after about 25 to 30 ejaculations, and aspermia must be confirmed by semen analysis. An alternative mode of contraception is advised until the sperm analysis confirms the patient is sterile. Complications from either procedure are uncommon. Vasectomy failures can be picked up by postoperative semen analysis, whereas failures of tubal ligation are detected only if a patient becomes pregnant. Each of these procedures is potentially reversible, although they are labeled as "permanent" sterilization. Tubal ligation can be reversed with a success rate of 40% to 85%. Success rates for reversal of vasectomy range from 37% to 90%.

POSTCOITAL CONTRACEPTION

Postcoital hormonal approaches include the use of Ovral or Lo-Ovral, with a dose of two Ovral pills taken within 72 hours of unprotected intercourse, followed by two more taken 12 hours later. A progestin-only product (Plan B) is also available for postcoital contraception. The primary side effect of emergency contraception is nausea (50%) and vomiting (20%). Antiemetic medication may be needed with these regimens. Bleeding should occur within 3 to 4 weeks. If pregnancy occurs, abortion should be discussed because of the possible teratogenic effects of the high-dose steroids. Emergency contraception prevents at least three of four pregnancies that would have occurred. Postcoital IUD insertion within 5 days after intercourse is also effective.

KEY POINTS

- More than half of the pregnancies in the United States are unintended.

- Natural family planning methods focus on abstinence around the time of ovulation but have a 20% failure rate.

- Barrier methods require significant patient motivation, but for highly motivated couples they can be effective.

- Condoms can be combined with other methods of contraception and can help prevent STD.

- The most effective methods of contraception are IUDs, hormonal contraception, and surgical sterilization.

- Hormonal contraceptives are highly effective when used correctly and are available in oral, injectable, transdermal, implantable, vaginal, and intrauterine forms.

- Benefits of combined hormonal contraception include a reduced risk of ovarian and uterine cancer, lower incidence of anemia, dysmenorrhea, osteoporosis, and benign breast disease.

- Serious complications from hormonal contraception occur most commonly in smokers over 35 and includes pulmonary embolism, stroke, and DVT.

- Both vasectomy and tubal occlusion are highly effective means of birth control. Sterilization procedures should be considered permanent and largely irreversible. Vasectomy is a less invasive, safer, and more easily reversed procedure than female sterilization.

- The method of contraception should be tailored to the individual patient.

63 | Vaginitis

Characterized by a vaginal discharge that is unusual in amount and/or odor, or by symptoms, such as itching or burning, vaginitis is one of the most common reasons for women to see a family physician. Most women experience at least one episode of vaginitis over their lifetime, and about half are plagued with recurrent symptoms.

PATHOGENESIS

The normal vaginal environment includes secretions, cellular elements, and microorganisms. Normal physiologic vaginal secretions are typically clear to opaque, containing primarily mucus and exfoliated cells. Physiologic vaginal secretions vary with age, stage of the menstrual cycle, pregnancy, and use of oral contraceptives. Normal vaginal flora contains numerous bacteria, with **lactobacilli** being the most prevalent. The lactobacilli produce hydrogen peroxide, which is toxic to pathogens and maintains the normal vaginal pH between 3.8 and 4.5. Vaginitis occurs when the vaginal flora is altered by the introduction of pathogens or changes in the vaginal environment.

Antibiotics, contraceptives, sexual intercourse, douching, and the introduction of sexually transmitted organisms are common factors that can disrupt the normal vaginal environment. These events can change the acidic pH of the vagina, leading to an overgrowth of different organisms. The most common organisms causing symptoms include *Candida*, *Trichomonas*, and *Gardnerella*.

CLINICAL MANIFESTATIONS

HISTORY

Most women with vaginitis complain of vaginal discharge, itching, and/or burning. The patient should be asked about the onset and duration of symptoms, previous episodes of vaginitis, and treatments. A general medical review, dermatologic review, and contraceptive history can be helpful. Illnesses such as diabetes and HIV and medications such as antibiotics or corticosteroids are associated with candidiasis. It is important to inquire about pelvic pain, fever, and possible pregnancy.

A sexual history can help identify patients at risk for STDs. Inquiry about the use of bubble baths, douches, deodorants, and spermicide preparations may identify individuals with irritant or contact vaginitis.

The amount, consistency, color, or odor may also suggest the cause. *Candida* usually causes itching and a thick white discharge, sometimes described as cottage-cheese-like. Other typical symptoms include vulvar itching, burning, dysuria, and dyspareunia. Symptoms of *Trichomonas* include itching associated with a profuse, frothy discharge with an unpleasant odor. The discharge can vary in color and may be yellow, gray, or green. Vaginitis caused by *Gardnerella* is commonly known as bacterial vaginosis or BV. Patients with BV may be asymptomatic or have a slight increase in discharge. Some patients report a profuse discharge often accompanied by a fishy odor but have only minimal itching.

Dysuria is also a common symptom of vaginitis and usually occurs when the urine touches the vulva. In contrast, internal dysuria, defined as pain inside the urethra, is a sign of cystitis.

PHYSICAL EXAMINATION

Inspection of the external genitalia for inflammation, masses, lesions, enlarged lymph nodes, and abnormal tissue is important. The pooled vaginal discharge should be assessed for color, consistency, volume, and adherence to the vaginal wall. Typically,

Candida produces a thick discharge that adheres to the vaginal wall, whereas BV or *Trichomonas* causes a thin discharge that pools in the vaginal vault and is easily swabbed off the vaginal wall. A bimanual examination is important to check for cervical, uterine, or ovarian tenderness or enlargement.

DIFFERENTIAL DIAGNOSIS

Approximately 90% of vaginitis cases are secondary to BV, candidiasis, or *Trichomonas*. Viral infections, such as HSV and HPV, sometimes cause vaginal irritation and discharge. Cervicitis, related to a chlamydial or gonorrheal infection, can also cause a vaginal discharge.

If no infection is identified, other causes of vaginitis—such as an allergic reaction, topical irritation, hormonal changes, and foreign bodies such as a forgotten tampon or condom—should be considered. Other noninfectious causes of vaginitis include skin conditions such as lichen sclerosis or early vulvar cancer. Atrophic vaginitis is common in menopausal women.

DIAGNOSTIC EVALUATION

A speculum examination is necessary to rule out neoplasm or foreign bodies and to determine whether the discharge is from vaginitis or cervicitis. A mucopurulent discharge from the cervix and cervical bleeding induced by swabbing the endocervical mucosa suggest cervicitis. Risk factors for cervicitis include age <24 years and a new sexual partner within the past 2 months. In suspected cases of cervicitis, obtain tests for *Chlamydia* and *Neisseria gonorrhoeae*.

If the history and physical examination are consistent with vaginitis, obtain a sample of the discharge. Standard office examinations include a wet mount preparation, a pH measurement, a whiff test to detect amines, and a slide prepared with 10% KOH. A positive whiff test is seen in BV when a fishy odor develops after 10% KOH is added to a slide. The odor results from the liberation of amines and organic acids produced by the alkalinization of anaerobic bacteria. A KOH preparation also dissolves most cellular material except filamentous hyphae and budding forms of yeast, aiding the detection of fungal tangles and spores (Fig. 63-1). While a Gram stain of vaginal secretions is more sensitive for identifying yeast infections most family physicians do not do this in the outpatient setting.

The wet mount is useful for detecting clue cells, *Trichomonas*, and polymorphonuclear leukocytes. Clue cells are vaginal epithelial cells that are coated with coccobacilli and are seen in BV (>20% of epithelial cells) (Fig. 63-2). They have a sensitivity and specificity of up to 98% for the detection of BV. Scanning several microscopic fields for *Trichomonas* has a sensitivity of 60% and a specificity of up to 99%. The *Trichomonas* protozoon is slightly larger than a WBC with three to five flagellae (Fig. 63-3). A wet mount may also detect fungal hyphae, increased numbers of polymorphonuclear cells (seen in *Trichomonas* infection), or round parabasilar cells (seen in atrophic vaginitis).

The pH can be determined by placing litmus paper in the pooled vaginal secretions or against the lateral vaginal walls. A pH >4.5 is found in 80% to

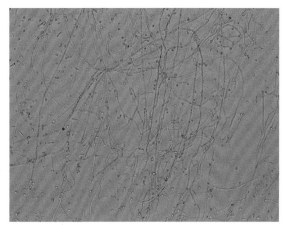

FIGURE 63-1. Microscopic view of fungal organism. (From Edwards L, Lynch P. *Genital Dermatology Atlas*. 2nd ed. Philadelphia, PA: Lippincott Williams & Wilkins; 2011.)

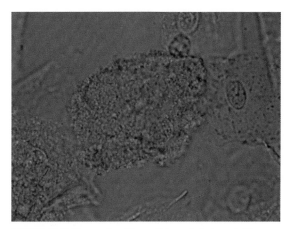

FIGURE 63-2. Clue cells. (From Edwards L, Lynch P. *Genital Dermatology Atlas*. 2nd ed. Philadelphia, PA: Lippincott Williams & Wilkins; 2011.)

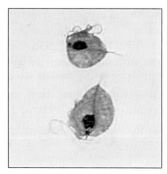

FIGURE 63-3. *Trichomonas* organism. (From https://www.cdc.gov/std/trichomonas/STDFact-Trichomoniasis.htm.)

90% of patients with BV and frequently in patients with *Trichomonas* vaginosis. The pH level is also high in atrophic vaginitis.

A vaginal culture for candidiasis using Sabouraud or Nickerson medium is helpful if microscopy is negative and *Candida* is still suspected. Alternatively, many clinicians will use a trial of antifungal therapy. Culture for *Trichomonas* increases the sensitivity of diagnosis. Because BV is a polymicrobial infection, culturing vaginal secretions is not recommended.

TREATMENT

Treatment for candidal vaginitis includes topical therapy with one of the azole agents, such as miconazole, clotrimazole, or terconazole. Miconazole (Monistat) is available as an OTC preparation. Nystatin suppositories and gentian violet are also effective. Fluconazole, given as a single 150-mg oral dose, is as effective as a topical regimen and in its generic form less expensive. Colonization with yeast is present in 20% of women, and the incidental finding of yeast on a Pap smear does not necessitate treatment if there are no symptoms. Recurrent yeast infections may respond to longer courses of topical treatment, ketoconazole for 1 to 2 weeks or fluconazole weekly.

Trichomonas can be treated with 500 mg of metronidazole twice a day for 7 days or 2 g in a single dose. Tinidazole 2 g in a single dose is another alternative. Metronidazole has the potential for a disulfiram (Antabuse)-like reaction, so patients need advice about not drinking alcohol while taking metronidazole. The most common side effects of metronidazole include nausea, abdominal cramps, and an unpleasant metallic taste. Treatment of the sexual partner is important, because 70% of sexual partners are asymptomatically colonized with *Trichomonas*. Treatment for BV usually consists of either 500 mg of metronidazole twice a day for 7 days or 300 mg of clindamycin three times a day for 7 days. Single-dose therapy with 2 g of metronidazole can be considered when compliance may be a problem. Both clindamycin and metronidazole are available as intravaginal preparations and offer an effective alternative.

KEY POINTS

- Most cases of vaginitis in women of childbearing age are due to infection from *Candida*, *Trichomonas*, or BV.

- Laboratory evaluation of vaginal discharge consists of a wet mount, KOH preparation, whiff test, and pH determination.

- A thick, cottage-cheese-like discharge suggests *Candida*, whereas a profuse, malodorous, gray–green frothy discharge is more consistent with *Trichomonas*.

- BV is a polymicrobial infection.

- Metronidazole is effective for *Trichomonas* and bacterial vaginitis.

64 | Preconception Counseling and Prenatal Care

Preconception counseling is a set of interventions aimed at identifying and modifying biomedical, behavioral, and social risks to a woman's health or pregnancy outcome through prevention and management. The goal is to ensure that the a woman is as healthy as possible before conception to promote her health and the health of her future children. It reduces maternal and fetal morbidity and mortality by optimizing management of medical diseases and enhancing the chances of conception when pregnancy is desired. It includes providing contraceptive counseling to help prevent unintended pregnancies and counseling about social and lifestyle modification, which includes exercise, cessation of smoking, alcohol and substance abuse. Preconception counseling should begin before a woman of childbearing age desires pregnancy. Opportunities for preconception counseling exist during routine office visits, especially for physicals, pap smear testing or STD screenings.

GENETIC COUNSELING

Screening for genetic diseases such as sickle cell anemia, cystic fibrosis, thalassemia, and Tay–Sachs disease depends on the parents' ethnic background, medical history, family history, and desire to have this information in advance. A family history of cystic fibrosis or congenital hearing loss also merits an offer of genetic testing. An important component of genetic counseling is presenting parents with options to continue or terminate a pregnancy based on the information given. Parents who do not wish to terminate for any reason may forego genetic testing or may use the information from genetic tests to prepare for the possibility of having a child with special needs.

In healthy pregnancies with no prior history of neural tube defect (NTD), daily supplementation of 400 µg of folate for at least 1 month before conception and at least 4 months into the pregnancy are recommended. Patients at risk for having babies with NTD should take 4 mg of folic acid to prevent NTD in a subsequent pregnancy. The risk factors are prior history of a pregnancy with NTD, taking antiseizure medications (valproate, carbamazepine), and personal history of diabetes. Periconceptional supplementation reduces the risk of recurrent NTDs by about 70%.

MEDICAL ASSESSMENT

A woman with a medical condition such as diabetes, hypertension, DVT, seizures, depression, or anxiety is at high risk for complications to herself and/or her fetus. Optimal preconception control of blood sugar with diet, exercise, and possibly with medication decreases the risk of congenital anomalies, spontaneous abortion, and fetal demise as pregnancy progresses. The other risks of diabetes in pregnancy include macrosomia, shoulder dystocia, operative vaginal delivery, cesarean delivery, and hypoglycemia in the newborn.

Optimal BP control decreases the risk of preeclampsia, renal insufficiency, and fetal growth restriction in hypertensive women. Alpha-methyldopa, labetalol, nifedipine, and hydralazine are considered "safer" antihypertensive medications in pregnancy. It is important to avoid ACE inhibitors and ARBs in all stages of pregnancy because of the risk of causing oligohydramnios, renal failure, anuria, or other birth defects in the fetus.

If possible, women with epilepsy should optimize seizure control with the lowest dose of a single medication. No single agent is the drug of choice for seizures in pregnancy. Antiseizure medications like valproic acid are strongly linked with NTD. Pregnancy is a risk factor for DVT; women who are on warfarin (Coumadin) for a previous history of thrombosis should have anticoagulation therapy continued, but it should be switched to heparin (low molecular weight or unfractionated) because of the teratogenic effects of warfarin. If there is a personal or family history of thromboembolic disease, screening for a clotting disorder may be advised before conception. Women with depression or anxiety may continue antidepressant therapy with SSRIs if necessary, but benzodiazepines should be avoided because of their rare teratogenic effects.

SCREENING

High-risk patients should be evaluated for HIV and syphilis. Hepatitis B and, if necessary, rubella and varicella immunizations should be updated before a planned pregnancy. Pregnancy should be avoided for 1 to 3 months following rubella and varicella immunizations because they are live attenuated vaccines. The risk of toxoplasmosis decreases by avoiding cat litter, garden soil, and raw or undercooked meat. Frequent hand washing and universal precautions for child care and health care workers decrease the risk of contracting CMV and parvovirus B_{19} (fifth disease).

ENVIRONMENTAL TOXINS

Occupational exposures and household chemicals such as paint thinners, strippers, other solvents, and pesticides should be avoided. Smoking cessation, avoiding alcohol, limiting tuna and swordfish consumption, and screening for illicit drugs are also important to decrease risk to mother and fetus.

LIFESTYLE

Patients should be counseled to control weight, engage in regular moderate exercise, prevent overheating during pregnancy by avoiding the use of a hot tub or sauna, limit caffeine to two cups of coffee or six glasses of soda a day, and to avoid overuse of vitamin A. Vitamin D deficiency is on the rise, and supplementation is recommended in pregnant women with 600 IU daily of vitamin D. Nutritional screening includes assessment for iron, calcium, and protein deficiencies as well as lactose intolerance. Women should also be screened for intimate partner violence.

PRENATAL CARE

Prenatal care encompasses care for the pregnant mother, fetus, and family. The ultimate objective of prenatal care is a healthy mother and a healthy infant, which include the following: reduction of maternal morbidity and mortality, reduction of fetal morbidity, enhancement of fetal health, and education about good parenting skills and infant care for the early childhood years. The timing of prenatal visits for low-risk pregnancies is listed in Box 64-1.

Accurate estimation of gestational age is critical to prevent unnecessary inductions and to allow for interventions and monitoring of fetal growth. An expected date of delivery (EDD) is established using Naegele's rule, assuming a woman with 28-day menstrual cycles. This is done by subtracting 3 months and adding 7 days to the first day of the last menstrual period (LMP). If the menses are irregular or uncertain, then sonographic estimation of gestational age must be obtained between 7 and 10 weeks. Measurement of crown-rump length (CRL) at 7 to 10 weeks of gestation is the most accurate biometric parameter for pregnancy dating (± 3 days). Ultrasound estimation of EDD in the first half of pregnancy is superior to dating based on LMP or physical examination, and is most accurate in the first trimester.

INITIAL PRENATAL VISIT

Often, the evaluation, education, and planning that should be discussed before pregnancy take place during the first prenatal visit. A thorough physical examination of the thyroid, heart, breasts, and pelvis is important. The pelvic examination should assess the bony architecture, uterus, adnexae, any abnormal vaginal discharge, and possible genital lesions. At this time, a Pap smear (for patients over age 21) and cultures (for *Neisseria gonorrhoeae* and *Chlamydia*) should be obtained. Blood tests include a CBC, rubella titer, hepatitis B surface antigen, ABO blood group,

BOX 64-1. Prenatal Visit Schedule for Low-Risk Pregnancies

> **Preconception Visit**
> Up to 1 year before conception
>
> **First Prenatal Visit**
> 6–8 weeks after missed menses
>
> **Every 4 Weeks**
> Up to 28 weeks gestational age
>
> **Every 2 Weeks**
> Up to 36 weeks' gestational age
>
> **Every Week**
> Until delivery

Rh type and antibody screen, serologic test for syphilis (VDRL), and HIV test. A clean-catch urine specimen for urine culture should be obtained to check for asymptomatic bacteriuria, which should be treated if present. ACOG and American College of Medical Genetics reaffirmed prenatal and preconception carrier screening for cystic fibrosis in all patients. Screening is most efficacious in non-Hispanic white and Ashkenazi Jewish populations.

SUBSEQUENT PRENATAL VISITS

An interval history and physical examination are performed at each visit to determine the mother's BP, state of physical and emotional health and nutrition, the presence of fetal movement, vaginal discharge or bleeding, and growth progress. The assessment of estimated fetal growth is an important part of the prenatal visit and is performed by measuring fundal height starting after 20 weeks of gestation. Box 64-2 gives an expected weight gain during pregnancy. A urine specimen should be obtained at each visit in order to check for proteinuria and glycosuria. Flu vaccine is recommended for all pregnant women at any gestational age during flu season. Tdap is given at 28 to 36 weeks of gestation to all women in order to confer passive immunity on the infant. RhoGAM is provided to mothers who are Rh negative at 28 weeks of gestation. Live attenuated vaccines are avoided in pregnancy (MMR, IPV, and Varicella).

Routine laboratory tests are listed in Box 64-3.

BOX 64-3. Routine Prenatal Laboratory Tests

Initial Visit
Pap smear, cervical culture, urine culture, CBC, rubella titer, hepatitis B surface antigen, ABO blood group, Rh type and antibody screen, serologic test for syphilis (VDRL), HIV, and offer CF testing.

15th–20th Week of Gestation
Offer MSAFP/triple-marker screen to test for NTDs, Down syndrome as well as other genetic and congenital anomalies.

24th–28th Week of Gestation
1-hour glucose challenge test for gestational diabetes mellitus.
Hemoglobin to screen for anemia.

28th–32nd Week of Gestation
VDRL and HIV testing.

35th–37th Week of Gestation
Group B streptococcus anogenital cultures; if positive, treat with antibiotics during labor to prevent transmission to neonate.

MSAFP; maternal serum alpha-fetoprotein screening (triple screen, AFP, beta-hCG, estriol)

BOX 64-2. Expected Weight Gain in Pregnancy

Prepregnancy BMI (kg/m²)	Category	Total Weight Gain Range in kg	Total Weight Gain Range in lb	Weight Gain Per Week in kg in Second and Third Trimester (range)	Weight Gain Per Week in lb in Second and Third Trimester (range)
<18.5	Underweight	12.5–18	28–40	0.51 (0.44–0.58)	1 (1–1.3)
18.5–24.9	Normal weight	11.5–16	25–35	0.42 (0.35–0.50)	1 (0.8–1)
25–29.9	Overweight	7–11.5	15–25	0.28 (0.23–0.33)	0.6 (0.5–0.7)
>30	Obese	5–9	11–20	0.22 (0.17–0.27)	0.5 (0.4–0.6)

Source: Adapted from weight gain during pregnancy: reexamining the guidelines. http://nationalacademies.org/hmd/~/media/Files/Report%20Files/2009/Weight-Gain-During-Pregnancy-Reexamining-the-Guidelines/Resource%20Page%20-%20Weight%20Gain%20During%20Pregnancy.pdf, 2009. Adapted from Weight gain during pregnancy: reexamining the guidelines. http://nationalacademies.org/hmd/~/media/Files/Report%20Files/2009/Weight-Gain-During-Pregnancy-Reexamining-the-Guidelines/Resource%20Page%20-%20Weight%20Gain%20During%20Pregnancy.pdf. Reprinted with permission from the National Academies Press. Copyright 2009, National Academy of Sciences.

KEY POINTS

- Preconception counseling should cover genetic screening, medical assessment for chronic diseases, screening for infectious disease, and updating of immunizations; it should also provide advice on proper nutrition and exercise, help with quitting unhealthy habits, and advice on avoiding environmental hazards.

- Prenatal care includes care of the pregnant mother, the fetus, and the family and growing infant for up to 1 year. The aim of prenatal care is to decrease morbidity and mortality of the mother and fetus, enhance family bonding, foster parenting skills, and decrease family violence.

65 | Common Medical Problems in Pregnancy

Pregnancy generally occurs during a healthy period of a woman's life. However, many women have medical concerns or develop acute medical conditions during pregnancy. In addition, women with chronic medical conditions may be at increased risk for complications of pregnancy. The most common medical problems that develop during pregnancy involve but are not limited to the digestive, cardiopulmonary, genitourinary, hematopoietic, and endocrine systems (Table 65-1).

DIGESTIVE SYSTEM

Pregnancy has a major effect on the motility of the GI tract because of increased levels of female sex hormones. These hormonal changes relax or slow down the GI tract. Some common GI issues are discussed here.

Nausea with or without vomiting is very common in early pregnancy. Up to 90% of pregnant women suffer nausea and/or vomiting, and 50% have vomiting alone. Severe vomiting resulting in dehydration and weight loss is called hyperemesis gravidarum, which occurs in about 1% of pregnancies. The exact cause is unknown but psychological, and hormonal changes, along with slowed gastric motility have been postulated in the etiology of vomiting. The mean onset of symptoms is at 5 to 6 weeks of gestation, peaks at about 9 weeks, and usually abates by 16 to 20 weeks of gestation; however, symptoms may continue until the third trimester in 15% to 20% of women and until delivery in 5%. Nonpharmacologic measures such as avoiding offending foods, frequent small meals, drinking liquids apart from meals, and keeping dry crackers at the bedside generally suffice for treatment. Pyridoxine alone or in combination with antiemetics, such as doxylamine, meclizine, promethazine, or ondansetron can be used. In extreme cases, such as in hyperemesis gravidarum, where there is dehydration, electrolyte imbalance, and weight loss, hospitalization is usually required.

Gastroesophageal reflux is also common during pregnancy occurring due to hormonal changes and increases in abdominal pressure as the uterus enlarges. Behavioral measures such as avoiding food at least 2 hours before bedtime, avoiding lying down 1 hour after food, avoiding smoking, and elevation of head end of the bed is helpful. Antacids can be used for symptom relief; in some cases, H_2 blockers such as famotidine or ranitidine may be necessary. PPIs may be required in cases refractory to H_2 antagonists.

Constipation, due to progesterone-induced alterations in bowel transit, is also common during pregnancy. Dietary management through increased consumption of fluid and fiber is the initial means of treatment. Medications such as polyethylene glycol (Miralax), bisacodyl (Dulcolax), or psyllium (Metamucil) can be used, but chronic laxative use and regular use of enemas should be discouraged.

Hemorrhoids are particularly common in the last trimester of pregnancy and immediately postpartum. Approximately 30% to 40% of pregnant women are affected by hemorrhoidal discomfort such as pruritus, bleeding, and occasional pain or discomfort. Constipation can exacerbate the symptoms.

CARDIOPULMONARY SYSTEM

Dizziness, presyncope, and syncope are a common and usually benign occurrences. These symptoms arise in response to hormone-induced vasodilatation and alterations in venous return, resulting from mechanical compression by the uterus that limits venous return. Women with these symptoms should be evaluated to rule out more serious problems such as dehydration, anemia, or a cardiac etiology as the cause.

Hypertension (HTN) and deep vein thrombosis (DVT) are two serious conditions related to pregnancy. Each of these conditions can cause maternal morbidity and mortality as well as fetal compromise. HTN is present when the BP is >140 systolic and/or 90 diastolic. HTN may be preexisting or gestational, with onset during pregnancy.

Gestational hypertension is defined by the new onset of hypertension (systolic blood pressure ≥140 mmHg and/or diastolic blood pressure ≥90 mmHg) at ≥20 weeks of gestation in the absence of proteinuria. The blood pressure readings should be documented on at least two occasions at least 4 hours apart. The diagnosis is changed to preeclampsia when proteinuria (>300 mg/24 hour) occurs. About 10% to 50% of women with gestational hypertension develop preeclampsia.

Preeclampsia can become severe if the systolic BP is >160 or diastolic BP >110 or symptoms such as headache, visual changes, and/or abdominal epigastric pain occur. Maternal complications include eclampsia (seizures), renal compromise, hepatic injury, and thrombocytopenia. Fetal complications include growth restriction, oligohydramnios, abruption, and fetal death. Patients with chronic HTN are at increased risk for superimposed preeclampsia. The ACOG and USPSTF recommend the use of low-dose aspirin (81 mg/day) as a preventive medication after 12 weeks of gestation in women who are at high risk for preeclampsia. Patients with preeclampsia warrant close monitoring, and delivery is usually induced when complications arise or at 37 weeks of gestation. A full discussion of preeclampsia and its treatment is beyond the scope of this chapter.

Pregnancy and the puerperium are well-established risk factors for DVT and pulmonary embolus (PE), which are collectively referred to as venous thromboembolic disease (VTE). Pregnancy causes venous pooling, changes in coagulation factors, and mechanical impedance to venous return. These factors contribute to the increased risk of VTE associated with pregnancy. In addition, patients with previously unrecognized hypercoaguable states such as factor V Leiden mutation, protein C or S deficiency, and antiphospholipid antibodies may first present during pregnancy. Diagnosis of DVT is generally made using venous duplex scans of the lower extremities. Patients suspected of PE may require V/Q scanning or computed-tomographic pulmonary angiography (CTPA) to establish the diagnosis. Warfarin crosses the placenta and is a known teratogen that is contraindicated during pregnancy. Subcutaneous (SQ) low molecular weight heparin (LMWH) is preferred over IV unfractionated heparin (UFH) or SQ UFH in most patients because it is easier to use and it appears to be more efficacious with a better safety profile. In contrast, IV UFH is preferred in patients who have a markedly elevated risk of bleeding or persistent hypotension caused by PE. Therapeutic dosing is maintained by measuring Anti-Xa levels and adjusting dosages for patients using LMWH and by measuring aPTT values and adjusting dosages in those using IV or SQ heparin. Anticoagulation is usually stopped 24 hours before expected delivery.

Asthmatic patients may improve, worsen, or remain unchanged during pregnancy. Management generally follows the guidelines as in nonpregnant patients. Patients with asthma are at increased risk for preterm labor and preeclampsia. Fetal surveillance to monitor for fetal growth and well-being is recommended. For patients with asthma who require prostaglandin treatment for termination of pregnancy, cervical ripening, induction of labor, or control of uterine hemorrhage; the recommendation is to use prostaglandin E1 or E2 (like Misoprostol), rather than analogs of prostaglandin F2-alpha (like Carboprost) because of the risk of bronchoconstriction associated with the latter agent.

About one in five women smoke during pregnancy. Smoking can aggravate existing cardiopulmonary diseases and has been associated with a number of problems such as low birth weight, spontaneous abortion, premature delivery, intrauterine growth restriction, placental abruption, placenta previa, and ectopic pregnancy. Smoking cessation during pregnancy results in birth weights similar to those of nonsmoking women. Therefore, counseling about cessation of smoking should be included in the prenatal care.

GENITOURINARY SYSTEM

A moderate increase in vaginal discharge is common with pregnancy and may not signify an underlying disorder. Evaluation for vaginitis and STDs should be performed, as discussed in Chapters 53 and 63.

Unlike in nonpregnant woman, asymptomatic bacteriuria is treated during pregnancy. The prevalence is about 10%. Screening for asymptomatic bacteriuria is recommended by ACOG in all pregnant women by urine culture at the first prenatal visit. Urinary tract infection occurs because pregnancy causes ureteral dilatation, urinary stasis, glycosuria, and vesicoureteral reflux. Untreated asymptomatic bacteriuria increases the incidence of pyelonephritis. Pyelonephritis is associated with increased risk for low birth weight and preterm labor. Evaluation should include US assessment for obstruction, along with UA and cultures. Treatment with antibiotics, such as beta-lactams (amoxicillin, amoxicillin-clavulanate) or a cephalosporin (cephalexin, cefpodoxime, and cefazolin) or nitrofurantoin in penicillin-allergic patients, should be initiated and then modified as necessary by culture results. Fluoroquinolones and sulfa drugs in the last trimester are contraindicated. Follow-up cultures after therapy are warranted to document bacterial eradication. In those with persistent bacteriuria, retreatment followed by chronic suppressive antibiotics throughout pregnancy is warranted. In addition, suppressive therapy is generally recommended for those treated for pyelonephritis.

HEMATOPOIETIC SYSTEM

Anemia is the most common hematologic problem encountered during pregnancy. Hemodilution, due to expansion of plasma volume relative to increase in RBC mass, occurs during normal pregnancy; thus, anemia during pregnancy is defined as a hemoglobin of <11 g/dL (World Health Organization). Women are more susceptible to iron deficiency anemia during pregnancy because of the increased maternal RBC mass, fetal needs, and blood loss that occurs with delivery. Iron supplementation (ferrous sulfate) of 325 mg/day is recommended when the hemoglobin is >10 g/dL; this dose may be taken two to three times daily by iron-deficient women with lower hemoglobin values. (The recommended daily dose for the treatment of iron deficiency in most adults is in the range of 150 to 200 mg of elemental iron daily.) Evaluation of the pregnant woman with anemia should proceed as described in Chapter 36. For those with megaloblastic indices, vitamin B_{12} and folate levels should be obtained; for those with microcytic indices, iron studies should be checked. In those with a history or family history of hemoglobinopathy, confirmation by hemoglobin electrophoresis is advised. In women at risk, genetic counseling and fetal diagnostic testing with chorionic villous sampling or amniocentesis may be warranted.

ENDOCRINE SYSTEM

Hypothyroidism is commonly present before pregnancy but may also develop during pregnancy. The most common cause of hypothyroidism during pregnancy is Hashimoto thyroiditis. The evaluation and treatment of hypothyroidism are discussed in Chapter 48. The universal screening of asymptomatic pregnant women for hypothyroidism in pregnancy is controversial. Because of insufficient evidence to support universal TSH screening, most professional societies, including the American Thyroid Association (ATA) and ACOG recommend targeted screening by measurement of serum TSH in areas of known moderate-to-severe iodine insufficiency, a family or personal history of thyroid disease, known presence of thyroid peroxidase antibodies (TPOAb), type 1 diabetes, history of preterm delivery or miscarriage, history of head or neck radiation, morbid obesity, or age >30 years. In pregnancy, the thyroid-binding globulin increases and hence the dosage of thyroid hormone (levothyroxine) replacement may need adjustment.

Hyperthyroidism is discussed in Chapter 47. Graves disease is the most common cause of hyperthyroidism during pregnancy. In the past, propylthiouracil (PTU) was considered the preferred drug of choice but has been linked to hepatic toxicity, and hence, the ATA recommends the use of PTU in the first trimester and switching to methimazole at the start of the second trimester. Surgery is an option for those not controlled with medication. Radioactive iodine is contraindicated owing to risks of ablation of fetal thyroid tissue.

Gestational diabetes (GD) is defined as carbohydrate intolerance with onset during pregnancy. GD is caused primarily by placental secretion of diabetogenic hormones including growth hormone, corticotropin-releasing hormone, placental lactogen, and progesterone. It affects 2% to 5% of all pregnancies and is associated with hydramnios, preterm labor, macrosomia, shoulder dystocia, maternal and infant birth trauma, hypertensive disease, operative deliveries, fetal hypoglycemia, and hyperbilirubinemia. Risk factors for developing gestational diabetes include personal history of gestational diabetes, birth of previous baby >9 lb, previous unexplained perinatal loss, family history of type 2 diabetes, advanced maternal age, obesity, and non-Caucasian ethnicity. Screening for diabetes is recommended for all pregnancies between 24 and 28 weeks of gestation using a 50-g glucose load followed an hour later by measurement of the glucose level. A value >140 mg/dL indicates the need for a confirmatory 3-hour glucose tolerance test (GTT). Gestational diabetes is diagnosed if two values of the 3-hour GTT is abnormal.

TABLE 65-1. Common Medical Conditions During Pregnancy

	Condition	Symptoms	Timing During Pregnancy	Treatment
Gastrointestinal	Hyperemesis gravidarum	Nausea/vomiting	First trimester	Avoiding offending foods, small frequent meals, antiemetics, pyridoxine
	Gastroesophageal reflux	Heartburn, waterbrash reflux, cough	Worsens as uterus enlarges	Modified diet, antacids, H_2 blockers, PPIs
	Constipation	Abdominal discomfort, hard and difficult to pass stools, worsening hemorrhoids	Throughout pregnancy	Increase fluids, fiber, and judicious use of laxatives
Cardiovascular	Hypertension	Elevated blood pressure, headache, abdominal pain	Chronic hypertension-first trimester; gestational hypertension >20 weeks without proteinuria; preeclampsia/eclampsia >20 weeks with proteinuria	Aspirin 81 mg/day; alpha-methyldopa, nifedipine, labetalol; close monitoring and potential early delivery
	Venous thromboembolic disease	Lower extremity pain, edema; shortness of breath, palpitations, chest pain with pulmonary embolus	Throughout pregnancy	SQ LMWH or UFH; IV UFH in peripartum period
Genitourinary	Urinary tract infections/ asymptomatic bacteriuria	Asymptomatic, dysuria, urinary frequency	Throughout pregnancy	Antibiotics
Hematologic	Anemia (hemoglobin <11 g/dL)	Fatigue, weakness, pica	Second, third trimesters	Iron; folate or B_{12} if deficient
Endocrine	Hypothyroidism	Asymptomatic, fatigue, constipation	Preexisting; incidental during pregnancy, postpartum following thyroiditis	Levothyroxine; iodine in deficient regions
	Hyperthyroidism	Asymptomatic, anxiety, palpitations	Preexisting; Graves during pregnancy; as part of postpartum thyroiditis	Propylthiouracil, methimazole, beta blockers
	Diabetes mellitus	Polyuria, polydipsia, asymptomatic	Preexisting; second/ third trimester	Insulin, metformin, sulfonylureas, diet

PPI, proton pump inhibitor; SQ LMWH, subcutaneous low-molecular-weight heparin; UFH, unfractionated heparin.

Patients diagnosed with gestational diabetes are counseled to monitor their diet, weight gain, and fasting and postprandial glucose values. Moderate exercise is safe in women without medical or obstetric complications. Absolute contraindications for exercise during pregnancy include significant cardiopulmonary disease, incompetent cervix, premature labor or ruptured membranes, placenta previa, persistent bleeding, preeclampsia, or pregnancy-induced HTN. Fasting glucose values >95 mg/dL and 2-hour postprandial values >120 mg/dL indicate a need for insulin therapy or the initiation of oral hypoglycemics, such as glyburide or metformin.

Fetal monitoring should begin at 28 weeks of gestation in poorly controlled patients or those with additional risk factors. US surveillance in the late second and third trimesters is also commonly used to monitor amniotic fluid volume and fetal weight. Patients with well-controlled gestational diabetes may be permitted to progress to term before induction of delivery is considered, whereas poorly controlled diabetics or those with abnormal testing (e.g., macrosomia) may require induction or cesarean section after 38 weeks or confirmation of fetal lung maturity.

Maternal glucose testing should be repeated postpartum, because hyperglycemia persists into the postpartum period in up to 10% of women with gestational diabetes. These women are also at increased risk for future diabetes and should be reassessed periodically.

KEY POINTS

- The most common medical problems that develop during pregnancy involve the digestive, cardiopulmonary, genitourinary, hematopoietic, and endocrine systems.

- The mean onset of nausea and vomiting is at 5 to 6 weeks of gestation, peaking at about 9 weeks, and usually abating by 16 to 20 weeks of gestation; however, symptoms may continue until the third trimester in 15% to 20% of women and until delivery in 5%.

- HTN and developing DVT are two serious conditions related to pregnancy. Each of these conditions can cause maternal morbidity and mortality as well as fetal compromise.

- The ACOG and USPSTF recommend the use of low-dose aspirin (81 mg/day) as preventive medication after 12 weeks of gestation in women who are at high risk for preeclampsia.

- Asymptomatic bacteriuria is treated in pregnancy to prevent low birth weight and preterm delivery. Urinary tract infection occurs in about 10% of pregnant women because of ureteral dilatation, urinary stasis, glycosuria, and vesicoureteral reflux.

- Hemodilution occurs during normal pregnancy; thus, anemia during pregnancy is defined as hemoglobin of <11 g/dL.

- Gestational diabetes affects 2% to 5% of all pregnancies and is associated with hydramnios, preterm labor, macrosomia, shoulder dystocia, maternal and infant birth trauma, hypertensive disease, operative deliveries, fetal hypoglycemia, and hyperbilirubinemia.

66 | Postpartum Care

The postpartum period, or puerperium, begins after delivery of the baby and placenta and until 6 to 8 weeks after delivery. During this time, most of the physiologic changes of pregnancy revert to the non-gravid state. Along with physiologic changes, there are emotional and psychosocial changes that can last up to 1 year resulting from the pregnancy, delivery, and the adjustment to caring for a newborn infant.

POSTPARTUM PHYSIOLOGIC CHANGES

Uterine changes begin immediately after delivery. First, there is denudation of the endometrium when placental detachment occurs. Contraction of the interlacing myometrial muscle bundles constricts the intramyometrial vessels and impedes blood flow, which is the major mechanism preventing hemorrhage. In addition, large vessels at the placental site thrombose, which is a secondary hemostatic mechanism for preventing blood loss. Bleeding does occur following delivery but diminishes to a reddish-brown discharge (lochia rubra) by the third day postpartum. The endometrium is infiltrated by leukocytes and begins restoration. A mucopurulent pinkish-brown discharge, (lochia serosa) is present for up to 3 weeks, followed by a yellow-white discharge (lochia alba) that may persist for up to 6 weeks. A brief period of bleeding may occur about 14 days following delivery because of sloughing of the endometrial eschar. At term, the pregnant uterus is 10 times larger and heavier than in the nongravid state. Within 2 weeks of delivery, the uterus is within the pelvis; by 6 weeks, it reverts to its normal size.

Prolactin elevation leads to suppression of ovarian function in the postpartum period. In women who do not breast-feed, prolactin levels will return to normal by the third week and ovulatory function returns on average by 10 weeks postpartum. In women who breast-feed, prolactin levels remain elevated and ovulation is suppressed for 6 months or more in over 90% of those who exclusively breast-feed.

POSTPARTUM CARE

The usual postpartum hospital stay is 2 days for vaginal deliveries and 3 to 4 days for cesarean section deliveries. During this time, the mother is able to learn how to care for her infant. Breast-feeding should be encouraged and rooming in of the infant permitted to facilitate feeding and promote maternal–infant bonding. An experienced mother with an uncomplicated delivery and good home support may be discharged earlier than 2 days. The American Academy of Pediatrics recommends follow-up of the infant within 3 to 5 days of discharge. It has been shown that early follow-up contributes to longer breast-feeding duration and may prevent complications such as failure to thrive and severe hyperbilirubinemia.

Typically for a normal vaginal delivery, postpartum follow-up is at 6 weeks and for a cesarean section at 1 to 2 weeks and then again at 6 weeks after discharge.

The patient should be counseled about the normal postpartum bleeding and discharge. If she has not had a laceration or episiotomy, she may use tampons with instructions to change them frequently. Patients who have had lacerations or episiotomies should be instructed to report any significant pain or fever. Care for perineal wounds include use of laxatives, regular bathing or showering, and pain medication. For those with significant edema, sitz baths may provide added relief.

Physical activity will vary by the individual but can be according to patient tolerance. For patients who have had cesarean section deliveries, driving and physical activity should be restricted until pain subsides. Sexual activity may be resumed in uncomplicated deliveries when bleeding subsides and patient comfort permits. For those with lacerations or episiotomies, sexual activity should be avoided for at least 3 weeks.

POSTPARTUM COMPLICATIONS

Many patients experience one or more problems in the postpartum period. The most common problems are perineal pain, lactation-related problems, incontinence, bleeding, infections, or depression. The most common problems requiring readmission to the hospital are excessive bleeding and infection.

Normal blood loss following vaginal delivery is <500 mL; amounts exceeding this are considered to represent postpartum hemorrhage. Postpartum hemorrhage is described as early (<24 hours) or late (>24 hours). Almost three-quarters of postpartum hemorrhages are secondary to uterine atony. Other causes of postpartum hemorrhage include vaginal and cervical lacerations, retained products of conception, placenta accreta, uterine rupture, and rarely thrombophilic disorders. (The causes can be remembered as 4Ts: Tone, Tissue, Trauma, and Thrombin.) A thorough examination must be performed when there is bleeding. While the cause is being determined, intravenous fluids should be administered and RBCs typed and cross-matched for possible transfusion. If no site of bleeding is identified and the patient is unstable, she should be taken to the operating room for further examination.

If a laceration is discovered, repair should be performed. For uterine atony, oxytocin, carboprost, and methylergonovine are administered along with uterine massage. If bleeding continues, a banjo curettage may be warranted for suspected retained products of conception. Patients with suspected placenta accreta or uterine rupture require exploratory laparotomy and surgical repair or hysterectomy.

Common causes of postpartum fever are UTI, endometritis, or mastitis. In patients with a perineal laceration or episiotomy repair, it is important to examine the site for infection. Patients with UTIs may complain of dysuria and suprapubic or back pain. A UA should be obtained along with urine culture. Antibiotics should initially cover gram-negative organisms and can be modified when culture results are available. Patients with endometritis most commonly present 2 to 5 days after delivery but can present a week or more following delivery with fever, malodorous vaginal bleeding, and uterine tenderness. Therapy includes use of broad-spectrum antibiotics until the patient has been afebrile for 48 hours and the WBC has normalized. Mastitis will present as a painful, tender breast with associated erythema, usually in the second or third postpartum week. The patient should be treated with antibiotics active against gram-positive organisms, including *Staphylococcus*, along with local moist heat and analgesics if needed. The patient may continue to breast-feed during therapy.

Urinary or fecal incontinence occurs in many women following delivery. Urinary incontinence occurs in up to 15% of women and anal incontinence in ~5%. Anal incontinence occurs more commonly after vaginal operative deliveries or deliveries associated with anal sphincter injury. Both conditions are generally self-limited and resolve within 6 months. Kegal exercises may be helpful in treating urinary incontinence. For those with persisting symptoms, further evaluation for neurologic or anatomic causes is warranted.

Lactation-related problems include breast engorgement, lactation failure, nipple confusion, and nipple soreness. Education in the prenatal and immediate postpartum periods can help to prevent these problems. Symptomatic breast engorgement occurs on the second to fourth days in those who do not breast-feed. In breast-feeding mothers, hot compresses before nursing may assist with the let-down of milk, and an increased frequency of feedings usually resolves this problem. Lactation failure may be treated in a similar fashion, along with assessment of technique. If lactation failure occurs in association with excessive vaginal bleeding, a rare complication called Sheehan syndrome (i.e., postpartum hypopituitarism) may be suspected. Nipple confusion will occur as a result of feeding infants from a bottle as well as the breast and can be prevented by breast-feeding exclusively. Nipple soreness requires a physical examination and evaluation of feeding technique. Proper positioning, frequent shorter feedings, and allowing the nipples to air-dry may assist with healing. Candida infection can cause nipple soreness and can be treated with topical nystatin.

Many patients complain of depressed mood following delivery. It is important to inquire about how the patient is adjusting to the newborn. During the initial 2 weeks, if the symptoms remain mild, observation and supportive care may be all that is necessary. This self-limited state is often referred to as the "postpartum blues." Up to 20% of women have more severe symptoms consistent with a major depression that requires treatment. If the patient has a past history of depression or of postpartum depression, the patient should be followed closely, being seen in the office 1 or 2 weeks after delivery. Postpartum depression can occur until 1 year after delivery, and postpartum depression screening with a tool such as the PHQ-9 (Fig. 66-1) is recommended for all patients (USPSTF, Grade B). For those diagnosed with moderate to major postpartum depression, medication and/or psychotherapy have been shown to be effective therapies.

Patient Health Questionnaire (PHQ-9)
Nine Symptom Depression Checklist

Name: _____   Date: _____

Over the *last 2 weeks*, how often have you been bothered by any of the following problems? (Please circle your answer.)

	Not at All	Several Days	More than Half the Days	Nearly Every Day
1. Little interest or pleasure in doing things	0	1	2	3
2. Feeling down, depressed, or hopeless	0	1	2	3
3. Trouble falling or staying asleep, or sleeping too much	0	1	2	3
4. Feeling tired or having little energy	0	1	2	3
5. Poor appetite or overeating	0	1	2	3
6. Feeling bad about yourself—or that you are a failure or have let yourself or your family down	0	1	2	3
7. Trouble concentrating on things, such as reading the newspaper or watching television	0	1	2	3
8. Moving or speaking so slowly that other people could have noticed. Or the opposite—being so fidgety or restless that you have been moving around a lot more than usual	0	1	2	3
9. Thoughts that you would be better off dead or of hurting yourself in some way	0	1	2	3

Add Columns, [_____] + [_____] + [_____]

Total Score*, [_____]   *Score is for healthcare provider incorporation

10. If you circled *any* problems, how *difficult* have these problems made it for you to do your work, take care of things at home, or get along with other people? (Please circle your answer.)

Not Difficult at All	Somewhat Difficult	Very Difficult	Extremely Difficult

A score of: 0–4 is considered non-depressed; 5–9 mild depression; 10–14 moderate depression; 15–19 moderately severe depression; and 20–27 severe depression.

PHQ-9 is adapted from PRIME ME TODAY™.
PHQ Copyright © 1999Pfour Inc. All rights reserved. Reproduced with permission. PRIME ME TODAY is a trademark of Pfour Inc.

FIGURE 66-1. PHQ-9 instrument for depression. (From McCarron RM, Xiong GL, Bourgeois JA, eds. *Lippincott's Primary Care Psychiatry*. Baltimore, MD: Lippincott Williams & Wilkins; 2009.)

POSTPARTUM CONTRACEPTION

Contraception is discussed in Chapter 62. In postpartum women who do not breast-feed, ovulation returns as early as 25 days after delivery. Although the first ovulation often occurs before the first menses, the return of menses cannot be used as a reliable marker for when to initiate contraception. The traditional practice of waiting for contraception use until postpartum follow-up is not required. The ACOG now recommends immediate postpartum long-acting reversible contraception (LARC) which includes IUDs and progestin implants as options that can reduce unintended and short-interval pregnancy. Women should be counseled about all forms of postpartum contraception in a context that allows informed decision making, and immediate postpartum LARC should be offered as an effective option for postpartum contraception. In women who are not breast-feeding, oral contraceptives can be started 2 to 3 weeks following delivery, though many physicians advise waiting for 6 weeks because of the associated thromboembolic risks. Combination oral contraceptives may suppress or diminish lactation and thus should not be started until the milk supply is established. Some authorities recommend progestin-only as the preferred method of hormonal contraception in those who wish to breast-feed. Diaphragm fitting should be performed at the 6-week postpartum visit, because a previously used diaphragm may no longer fit properly. Recommendations for condoms and sterilization techniques are unaffected by the postpartum state.

KEY POINTS

- During the 6-week postpartum period, the physiologic changes of pregnancy revert to the previously nongravid condition.
- Postpartum complications of bleeding and infection are the most common causes of hospital readmission.
- Postpartum depression affects up to 20% of women.
- Immediate postpartum LARC should be offered to women as a contraception option.

CLINICAL VIGNETTES

VIGNETTE 1

A 24-year-old female presents for a well woman examination.

1. Which of the following are indicated in this individual?
   a. Pap smear yearly
   b. Pap smear and HPV every 3 years
   c. Pap smear every 3 years
   d. She does not need Pap smears
   e. HPV testing only every 3 years

VIGNETTE 2

A 30-year-old female presents for a routine check-up and reveals that she is trying to get pregnant with her husband.

1. In counseling this patient, which of the following is recommended?
   a. Aspirin 81 mg daily
   b. Vitamin D 5000 IU daily
   c. Folic acid 400 µg daily
   d. Thiamine 100 mg daily

2. Two months later, the patient returns and has a positive pregnancy test confirmed. Which of the following is now indicated in this patient?
   a. Glucose testing
   b. TSH
   c. Tdap
   d. Urine culture
   e. RhoGAM

3. Following delivery, the patient comes for her postpartum visit at 6 weeks with no complaints. Which of the following screening tests should be part of this visit?
   a. Pap smear
   b. Depression scale
   c. Mammogram
   d. Glucose
   e. TSH

ANSWERS

VIGNETTE 1 Question 1

1. Answer C:

Screening Pap smears are recommended beginning at age 21. For ages 21 to 30, this would be in the form of cytology every 3 years. For those between the ages of 30 and 65, the Pap smear frequency can be lengthened by adding HPV cotesting to cytology every 5 years. Pap smear screening may be stopped at age 65 provided a woman has had adequate prior screening and at not at increased risk.

VIGNETTE 2 Question 1

1. Answer C:

Folic acid is an essential vitamin for DNA/RNA synthesis, and in nonpregnant individuals, a deficiency may be apparent as development of angular stomatitis or megaloblastic anemia. Folate in the developing child is needed for normal neural tube development. Folate intake >400 µg/day is recommended for women who are considering pregnancy. In those who are pregnant, the recommendation increases to 600 µg/day and is included in the prenatal vitamin. Vitamin D and calcium intake are important in all women and should increase during pregnancy because the developing newborn skeleton will take calcium from the mother. Vitamin D supplementation is recommended for pregnant women with 600 IU daily. Aspirin is not routinely recommended but may lower risk for preeclampsia in selected women during pregnancy. Thiamine is not recommended as a supplement for those attempting pregnancy.

VIGNETTE 2 Question 2

2. Answer D:

Urine culture is considered as part of routine prenatal labs that also include: CBC, rubella titer, hepatitis B surface antigen, ABO blood group, Rh type and antibody screen, serologic test for syphilis (VDRL), and HIV test. Pap smear testing is done in those over age 21 if indicated by no prior screening. Glucose testing is performed around 28 weeks of gestation, which is when Tdap and RhoGAM are provided. RhoGAM is provided only to those who are Rh negative. TSH is not routinely performed as a screening test during pregnancy.

VIGNETTE 2 Question 3

3. Answer B:

Screening for postpartum depression is indicated at the postpartum visit and screening tools such as the PSQ-9 can be helpful. Postpartum blues is a term used for very mild transient depressed mood that resolves within the first 2 weeks postpartum. Depression that is more severe or persistent warrants close follow-up, and treatment that may include therapy and medications. In those with a history of depression, the first postpartum visit should be within 1 to 2 weeks of delivery. Pap smear, mammogram, glucose, and TSH testing are not routinely performed without a specific indication in the postpartum period.

PART VI CARE FOR INFANTS, CHILDREN, AND ADOLESCENTS

67 | Preventive Care: Newborn to 5 Years

Preparing for a child is a time of both joy and anxiety for parents. Most families, especially first-time parents, need education, reassurance, and encouragement. Ideally, education should begin during pregnancy and continue throughout childhood starting with an initial prenatal visit for first-time parents, high-risk pregnancies, or if the parents desire one. The prenatal visit provides an opportunity to build rapport with the family, to screen for any risk factors, and to provide anticipatory guidance about home preparation for the newborn.

A "newborn" refers to a child within the first few days after birth. A "neonate" is defined as 0 to 28 days (loosely, the first month) of life. Hence, a "newborn" is also a "neonate." An "infant" is any child 1 month to <1 year of age. A "toddler" is between 1 and 5 years of age. A "school-aged" child is 3 to 5 years of age (preschool–KG) until adolescence (teenage years), followed by adulthood at 18 years of age.

After birth, both the American Academy of Family Physicians (AAFP) and the American Academy of Pediatrics (AAP) recommend the same schedule for well child visits with the first outpatient newborn within 48 to 72 hours of hospital discharge and then at either a 2 week or 1 month well child examination. Afterwards, routine well child examinations should be scheduled at 2, 4, 6, 9, 12, 15, 18, and 24 months of age followed by yearly examinations. In some instances, a 30-month well child visit may be required to ensure proper development for the child.

Between birth and 5 years, the most common causes of morbidity and mortality are diseases acquired in the perinatal period, congenital diseases, sudden infant death syndrome (SIDS; the leading cause of death until age 4 months), and accidents. Motor vehicle accidents cause the most accidental deaths after age 3. Drowning is the second leading cause of death followed by fires and burns. Before the introduction of vaccines, infectious diseases contributed significantly to infant and early childhood morbidity and mortality. Preventive care for infants, children, and adolescents includes physical examination and assessment of childhood development, administration of vaccines, screening for treatable congenital conditions, and counseling about safety issues.

NEWBORN TO 2 MONTHS OF AGE

A newborn needs a comprehensive examination within 24 hours after delivery with attention to antenatal risk factors such as maternal Group B streptococcus (GBS) status, TORCH titers, smoking, medications, as well as intrapartum factors such as prolonged rupture of membranes, shoulder dystocia, and ceasarean section. Breastfeeding should be encouraged with full lactation support in the hospital. A newborn should pass stool within 36 hours after birth and urinate within 24 hours of birth—failure to do so dictates an evaluation for diseases of the gastrointestinal or genitourinary systems.

After birth, the newborn should receive hepatitis B vaccine, vitamin K, and either erythromycin ophthalmic ointment or drops. Vitamin K prevents hemorrhagic disease of the newborn, and ophthalmic antibiotics prevents conjunctivitis caused by Neisseria gonorrhoeae, or *Chlamydia*, which may be acquired as the infant passes through the birth canal.

The first newborn office visit should be within 48 to 72 hours after hospital discharge and should include a comprehensive examination including screening for hip dysplasia, listening for murmurs, evaluating for jaundice, checking for hypospadias, and assessing weight. In addition to jaundice, benign rashes in the newborn such as mongolian spots, milia, erythema toxicum, and infantile seborrhea are common. Normal patterns of sleeping, feeding, stooling, and urination should be discussed with the family along with age appropriate guidance regarding SIDS, fever, reflux, colic, car seats and injury prevention.

The second visit should be around 2 weeks of age and should encompass the same as above.

SLEEP

Although sleep patterns vary among infants, a newborn often sleeps up to 20 hours/day. Infants should sleep on their backs, because prone and side-sleeping positions are associated with an increased risk for SIDS. Other SIDS risk factors include smoke exposure, cosleeping, and having objects in the crib such as extra blankets, toys, infant crib wedges, or guards. Pacifier use as the infant is falling asleep **decreases** SIDS risk; however, once the child is asleep pacifiers should be removed from the crib.

INFANT BEHAVIOR

All babies cry. Crying may be a sign of hunger, discomfort, a wet diaper, frustration, or a desire for attention. The average infant cries for 1 to 3 hours/day, and daily periods of crying can occur often in the afternoon or early evening. Rhythm rockers, pacifiers, swaddling, and cuddling are common methods to reduce crying. Paroxysmal crying or irritability characterizes infant colic in an otherwise healthy infant. The crying episodes can last for more than 3 hours/day and occur more than 3 days/week. Infantile colic generally has its onset by 3 weeks of age and almost 90% of cases resolve by 4 months of age. Uncontrollable, nonstop crying for 1 hour can be a sign of illness and merits emergent medical evaluation.

In addition to inconsolable crying, the infant who feeds poorly, shows signs of respiratory difficulty or exhibits skin color changes (e.g., cyanosis, jaundice) needs emergent evaluation. Although infants may not mount a fever with infection, the presence of fever (rectal temperature $\geq 38°C$ or $100.4°F$) mandates physician evaluation. The parents who are uncertain about how to measure temperature need instruction about proper methods for obtaining a rectal temperature.

BATHING

Sponge baths are recommended until the umbilical cord falls off and the circumcision heals (10 to 14 days of age); afterwards, the child can be immersed in a small tub in up to 3 to 4 inches of water. Although the umbilical cord stump remains attached, it should be washed with soap and water daily. Baths should be limited to every other day using baby soap to avoid dry skin. Water heater temperature should not exceed $115°F$ ($46°C$), and parents should never turn their attention away while bathing an infant.

ELIMINATION

Newborns usually urinate the number of wet diapers as their age in days until 6 days of age (i.e., 2-day old, 2 wet diapers) and then wet a minimum of 6 diapers per 24 hours thereafter.

Breastfed babies average between 3 and 8 stools a day. Formula-fed infants generally have fewer stools. Infants and toddlers normally have visible straining for passage of bowel movements. If the child passes soft stools, has bowel movements every 3 to 5 days, feeds adequately, and is otherwise well, the parents can be reassured if worried about constipation.

Diaper rashes are common due to moisture in the area and generally respond to keeping the skin clean and dry. Avoiding harsh soaps and leaving the diaper area open to air is helpful. Satellite lesions and involvement of the inguinal folds often identify a secondary infection with yeast, usually *Candida*. Treatment consists of zinc oxide cream or prescription antifungal preparations (e.g., nystatin or clotrimazole) along with frequent diaper changes.

SCREENING NEWBORNS

Universal newborn testing differ by state, but usually screening for cystic fibrosis, hypothyroidism, metabolic disorders such as phenylketonuria and galactosemia, and congenital adrenal hyperplasia. Early recognition and treatment of metabolic disorders can prevent irreversible damage. Ideally, the screening tests should be drawn 24 hours after delivery and before 7 days of age. Factors such as timing of blood draw, preterm delivery, transfusion, and parenteral nutrition can affect the accuracy. If a newborn screening test is abnormal, the first step is to reassess the infant and to repeat the screen.

A hearing screen should also be completed before discharge. If the newborn fails the hearing screen examination, the infant needs a follow-up outpatient-hearing test within 2 weeks. If there is a hearing deficit, the goal is to fit the child with hearing aids as soon as possible (preferably by 6 months of age) to prevent speech and language delays.

The newborn should be monitored for pathologic jaundice (occurs <24 hours of age), physiologic jaundice (>24 hours), and risk factors for hyperbilirubinemia. A transcutaneous or serum bilirubin after 24 hours of birth assesses risk. Plotting bilirubin levels using the Bhutani nomogram assesses the need for phototherapy or exchange transfusion.

NUTRITION

Either infant formula or breast milk can meet an infant's nutritional needs until 6 months of age. Breastfeeding is encouraged because of its nutritional value in meeting needs for infant growth, along with low cost, convenience, and associated mother–infant bonding. Breast milk contains immunoglobulins such as immunoglobulin A (IgA), which result in fewer enteric and respiratory infections in breastfed infants as well as a lower incidence of allergies and asthma as the child gets older. The AAP recommends supplementing nursing infants with 400 IU/day of vitamin D.

Although rare, contraindications to breastfeeding include metabolic diseases that require special formulas, maternal ingestion of medications transmissible in the breast milk that would be harmful to the infant, or maternal infectious disease such as HIV. Maternal hepatitis B is *not* a contraindication to breastfeeding as long as there are no cuts or sores on the breasts; however, certain medications taken by the mother preclude nursing.

Formula provides adequate infant nutrition and mothers who choose not to breastfeed should not be made to feel guilty. In the United States, formulas are iron-fortified and range from 20 to 24 cal/oz. Initially feeding the infant 1 to 2 oz of a 20 cal/oz formula preparation every 3 to 4 hours and on demand is appropriate. The best way to determine whether feeding is adequate is to monitor infant weight. Term newborns can lose up to 10% of extracellular fluid weight in the first 3 to 5 days of life but usually return to birth weight by 2 weeks of age if formula fed and by 3 weeks if breastfed.

Cereal is introduced at age 4 to 6 months using a spoon and vegetables and fruits are introduced one at a time at around 6 months. Water may supplement formula to assure adequate hydration. A cup can be introduced at 6 months with the goal of discontinuing the bottle by 12 months of age. By age 1, children should eat three meals with two snacks and drink about 16 to 24 oz of whole milk using a cup. The use of juices should be limited.

2 TO 18 MONTHS

Visits during this period usually coincide with vaccine administration. During this time, in addition to physical examination, the focus of well child visits is on addressing parental concerns, reviewing the infant's growth and development, administering vaccines, and providing appropriate anticipatory guidance. The provider should counsel parents about "childproofing" the home. Safety measures such as storage of hazardous or poisonous materials in a locked or out-of-reach cabinet, covering electric outlets, and providing the parents with a phone number for poison control.

Plotting growth (height, weight, head circumference) on a growth chart evaluates if growth is proceeding normally (Fig. 67-1A and B). After achieving birth weight at 2 weeks, infants should gain 30 g/day until 3 months, 20 g/day from 3 to 6 months, and 10 g/day from 6 to 12 months of age. Generally, an infant should double its birth weight by 4 months and triple it by 1 year of age. Afterwards, a child should gain approximately 2 kg/year and a child with a weight gain <1 kg/year merits a nutritional assessment.

Infants grow on average 10 inches from birth to 12 months of age, at a rate of 1-inch/month until 6 months and then 0.5 inches/month from 7 to 12 months of age. From 12 to 24 months, toddlers grow >4 inches/year; from 24 to 48 months, about 3 inches/year; and 48 months to 10 years, about 2 inches/year. A child reaches half-adult height by 24 to 30 months of age. Improper growth requires evaluation.

SCREENING AND PREVENTION

A questionnaire can assess the risk of lead exposure at 12 and 24 months of age and lead levels measured for those at risk.

The AAP recommends a screening hemoglobin level (or CBC) between 9 and 12 months of age to rule out iron deficiency anemia.

TB screening with an intradermal purified protein derivative (PPD) is recommended for all high-risk children at 12 to 15 months and is required by some preschools.

An autism screen (i.e., modified checklist for autism) is performed at 18 and 24 months of age.

Dental and vision screening are recommended starting at 1 and 3 years of age, respectively.

Fluoride supplementation is recommended for infants living in areas with an inadequately fluorinated water supply (i.e., well water) and should begin with tooth eruption. Most experts recommend weaning a child from the bottle or breast by age 12 months to reduce the risk of dental decay. Developmental screening questionnaire (i.e., "Denver Developmental

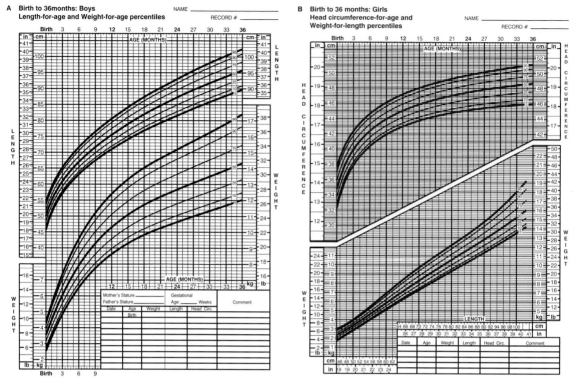

FIGURE 67-1. (A) Birth to 36 months: Boys—length-for-age and weight-for-age percentiles. Published May 30, 2000 (modified April 20, 2001). **(B)** Birth to 36 months: Girls—head circumference-for-age and weight-for-length percentiles. Published May 30, 2000 (modified October 16, 2000). (Developed by the National Center for Health Statistics in collaboration with the National Center for Chronic Disease Prevention and Health Promotion. 2000. http://www.cdc.gov/growthcharts.)

Screening Tool" or "Ages & Stages") at the 9, 18, and 24 or 30 months visits assesses development, but can also evaluate a child whenever there may be a concern for developmental delay. Childhood development can also be assessed by observing the child's behavior in office (Table 67-1).

2 TO 5 YEARS

During this interval, only an annual influenza vaccine is needed until the 5-year-old visit. Visits consist of a physical examination, including BP measurement starting at age 2 years, review of growth and development, and reinforcement of safety measures. Before school entry, children should have their vision and hearing checked. TB screening (PPD) is required for entry into most preschools, schools, and day care if at high risk.

The 5-year visit is important for assessing school "readiness." The average child should be able to tell stories, follow directions, engage in-group activities with other children while being able to separate from parents for a few hours. Parents should make sure their child knows his or her name, address, and telephone number as well as how to act around strangers for overall safety.

TABLE 67-1. Commonly Quizzed Developmental Milestones

Age	Gross Motor	Fine Motor and Vision	Language and Hearing	Social Interactions
Birth to 1 month	Raises head off table when prone	Hands in a fist; eyes cross due to lack of focusing ability	Alerts/startles to sound	Prefers to look at faces instead of objects
2 months	Lifts head *and* shoulders when prone	Hands often open; **visually fixes on an object** and tracks to 180°	Coos; makes reciprocal vocalizations	Social smile; recognizes parent
4 months	Lifts up to nipple line; **no head lag should be present;** rolls one way	Grasps with *both* hands together and reaches for objects; **failure to visually *track* objects is abnormal**	Laughs out loud; squeals	Initiates social interaction
6 months	Sits with support in tripod position; rolls in both directions	Transfers object from hand to hand; reaches with *either* hand	Babbles consonant sounds; **lack of turning to sound or voice is abnormal**	Recognizes strangers; blows "raspberries"
9 months	**Sits without support;** *starts* to crawl, pull to stand or cruise	Uses *immature* pincer grasp	Uses "dada/mama"—nonspecific; **lack of babbling is abnormal**	Plays pat-a-cake; recognizes objects and people; turns to own name; has stranger anxiety
12 months	Pulls to stand and cruises well. Starts taking independent steps	*Mature* pincer grasp. Throws, releases objects	Uses "dada/mama"—*specifically* along with one additional word	Imitates; comes when called
15 months	Walks well; stoops and recovers	Drinks from cup; builds two-cube tower; scribbles	3–6 specific words; follows one-step commands; points to things she or he wants	Plays ball; gives and takes toys
18 months	Runs; **lack of walking is abnormal**	Uses spoon; 3-cube tower	7–10 specific words; points to 1 or more body parts	Imitates household tasks; voices needs with words
24 months	Walks well up and down stairs; jumps with both feet off the floor	Uses spoon and fork; 4–6 cube tower; removes clothing	Combines 2–3 words; 50+ word vocabulary; uses pronouns ("I" "me"). Understands 2-step commands; stranger understands 50% speech. **Failure to use single words is abnormal**	Throws ball overhand; kicks ball

(continued)

TABLE 67-1. Commonly Quizzed Developmental Milestones (*continued*)

Age	Gross Motor	Fine Motor and Vision	Language and Hearing	Social Interactions
3 years	Can ride a tricycle	Helps in dressing and putting on shoes; 10-cube tower; copies a circle	5–8 word sentences; uses simple adjectives (i.e., thirsty); stranger understands 75% speech	Plays in a group; shares; knows age and gender
4 years	Alternates feet going downstairs; stands on 1 foot for 3 seconds	Dresses alone; copies a cross	Knows primary colors; stranger understands 100% speech	Catches ball; imaginative play with objects; has an imaginary friend
5 years	Skips alternating feet	Can tie shoes	Writes first name	Plays board games; understands consequences of broken rules

Bold items refer to when a child needs referral.
Source: Adapted from Marino BS, Fine KS. *Blueprints Pediatrics*. 3rd ed. Malden, MA: Blackwell Publishing; 2004:44. Copyright 2004, Blackwell Publishing. And "Chapter 1: Growth and Development: Part C. Developmental Milestones." American Academy of Pediatrics Board Content Specifications. 2010. www.abp.org. Accessed September 2012.

KEY POINTS

- Preventive health care in children begins with the prenatal visit.
- Safety counseling and appropriate anticipatory guidance is an important part of each visit.
- Breast milk contains immunoglobulins such as IgA, which result in fewer enteric and respiratory infections in breastfed infants.

- Contraindications to breastfeeding are rare; they include metabolic diseases that require special formulas, instances where the mother takes a medication that is passed in the breast milk and is harmful to the infant, or if the mother has a contagious illness such as HIV.

68 | Preventive Care: 5 to 12 Years

Health care visits for this age group generally occur episodically in association with illness, summer camp physicals, or preparticipation clearance for sports activities. When children change schools, advance from elementary to middle school, or enter high school, they may need an examination before entry. Thus, routine health care measures and counseling often have to be incorporated into visits for an illness or preparticipation examinations.

The leading causes of morbidity and mortality in this age category are accidents followed by homicide and suicide, both of which increase in prevalence as children enter adolescence. Also as children enter adolescence, increased risk-taking behavior and experimentation occurs. This frequently leads to the use of cigarettes or other substances and high-risk sexual activities. In addition to the physical examination, review of immunization status, growth and development, and counseling are important to include during these health care visits (Table 68-1).

TABLE 68-1. Preventive Care Ages 5 to 12 Years

Ages	Morbidity and Mortality	Testing/Vaccine	Counseling
5–6	Accidents	Blood pressure Vision Hearing Tuberculosis (high risk) Lipids (high risk) MMR IPV DTaP Pneumococcal vaccine[a] Influenza Varicella	Seatbelts Bicycle helmets Firearms Water safety Matches/poisons Exposure to violence Dental care Exercise Sun exposure
7–12	Accidents	Blood pressure Scoliosis Lipids (high risk) Tuberculosis (high risk) Tdap Meningococcal Human papillomavirus Annual Influenza Pneumococcal vaccine[a] HbA_{1C} (high risk)	Seatbelts Bicycle helmets Firearms Water safety Matches/poisons Exposure to violence Sun exposure Dental care Exercise Diet Tobacco/drugs/alcohol

[a]At-risk individuals.
DTaP, diphtheria, tetanus, acellular pertussis; IPV, injectable polio vaccine; MMR, measles, mumps, rubella.

5 TO 6 YEARS

The health care visit at this age may be the last scheduled well visit until the child enters junior high school. Accidents continue to be the leading cause of morbidity and mortality at this age. In addition to reviewing the past medical history, including growth and development, preventive services should focus on updating vaccinations and providing counseling and anticipatory guidance. Between ages 4 and 6 years, immunization with DTaP, MMR, IPV, and varicella are part of the recommended routine schedule. Annual influenza vaccination is recommended for all children more than 6 months of age. For children with chronic diseases, such as asthma or sickle cell disease, pneumococcal vaccination is recommended. The physical examination includes BP measurement, vision, and hearing testing. Those at risk, such as children living in poverty, those residing in areas where TB is prevalent, and those with history of TB exposure need TB screening. Lipid screening should be encouraged in children with family history of premature CAD or with parents who have cholesterol levels over 240 mg/dL. Routine UA is no longer recommended.

Counseling and anticipatory guidance are important parts of health care visits during childhood. Safety issues to discuss include the routine use of seat belts and bicycle helmets, firearm safety, safe storage of toxic substances (including matches and lighters), and rules regarding encounters with strangers. Parents should be encouraged to provide good role modeling and a healthy environment that is smoke-free, includes a healthy diet, and incorporates exercise as part of the family routine. Protection from excess sun exposure and use of sunscreen should be encouraged for the entire family. Regular teeth brushing, flossing, and visits to the dentist should be encouraged. Television viewing should be limited, reading encouraged, and exposure to violence monitored. Children should be encouraged to participate in age-appropriate activities and praised liberally for their positive actions.

7 TO 12 YEARS

The child may have no routinely scheduled health care visits during this age range, and preventive care and counseling may have to be incorporated into sick visits or preparticipation examinations. The physical examination includes BP measurement, assessment of growth and sexual development, and scoliosis screening. Having the child assume a diving position with the hands together and the trunk forward flexed can be used to screen for scoliosis. Asymmetry of the rib cage along the spine may be indicative of an abnormality. Immunization status should be updated if needed and annual influenza vaccination given. Pneumococcal vaccination should be administered to at-risk children. Routine immunization guidelines call for Tdap, meningococcal, and human papillomavirus vaccines for all 11- to 12-year-old children. Lipid screening can be offered for children with a strong family history of atherosclerosis. Vision and hearing screening are indicated if the history or physical examination suggests concerns about vision or hearing. HbA_{1C} should be checked if the child is obese, has a family history of diabetes, or signs of insulin resistance (acanthosis nigricans).

Counseling and anticipatory guidance should continue to emphasize accident prevention, addressing seat belt and bicycle helmet use and water safety, along with encouraging the child to learn to swim. Parents and their children should be educated regarding the importance of avoiding sunburns as well as the importance of using sunscreens and protective clothing to lower future risk of skin cancer. Additional questions to assess violence exposure, mood, and potential for engaging in high-risk behaviors should be incorporated into the visit. This portion of the interaction is best performed without the parents in the examination room. Reinforcement of healthful behaviors regarding exercise, sleep, and diet as well as abstinence from sexual activity, tobacco, drugs, and alcohol are important messages for the child to receive from the physician and his or her parents. Encouraging the parents to discuss these topics with their children is important, as is role modeling of the positive behaviors desired in the child.

KEY POINTS

- Accidents are a major cause of morbidity and mortality during childhood.
- As children enter adolescence, homicides and suicides are other leading causes of morbidity and mortality.

- In addition to accident prevention, counseling should be provided regarding risks associated with sun exposure, cigarette smoking, substance abuse, and sexual activity.

69 | Adolescent Medicine

Adolescence is a period of rapid physical, cognitive, and emotional change. Physically, adolescent patients are generally very healthy. As a result, health care visits by adolescent patients are infrequent, generally occurring in association with illness or a preparticipation evaluation for sporting activities. Illness-related visits are generally for respiratory, dermatologic, or musculoskeletal conditions. During the course of these examinations, many issues that might not necessarily fall within the scope of the visit should be addressed to provide comprehensive health care to this group of patients.

To obtain accurate information about the adolescent patient's habits and concerns, the patient and his or her parents must understand the need for confidentiality in all matters that do not pose an imminent threat to the patient's or others' lives. To also include the parents in their child's health care, the interview can be conducted in two phases, with the parents initially present and voicing their concerns, followed by a talk with the patient alone. Arrangements can be made with the parents that allow the adolescent to seek care when he or she feels it to be necessary, thus providing better access for care. In many states, adolescent patients can seek care on their own for STDs, pregnancy, contraception, and mental illness, including substance abuse. The ability to maintain this confidentiality may be compromised by the patient's limited resources and bills/insurance statements that are sent to the parents.

CLINICAL MANIFESTATIONS

HISTORY

In addition to eliciting parental concerns and the details surrounding these concerns, information regarding the past medical history, medication use, allergies, and family and social histories should be obtained. Immunization status should be reviewed. Additional history will have to be obtained directly from the adolescent patient without the parents' presence. Because of their increasing autonomy, emerging sexual identity, and the influence of peer groups, questions specific to adolescent patients are necessary (Table 69-1). Asking these questions in a nonthreatening way, such as "Some patients of mine . . ." or "Do any of your friends or the kids at school . . .," may allow for more candid responses. Although adolescent patients do not openly show concern about their health, studies suggest that many do have health concerns. Many of these concerns may be related to the issues they face regarding their changing bodies, sexuality, substance use, or peer pressure. Nonthreatening questions about their concerns can help to provide any needed reassurance or counseling.

PHYSICAL EXAMINATION

The physical examination should include BP measurement, assessment of growth and development (including sexual maturity), scoliosis screening, and a general physical examination. A pelvic examination (external observation or comprehensive examination) may be indicated for sexually active teens and for teens with genitourinary complaints. For those with visual or hearing complaints, appropriate screening should be performed.

Assessment of cognitive and psychosocial development can be difficult. During adolescence, thought processes should change from concrete in nature to the ability to think abstractly. Another task of adolescence is developing autonomy and a sense of personal and sexual identity. Success in courses such as algebra and geometry indicates an advancement from concrete to abstract thought processes. Less interest in parent/family activities and an increase in

TABLE 69-1. Sample Questions for Adolescent Patients

Environment

Who lives in your home?

Who are you closest to at home?

Have there been any recent changes at home?

How do you get along with others at home?

Do you feel safe?

Education/Activities

How is school?

What grade are you in?

How are your grades?

What do you want to do after you graduate?

What do you and your friends do for fun?

What extracurricular activities are you involved with?

What are your hobbies?

Have you had a job?

How much do you exercise in an average day/week?

Body Image/Mood

How do you feel about your weight?

Has your weight changed recently?

What do you like or do not like about your body?

Do you ever feel sad or down?

How do you make yourself feel better?

Have you ever tried to hurt yourself or kill yourself?

Sexuality

Do you have a boyfriend or girlfriend?

Have you ever had sex?

Have you used condoms or other types of contraception?

Have you ever been pregnant?

Have you ever had a sexually transmitted disease?

Drugs/Safety

Do you wear a seat belt?

Do you use a helmet for biking/rollerblading?

Do any of your friends smoke/drink/use drugs?

Have you ever smoked/drunk/used drugs?

Have you ever driven a vehicle after drinking/using drugs?

Have you ever ridden in a vehicle where the driver has used drugs or alcohol?

TABLE 69-2. The Adolescent Psychosocial History: HEADSS[a]

Home (family members, relationships, living arrangements)

Education (academic performance/educational goals)

Activities (peer relationships, work and recreational activities)

Drugs (substance use/abuse, including tobacco, alcohol, steroids, inhalants, and illicit drugs)

Sexuality (dating, sexual activity, contraception, sexual orientation)

Suicide (depression, anxiety, other mental health concerns)

[a]Some experts suggest that a second "E" should be added to remind physicians to screen for behaviors associated with **E**ating disorders and/or **E**xercise and that a third "S" should be included to prompt questions concerning **S**afety (the potential for abuse or violent behavior [e.g., gang membership, owning a firearm]). Source: From Marino BS, Fine KS. *Blueprints: Pediatrics*. 6th ed. Baltimore, MD: Lippincott Williams & Wilkins; 2013:44, Table 3.1.

peer pressure and interest in peer-related activities are part of adolescent development and increasing autonomy. As teens mature, boyfriend/girlfriend relationships indicate the formation of a personal and sexual identity and the diminishing importance of the peer group. The pneumonic HEADSS in Table 69-2 outlines the key features of the adolescent psychosocial history.

Determining sexual maturity (Table 69-3) can assist in providing counseling regarding menarche and concerns about maturity. Pubertal changes occur earlier in girls than in boys and are heralded by the formation of the breast bud. The first sign of puberty in boys is testicular enlargement. In girls, the growth spurt generally occurs around Tanner stage 3, whereas in boys it does not occur until Tanner stage 4. Menarche occurs near the end of the growth spurt, which is on average at 12.8 years of age.

SCREENING

A tetanus booster, utilizing Tdap to include pertussis, and meningococcal vaccines are recommended at 11 to 12 years of age. A meningococcal booster is also recommended from 16 to 18 years of age. Individuals who have not had chicken pox need vaccination. Many experts recommend that children with a family history of premature CAD or with parents whose cholesterol is above 240 mg/dL have lipid screening. A hemoglobin test is recommended for menstruating teenagers. Routine UA is no longer recommended.

TABLE 69-3. Tanner Stages of Sexual Maturity

1	Prepubertal stage Prepubertal penis and testicles (<1.5 mL volume) No pubic hair	Prepubertal stage No breast development No pubic hair
2	Penis unchanged Scrotum and testicles enlarge (1.6–6 mL) Small amount of fine, long pubic hair	Breast buds Small amount of fine, long pubic hair
3	Penis elongates Continued growth of testicles (6–12 mL) and scrotum becomes pendulous with thinning of skin Coarse and curly pubic hair	Breast tissue grows past areola, but areola is still part of the rest of the breast Coarse and curly pubic hair
4	Penis increased in length and diameter Testicular size 12–20 mL. Darkening of scrotum Adult hair texture over pubic area	Areola separate mound from breast tissue Adult hair texture over pubic area
5	Adult penis, scrotum Adult testes usually ≥20 mL volume Pubic hair extends to thighs	Adult breast contours Pubic hair extends to thighs

Accidents continue to be the leading cause of death in the adolescent population. Other causes that increase in importance as the child enters adolescence are homicides and suicides. In addition, increased risk-taking behavior occurs during this period, leading to experimentation with tobacco, drugs, alcohol, and sexual activities. Because adolescence is often the time when adult behaviors develop, it is important to lay the groundwork for a healthy lifestyle. Thus, counseling during this age should include not only emphasis on accident prevention but also inquiries into these other high-risk behaviors.

The incidence of depression increases throughout adolescence to ~10% at age 18. Over half of adolescent girls and nearly three-quarters of adolescent boys have sexual intercourse before they are 18 years of age. Thus, to have an impact on these common issues related to the adolescent period, identification of at-risk individuals, encouraging dialogue on these matters between adolescent and parent, and referring those in need of further therapy is beneficial. Discussion of the risks associated with the use of drugs, alcohol and tobacco should be part of the counseling. In addition, counseling adolescents about birth control, STDs, and responsible sexual activity is important. For sexually active individuals, examination and screening for STDs are also recommended. Vaccination against HPV should be provided to adolescent girls and boys between ages 11 and 12 years, but can be administered starting at 9 years of age.

KEY POINTS

- Parents can be included in the history but must respect the adolescent patient's need for confidentiality in receiving medical care.
- During adolescence, accidents, homicides, and suicides are leading causes of morbidity and mortality; counseling should be provided regarding these risks.
- Over half of the 18-year-olds are sexually active and should be screened for STDs.
- Appropriate immunizations should be given including Tdap booster, meningitis, and HPV vaccines.

70 | Common Medical Problems in Children

Many of the common medical conditions in children are covered in other chapters. Some additional conditions that are unique to children and that are discussed here include failure to thrive (FTT), stridor and croup, crying/colic, and seizure disorders (including febrile seizures).

FAILURE TO THRIVE

FTT is defined as "failure of the child to grow and develop at an appropriate rate." FTT describes a condition and not the cause for an aberrant growth pattern. FTT should be suspected and evaluated when the weight for height is <80% of predicted ideal weight, a persistent weight below the third percentile, a growth rate that is too slow (i.e., decreasing over two major percentile lines on growth chart), and when developmental or interactional milestones are delayed.

PATHOGENESIS

To grow and develop normally, children require oxygen, adequate nutrition/energy balance, hormonal balance, and love/nurturing. Adequate energy intake needs both to maintain basal metabolic requirements and to support the child's growth. Conditions leading to inadequate caloric intake, such as neglect or malabsorptive digestive disorders, can slow growth. Conditions that increase caloric expenditure or impair the efficient use of calories, such as chronic infections or chronic pulmonary diseases, make it difficult to meet caloric needs for growth. Finally, neglected children, even when provided with adequate calories and nutritional intake, may not grow at a normal rate because of their unmet needs for emotional support and nurturing. The exact reason for why emotional deprivation causes FTT remains uncertain but demonstrates the need for love and nurturing of children.

CLINICAL MANIFESTATIONS

History

The history should ask about events related to birth, social environment, and family support systems. A detailed review of systems should assess respiratory, gastrointestinal, and neurodevelopmental milestones. The pregnancy history should be reviewed, including whether it was planned, maternal illnesses, substance abuse in the home and whether the child delivered at term or prematurely. Parental stature is also an important consideration in evaluating a child's growth.

A detailed diet history is essential including the type and amount of foods offered to the child, how much and how often the child eats, and who feeds the child.

Physical Examination

In addition to a thorough physical overview, the physical examination should assess growth parameters. Particular attention should be on recognizing dysmorphic features that may warrant referral for genetic evaluation. Any identified abnormalities, such as heart murmurs, should be evaluated. Social interactions with the examiner and developmental achievements can provide clues to nonorganic causes.

DIAGNOSTIC EVALUATION

Laboratory evaluation includes a CBC, metabolic profile, UA with culture, and evaluation of the stool for reducing substances, occult blood, and in selected cases ova and parasites. Clues provided by the history and findings on physical examination should direct further investigations. In general, organic FTT does not present with isolated growth failure, other signs and symptoms are evident with a detailed history and physical. The majority of FTT cases (80%) are from nonorganic causes such as improper feeding techniques, nutritional misconceptions, economic issues, neglect, emotional deprivation, and child abuse or caregiver depression. However, finding an organic cause does not rule out nonorganic causes as a contributing factor because the two are not mutually exclusive.

TREATMENT

Management includes a psychosocial assessment of the home environment and frequently requires social service assistance to uncover social needs or parenting issues. Enrollment in public assistance programs, such as the Special Supplemental Nutrition Program for Women, Infants, and Children (WIC), may be of benefit. The Child Protective Services should be contacted to assess the suitability of the child's home environment in cases of suspected neglect or abuse. In cases of severe malnutrition, hospitalization may be required for further assessment and to monitor growth and nutritional intake.

COLIC AND CRYING

Crying is a form of communication for an infant and may be normal or excessive. At 2 weeks of age, normal infants cry on average for 1¾ hours/day. Peak crying activity occurs at around 6 weeks of age and averages 2¾ hours/day. By 3 months of age, crying time in normal infants decreases to an average of 1 hour daily. Excessive crying is defined as crying more than 3 hours/day for more than 3 days/week. Excessive crying may be secondary to distress or disease but can be idiopathic. Idiopathic excessive crying is termed colic and resolves in most infants by 3 to 4 months of age.

PATHOGENESIS

Although many theories seek to explain the cause of colic, no data support one over another. Infants with colic may have a heightened sensitivity to environmental stimuli causing them to respond by crying excessively. Parental responses to crying and anxiety are controversial contributing factors that can either be a primary cause or aggravate the excessive crying. Some theories propose GI motility, excess intestinal gas, food allergies, or lactose sensitivity as contributing factors. Most likely colic results from a combination of factors and not from a single cause. Box 70-1 lists some common causes for excessive crying.

CLINICAL MANIFESTATIONS

History

When parents bring their child in for evaluation of crying, a thorough history and physical examination are warranted. The birth history, prior history of any medical concerns, social history, and supports should all be noted. The onset of crying, parental responses, and specific parental concerns help in evaluating the infant. Infant feeding, bowel movements, and sleep behaviors should be assessed.

Physical Examination

A thorough physical examination is important for identifying underlying causes of an infant's crying. Appendages should be examined for a hair tourniquet with may strangle a finger or toe, the eyes checked for a corneal abrasion or foreign body, the mouth for problems such as stomatitis, the ears for an occult otitis media, the testes for torsion, and a musculoskeletal examination for signs of trauma or joint tenderness. A careful GI examination may help provide a clue to problems such as an incarcerated hernia or anal fissure. Weight gain and growth are important parameters to monitor. Colic is a diagnosis of exclusion and conditions such as those listed in Box 70-1 should be eliminated. Laboratory evaluation may include UA and culture but otherwise directed by the history and findings on physical examination.

TREATMENT

Colic is distressing, and parents need physician reassurance that crying is a normal infant/child behavior, that crying does not harm the child, and that the behavior peaks at 6 weeks of age and wanes after 3 to 4 months of age. Although common, colic is a diagnosis of exclusion and requires eliminating serious problems such as infection or physical injury. After eliminating a correctable cause, management includes developing parental strategies to respond to their infant or child and how to address the forms of distress that may cause crying. Parents need guidance to develop a set

---

BOX 70-1. Common Causes for Excessive Crying

Idiopathic (colic)
Anal fissure
Child abuse (fracture, Shaken Baby syndrome)
Constipation
Corneal abrasion/foreign body
Dermatitis
Gastroesophageal reflux
Otitis media
Urinary tract infection
Sickle cell disease
Stomatitis
Tourniquet injury to digit/penis (hair or fiber)

of responses to comfort the child. For example, they may cuddle and hold or rock the child initially. If crying persists, then changing and feeding the child may be tried. If crying persists, then changing the environment, such as going for a walk, may be helpful.

Parental frustration and child safety should be determined. Involving both parents and trusted friends or relatives may be important in providing respite for parents who feel particularly stressed.

STRIDOR AND CROUP

"Stridor" refers to audible, turbulent airflow due to narrowing of the larger airways. "Croup" refers to stridor in combination with hoarseness, a barking cough, and some degree of respiratory distress.

PATHOGENESIS

Swollen or narrowed upper airways (subglottic region, vocal cords, and pharynx) can cause harsh, adventitious respiratory sounds during inspiration. The word croup derives from the Scottish word for a raven's croak, which reflects its characteristic sound. When the obstruction occurs at the cricoid cartilage or below, stridor can occur during expiration as well as during inspiration. Children more commonly experience stridor because of the smaller caliber of their airways. Causes of stridor may be infectious, anatomic, functional, or due to foreign bodies. Common infectious etiologies include viral croup, bacterial epiglottitis, tracheitis, severe pharyngitis, and bronchitis. Anatomic causes may be congenital (vascular rings, laryngeal webs, and choanal atresia) or secondary to airway injury or scarring, as may occur from trauma, caustic ingestions, or intubation. Functional causes include laxity of the trachea or larynx (tracheomalacia and laryngomalacia) that resolve as the infant matures and the airways grow in diameter.

Croup generally affects children between 6 months and 3 years of age, because of the narrower diameter of the airway with a peak incidence of 2 years of age. Croup is typically infectious due to parainfluenza, respiratory syncytial, or influenza viruses. Spasmodic croup is a variant of croup that may be associated with viral upper respiratory infections or allergies and generally occurs at night, develops suddenly, and is recurrent.

CLINICAL MANIFESTATIONS

History

Assessment of children with stridor and croup should note the onset of symptoms; associated respiratory symptoms or fever, and the presence of respiratory distress. Viral croup typically presents with a prodrome of mild URI symptoms such as nasal congestion and low-grade fever that progress to hoarseness, barking cough, and inspiratory stridor. Symptoms usually peak at around 2 to 4 days into the illness. Stridor associated with a choking event suggests a foreign body. An abrupt onset associated with fever and drooling are characteristics of epiglottitis.

Physical Examination

The physical examination includes an assessment of the child's general appearance, vital signs, and throat and lung examinations. An ill appearing child, who leans forward and cannot control their secretions (drools), suggests possible epiglottitis. In contrast, a child with croup often sounds worse than they look. Throat examination should note size and appearance of the tonsils. On occasion, the epiglottis may be visible, but avoiding aggressive attempts at visualization is important because this may upset the child and worsen any tissue trauma or airway edema that is present. Stridor may be heard on lung examination as a harsh inspiratory sound that is maximal over the laryngeal region and transmitted to the lungs. With significant airway narrowing, inspiratory and expiratory phases may be audible. Note should be made of the respiratory effort as evidenced by intercostal retractions and respiratory rate.

DIAGNOSTIC EVALUATION

In most cases, imaging or blood testing is not indicated unless the diagnosis is uncertain. However, in suspected cases of bacterial infection, a CBC, blood culture, and imaging may be helpful. The WBC is elevated with epiglottitis but generally normal or minimally elevated with viral causes. Soft-tissue neck x-rays reveal subglottic narrowing with viral croup, often referred to as the "steeple sign," whereas enlargement of the epiglottis supports the diagnosis of epiglottitis. A widened retropharyngeal space suggests a retropharyngeal abscess. Many foreign bodies are also visible on x-ray evaluation. CT of the neck and thorax and barium swallow studies may be helpful in evaluating children with stridor and suspected congenital anomalies.

TREATMENT

Patients with croup and stridor at rest, significant retractions, and decreased air movement warrant close monitoring and if in respiratory distress hospitalization. Treatment of croup includes the use of humidified oxygen or mist therapy and maintaining hydration. For children with mild-to-moderate symptoms and with reliable caregivers, oral dexamethasone with close follow-up can be an effective option. Steroids have an onset of improvement in 6 hours that persists for at least 12 to 24 hours. For those with more severe disease, dexamethasone can be provided orally or parenterally in the hospital. Racemic epinephrine can benefit those with moderate-to-severe disease, but patients who receive this treatment need monitoring for 4 hours to assess for "rebound" after the effects of the medication wear off. Children who fail to improve with nebulized epinephrine or who need more than two doses usually merit hospital admission. Severe disease warrants monitoring in an intensive care unit (ICU) because up to 10% of these children require intubation. Antibiotics have no role in uncomplicated croup because most cases are of viral etiology. Antitussives such as codeine have no proven effect and may increase sedation interfering with assessment.

Hospitalization is advisable when epiglottitis or bacterial tracheitis is suspected. Intravenous antibiotics, close monitoring, and—in many cases—intubation are required for successful treatment of these conditions.

Otolaryngology referral is recommended for those patients with stridor and congenital anomalies, foreign body, caustic ingestion, or trauma.

SEIZURE DISORDERS

Seizures occur from abnormal neuronal brain activity that occurs focally (focal seizure), focally with evolution to generalized convulsive activity or diffusely throughout the brain (generalized seizure). Seizures may occur as part of systemic condition, such as a febrile illness, brain injury, or metabolic abnormalities, or they may be primary congenital disorders. Febrile seizures are generalized tonic–clonic seizures associated with a rapid rise in temperature due to viral or bacterial non-CNS infection and are the most common form of childhood seizures. Febrile seizures affect up to 5% of children, most commonly between the ages of 6 months and 5 years. Nonfebrile seizures affect 0.5% to 1.0% of children and are classified as outlined in Box 70-2. The diagnosis of epilepsy requires at least two or more unprovoked seizures. A child with a seizure that occurs in the context of an acute abnormality,

BOX 70-2. Classification of Seizure Types

Generalized
Absence
Myoclonic
Atonic
Tonic–clonic
Syndromes (e.g., infantile spasms, Lennox–Gastaut)

Focal
Without alteration in consciousness
With sensory or psychic symptoms
With impairment of consciousness
Evolving to bilateral generalized convulsive seizure activity

Febrile
Unknown

such as trauma or fever, does not meet the criteria to diagnose epilepsy unless the seizures recur after correcting the underlying abnormality.

CLINICAL MANIFESTATIONS
History
In evaluating a child suspected of having had a seizure, an eyewitness description of the event is very helpful. Older children may be able to describe an aura preceding an event. The child's level of alertness and associated motor activity helps distinguish focal from generalized seizures. Recurrent episodes of staring or inattention may signify absence seizures. Incontinence, injury, and postictal drowsiness are characteristics associated with seizure activity. A review of systems should focus on neurologic and infection.

Past medical history should be reviewed in detail including birth history, childhood development, and history of CNS injury or infections. Family history of febrile and afebrile seizures is associated with an increased risk of seizures in those with affected first-degree relatives.

Physical Examination
The physical examination should note the child's alertness and activity following the event. Temperature elevation may suggest febrile seizure as the diagnosis. Individuals experiencing a seizure need a complete physical examination with attention to identifying sources of infection and focal neurologic deficits. Appropriate developmental milestones should be determined as well.

DIAGNOSTIC EVALUATION

In older children suspected of having had a simple febrile seizure (one generalized seizure, lasting <15 minutes) who have an obvious source of infection and a normal postictal neurologic examination, no further workup may be necessary. Since seizures are the presenting sign of meningitis in about 15% of patients and about one-third may not have meningeal signs, AAP guidelines strongly recommend an LP in children <12 months and an LP for those aged 12 to 18 months. Complex febrile seizures are those that are focal or focal with generalization, last longer than 15 minutes, or occur repetitively. Complex febrile seizures require neuroimaging, lumbar puncture, and EEG to be fully evaluated. Patients with nonfebrile seizures need neuroimaging and EEG evaluation. Testing fails to identify an underlying cause in 60% to 80% of children with recurrent seizures. A child's age, clinical evaluation, and past medical history directs the need for further testing. Glucose testing is generally warranted, and infants with new-onset seizures should undergo screening for metabolic disorders.

TREATMENT

Treatment for febrile seizures consists of antipyretics at the onset of an illness to lessen the rapidity and extent of temperature rise and to prevent seizure activity. Most febrile seizures spontaneously abort but diazepam can be used for serial seizures or those lasting more than 5 minutes. One-third of children with a febrile seizure experience a recurrence. Parental education and reassurance are also very important aspects of care in these cases. Therapy for nonfebrile seizures consists of anticonvulsant therapy, generally in consultation with a neurologist. Monitoring seizure control and childhood development are important aspects of care. Two-thirds of children with seizures have a good prognosis developmentally. Some seizure types are associated with a poor prognosis for normal development regardless of the success in controlling seizures, whereas in others prognosis may depend on the degree of seizure control.

KEY POINTS

- To grow and develop normally, children require oxygen, adequate nutrition/energy balance, hormonal balance, and love/nurturing.

- Excessive crying is defined as crying more than 3 hours/day for more than 3 days/week. Excessive crying may be secondary to distress or disease or may be idiopathic.

- Causes of stridor may have an infectious, anatomic, or functional cause or be due to a foreign body. Common infectious etiologies include viral croup, bacterial epiglottitis, tracheitis, severe pharyngitis, and bronchitis.

- Febrile seizures affect up to 5% of children, most commonly between 6 months and 5 years of age. Nonfebrile seizures affect 0.5% to 1.0% of children.

71 | Behavioral Issues in Children

Childhood is a critical time for behavior and personality development. Family physicians should understand normal behavioral development in children and know how to respond to challenges that parents of young children are likely to face.

BIRTH TO 2 MONTHS

Understanding normal development helps clinicians to distinguish normal from abnormal (Table 71-1). From birth to 2 months, a healthy infant learns to look around, to follow faces, to smile spontaneously, to gaze at black and white objects, to discriminate mother's voice, to cry out in distress, and to coo. Explaining normal behavior and development to the parents is crucial so that they can recognize abnormal behavior and alert the provider about their concerns during well-child visits. In addition, it helps parents celebrate each milestone achieved.

BONDING AND ATTACHMENT

At birth, bonding occurs as unidirectional feelings of love from the parents to the child. Over the first year, parents and child develop reciprocal feelings toward each other, known as attachment. Strong bonding and attachment are essential for normal, healthy behavioral development and should be actively encouraged. It is important to encourage parents to interact with their children in positive ways. It is also equally important for parents to allow time for themselves, so that they will be more capable of positive interactions.

TEMPERAMENTS

Infants may display a wide range of temperaments that are partially hardwired and partially environment related. Understanding what constitutes a normal temperament helps physicians to reassure parents and monitor for truly abnormal behavior.

Approximately 40% of infants are considered "easy." They sleep, eliminate, and feed on a relatively regular schedule. They react positively to new stimuli, adapt well to new environments, and are generally happy. Around 10% of infants are classified as "difficult." Their sleeping, eating, and elimination schedules are irregular. These infants tend to withdraw from new stimuli, adapt poorly, and are more often in a negative mood. "Slow-to-warm-up," cranky infants make up 15% of children and are known to have a low activity level. All other normal children display a mix of one or more of these temperaments.

CRYING

Crying is essentially the mode of communication by an infant. Healthy children cry on average nearly 3 hours/day at 6 weeks of age. Most often, crying is used to convey distress; the infant is either wet, tired, hot, cold, hungry, needs a diaper change, or just wants to be held. However, many infants will still have periods of 15 minutes to an hour every day where they cry for no apparent reason. During these periods, encourage parents to continue to hold the crying baby to let them know that they are responding to the infant's distress. Over time, parents will recognize these normal bouts of crying and be able to distinguish them from crying that signifies a true emergency. Inconsolable crying for more than 2 hours straight may indicate something more serious and warrants further evaluation. Unexplained bouts of crying for more than 3 hours/day, and more than 3 days/week, can be very hard on parents. A common reason for frequent bouts of crying is colic. Physicians should let frustrated parents vent about the crying, educate them about normal crying patterns, and help them determine whether their child is truly colicky. They should also be reassured that colic typically resolves by 3 months of age.

TABLE 71-1. Typical Developmental Milestones

Age	Gross Motor	Fine (Visual) Motor	Language	Social/Adaptive
Birth–1 month	Raises head slightly in prone position	Follows with eyes to midline only; hands tightly fisted	Alerts/startles to sound	Fixes on face (at birth)
2 months	Raises chest and head off bed in prone position	Regards object and follows through 180° arc; briefly retains rattle	Coos and vocalizes reciprocally	Social smile; recognizes parent
4 months	Lifts onto extended elbows in prone position; steady head control with no head lag; rolls over front to back	Reaches for objects with both hands together; bats at objects; grabs and retains objects	Orients to voice; laughs and squeals	Initiates social interaction
6 months	Sits, but may need support; rolls in both directions	Reaches with one hand; transfers objects hand-to-hand	Babbles	Recognizes object or person as unfamiliar
9 months	Sits without support; crawls; pulls to stand	Uses pincer grasp; finger-feeds	Imitates speech sounds (nonspecific "mama," "dada"); understands "no"	Plays gesture games ("pat-a-cake"); understands own name; object permanence; stranger anxiety
12 months	Cruises; stands alone; takes a few independent steps	Can voluntarily release items	Discriminative use of "mama," "dada," plus 1–4 other words; follows command with gesture	Imitates; comes when called; cooperates with dressing
15 months	Walks well independently	Builds a two-block tower; throws ball underhand	4–6 words in addition to above; uses jargon; responds to one-step verbal command	Begins to use cup; indicates wants or needs
18 months	Runs; walks up stairs with hand held; stoops and recovers	Builds a three-block tower; uses spoon; spontaneous scribbling	Uses 10–25 words; points to body parts when asked; uses words to communicate needs or wants	Plays near (but not with) other children
24 months	Walks unassisted up and down stairs; kicks ball; throws ball overhand; jumps with two feet off the floor	Builds four- to six-block tower; uses fork and spoon; copies a straight line	Uses 501 words, two- and three-word phrases; uses "I" and "me"; 50% of speech intelligible to stranger	Removes simple clothing; parallel play
36 months	Pedals tricycle; broad jumps	Copies a circle	Uses 5–8 word sentences; 75% of speech intelligible to stranger	Knows age and gender; engages in group play; shares

TABLE 71-1. Typical Developmental Milestones (*continued*)				
Age	**Gross Motor**	**Fine (Visual) Motor**	**Language**	**Social/Adaptive**
4 years	Balances on one foot	Copies a cross; catches ball	Tells a story; 100% of speech intelligible to stranger	Dresses self; puts on shoes; washes and dries hands; imaginative play
5 years	Skips with alternating feet	Draws a person with six body parts	Asks what words mean	Names four colors; plays cooperative games; understands "rules" and abides by them
6 years	Rides a bike	Writes name	Identifies written letters and numbers	Knows right from left; knows all color names

Source: From Marino BS, Fine KS. *Blueprints: Pediatrics*. 6th ed. Baltimore, MD: Lippincott Williams & Wilkins; 2013:257, Table 15-1.

2 MONTHS TO 1 YEAR

From 2 months to 1 year, a baby undergoes tremendous transformations and rapid development. At 2 months, the child learns to smile socially in response to parents and known faces. When social smiling appears, the positive parental response reinforces the behavior and the infant's learning.

As the infant learns to crawl and walk, their curiosity and desire to explore and learn can make parents anxious. Counsel parents on child safety but encourage them to allow their child to explore in a safe setting, so that he or she can continue to learn and develop social and behavioral skills through interactions with the environment.

At the age of 8 to 9 months, children learn object permanence. This is also the time when they will experience separation anxiety as they learn that parents still exist even though they cannot be seen. This realization of separation from the primary caregiver is very stressful for children. Parents should work to reduce this stress, while continuing to encourage active exploration and the development of independence and identity.

1 YEAR THROUGH PRESCHOOL

DISCIPLINE

From 1 to 3 years of age, toddlers learn to walk and talk and become very much their own persons. They exert their independence by learning to say "no" and by exploring and testing new behaviors along with pushing their boundaries to see what they can get away with. Some parents may react negatively by scolding, threatening, or punishing the child physically by spanking, hitting, or other means. This kind of discipline is harmful to the child's self-esteem and

sense of security, and may provoke retaliatory behavior. Negative reinforcement should be discouraged to prevent the child from repeating similar behaviors when disagreeing or when upset with others.

Positive discipline is taught by setting boundaries while still allowing freedom of expression and exploration. Behaviors such as hitting, kicking, and biting must be dealt with quickly and appropriately so that they do not continue. The physician should help parents set up reasonable rules, develop ways to present these rules and the consequences for disobedience to their child. One way to modify behavior is with the "time-out" rule. When the child is breaking a rule, he or she should be removed from the situation and placed in a quiet place. The maximum time out should be 2 minutes per year of age. Lecturing to or reasoning with the child is not helpful and should be avoided, because the child does not understand.

Imposing strict boundaries or limits on exploration of the environment may cause restlessness in a child and can provoke temper tantrums, which are a normal part of development. Temper tantrums peak between 2 and 5 years of age and must be dealt with calmly and consistently using time-outs, ignoring the behavior, distracting the child with another activity, or holding the child calmly to help control the tantrum. Although discipline should be started at an early age, the child will continue to act out and test boundaries throughout preschool, elementary school, and into adolescence.

TOILET TRAINING

One of the most significant milestones for a toddler is toilet training. The age of toilet training varies widely by culture, but in the United States it is generally accepted to be between 24 and 48 months of age. Discussions regarding toilet training should be

BOX 71-1. Signs of Readiness for Toilet Training

Developmental
Ability to ambulate
Stability while sitting
Ability to remain dry for several hours
Ability to pull up pants
Ability to follow two-step commands
Ability to communicate need to eliminate

Behavioral
Ability to imitate
Ability to put things in proper places
Demonstration of independence by being able to say "no"
Interest in toilet training
Desire to please
Desire for independence and control of functions of elimination
Diminished frequency of power struggles

initiated early between the parents and the provider to ease transition. Parents need to be educated to look for signs of child "readiness," and should not initiate toilet training until then (Box 71-1). Power struggles between parent and child should be minimized, because these could lead to stool withholding by the child and cause chronic constipation. Table 71-2 outlines an approach to toilet training that parents may use. Once toilet training commences, the child should be positively reinforced to encourage the behavior.

SLEEP DISTURBANCES

Children often have nightmares and may either wake up screaming or come to the parents' room crying. The child should be reassured that he or she is safe, and taken back to his or her room to reassure him or her that there are no dangers such as monsters hiding under the bed or in the closet. It is acceptable to let the child stay in the parent's bed for a short time, but doing this continuously will make it difficult for the child to sleep alone and could disturb his or her regular sleeping pattern.

Night terrors are events where a child partially awakens crying or screaming for a short period of time and is inconsolable. The child will then return to sleep and have no recall of the event. Night terrors are a variant of sleepwalking and occur during deep (stage 4) sleep, whereas nightmares occur during rapid eye movement (REM) sleep. They typically occur between 4 and 12 years of age.

Children with chronic sleep disturbances should be evaluated for medical problems that interfere

TABLE 71-2. A Sample Approach for Parents to Toilet Training	
Vocabulary	Pick the words to use for elimination and then be consistent.
Buying the potty chair	Let the child pick out the chair or have him or her draw on it or write his or her name on the chair. Potty chairs are better than over-the-toilet covers.
Accessibility	Place the potty in an easily accessible location so that the child can see it and become comfortable with it.
Comfort level	Place child on the potty chair fully clothed at first, with toys to play with and books to read. Encourage the child to imitate you by having the child on the potty chair while using the toilet yourself.
Making the connection	After a week of fully clothed potty sitting, encourage child to sit naked on the chair. Place soiled diapers in the potty chair to help the child make the connection. Once the child connects elimination with the potty chair, demonstrate disposal of feces in the adult toilet. The flushing of feces down the toilet can scare a child; so, first let the child flush with pieces of toilet paper or wave bye-bye to feces.
Practice and encouragement	Praise the child each time he or she indicates the need to go potty. The child should be led to the chair and encouraged to eliminate. Also praise the child for successful potty attempts. Avoid punishing the child if potty attempts are not successful, because negative reinforcement can lead to numerous elimination problems later on.
Transition to toilet-training pants or underwear	After success with using the potty for at least 1 week, transition the child to training pants or cotton underwear. If the child cannot remain dry, return to diapers. Do not rush the child out of diapers. Continue positive reinforcement each time the child uses the potty successfully.

with sleep, such as obstructive sleep apnea and enuresis. Once medical conditions have been ruled out, the physician should encourage the parents to set up a nightly routine, limit vigorous activity in the evening, limit fluid intake after dinner, and limit television watching and video game playing before bedtime. If these measures do not alter the behavior, referral to a sleep specialist may be considered.

PRESCHOOL AND ELEMENTARY SCHOOL

Most elements of behavioral development that begin as toddlers continue into preschool and elementary school. However, some new behaviors and concerns also arise.

ENURESIS

Children are often in the process of toilet training during their preschool years and should be toilet trained by the time they reach kindergarten or the first grade. However, many will still have enuresis. Enuresis is defined as urinary incontinence at any age at which urinary continence is considered normal. A child who has never been continent for more than a 3- to 6-month period is considered to have primary enuresis, whereas a child who was continent for 3 to 6 months and is wetting again is considered to have secondary enuresis. The most common type of enuresis is primary nocturnal enuresis, or bedwetting.

A medical workup can rule out organic causes of enuresis, such as infection. After eliminating organic causes, the presumed diagnosis is behavioral enuresis. Treatment is usually not initiated until 6 years of age, owing to the high rate of spontaneous resolution. From 6 years of age onward, spontaneous cure rates are still high for both primary and secondary enuresis without an organic cause. Still, treatment may be useful at this age. Common treatments include behavioral modification, bedwetting alarms, and pharmacologic management with desmopressin acetate (DDAVP) or imipramine. DDAVP acts by concentrating the urine, and, if given in the evening, lessens urine production, reducing the risk of bedwetting. Because of its risk of side effects, its use is often limited to special situations like sleepovers or overnight camp. Bedwetting alarms work by waking a child when they start to urinate, eventually conditioning the child to wake up and empty his or her bladder before wetting the bed.

Behavioral modification works in part by raising awareness in the child and getting the child involved. First, reassure parents that bedwetting has an excellent cure rate, and talk to the child about the bedwetting experience and how he or she can help make it better. Have parents help the child to keep a calendar of wet and dry nights, and to urinate before bedtime; also have the child participate in changing the wet clothes and sheets. Parents should not react angrily when the child does wet the bed. Instead, they should offer praise or other positive reinforcement for each dry night. Techniques, such as restricting fluid intake after dinner, regular voids, and positive reinforcement, help tremendously.

SOCIAL PLAY

Infants and very young children engage in what is called "parallel play," where each child plays in his or her own fantasy world alongside other children, they play together but not with each other. During preschool and elementary school, children learn to interact and play more with each other, developing friendships and learning valuable social skills. At this age, parents should teach their children about the value of sharing, as well as continuing to enforce limits and boundaries as deemed appropriate.

SPECIFIC BEHAVIORAL TOPICS

ATTENTION DEFICIT HYPERACTIVITY DISORDER

Attention deficit hyperactivity disorder (ADHD) is characterized by inattentiveness, impulsivity, and overactivity. The child is easily distracted and impulsive to a point where the behavior hampers him or her socially and academically. The inattentiveness is often picked up by teachers when the child fails to complete tasks once they are begun, fails to grasp directions, and makes mistakes because of inattentiveness as opposed to not understanding the task at hand. The impulsiveness manifests itself as shifting quickly from one activity to another and exhibiting the right behavior at the wrong time. Overactivity can be seen in children as they constantly move around and fidget in their seats. ADHD affects about 5% to 7% of children and is more common in boys.

The issue of ADHD often first arises when a parent brings a child in for a visit and relates that the child's teacher has made a "diagnosis" of ADHD. A careful examination of the history of the child's behavior, along with observation of the child in the examining room, is important in establishing the diagnosis. ADHD is a clinical diagnosis with set criteria. Symptoms must be present by age 7, persist for at least 6 months, and observed in multiple environments. School performance and self-esteem often suffer. Detailed investigations and neurologic workups are generally not fruitful unless an underlying medical condition, such as seizures, is suspected. However, up to 25% of children with ADHD have a concomitant learning disability, and an educational assessment should be considered for students having trouble with school.

A combination of medical and behavioral interventions is necessary for appropriate treatment of ADHD. Stimulants (e.g., dextroamphetamine and methylphenidate), nonstimulants (e.g., atomoxetine), antidepressant medications (e.g., bupropion), and antihypertensive medications (e.g., clonidine) are the most commonly prescribed medications for ADHD. The stimulants work by increasing availability of dopamine and norepinephrine. Side effects include insomnia, increased blood pressure, loss of appetite, and nausea. Nonstimulants help when a child cannot tolerate a stimulant, if a stimulant was ineffective, or, in some, in combination with a stimulant drug to enhance effectiveness. Nevertheless, a structured environment with regular schedules is an equal, if not an even more essential, part of treatment. Over time, many symptoms improve as the neurologic system matures. However, adolescents and young adults with a childhood history of ADHD tend to have more difficulty with social interaction and depression. For such individuals, continued medical management and routine monitoring may be necessary.

LEARNING DISABILITIES

Approximately 5% to 15% of school-age children are diagnosed with learning disabilities. These problems are usually not apparent until the child enters elementary school. Screening tests, such as the Ages and Stages Questionnaire, are useful tools in the primary care setting to help identify children needing further assessment and should be used routinely. Children needing an assessment for learning disabilities merit vision and hearing testing, because sensory abnormalities can limit perception and impede learning. If those are normal, an extended neurologic examination along with an expanded neurodevelopment examination will be useful in describing the child's strengths and weaknesses. Teachers should be informed of the results of such an evaluation and should participate with the parents and physician to develop an appropriate learning environment for the child.

PARENTAL DIVORCE/DEATH OF A PARENT

As of 2014, the divorce rate in the United States was an estimated 40% of all marriages. Divorce or death of a parent is extremely stressful for a child. Young children are often not aware of problems between parents until separation occurs and one parent leaves the home, whereas older children may be aware of the tension and fighting for years before separation occurs. The departure of a parent is very disruptive to a child. In addition to the loss or decreased contact with a parent, financial consequences can add to the toll. The family may have to relocate, or stay-at-home moms need to leave the home to work, causing the child an additional loss.

A child's initial response to divorce depends mainly on his or her age. Children 2 to 5 years of age often regress, become irritable, or have trouble sleeping. The physician should encourage the stabilization of household and bedtime routines, maintaining contact with the absent parent, and encouraging the parents to reassure their children that the divorce was not their fault. Children 6 to 8 years of age often grieve openly and feel rejected. In their case, reassurance and supporting continued connection to both parents is important. At 9 to 12 years of age, children may be frightened or angry with one or both parents. The physician should be available to the children and provide opportunities to talk or vent. Adolescents likewise become angry and often depressed. For them, the physician should encourage private discussion of the situation. Children who fare better are those who are given specific details about living arrangements and daily routines after the separation, are reassured repeatedly that the divorce is not their fault, are allowed to vent their sadness and frustration, and have the support of grandparents, family, and friends.

Death of a parent at a young age is less common, but the emotional fallout for a child is as serious or worse. The surviving spouse is grieving for the loss and may be emotionally unable to address the needs of the child. If the death was sudden, the family will likely be in a state of shock. The involvement of a social worker and psychological counseling are important aspects of helping the family grieve and adjust to life without the loved one.

KEY POINTS

- Positive discipline is taught by setting boundaries while still allowing freedom of expression and exploration.

- Approximately 5% to 15% of school-aged children are diagnosed with learning disabilities.

- These problems are usually not apparent until the child enters elementary school.

- In dealing with the issue of divorce, the physician should encourage the stabilization of household and bedtime routines and maintaining contact with the absent parent.

72 | Fever in Children

Normal body temperature varies between 97°F and 99.3°F (36.1°C and 37.4°C) rectally, with a diurnal variation of lower temperatures in the mornings and higher ones in the evenings. Fever is defined as a rectal temperature greater or equal to 100.4°F (38.0°C). Most pediatric patients presenting with fever will have an identifiable source, such as a viral upper respiratory infection, otitis media, or gastroenteritis. However, the source of infection is not always obvious and fever is not always due to infection. For example, fever can also occur with malignancies and connective tissue diseases. A thorough history and physical examination is crucial in evaluating children with fever. Children without an apparent source for fever, after a comprehensive history and physical examination, warrant close monitoring or further evaluation. Since sources of fever, organisms causing infections, and host immune responses to infection vary by age, the clinical approach to fever in children also varies by age. An age-dependent approach typically groups the children into the following categories: birth to 3 months, 3 months to 3 years, and 3 years and older. A fever that persists for longer than 14 days in a child without an identifiable cause is defined as a fever of unknown origin.

PATHOGENESIS

Fever is caused by the release of endogenous pyrogenic cytokines (e.g., interleukins, tumor necrosis factor, and interferons), in response to exotoxins from gram-positive organisms, endotoxins from gram-negative organisms, endogenous immunologic stimuli (e.g., malignancy), or medications. Monocytes, macrophages, and endothelial cells are the major cell types responsible for releasing these cytokines, also known as pyrogens. These pyrogens stimulate release of prostaglandins from the central hypothalamus, which then act on the preoptic and anterior hypothalamus to increase the thermoregulatory set point. Raising this set point increases heat production and conservation, thus elevating the body temperature. Medications used to treat fever either target prostaglandin production (NSAIDs) or blunt the hypothalamic response to changes in the thermoregulatory set point (acetaminophen). Rigors or shaking chills occur when the hypothalamic set point raises rapidly. Cutaneous vasoconstriction raises the core temperature in fever, causing cold receptors in the skin to sense "cold" and cause chills; hence many patients bundle up with blankets despite having a fever. Defervescence happens when cutaneous vasodilatation occurs, which lowers the fever and can result in sweats.

CLINICAL MANIFESTATIONS

HISTORY

A detailed history remains a key element in determining the source of fever. Parents should be questioned regarding the onset of the fever, how the temperature was taken, and the height of the fever. In addition, associated symptoms—such as vomiting, diarrhea, rhinorrhea, respiratory difficulty, cough, and presence of rash—should be elicited. Inquiry into the child's behavior is an important part of the history. For example, pulling on an ear may indicate an ear infection, decrease in oral intake and number of wet diapers may indicate early dehydration, and refusal to walk may indicate a joint or extremity as a source of pain or infection. The child's activity level and oral intake help assess the severity of illness. History of travel or exposure to illness and a thorough past medical history, birth history, immunization history, and review of systems should be included.

PHYSICAL EXAMINATION

The physical examination will often direct the intensity and direction of further workup of the febrile child. Temperature, vital signs, and weight should be recorded. Temperature in infants and toddlers should be obtained rectally, whereas older children may have their temperature taken orally or in their ear canal. Tachycardia or tachypnea out of proportion to the temperature elevation suggests the presence of sepsis, dehydration, or a primary cardiac (e.g., myocarditis, pericarditis) or respiratory (e.g., pneumonia, bronchiolitis) condition.

Examination of the child should include an assessment of his or her general appearance, including alertness, irritability, and respiratory effort. Auscultation is often an initial part of the examination and can be performed while the parent is holding the child. The abdomen, skin, and extremities—including range of motion—should be examined. Testing for meningismus and palpation of the fontanelles should be performed. Finally, inspection of the ears and oropharynx is important and, usually done after other parts of the examination that require the patient to be quieter or more cooperative. A skin rash may provide clues to the cause of a fever.

DIFFERENTIAL DIAGNOSIS

The first and foremost consideration in the initial evaluation of the child with fever is an infectious etiology. The history and physical examination often determines the likely cause. For example, the parents may report a history of vomiting and diarrhea, suggesting gastroenteritis as the cause. The patient may have rhinorrhea or an erythematous, bulging tympanic membrane on physical examination, establishing the diagnosis of an URI or otitis media. However, it is not uncommon for a child to present without localizing symptoms, in which case a broader differential diagnosis must be entertained. Table 72-1 outlines the most common causes of fever in children. When the fever persists and is classified as fever of unknown origin (>14 days), additional diseases must be considered (Table 72-2).

DIAGNOSTIC EVALUATION

The approach to the child with fever varies depending on the child's age. For example, clinical assessment of infants between birth and 3 months of age cannot

TABLE 72-1. Common Causes for Pediatric Fever

Systemic Viral Infections

Fifth disease
Rubeola
Mumps
Measles
Rubella
Infectious mononucleosis

Occult Bacteremia

Respiratory Infections

Upper respiratory infections
Pharyngitis
Otitis media
Sinusitis
Bronchiolitis
Croup
Pneumonia

Gastrointestinal

Viral gastroenteritis
Bacterial gastroenteritis
Viral hepatitis

Nervous System

Viral meningitis
Bacterial meningitis
Encephalitis

Genitourinary

Pyelonephritis
Pelvic inflammatory disease

Musculoskeletal/Skin

Osteomyelitis
Septic joints
Cellulitis

reliably distinguish those with serious infections from those with less serious causes of fever. The approach to infants in this age group often involves a full septic workup, including a CBC, blood cultures, CXR, UA, urine culture, and lumbar puncture to ensure detection of serious infections.

Children between 3 months and 3 years of age are more likely to have an identifiable source of fever, and the clinical assessment is more reliable in establishing the severity of illness. Table 72-3 provides some clues that suggest a serious infection. Children without a source of their fever can be classified based on their clinical appearance (toxic vs. nontoxic) and the height of the temperature.

TABLE 72-2. Causes for Fever of Unknown Origin

Infectious

Endocarditis
Sinusitis
Abscess
Tuberculosis
Infectious mononucleosis
Viral hepatitis
Cytomegalovirus
Malaria
Rheumatic fever
AIDS

Collagen/Vascular

Juvenile rheumatoid arthritis
Lupus erythematosus
Vasculitis

Gastrointestinal

Ulcerative colitis
Crohn disease

Malignancy

Lymphoma
Leukemia
Neuroblastoma
Wilms tumor

Other

Drug-induced fever
Kawasaki syndrome
Hyperthyroidism
Environmental
Factitious

TABLE 72-3. Clues to Serious Infections in Children

Toxic appearance

Lethargy

Cyanosis

Hypotension

Respiratory distress

Tachycardia

Tachypnea

Petechial rash

Meningeal signs

Poor peripheral perfusion

Decreased urinary output

Inconsolability

Parental concerns

Toxic-appearing children need hospital admission and complete evaluation, including blood cultures, UA, urine culture, and CXR. Children with clinical signs of meningitis or those who appear seriously ill without an established diagnosis warrant lumbar puncture and empiric antibiotic coverage pending culture results. Less ill children without an identified source of fever and a temperature below 102°F (39°C) may be followed clinically as outpatients. Children with temperatures above 102°F (39°C) are at increased risk for occult bacteremia and an underlying bacterial illness, and a partial workup should be considered to help direct management. One approach to these children is to obtain a CBC. Those with WBCs greater than 15,000 merit admission, with urine and blood cultures ordered. A CXR is indicated in those with respiratory symptoms.

In children above age 3, occult bacteremia is significantly less common and clinical evaluation, including a thorough history and physical examination, can usually identify the source of fever. Since the introduction of pneumococcal vaccine, the rate of occult bacteremia has fallen to <1% in healthy, immunized infants. Clinical findings direct the laboratory evaluation in these older children.

TREATMENT

For neonates (age birth to 1 month) and ill-appearing infants 1 to 3 months of age, hospitalization and empiric antibiotic coverage are indicated to cover the most common bacterial pathogens encountered in this age group, until culture results are available. Infants 1 to 3 months of age, who appear well, have normal laboratory studies, and have a WBC between 5000 and 15,000 may be discharged with an outpatient follow-up visit in 24 hours. Empiric antibiotic coverage (e.g., ceftriaxone IM) is commonly provided pending follow-up and culture results.

Children in whom cultures are obtained should generally receive empiric antibiotic coverage until the culture results are available. Children between 3 months and 3 years of age with temperatures above 102°F (39°C) should have follow-up the next day.

KEY POINTS

- Fever is defined as rectal temperature of 100.4°F (38°C).

- Most children with fever will have a common identifiable source, such as upper respiratory infection, otitis media, or gastroenteritis.

- Important factors in evaluating febrile children without an apparent source include the age of the child, height of the fever, and appearance of the child.

- Febrile children from birth to 3 months of age warrant a laboratory evaluation including CBC, cultures, CXR, and often lumbar puncture.

- The clinical appearance of the child and height of the fever dictate the workup of febrile children from age 3 months to 3 years.

- Clinical assessment will usually identify the source of fever in children over 3 years of age.

73 | Otitis Media

The term "otitis media" encompasses four conditions: acute otitis media (AOM), recurrent otitis media (ROM), otitis media with effusion (OME), and chronic suppurative otitis media (CSOM). AOM is defined as the presence of a purulent middle ear effusion characterized by fever and ear pain. AOM is more common in the winter months, often occurring in association with a viral URI. The highest incidence of AOM occurs in children between 6 and 24 months of age. By age 2, 90% of all children in the United States have had at least one ear infection, and about 50% experience at least three episodes. Risk factors include bottle-feeding, prematurity, Native-American ethnicity, exposure to passive smoke, and day care attendance. ROM is defined as three episodes of AOM within 6 months or four episodes within 1 year, with normal examinations between infections. OME is diagnosed when there are no signs and symptoms of infection, but the physical examination reveals fluid behind the tympanic membrane (TM). AOM often precedes OME. OME is generally asymptomatic, but may manifest as hearing loss. CSOM is characterized by chronic middle ear mucosal inflammation with TM perforation and persistent otorrhea (discharge persisting for a minimum of 2 to 6 weeks).

PATHOGENESIS

For anatomic reasons, children <2 years of age are more likely to develop OM. The eustachian tube in these children is shorter and is more horizontal than in adults, allowing easier passage of bacteria from the nasopharynx into the middle ear. Furthermore, the canal of the eustachian tube is narrower and more prone to occlusion by the surrounding adenoids and lymphoid follicles. Even mild URIs can cause the lymphoid tissue to enlarge and obstruct the drainage of fluid from the middle ear. URIs also damage the ciliated epithelium of the eustachian tube, which increases the likelihood of bacteria adhering to the mucosa predisposing the individual to a superimposed bacterial infection. Ear pain results from increasing pressure due to fluid accumulation and inflammation.

The most common bacteria associated with otitis media are *Streptococcus pneumoniae*, *Haemophilus influenzae*, and *Moraxella catarrhalis*. About 30% of cases of AOM are due to viruses such as respiratory syncytial virus (RSV), parainfluenza, and rhinovirus. AOM is often followed by OME, which usually resolves over 4 to 12 weeks. OME that is persistent or interferes with normal hearing requires evaluation and treatment.

CLINICAL MANIFESTATIONS

HISTORY

The presenting complaint of AOM varies depending on the age of the child. Ear pain is the most common complaint in children old enough to complain of pain. Younger children may present with irritability, sleep disturbances, fever, excessive crying, or a history of pulling on the affected ear. Otitis media may also cause nausea, vomiting, and diarrhea. Older children may complain of hearing loss; in younger children, this may manifest itself as inattention, loss of balance, dizziness, or tinnitus. However, clinical history alone is poorly predictive of the presence of AOM, especially in younger children.

PHYSICAL EXAMINATION

AOM is usually associated with a URI. The examination of the ear should focus on the color and appearance of the TM and the presence of pus or air bubbles behind the TM. The affected TM may be dull or erythematous, and in cases of AOM maybe

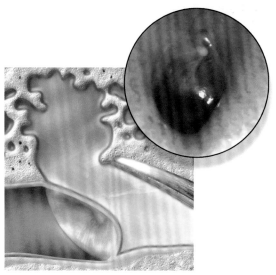

FIGURE 73-1. Serous otitis with effusion. (From Anatomical Chart Company. *Middle Ear Conditions Anatomical Chart*. Alphen aan den Rijn, The Netherlands: Wolters Kluwer; 2009.).

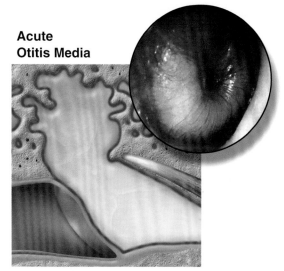

Acute Otitis Media

Infected fluid in the middle ear, of rapid onset and short duration.

FIGURE 73-2. Acute otitis media. (From Anatomical Chart Company. *Middle Ear Conditions Anatomical Chart*. Alphen aan den Rijn, The Netherlands: Wolters Kluwer; 2009.)

bulging or retracted (Fig. 73-2). The TM can perforate with AOM and cause an otorrhea that obscures the TM. Decreased mobility of the TM, assessed with a pneumatic otoscope, can be seen in both AOM and OME. In OME, there is no fever or other sign of infection, and the TM may appear dull or normal, but not erythematous (Fig. 73-1). Children with CSOM will have otorrhea, which may be foul-smelling. They are also likely to have hearing loss, and examination of the TM usually demonstrates a perforation.

DIFFERENTIAL DIAGNOSIS

Vigorous crying may cause a reddened TM and result in an abnormal examination. Infectious causes of a hyperemic TM include AOM, ROM, or CSOM. Other causes of ear pain may include otitis externa, TMJ dysfunction, and pain referred from pharyngitis or a dental source.

DIAGNOSTIC EVALUATION

The diagnosis of OM is based on the history and physical examination, and rarely requires laboratory studies. However, if the child is <6 weeks old and has a fever, a full sepsis workup is indicated. If symptoms persist despite the use of different antibiotics, tympanostomy to obtain fluid for culture and sensitivity may be needed to direct antibiotic therapy.

It is also important to differentiate otitis externa from OM. In otitis externa, the ear canal may appear red, with purulent material in the canal, and is tender to touch. The ear canal is neither erythematous nor tender to the touch with AOM. OME is diagnosed when there are no signs of infection, but pneumatic otoscopy shows TM immobility indicating fluid behind the TM. Tympanometry can help confirm the presence of fluid in the middle ear with both AOM and OME. In children with OME, a hearing evaluation may be warranted to document the impact of the fluid on the child's hearing. A chronic history of ear discharge along with the physical finding of perforated TM with visible discharge suggests the presence of CSOM.

TREATMENT

Many infections of the middle ear resolve spontaneously, requiring observation and supportive care only. The decision to prescribe antibiotics depends on the child's age, the certainty of the diagnosis, and the severity of illness (Table 73-1). The goals of treatment are to prevent recurrent infections that can lead to chronic otitis media and persistent OME. Persistent OME may affect a child's hearing and thus language development.

Antibiotic therapy is recommended for children <6 months of age and those with moderate or severe otalgia, otalgia for >48 hours, temperature >39°C (102.2°F), and those with bilateral AOM who are <2 years of age. Either antibiotic treatment or observation with

TABLE 73-1. Therapy for Otitis Media			
Antibiotics indicated	Otorrhea; toxic appearance; temperature >39°C; pain > 48 hours; age < 6 months; bilateral disease < 2 years of age; uncertain follow-up	First line: Amoxicillin; amoxicillin-clavulanic acid	Alternative: Ceftriaxone; cefdinir; cefuroxime; cefpodoxime/clindamycin
Option of observation	Unilateral disease > 6 months of age without otorrhea; bilateral disease > 2 years of age without otorrhea		

close follow-up can be recommended for children over 6 months of age with unilateral AOM without otorrhea or severe signs/symptoms, OR children older than 24 months with unilateral or bilateral AOM without otorrhea or severe signs/symptoms.

Children <6 months of age are at a higher risk of developing serious infectious complications like meningitis or sepsis, making them appropriate candidate for antibiotic therapy for AOM. Children above 6 months of age may be treated more conservatively as long as follow-up with the clinician is reliable. For less severely ill children, observation for 48 to 72 hours will give the child a chance to improve on his or her own. If symptoms worsen or do not improve after 48 to 72 hours, the drug of choice is amoxicillin (80 to 90 mg/kg/day) for 10 days. For patients who have taken amoxicillin within the past month, who have had repeated courses of antibiotics, or who are penicillin allergic, alternative antibiotics must be selected. A clinical sign of Haemophilus infection, which has high rates of penicillinase production, is a concomitant purulent conjunctivitis. These patients should also receive either high-dose amoxicillin-clavulanic acid or a cephalosporin with *H. influenzae* activity (e.g.,

cefdinir, cefuroxime, cefpodoxime). Ceftriaxone intramuscularly or intravenously is an alternative in children who cannot take or keep down oral medicines. Children with persistent symptoms despite multiple courses of antibiotics merit tympanocentesis with culture and sensitivity testing. Also, immunocompromised children may require a tympanocentesis before starting antibiotics.

Supportive therapy including antipyretics (acetaminophen or ibuprofen), topical anesthetic drops (Benzocaine), and local heat may help relieve pain. Parents should be advised not to expose children to passive smoking and to avoid supine bottle-feeding.

Patients with ROM may benefit from prophylactic antibiotics, such as amoxicillin 20 mg/kg at bedtime for 6 months or sulfisoxazole in penicillin-allergic patients. If this fails, the child should be referred to an otolaryngologist for possible tympanostomy tube placement. Children with OME that persists for more than 4 to 6 months despite antibiotic therapy may benefit from myringotomy and tympanostomy tube placement. If there is significant hearing loss, tympanostomy may be performed earlier.

KEY POINTS

- AOM is diagnosed when there is a rapid onset of symptoms, middle ear effusion, and a hyperemic TM with decreased mobility.

- ROM is defined as three episodes within 6 months or four or more episodes within a year.

- The most common bacterial pathogens are *S. pneumoniae*, *H. influenzae*, and *M. catarrhalis*.

- The drug of choice is amoxicillin (80 to 90 mg/kg/day), unless infection with a resistant organism is suspected or the child is allergic to penicillin.

- Myringotomy and tympanostomy tube placement are indicated for recurrent infections despite antibiotic prophylaxis or for persistent effusion associated with hearing loss.

74 | Preparticipation Evaluation

Over 30 million children participate in organized sports, and many more adults and children participate in unorganized sporting activities. Sports promote physical fitness, provide opportunities for psychosocial growth, promote self-confidence, and foster healthful lifetime habits and hobbies. The physician's role in sporting activities is to provide preparticipation health examinations (PPEs), counseling regarding appropriate participation, and care for injuries and illnesses. The purpose of the PPE is to identify medical conditions that may interfere with athletic performance, as well as possible life-threatening conditions that may prevent an athlete from safely participating in his or her sport. The PPE also gives the physician a chance to evaluate healthy individuals who may not otherwise seek medical care, thus providing an opportunity to assess an athlete's general health and offer counsel about preventive issues such as tobacco avoidance and safe sex practices. A recent emphasis is the PPE's role in identifying athletes at risk for sudden cardiac death defined as a nontraumatic, nonviolent, unexpected event resulting in sudden cardiac arrest within 6 hours of a previously witnessed state of normal health. The estimated incidence of sudden cardiac death among high school and college athletes is 1 in 200,000, with only about 50 such deaths occurring annually in the United States. Although sudden cardiac death occurs infrequently, it can devastate the community, family, and medical personnel associated with such an event.

PATHOGENESIS

Physicians generally recommend that individuals participate in some form of physical exercise. However, physical exertion stresses the body and can exacerbate an underlying medical condition and place the participating individual at risk for harm. For example, the risk of injury to a solitary kidney or enlarged spleen may preclude such an individual from participating in contact sports. The presence of CAD or asymmetric hypertrophic cardiomyopathy may prevent any sports participation until completing further evaluation or initiating therapy. In determining an athlete's risk for sports participation, the physician must decide which types of activities may be appropriate for that individual.

Dynamic activity is highly aerobic and includes activities such as running, cross-country skiing, and swimming. These athletes must maintain an elevated cardiac output for an extended period of time, which leads to an increase in the thickness of the left ventricular wall and the volume of the left ventricle. Athletes who regularly engage in dynamic activity often have an increase in baseline vagal tone and may have resting pulses as low as 30 beats/minute.

Static or isometric exercise includes activities such as weight lifting. This type of exercise involves a tremendous but brief increase in cardiac output against elevated peripheral resistance. Athletes who frequently engage in isometric exercise develop symmetric left ventricular thickening, in contrast to asymmetric thickening, which indicates possible pathology. Activities are then sorted by the level of dynamic and static activities (e.g., billiards is low dynamic and low static; football is high dynamic and high static).

In addition, activities may also be categorized according to type of interaction with other athletes. For example, football, lacrosse, and rugby are examples of collision sports, whereas contact sports include soccer, basketball, wrestling, and others. Noncontact sports typically include tennis, track, golf, and swimming.

In adults over the age of 40 and in those with a family history of heart disease, CAD is the most common cause of sudden cardiac death. In association with physical exertion, individuals with CAD are vulnerable to MI or ischemia resulting from atherosclerotic plaque rupture. Hypertrophic cardiomyopathy is the most common cause of sudden death in athletes below 35 years of age, accounting for roughly 40% of cases. Hypertrophic cardiomyopathy is an autosomal dominant trait with variable expression; thus, not everyone with the gene expresses the trait. Mutations of the beta cardiac heavy myosin chain result in asymmetric thickening of the left ventricular wall, which, with significant physical exertion, predisposes individuals to arrhythmias.

CLINICAL MANIFESTATIONS

HISTORY

The history can identify many athletes at risk for sudden cardiac death, as well as those with medical conditions that might place them at an increased risk when participating in athletics. The patient's age, complete past medical history including previous surgeries and injuries, medications, history of a heart murmur or rheumatic fever, and previous athletic experience should be documented. Patients should be asked specifically about episodes of chest tightness, chest pain, palpitations, shortness of breath with little or no exertion, light-headedness, head trauma/concussions, seizures, and syncope. Family history of sudden cardiac death before the age of 40, cardiomyopathy, Marfan syndrome, and prolonged QT syndrome should be assessed. In women, menstrual history is important. Female athletes should be asked about regularity of menses, and in those with amenorrhea or oligomenorrhea, inquiry into eating habits and weight loss should be pursued. The use of illicit drugs such as cocaine and anabolic steroids should also be asked about.

PHYSICAL EXAMINATION

The patient's vital signs, height, and weight should be reviewed. General inspection should observe for body habitus consistent with Marfan syndrome (usually marked by greater than normal height, arm span greater than height, pectus excavatum, myopia, and displaced lenses). BP should be checked; if it is elevated, serial measurements should be taken to assess for HTN. Funduscopic examination is indicated in those with HTN. Cardiovascular assessment includes

femoral and radial pulses to screen for coarctation of the aorta. Careful cardiac auscultation is important to detect murmurs, and, if present, how they change with respiration and in the standing and sitting positions should be noted. Benign flow murmurs may increase with lying down or squatting, but typically diminish or do not change with the Valsalva maneuver or upon standing. Murmurs associated with asymmetric hypertrophic cardiomyopathy will decrease in the supine or squatting positions and increase with Valsalva and standing. Any extra heart sounds or clicks should be documented. The abdominal examination should note surgical scars and the presence of hepatomegaly or splenomegaly. The male genital examination should note developmental state, bilateral descent of the testicles, and the presence of an inguinal hernia.

The musculoskeletal examination is another area of importance. Assessment of the neck, spine, shoulders, elbows, wrists, fingers, hips, knees, ankles, and feet for ROM and stability should be performed. Asymmetry should be noted and, if present, lead to a more focused examination. The spine should be examined for kyphoscoliosis. Upper extremity strength should be assessed by testing the different muscle groups; duck walking while squatting down can be performed to assess the lower extremities.

DIAGNOSTIC EVALUATION

The history and physical examination are sufficient evaluation for most people who undergo sports PPEs. Routine screening ECGs and echocardiograms are not cost-effective interventions because of the low incidence of cardiac abnormalities in this group.

In patients with suspected hypertrophic cardiomyopathy, a CXR, ECG, and echocardiogram are indicated. In patients with a history of syncope and no murmurs on physical examination, an event monitor or 24-hour Holter may help in addition to the ECG and echocardiogram. A stress test is useful for older patients who complain of chest pain with exertion or those with significant risk factors for heart disease. Radiographs are not routinely indicated, but may be indicated in patients with joint complaints or findings. Cervical radiographs can help detect cervical instability in those with Down syndrome. Laboratory evaluation may be useful in patients with ongoing medical conditions, such as hepatitis or diabetes, but is seldom indicated otherwise.

TREATMENT

Most athletes seen in PPEs are cleared to play. In deciding not to allow an athlete to participate, the rationale for exclusion must be thoroughly discussed with the athlete, family, coaching staff, and other medical staff, with the emphasis on the activities in which the athlete can participate.

Athletes with active contagious infections should be excluded from all sports until their infections resolve. Participants with skin lesions such as tinea corporis, impetigo, or herpes simplex should not participate in contact sports. Individuals with joint injuries should rehabilitate the joint prior to returning to participation. Individuals with medical conditions such as recent concussion or splenomegaly should avoid sports that may involve collision contact. Patients with Down syndrome should not participate in collision sports, and those with cervical instability should avoid specific sports that may cause excessive motion at the cervical spine (e.g., gymnastics).

In athletes with an active medical illness such as uncontrolled diabetes or asthma, appropriate tests and treatment are recommended before allowing participation. In patients with certain congenital or acquired conditions, referral to the appropriate specialist (e.g., nephrologist with solitary kidney, neurologist with seizure disorder) may assist in providing additional counseling regarding all the risks associated with participating in athletics. In patients with HTN, diet, lifestyle modification, and possibly medications to lower BP may be warranted before allowing participation. Certain antihypertensive medications are banned by the National Collegiate Athletic Association (NCAA) and U.S. Olympic Committee, which is important to keep in mind for evaluating high-level athletes.

Finally, people with a worrisome past medical history, significant family history, or an abnormality on cardiovascular examination or testing, may warrant cardiology consultation to provide additional information regarding safe sports participation.

KEY POINTS

- The purpose of the PPE is to identify (a) medical conditions that may interfere with athletic performance and (b) possible life-threatening conditions that may prevent an athlete from participating in his or her sport safely.

- The history and physical examination are sufficient evaluation for most of those who undergo sports PPEs.

- In patients with suspected hypertrophic cardiomyopathy, a CXR, ECG, and echocardiogram are indicated.

- In deciding to not allow an athlete to participate, the rationale for exclusion must be thoroughly discussed with the athlete, family, coaching staff, and other medical staff; emphasis should be placed on the activities in which the athlete *can* participate.

CLINICAL VIGNETTES

VIGNETTE 1

A 3-week-old infant presents with a temperature of 101°F. The child has not been feeding quite as well but has no other focal findings reported by the parents. He has been having normal amounts of urine and stool and has thus far gained weight appropriately.

1. Appropriate management would now include which of the following?
   a. Observation
   b. Follow-up in the office in 24 hours for recheck
   c. Oral antibiotics and follow-up in 1 week
   d. Urine and blood culture with IM antibiotics and follow-up in 2 days
   e. Inpatient sepsis workup and intravenous antibiotics

VIGNETTE 2

A 2-year-old male presents with an URI and temperature to 100.8°F. He has rhinorrhea but is in no respiratory distress. He is active and eating normally. On examination, he has an erythematous tympanic membrane on the left, rhinorrhea, and clear lungs and skin.

   1. Management for this child would include which of the following?
     a. No antibiotic therapy
     b. Amoxicillin
     c. Ceftriaxone
     d. Azithromycin

VIGNETTE 3

A 16-year-old female presents for a well-child visit with no complaints. She is current on immunizations and denies smoking, substance use, or sexual activity.

   1. Which of the following is indicated as a screening test for this patient?
     a. Pap smear
     b. Scoliosis screen
     c. Lipid panel
     d. Blood pressure
     e. Depression scale

ANSWERS

VIGNETTE 1 Question 1

1. Answer E:

The source of infection is often less apparent in neonates (birth to 1 month of age) and in those <3 months of age. In older children, the source of infection is generally more apparent, and usually can be determined based on history and/or physical examination findings.

    Thus, for neonates and ill-appearing infants 1 to 3 months of age, hospitalization and empiric antibiotic coverage are indicated to cover the most common bacterial pathogens encountered in this age group, until culture results are available. Infants 1 to 3 months of age, who appear well, have normal laboratory studies, and have a WBC between 5000 and 15,000, may be discharged with an outpatient follow-up visit in 24 hours. Empiric antibiotic coverage (e.g., ceftriaxone IM) is commonly provided pending follow-up and culture results.

    Children in whom cultures are obtained should generally receive empiric antibiotic coverage until the culture results are available. Children between 3 months and 3 years of age with temperatures above 102°F (39°C) should have follow-up the next day.

VIGNETTE 2 Question 1

1. Answer A:

Indications for antibiotic therapy for acute otitis media in guidelines published by the American Academy of Pediatrics include the following: presence of otorrhea, toxic appearance of the child, temperature >39°C (102°F), pain >48 hours, age <6 months, bilateral disease in a child <2 years of age, and uncertain follow-up. The option of observation can be provided to select groups of children and include the following: unilateral disease in a child >6 months of age without otorrhea and bilateral disease in a child >2 years of age without otorrhea; in both instances, this assumes a temperature less than 39°C, a nontoxic appearance, and pain <48 hours.

VIGNETTE 3 Question 1

1. Answer E:

The USPSTF recommends screening adolescents for depression if there are systems in place to provide further assessment and therapy. Screening could be provided with use of one of several screening scales. There is indeterminate evidence to support or refute testing for lipids or BP as screening tests for adolescents. The USPSTF recommends against providing screening Pap smears or scoliosis screening in this age group.

75 | Preventive Care: 65 Years and Older

A loss of independence is not an inevitable consequence of aging. Routine health assessments of older adults can identify and treat potential problems before they significantly affect function. Life expectancy has increased over the past century and the number of adults living active lives into their 80s and 90s has also increased. The average life expectancy in the United States is 76 years for men and 81 years for women. However, a 75-year-old can expect to live past his or her mid-80s, although the expected life span of older patients with significant underlying medical conditions—such as severe COPD, cancer, or heart disease—may be considerably less. Preventive strategies should be tailored to an individual's health status and his or her personal preferences. For example, many patients in their 80s and 90s may consider undergoing aggressive treatments, such as major abdominal or heart surgery, but others may refuse screenings for diseases that would require intensive treatment. Involving patients and their families in decisions about the overall approach to the patient's care can help guide physicians to personalize the approach to an older patient.

The most common causes of morbidity and mortality in the adult over age 65 are cardiovascular disease, cerebrovascular disease, cancers, and lung disease. Cardiovascular disease is the leading cause of death in the United States and is more prevalent with increasing age. Many types of cancer are also more prevalent in older populations. COPD is primarily a smoking-related disease with significant morbidity and mortality among the elderly. Pulmonary infections in older adults have a higher morbidity and mortality rate than in younger individuals.

CLINICAL CONSIDERATIONS

HISTORY

Most physicians recommend annual preventive care visits for older patients. Screening guidelines are presented in Table 75-1. In addition to preventive issues common to all age groups, the visits should focus on functional issues. Inquiries into exercise should be made. Routine exercise recommendations consist of aerobic activity five times per week for 30 minutes, but may need modification for an older, frailer adult. Weight training or resistance exercises are important to maintain strength. Stretching and flexibility activities should be done prior to and after exercise. Balance training (Tai Chi or yoga) also improves a patient's flexibility, and research indicates that balance exercises combined with strength training prevent frequent falls.

Substance abuse is a common problem among geriatric patients, and the prevalence is underestimated because of age bias. About 10% of patients over age 65 have problems with alcohol. The CAGE questionnaire screens for alcohol abuse. A positive screen indicates the need to provide counseling and possibly a referral. Regular ongoing counseling to stop smoking is important, because patients benefit from smoking cessation even after years of smoking. Counseling and close follow-up combined with pharmacotherapy increase quit rates.

Regular medication reconciliation for drug completeness, efficacy, and adherence is a key part of preventive care. Although the elderly comprise 13% of the population, they receive about one-third of dispensed medications. Each year, older adults take an estimated 17 to 20 drugs. Age-related physiologic changes and drug interactions make the elderly adult more susceptible to an adverse drug reaction. Paying careful attention to specific drugs that have a high-risk profile, such as psychotropic, analgesic, antidiabetic, anticholinergic, anticoagulant, NSAIDs, antihypertensive, and heart medications, helps avoid drug-related problems.

Discussion concerning advanced directives should be noted and documents such as an up-to-date living will placed in the chart. Evaluation for depression, cognition, and assessing psychosocial support systems are important, because these all may influence advance directives.

Falls are the most common cause of injury-related death and hospitalization. An environmental assessment and education are elements of fall prevention. Walkways at home should be uncluttered, well lit, and free of throw rugs. Reinforcement of healthy behavioral measures should also be incorporated into the visit. These discussions can include topics such as seat belt use, bicycle helmet use, firearms and water safety, smoke detectors, and training in cardiopulmonary resuscitation (CPR) for household members.

The driving ability of older adults, especially the frail elderly, needs review. Visual problems, hearing difficulty, and cognitive impairment occur more frequently in the geriatric population and may compromise driving ability. If there are concerns about driving safety, referral for testing may be warranted.

PHYSICAL EXAMINATION AND TESTING

The USPTFS recommends checking BP annually to screen for HTN. Treating HTN provides substantial benefit in the elderly, reducing the incidence of strokes and cardiovascular events. When initiating antihypertensive medication, monitoring BP both at home and in the office helps ensure that treatment achieves BP targets. Monitoring orthostatic BP, renal function, and electrolyte imbalances minimizes side effects.

Adequate nutrition is essential in the geriatric population who are at greater risk for being either malnourished or obese than younger adults. Measuring height and weight along with a dietary history can identify obesity and malnutrition. An involuntary weight loss of 10% or more per year should trigger an assessment of possible medical or medication-related causes. The physician should investigate the patient's appetite, caloric intake, swallowing ability, dietary restrictions, and use of nutritional supplements. Counseling to promote a healthy diet, including appropriate amounts of calories, fat, vitamins, and fiber, is important. The dietary calcium of many older

individuals is insufficient; many experts recommend supplemental calcium and 800 international units of vitamin D.

Most experts recommend screening vision and hearing annually. The whisper test and simple screening questions such as "Do you have trouble hearing?" can identify hearing problems. Patients who fail a hearing screen can be referred for more formal audiometric testing. Visual loss is associated with cognitive decline, functional impairment, and falls.

Although the USPSTF concludes that the current evidence is insufficient to support screening for cognitive impairment, many experts recommend a Mini-Cog screening test to assess cognitive function. Additional history from family members can supplement the patient history, because some individuals may be unaware of memory or depressive issues. A Folstein Mini-Mental State Exam helps assess patients with complaints of memory loss or individuals with new functional impairments.

Depression is common in the elderly population, and men over age 65 have among the highest rate of completed suicide attempts. Two basic questions screen for depression: (1) During the past month, have you been bothered by feeling down, depressed, or hopeless? (2) During the past month, have you often been bothered by having little interest or pleasure in doing things? A positive response to either question can be followed with a more formal depression evaluation using the PHQ-9 depression survey.

If the patient's history indicates a risk for falls, gait, and balance the "Get Up and Go Test" (see Fig. 76-1) tests balance and gait. If the patient uses an assistive device to ambulate, the provider can check to ensure the device is set at the correct height and that the assistive device is appropriate for the patient's impairment. Physical therapy can reduce the incidence of falls.

Lipid screening and treatment is recommended for patients whose CAD risk exceeds 10% over 10 years. Low-dose aspirin reduces cardiovascular morbidity and mortality, and its benefits outweigh the risks for individual at high risk for CAD. Anticoagulation for elderly patients with atrial fibrillation reduces the risk of strokes, and the benefits of anticoagulation outweigh the risks for most patients with atrial fibrillation. Diabetic screening is indicated in patients with a BMI greater than 25 kg/m^2, or in those who have coexisting hypertension or hyperlipidemia. The incidence of hypothyroidism in women increases after age 65, and many guidelines recommend TSH testing annually. PSA testing recommendations are controversial and options for testing should be

TABLE 75-1. Screening Guidelines for Geriatric Patients

History:	
Incontinence	Type, therapy, prior evaluation
Falls/fall risk	Fractures; assistive devices; exercise; vitamin D
Social supports	Financial and, if needed, caregiving
Alcohol/substance use	Quantity and screen for dependence
Smoking status	Current/former
Advanced directives	Resuscitation and care preferences; power of attorney for finances and healthcare
Medications:	
Review current medications	Reference Beer's criteria
Aspirin	Low-dose aspirin for men aged 45–79 at risk for myocardial infarction and women aged 55–79 at risk for ischemic stroke
Vitamin D/calcium	Diet plus supplement of 800 IU/1200 mg or more
Immunizations:	
Pneumonia	13-Valent at age 65 followed in 1 year by 23-valent for average-risk persons
Influenza	Annual
Tetanus	Tdap once in place of every 10 years Td
Shingles	After age 50 years
Examination:	
Vision	Snellen chart
Hearing	Screen with whisper test or screening questions
Mental Status	Mini-Cog and/or Mini-Mental State Exam testing
Depression	PHQ-9
Gait	Get Up and Go test
Testing:	
Lipid profile	Helps assess cardiovascular risk status
Glucose/hemoglobin A_{1c}	Diabetes screen
Mammogram	Biennial after age 50–75 years
Pap smear	Every 5 years with HPV testing and stopping at age 65 years if prior results normal past 10 years
Colon cancer screen	Beginning at age 50, colonoscopy every 10 years, if normal; stopping at age 75
	Recommended until age 75 or a life expectancy <10 years
Chest CT scan	Annual for ages 55–80 with 30-pack year history and quit within past 15 years
DEXA scan	Women age 65 years and older; repeat testing uncertain
AAA screen	Men over age 65 who have ever smoked (one time)

DEXA, dual-energy x-ray absorptiometry; HPV, human papillomavirus; PHQ-9, Patient Health Questionnaire-9.

discussed and individualized. Most guidelines recommend against PSA testing in individuals over age 75 or with a life expectancy <10 years.

The USPSTF recommends one-time ultrasound screening for abdominal aortic aneurysm in men between the ages of 65 and 79 years old who have ever smoked. The USPSTF recommends selective screening for men, who have never smoked, based on additional risk factors for abdominal aortic aneurysm. The USPSTF does not recommend aortic aneurysm screening for women.

Bone density screening for osteoporosis begins at age 65 for women. Consider screening men with a history of a previous fracture, loss of height, hyperthyroidism, or for men taking androgen deprivation medication. Incontinence screening is appropriate for older adults because of increased prevalence, and begins with the simple question, "During the last 3 months, have you leaked urine, even a small amount?" The at-risk patient population includes older women and those with immobility, impaired cognition, depression, certain medication usage (e.g., diuretics and anticholinergics), stool impaction, environmental barriers, diabetes, and estrogen depletion. An evaluation should begin with a history to assess the type of incontinence (stress, urge, or overflow) and a medication review, followed by a genitourinary examination, and urine analysis.

CANCER SCREENING

Cancer screening continues to be a major focus of health screening in the geriatric population, although tempered to some degree by the presence of comorbid disease, a patient's life expectancy, potential procedural complications, the patient's past screening history, and the patient's preferences regarding continued screening.

Cancer screening in women includes Pap smears and mammograms. ACOG recommends discontinuing Pap smears at or after the age of 65 in women with a history of three consecutive normal Pap smears within a 10-year period. Cervical cancer screening may be discontinued earlier after hysterectomy for benign indications. The incidence of breast cancer increases with age. However, most breast cancers diagnosed after the age of 75 are localized and can be cured with less radical surgery. As long as a woman's life expectancy is at least 10 years, yearly mammography screening should be continued.

The USPSTF recommends annual low-dose CT (LDCT) scanning of the chest to screen for lung cancer between 55 and 80 years of age for individuals with a 30 pack-year history of smoking, who continue to smoke or have quit within the past 15 years. Screening may be stopped if more than 15 years have elapsed since the patient stopped smoking. Individuals with a limited life expectancy or those who are not candidates for surgery to evaluate abnormal LDCT findings do not need screening.

Colorectal cancer screening options include annual fecal occult blood testing, flexible sigmoidoscopy screening every 5 years with stool for occult blood, or colonoscopy screening every 10 years. Screening intervals may shorten depending on results. The USPSTF recommends that in average-risk individuals colon cancer screening begin at age 50 and stop at age 75 or if life expectancy is <10 years. Colon cancer screening between the ages of 75 and 85 may be considered if the patient has never been screened and has no significant comorbidities.

IMMUNIZATIONS

Tetanus immunization (dT) needs updating every 10 years with Tdap substituting for one of these as an adult. All patients over 65 years of age should receive PCV13 followed by PPSV23 1 year later. Individuals over age 65 are among those who benefit the most from annual influenza vaccination. TB screening is routinely recommended for patients residing in long-term-care facilities and others at high risk. If previously unimmunized, patients at risk because of travel can be given hepatitis A or B vaccines. The CDC recommendeds a recombinent vaccine to prevent shingles (Shingrix) be given at age 50 or older in two doses separated by two to six months. This appears to be more effective than the older vaccine and should be offered to those previously vaccinated.

KEY POINTS

- The most common causes of death in adults over age 65 are cardiovascular disease and cancer.
- In addition to recommendations common to all age groups, increasing focus in geriatric preventive care on functional issues and future care should be incorporated into the visits.

- Substance abuse and depression are common problems among geriatric patients.
- Along with assessment of vision and gait, an environmental assessment and education of the family should be included to help with the prevention of falls.

76 | Geriatric Assessment

Geriatric assessment is a multidisciplinary approach to the evaluation of an older individual's physical limitations, psychosocial impairments, and functional disabilities. Geriatric assessment uses a team approach that recognizes the complex medical and social problems facing many elderly individuals, and requires sensitivity to their concerns and an awareness of the many unique aspects of their medical problems. Besides the physician, the evaluation team often includes a social worker, nutritionist, nurse coordinator, and physical and occupational therapists.

In the elderly, quality of life and maintaining function are critically important. Although disease in general is more common in older adults, treating an illness should not reflexively be dismissed because of age. Although diseases should be diagnosed and assessed, maintenance or restoration of function may be more important than curative treatment. Treating an illness always requires a detailed analysis of risk versus benefits.

FUNCTIONAL ASSESSMENT

Functional assessment measures an individual's ability to manage everyday life. Typically these assessments focus on an individual's ability to provide self-care, known as activities of daily living (ADLs) and instrumental activities of daily living (IADLs) (Table 76-1). ADLs include daily self-care activities, such as dressing, eating, bathing, ambulating, and maintaining bladder and bowel function. IADLs assess the ability to function independently by evaluating higher level functions, such as managing bill payments, using a phone, taking medications correctly, cleaning one's home, and preparing meals.

Geriatric assessment is important because of the high prevalence of disability among the elderly. In practice, a geriatric assessment involves assessment

TABLE 76-1. Activities of Daily Living and Instrumental Activities of Daily Living

Activities of Daily Living
Bathing
Dressing
Grooming
Eating
Toileting
Transferring

Instrumental Activities of Daily Living
Housekeeping
Preparing meals
Using the telephone
Shopping
Managing one's transportation
Managing finances
Taking medications

and developing recommendations as well as plans for implementation. Measurement tools are often used as part of the assessment. Mobility is an important consideration, and observing the patient provides invaluable insight. Watching whether the patient can get up easily from a chair, walk steadily, turn around, walk back, and sit down provides significant information about functional status (Timed Up and Go test, Fig. 76-1). Fall risk can be decreased with physical therapy and vitamin D supplementation.

A geriatric assessment includes an evaluation of which ancillary support services and disciplines might benefit the patient. For example, occupational therapy might make specific recommendations about environmental modifications to enhance safety and functional ability, and speech pathology might help someone with difficulty swallowing. Finally, the functional assessment should include a discussion of the patient's preferences and expectations, combined

Purpose: To assess mobility.

Equipment: A stopwatch.

Directions: Patients wear their regular footwear and can use a walking aid if needed. Begin by having the patient sit back in a standard arm chair and identify a line 3 meters or 10 feet away on the floor.

Instructions to the patient: When I say **"Go,"** I want you to:

1. Stand up from the chair

2. Walk to the line on the floor at your normal pace

3. Turn

4. Walk back to the chair at your normal pace

5. Sit down again.

On the word **"Go,"** begin timing. Stop timing after the patient has sat back down and record time.

Time: _____ seconds

An older adult who takes 12 seconds to complete the TUG is at high risk for falling.

Observe the patient's postural stability, gait, stride length, and sway.

Circle all that apply:

Slow tentative pace	Steadying self on walls
Loss of balance	Shuffling
Short strides	En bloc turning
Little or no arm swing	Not using assistive device properly

FIGURE 76-1. The Timed Up and Go (TUG) test. (For relevant articles, go to Centers for Disease Control and Prevention National Center for Injury Prevention and Control. www.cdc.gov/steadi.)

with the family's expectations and willingness to provide care. It is of paramount importance that the patient's preferences receive the highest priority and to recognize that these may be in conflict with those of the family. Unrealistic expectations, inability to provide support, or reluctance of the family to help can doom a care plan to failure. A home visit often provides additional information about issues discovered during an office evaluation or to clarify conflicting information from the patient and family members.

HISTORY

Several common problems can make history taking more challenging in the elderly. Impaired hearing and vision are common and can interfere with effective communication. Eliminating extraneous noise, facing the patient, speaking slowly in deep tones, and providing good lighting can help.

Many elderly patients ignore symptoms because of their cultural backgrounds or because they may believe their symptoms are a normal concomitant of aging. Fear of illness may lead to denial and underreporting of symptoms. Altered responses to illness are common and can lead to vague or absent symptoms (e.g., a painless MI). Impaired memory or cognitive function can also work against obtaining an accurate history.

At the other end of the spectrum are those elderly patients with multiple complaints. Sorting through multiple symptoms and getting to know the patient may take time. By being alert to new or changing symptoms, the physician will be better able to detect potentially treatable conditions and avoid overlooking important issues.

The past medical history should include previous surgeries, major illnesses, and hospitalizations. As a rule, surgeries or illnesses occurring within the previous 5 years are more relevant than remote events such as childhood illnesses. Immunization status and a review of past results of TB testing are also important but frequently overlooked. Treatment of diabetes, hypertension, and CAD reduces the risk of future disability. Cancer screening may allow for early detection and curable situations. Inquiring about markers of frailty (see Table 76-2) is important, and helps identify those at an increased risk for functional limitations, hospitalization, and death. These patients commonly benefit from coordination of care and expertise across disciplines.

Of paramount importance is reviewing all medications, including prescription, over the counter, supplements, and herbal medications. Elderly patients are more vulnerable to side effects, and nonprescription medications can cause significant side effects that may be overlooked unless specifically asked about. The "brown bag" technique, where the patient collects all his or her medications in a paper bag and brings them to the office, can be useful. It is also important to assess patients' knowledge of their medication regimes and their adherence to them.

Additional historic information should include evaluation of nutrition and weight loss, vision, hearing, incontinence issues, balance, recent falls, osteoporosis, and medical treatments of diseases.

PHYSICAL EXAMINATION

The complete physical examination is similar to that performed on younger individuals, with some special emphasis on physical performance and mental status. Successful function requires intact cognitive skills, and a Mini-Cog or a Mini-Mental State examination is useful to screen for cognitive impairment. Formal cognitive testing may help if a patient appears to be impaired despite a normal screening examination. The patient's general appearance and grooming provide clues to functional problems, and poor hygiene may indicate a need for intervention.

Blood pressure should routinely be checked, both sitting and standing, because elderly individuals often have significant orthostatic changes that contribute to falls. It is not uncommon for the elderly to have mild asymptomatic irregularities in their pulse; an asymptomatic finding seldom needs extensive workup or treatment. Sensory loss is common and many experts recommend hearing and vision screening even though the USPSTF gives both an "insufficient evidence to recommend for or against" recommendation.

Careful inspection of the oral cavity is part of the nutritional assessment. Poor nutrition is common, and an involuntary weight loss greater than 5 lb/month or losses in excess of 10 lb over 3 months merit investigation for underlying disease. Rapid weight gain suggests edema or ascites. Many older persons have mineral and/or vitamin deficiencies because of a poor diet or medical conditions such as pernicious anemia or malabsorption. Supplements of vitamins A, B_{12}, C, and D, calcium, iron, zinc, and magnesium may be necessary. Hearing loss is a common condition in older patients. Hearing may be assessed by the "whispered voice test," where the examiner stands about 3 feet behind the patient and whispers a series of numbers and letters. Inability of the patient to repeat the sequence indicates hearing loss and should prompt a more formal evaluation for possible hearing aids.

Urinary incontinence is associated with both psychosocial and physical implications. Patients with incontinence are more likely to suffer from depression, social isolation, and feelings of loss of control and poor self-esteem. Urinary incontinence is also associated with recurrent urinary tract infections, acute kidney injury, poor healing of decubitus ulcers, and increased overall mortality. A careful rectal and genitourinary examination is important for helping to assess bowel and bladder

TABLE 76-2. Markers of Frailty
Self-reported exhaustion
Inactivity
Immobility or slowness
Involuntary weight loss
Muscle weakness

function and detecting uterine prolapse, hernias, and testicular atrophy.

Polypharmacy is common in older persons and can result in mental status changes, falls, and other adverse drug effects. Beer's criteria attempt to reduce adverse side effects by listing medications and medication classes to avoid in older adults. The USPSTF recommends screening patients for depression. A single affirmative answer to a two-question screening tool, "During the past month have you been bothered by feelings of sadness, depression, hopelessness?" and "Have you been bothered by a lack of interest or pleasure in doing things?" indicate the need for a more thorough evaluation for depression.

Assessing memory is part of a geriatric assessment and the Mini-Mental State Exam is one useful screening tool. Often, family members are more aware of the patient's memory impairment than the patient. Appropriate early diagnosis of dementia presents an opportunity to offer patients medications that may reverse, slow down, or stabilize the memory impairment. Coexisting situations such as denial, depression, and loss of independence can also be discussed with the patient and family. Careful assessment may identify social or physical evidence that a patient is at risk for elder abuse. Signs of abuse include trauma, burns, and weight loss.

DIAGNOSTIC EVALUATION

Preventive services recommended by the US Government Site for Medicare include a "Welcome to Medicare" visit at 65 years of age that reviews recommended evaluations, education, and treatment services. Medicare also recommends a yearly preventive visit after age 65 years to assess potential medical problems and when possible to initiate early interventions.

If not recently available, most patients benefit from basic testing such as a CBC, chemistry profile, UA, and TSH. Mammography and colon cancer screening are recommended for patients until age 75, depending on patient preference and expected life span. Pap smear screening can be discontinued at age 65 if there has been regular testing and a normal Pap smear within the previous 3 years. Other tests should be ordered as clinically indicated.

Although abnormal laboratory findings occur regularly in an elderly population and are often attributed to aging, few are truly the result of advanced age. Misinterpretation can lead to either underdiagnosis or overtreatment. Table 76-3 lists some commonly abnormal laboratory tests in older adults.

TABLE 76-3. Commonly Abnormal Laboratory Values in Older Adults	
Laboratory Test	**Finding**
Albumin	Frequently low in the elderly; can be a sign of poor nutrition
Alkaline phosphatase	Mild asymptomatic elevations are common. Liver or bone disease should be considered when values exceed 1.5 times normal.
Calcium	Unchanged in aging; abnormalities should prompt further evaluation. Need to correct for low albumin levels.
Chest x-ray	Mild interstitial changes or findings consistent with early COPD are common. A calcified aortic arch, old granuloma, and vertebral osteopenia are common age-related findings that are not a normal consequence of aging.
Creatinine	Low in the elderly due to decreases in lean body mass; high-normal and mildly elevated values may indicate significant renal impairment.
ECG	Nonspecific ST and T wave changes, PVCs, conduction abnormalities, and atrial arrhythmias are common in asymptomatic elderly and may not need further evaluation and treatment.
Electrolytes	Unchanged in aging; abnormalities should prompt further evaluation.
Iron/TIBC	Abnormal values are not due to aging and may indicate GI blood loss, poor nutrition, or chronic disease.
Glucose	Prevalence of glucose intolerance and type 2 diabetes increases with age.
Hemoglobin	Does not change with aging, but mild anemias because of chronic disease are often present. An acute drop or unexplained values under 12 g/dL generally merit investigation.
LFTs	Unchanged in aging; abnormalities should prompt further evaluation.

TABLE 76-3. Commonly Abnormal Laboratory Values in Older Adults (*continued*)

Laboratory Test	Finding
Platelet count	Unchanged in aging; abnormalities should prompt further evaluation.
PSA	Often elevated due to BPH, but marked elevations or increasing values suggest possible prostate cancer. Further evaluation of patients with possible prostate cancer should be undertaken only if the diagnosis would result in a change in management.
RA and ANA	Positivity in low titers often common and rarely indicative of disease.
Sedimentation rate	Mild elevations may be age-related. Levels >50 are more likely associated with disease.
TSH	Unchanged in aging; abnormalities should prompt further evaluation.
UA	Asymptomatic bacteriuria is common and does not merit treatment. Hematuria is never a normal finding and generally merits investigation.
WBC	Unchanged in aging; abnormalities should prompt further evaluation.

ANA, antinuclear antibodies; BPH, benign prostatic hypertrophy; COPD, chronic obstructive pulmonary disease; ECG, electrocardiogram; GI, gastrointestinal; LFTs, liver function tests; PSA, prostate-specific antigen; PVC, premature ventricular contraction; RA, rheumatoid arthritis; TIBC, total iron-binding capacity; TSH, thyroid-stimulating hormone; UA, urinalysis; WBC, white blood cell.

KEY POINTS

- Geriatric assessment is a multidisciplinary approach to the evaluation of an older individual's physical and psychosocial impairments and functional disabilities.

- The functional assessment should include a discussion of the patient's preferences and expectations combined with the family's expectations and willingness to provide care.

- Patients should also have a comprehensive evaluation including history, physical examination, and laboratory testing such as a CBC, chemistry profile, lipid profile, urine analysis, TSH, and other tests as indicated after patient evaluation.

- The types of treatments often of value in an older population include physical therapy, occupational therapy, speech therapy, and the services of psychologists, case managers, dieticians, and nurses.

77 Common Medical Problems in Older Adults

SENSORY IMPAIRMENT

HEARING LOSS

Hearing loss or difficulty hearing is the most common sensory impairment of old age and ~40% of elderly individuals experience some type of hearing loss. Age is the most important risk factor, and by age 85, more than 80% of individuals suffer from a hearing problem. Men usually experience greater hearing loss and have an earlier onset compared to women. Presbycusis or age-related hearing loss is the most common type of hearing loss, and is a bilateral sensorineural impairment of the higher frequencies that may compromise speech comprehension. Other causes of hearing loss include ototoxicity from medications, otosclerosis, Ménière disease, and cerumen impaction.

Hearing impairment can be evaluated clinically by the whispered voice test, by testing with a hand-held audiometer or by using a single-item screening question: "Do you have difficulty with your hearing?" Patients, who fail screening or admit to difficulty hearing, should be referred for more formal testing and treatment when indicated.

Hearing aids are usually worn in the ear and amplify sound. Hearing aids can minimize the effect of hearing loss and improve daily functioning. They are most effective in peripheral hearing loss and less helpful in those with a central auditory processing defect. Conduction loss from cerumen impaction may aggravate all forms of hearing loss, and cerumen should be removed either manually or with ceruminolytic agents.

VISION LOSS

Presbyopia is age-associated loss of the eye's ability to accommodate, and most individuals need glasses for reading by their 50s. The four most common ophthalmologic diseases encountered in the elderly are cataracts or lens opacification, macular degeneration, open-angle glaucoma, and diabetic retinopathy. Risk factors for cataracts include sun exposure, smoking, steroid use, and diabetes mellitus. Treatment consists of surgical removal of the lens and is indicated if the corrected acuity is 20/50 or worse, and/or if there is significant functional impairment from the cataract.

Macular degeneration is the atrophy of cells in the central macula. It is the most common cause of visual impairment in Caucasian elderly, whereas glaucoma is the most common cause in African Americans. There are two types of macular degeneration, wet and dry. Wet macular degeneration is less common (10% of cases) and is characterized by rapid vision loss from abnormal blood vessel growth and leakage underneath the retina. Laser photocoagulation or newer intravitreal antiangiogenic antibody injections may help individuals with wet macular degeneration. The dry form is more common (90% of cases), and is associated with a slow onset of vision loss with characteristic yellow white retinal deposits known as drusen. Patients with macular degeneration should be monitored daily for visual changes with an Amsler grid. Antioxidant supplement therapy is useful for reducing the risk of progression.

Glaucoma is an optic neuropathy characterized by an elevated intraocular pressure and an increased optic cup-to-disc ratio. If untreated, glaucoma can lead to a loss of peripheral vision and eventually blindness. Treatment is indicated when pressures are elevated (>25 mmHg), or in the presence of optic nerve atrophy or visual field loss. Pharmacologic treatment with drops that either decrease aqueous production (e.g., beta blockers, adrenergic agents) or increase aqueous drainage (e.g., miotics) can lower pressure. Surgery is indicated when pressures are poorly controlled by topical agents or visual loss progresses.

COMMON DISORDERS

WEIGHT LOSS

Involuntary weight loss in the elderly is a serious problem. An involuntary weight loss of >10 lb is significant, and even a loss as small as 5% over 3 years is associated with increased mortality. Several screening tools can help identify patients at risk for poor nutrition. The causes of weight loss in older patients are similar to those in middle-age adults and include depression and cancer, especially gastrointestinal and lung malignancies. Other medical conditions that can cause weight loss include gastrointestinal disorders (dysphagia, peptic ulcer disease, reflux, ischemic bowel, celiac disease), endocrine disorders (new-onset diabetes, hyperthyroidism), end organ disease (congestive heart failure, end-stage renal disease, chronic obstructive lung disease, hepatic failure), neurologic disease (Parkinsonism, dementia, stroke), rheumatologic disorders (fibromyalgia, rheumatoid arthritis, polymyalgia rheumatica), alcohol or drug abuse, and medication side effects.

Elderly patients may also have reduced dietary intake from oral problems, such as poorly fitted dentures, functional impairment because of stroke or arthritis, difficulty swallowing, or social isolation. Access issues such as having insufficient resources to purchase food or the inability to shop or prepare meals may also limit adequate nutrition. Collaboration with a social worker may be needed to identify services that address access needs or to provide meal assistance.

If a complete history, physical examination, assessment of appetite, and dietary intake fail to suggest the diagnosis, laboratory testing including CBC, sedimentation rate, comprehensive metabolic panel, urinalysis, TSH, CXR, PSA, and HIV testing (in those at risk) help screen for organic disease. If no cause for the weight loss is found on initial evaluation, chest/abdomen/pelvic CT scan with and without contrast could be considered. Treatment depends on the underlying cause. In about 25% of cases, no cause for an involuntary weight loss is identified.

Nutritional supplements to increase caloric intake often benefit patients regardless of cause. Increasing the fat content of foods and snacks between meals can also help. A daily multiple vitamin with mineral supplement is indicated in patients with reduced caloric intake because these individuals are often deficient in vitamin B_{12}, vitamin D, and calcium intake. Few studies exist that examine appetite stimulants in older patients with weight loss without a diagnosis of cancer but, megestrol acetate can improve weight gain in patients with cancer. Oral prednisone increases appetite and weight, but has significant long-term side effects. Mirtazapine is associated with weight gain and may be a good choice for depressed individuals who might benefit from an enhanced appetite. However, no studies support its use in patients with weight loss without depression.

OSTEOARTHRITIS

Osteoarthritis is one of the most common chronic diseases among older adults, with over 95% of those over age 65 demonstrating some evidence of osteoarthritis. Women are affected more than men, and the most commonly affected joints are the hands, lower extremities, and spine. Classic symptoms of osteoarthritis include joint pain and stiffness that tend to worsen with activity, decreased range of motion, and in more advanced disease joint locking and joint deformities. Osteoarthritis is a degenerative disease of the joint cartilage accompanied by a reactive overgrowth of the periarticular bone. In most cases, the diagnosis can be made clinically with x-ray imaging to confirm the diagnosis. Inflammation markers (sedimentation rate, CRP) and other laboratory testing are usually normal. Immunologic testing for lupus or rheumatoid arthritis is indicated when there is evidence of joint inflammation. In cases of suspected gout, a serum uric acid level aids in the diagnosis. Negatively birefringent crystals seen in aspirated joint fluid confirm the diagnosis of gout.

Treatment focuses on relieving pain and maintaining function. Regular exercise that does not aggravate the pain helps stabilize joints and preserves function. Consultation with physical therapy to recommend an exercise program or participation in a supervised exercise program can be beneficial. Acetaminophen is considered first-line therapy for mild osteoarthritis because of its safety profile. NSAIDs are superior to acetaminophen for treating moderate to severe osteoarthritis but have more side effects. Although there is mixed evidence to support their use, some patients benefit from topical therapies such as capsaicin or supplements containing glucosamine with chondroitin. One option is a therapeutic trial period of at least 3 months to assess the benefit in an individual patient. Corticosteroid joint injections for acute exacerbations can be considered. Intraarticular hyaluronic acid injections also offer modest temporary relief of knee osteoarthritis. Patients with continued pain or disability after maximum medical therapy may be candidates for total joint replacement. Narcotic pain medication should be used sparingly and limited to patients with severe symptoms with ongoing reevaluation of risks versus benefits.

TREMOR

Tremor is an involuntary movement disorder that is most common among middle-aged and older adults. Determining the underlying cause is important because prognosis and specific treatment plans depend on the cause of the tremor. Common causes in the elderly include enhanced physiologic tremor, essential tremor, the tremor of Parkinsonism, drug and metabolic–induced tremors, and psychogenic tremor.

Enhanced Physiologic Tremor

Enhanced physiologic tremor occurs at rest and is not worsened by movement. The tremor is often more pronounced by stress, anxiety, and certain medications. A mild tremor that worsens with anxiety, medication use, caffeine intake, or fatigue does not need further evaluation.

Essential Tremor

Essential tremor is often called familial tremor because about 50% of cases are thought to be inherited in an autosomal dominant fashion. Essential tremor progresses in severity as the patient ages. It most commonly affects the hands and wrists when the patient holds their arms out in front of themselves. An essential tremor improves with alcohol use, and some patients will self-medicate with alcohol. First-line medications used to treat essential tremor are propranolol and/or primidone. Gabapentin and topiramate are often used if first-line medications are ineffective.

Parkinson Tremor

Parkinson disease (PD) is a clinical syndrome consisting of tremor at rest, rigidity, bradykinesia, and gait disturbance that affects about 1% of individuals over age 60. Patients often have micrographia, masked facies, and abnormal heel-to-toe testing. Idiopathic Parkinsonism is the most common form of the disease. Other causes include brainstem infarction, multiple system atrophy, and medications that block or deplete dopamine (methyldopa, metoclopramide, haloperidol, and risperidone).

Idiopathic PD is a degenerative disorder of the substantia nigra and ventral tegmental area of the brain, resulting in a depletion of striatal dopamine. On autopsy, individuals with PD have Lewy bodies (LBs), which are intracytoplasmic inclusion bodies in the nigral neurons. LBs are also found in the cerebral cortex, which may explain why about one-third of PD patients develop dementia later in the course of the disease.

PD may be confused with essential tremor because the incidence of both increase with age. However, unlike the parkinsonian resting tremor that decreases with activity, essential tremor increases with movement and decreases with rest. Stroke-related tremor is sometimes confused with PD. However, in PD other features such as cogwheel rigidity and bradykinesia are present, whereas stroke-related defects such as weakness, decreased sensation, and abnormal reflexes are absent. Multiple small strokes can also mimic PD, but an MRI showing multiple small strokes in the basal ganglia and a poor response to levodopa usually distinguish the two.

No cure is available for PD, but symptomatic pharmacologic treatment is helpful when symptoms begin to interfere with the patient's occupational and social functioning. Drugs for PD are listed in Table 77-1.

Levodopa remains the mainstay of therapy. Combinations of levodopa and carbidopa are the most effective ways to get dopamine into the brain. Dopamine is ineffective because it does not cross the blood–brain barrier; however, levodopa is able to cross, and once in the brain is converted to dopamine through decarboxylization. Carbidopa inhibits the peripheral decarboxylation of levodopa and lessens side effects by enhancing the central availability of levodopa and making it possible to reduce the therapeutic dose. Levodopa/carbidopa is available in a wide range of formulations; so, dosing can be titrated to an individual's needs. Levodopa is usually most effective for bradykinesia and rigidity and less so for tremors. If patients with suspected PD fail to respond at all to levodopa, one of the atypical PD states such as Wilson disease or a hereditary condition should be considered.

For younger patients with mild symptoms, anticholinergic or dopamine agonist medications may be adequate therapy. Anticholinergics are more effective for tremor than for rigidity or bradykinesia. The effectiveness of levodopa diminishes and the incidence of adverse effects increases over time with use of levodopa. For patients that require higher doses of levodopa, dopamine agonists can be added as adjunctive therapy.

Medication/Metabolic Tremors

Patients with new-onset tremor need a complete medication review because several medications can cause tremor. Medications most commonly causing tremor

TABLE 77-1. Pharmacologic Therapies for Parkinson Disease

Drugs	Comment	Side Effect
Dopamine precursors Levodopa/carbidopa (Sinemet)	Mainstay of PD therapy	Gastrointestinal, dizziness, confusion, common dyskinesia
Anticholinergics Trihexyphenidyl (Artane) Benztropine (Cogentin)	Effective for tremor/drooling	Confusion, constipation, urinary retention, dry mouth; side effects more common in elderly
Dopamine agonists Amantadine Bromocriptine (Parlodel) Pergolide mesylate (Permax) Pramipexole (Mirapex) Ropinirole (Requip)	Expensive, may be effective as single agent in early PD. Not as effective as Sinemet. Also used as adjunct in later stages. Effect of amantadine disappears in a few months.	Nausea, dizziness
Monoamine oxidase type B inhibitor Selegiline	Symptomatic benefit limited. Controversial but may have protective effect in early PD. Expensive.	
Catechol-O-methyltranferase inhibitors Tolcapone (Tasmar) Entacapone (Comtan)	Enhances levodopa therapy	Dizziness, diarrhea, dyskinesia; use of tolcapone requires monitoring of liver function tests.

are those that stimulate the sympathetic nervous system (amphetamines, terbutaline, and pseudoephedrine) and psychoactive medications (tricyclic antidepressants, allopurinol, and fluoxetine). Other common offenders are caffeine, hypoglycemic agents, theophylline, thyroid hormones, and valproic acid. Metabolic causes of tremor include hypocalcemia, hypoglycemia, hyponatremia, hyperthyroidism, hyperparathyroidism, vitamin B_{12} deficiency, and hypomagnesemia.

Cerebellar/Psychogenic Tremors
Cerebellar tremor usually presents as a slow intention tremor associated with postural difficulties. This can be caused by brain stem tumors, previous multi-infarct strokes, inherited disorders, chronic alcoholism, and multiple sclerosis. Psychogenic tremors are usually associated with stressful life events. These tremors often have an abrupt onset with spontaneous remission. Typically, they occur in patients with multiple undiagnosed conditions, in the presence of psychiatric disease, and often are unresponsive to antitremor medications.

SKIN DISORDERS

XEROSIS
Xerosis (dry skin) is related to a decrease in sebum production and an increase in water vapor permeability. Treatment includes the frequent use of emollients and moisturizers, up to four times a day.

Pruritis, which is often due to xerosis, is most common in the winter and may be exacerbated by excessive bathing and harsh soaps or medications. Other causes include stress and systemic diseases such as renal insufficiency, hypothyroidism, hepatitis, anemia, diabetes, and malignancy. Therapy should be directed at the underlying cause. Symptomatic treatment includes emollients, nonmedicated soaps, limitation of soap usage to the axillae and genital areas, and the use of topical steroids and systemic antihistamines.

SEBORRHEIC KERATOSIS
Seborrheic keratosis, is a form of a benign skin condition, present in more than 90% of older adults. It typically varies in color from tan to dark brown, and ranges in size from lesions barely visible to several centimeters. It often has the appearance of being stuck on the skin. Removal of seborrheic keratoses may be indicated when they cause discomfort because of their location or if they cause cosmetic concerns. They may be removed using cryotherapy or shave biopsy excision.

ACTINIC KERATOSES
Actinic keratoses are precancerous lesions primarily seen in the middle-aged and elderly population. These lesions are induced by ultraviolet light damage and are more common in fair-skinned individuals. Untreated, they have about a 1% per year risk of developing into squamous cell carcinomas. Actinic keratoses are asymptomatic, red, rough, scaly lesions

on sun-exposed sites such as the face, hands, and arms. Treatment consists of local destruction by one of several methods including cryotherapy or shave biopsy excisions. Extensive lesions may be treated with a topical agent such as 5-fluorouracil.

SKIN CANCERS

Basal Cell Carcinoma

Basal cell carcinoma (BCC) is the most common human malignancy. Risk factors include fair skin, history of sunburn, family history of skin cancer, and outdoor occupation. Approximately 80% of these lesions occur on sun-exposed areas of the head and neck. The typical appearance is a pink nodule with a translucent or pearly quality with overlying telangiectatic vessels (Fig. 77-1). Basal cell cancer rarely metastasizes but can become locally invasive and destructive over the course of years. The diagnosis relies on clinical suspicion followed by biopsy of the lesion. The most common form of therapy is surgical excision.

Squamous Cell Carcinoma

The incidence of squamous cell carcinoma, like BCC, is increasing. Risk factors for squamous cell carcinomas include sun exposure, past psoriasis treatment, history of actinic keratoses, and smoking. Squamous cell carcinomas that arise from actinic keratoses are more thickly scaled with a raised erythematous bed. Lesions can often develop a keratin horn. Usually, there is an ulcerated center of the lesion from the patient scratching the lesion. Squamous cell cancers

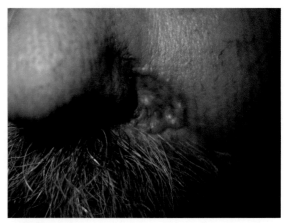

FIGURE 77-1. Basal cell carcinoma. (From Dr. Barankin Dermatology Collection.)

are more aggressive than basal cell cancers and have metastatic potential. Treatment begins with a shave biopsy for diagnosis and excisional biopsy for cure.

Malignant Melanoma

Malignant melanoma is a neoplasm especially important to diagnose because it is one of the few potentially fatal skin diseases. Patients at greater risk include those with fair complexions and light hair and eyes, and those with excessive sun exposure. The diagnosis of malignant melanoma requires an excisional biopsy of clinically suspicious lesions. Management should be individualized for each patient, especially for the elderly individual. Survival is most closely related to the depth of tumor invasion.

KEY POINTS

- Hearing loss is the most common sensory impairment of old age; ~40% of elderly individuals have some type of hearing loss.

- The four most common ophthalmologic diseases encountered in the elderly are cataracts or lens opacification, macular degeneration, open-angle glaucoma, and diabetic retinopathy.

- Involuntary weight loss in the elderly is a serious problem; a 1-year documented weight loss of >4% is the best single predictor of death within 2 years.

- PD is a clinical syndrome consisting of tremor at rest, cogwheel rigidity, bradykinesia, and shuffling gait disturbance that affects about 1% of individuals over age 60.

- Tremor occurs more commonly with age and can lead to progressive disability. Evaluation should reveal the cause and then treatment for tremor control.

- BCC is the most common human malignancy. Approximately 80% of these lesions occur on sun-exposed areas of the head and neck. They rarely metastasize but can become locally invasive and destructive over the course of years.

- Malignant melanoma is a neoplasm that is especially important to diagnose because it is one of the few potentially fatal skin diseases.

78 | Dementia

Dementia is a progressive decline in memory, accompanied by a loss of intellectual capabilities severe enough to interfere with social or occupational function. In addition to memory loss, associated cognitive impairment can affect language, judgment, cognition, visuospatial skills, and personality.

The prevalence of dementia increases significantly with age, with roughly 1% of the population affected by age 60 and almost 50% after age 85. By the year 2030, nearly 20% of the population will be over age 65 and the societal burden of dementia will become an even greater concern. Although most cases of dementia are irreversible, family physicians must be aware of the reversible causes, methods of diagnosing the various causes of dementia, and treatment options for both the patients and their families.

PATHOGENESIS

Alzheimer disease (AlzD) is the most common cause of dementia and accounts for over half of all cases. Every year, 10% to 15% of patients with mild cognitive impairment develop AlzD. AlzD is progressive and, on average, patients with AlzD live 8 to 10 years from diagnosis with the most common cause of death being pneumonia. The incidence of AlzD is increasing and the CDC reports AlzD as the fifth leading cause of death in the United States.

Postmortem analysis of patients with AlzD demonstrates brain atrophy, enlarged ventricles, and minimal evidence of vascular disease. Histologic findings usually located in the frontotemporal lobes include intracellular neurofibrillary tangles comprising tau proteins and extracellular plaques consisting of beta amyloid protein. These changes lead to neuronal loss and subsequent disturbances in the cholinergic system, which accounts for the progressive cognitive decline. Although there is a rare autosomal dominant form of the disease involving the gene for the amyloid protein, most cases are sporadic.

Risk factors for AlzD include advanced age, female gender, family history of AlzD, chronic anticholinergic use, cerebrovascular comorbidities, and lower educational level. The apolipoprotein APO-E4 gene on chromosome 19 is associated with an increased risk for AlzD. However, testing for APO-E4 is neither sensitive nor specific enough to justify its use as a screening test.

Vascular dementia is the second most common cause of dementia and results from tissue damage because of cerebral ischemia and hypoxia. Patients with HTN, diabetes, a history of smoking, and known arterial disease are at risk. Multiinfarct dementia due to a series of small-vessel infarctions known as lacunar strokes is one type of vascular dementia. The multiple infarcts typically cause patients to experience discrete episodes of worsening cognition that occur in a stepwise manner. In older patients, AlzD and vascular dementia may occur together.

Severely depressed patients may present with cognitive slowing and poor memory, a condition termed pseudodementia, which mimics dementia. These individuals usually improve once treatment is initiated. Depression is also common in patients with an underlying dementia, particularly early in the course of the disease.

Lewy body (LB) dementia is characterized by the presence of LBs, or intracytoplasmic inclusions, and by decreased neuronal density in the hippocampus, amygdala, cortex, and other portions of the brain. Patients with LB dementia typically have a more rapid clinical decline than those with AlzD. Visual hallucinations, episodic delirium, and extrapyramidal motor signs are commonly present and help differentiate LB from AlzD.

Space-occupying lesions such as subdural hematoma and tumor, infections such as syphilis and HIV, and other neurologic disorders such as MS,

PD, and Huntington disease may disrupt neural pathways involved with cognition and memory. Normal pressure hydrocephalus is characterized by ataxia, incontinence, and dementia and occurs due to diminished absorption of CSF, resulting in compression of the affected neural pathways. Medical disorders such as hypothyroidism, hypercalcemia, vitamin B_{12} or folate deficiency, and acute intoxication can lead to memory impairment. Medications such as sedatives, opiates, antihypertensives, and neuroleptics may cause or exacerbate the mental status changes associated with dementia.

CLINICAL MANIFESTATIONS

HISTORY

Because most patients with dementia lack objective insight into their condition, the history is often best obtained through family members, friends, and caregivers. Dementia may also be suspected during a routine evaluation if a patient has difficulty recalling medications, recent events, and medical history. Questions should be asked about patient orientation, episodes of forgetfulness, ADLs, and job duties. Early dementia can be difficult to recognize. Examples of symptoms include instances of patients getting lost; forgetting words, names, or recipes; neglecting personal hygiene; and not knowing common facts such as their own address and current events. Episodes of social withdrawal, frustration with emotional outbursts, and difficulty driving are common in patients with dementia and need to be asked about. The time course of symptoms (e.g., abrupt vs. gradual), duration, and course (e.g., continuous, fluctuating, or stepwise) help determine the type of dementia. Past surgical and medical history should focus on episodes of head trauma, previous vascular surgery, meningitis, and other neurologic diseases.

All medications must be reviewed and alcohol intake and nutrition assessed. Sexual history determines risk for HIV and syphilis. Review of systems should also focus on signs of depression, thyroid disorder, and other neurologic disorders.

PHYSICAL EXAMINATION

The physical examination should include mental status evaluation, neurologic examination, and a general examination aimed at identifying illness that may be contributing to the patient's cognitive decline. A general assessment provides information about hygiene, nutritional status, and attentiveness. The physical examination can also identify problems such as hearing or vision loss and orthopedic problems that may interfere with ADLs.

During the initial visit, quick assessment tools can be used to assess the need for a more detailed cognitive evaluation. A verbal fluency test is one example. The patient is given 1 minute to name as many animals as possible and scores one point for each animal named. A score of <15 suggests dementia and the need for further testing. A "passing" score may be lowered to <12 if the patient has <7 years of formal education. Another screening test is the Mini-Cog Assessment tool. The patient is given three words to repeat and remember, then asked to draw the face of a clock with hands to a time (e.g., 10 past 11), and then asked to recall the three words. The patient gets one point for each word remembered and two points for a correct clock drawing. A score of two or less makes dementia likely. The Mini-Mental State Exam (MMSE) is a more detailed standardized test useful for confirming the presence of dementia if a screening test implies dementia. Specifically, the MMSE provides insight into patient orientation, recall, attention, language ability, visuospatial ability, and executive functioning. The score can be corrected for the level of education and followed over time.

A complete neurologic examination can detect abnormalities suggesting prior stroke, a mass, or evidence of PD. Abstract reasoning can be assessed by asking the meaning of proverbs such as "People in glass houses shouldn't throw stones" or "A stitch in time saves nine." Psychiatric assessment determines the presence of depression and other psychiatric disorders. Neuropsychiatric testing can also be done to differentiate the type of dementia and to characterize its extent.

DIFFERENTIAL DIAGNOSIS

Box 78-1 lists the causes of dementia. AlzD accounts for about 50% of cases, and about 15% have a vascular dementia. Other patients may have a mixed dementia, which is caused by a combination of AlzD and vascular disease, LB dementia (10% to 15%), and frontotemporal dementia (5% to 10%). Dementia must also be distinguished from other causes of mental confusion, such as depression and delirium.

Delirium, or an acute confusional state, affects memory and cognition. Delirium typically occurs rapidly over hours to days and is associated with a clouding of consciousness and disruption of the sleep cycle. Unlike dementia, delirium is often reversible. Patients with dementia are at increased risk for

BOX 78-1. Differential Diagnosis for Dementia

Alzheimer disease
Multiinfarct dementia
Lewy body dementia
Depression (pseudodementia)
Normal pressure hydrocephalus
Thyroid disorder
B_{12} deficiency
Folate deficiency
Syphilis with CNS involvement
HIV with CNS involvement
Subdural hematoma
Medications
    Opiates
    Neuroleptics
    Antidepressants
    Anticholinergics
Multiple sclerosis
Parkinson disease
Huntington disease
Down syndrome
Intoxication

developing delirium. Acute changes in mental status merit ruling out a toxic reaction to a medication as well as physical illnesses such as infection, dehydration, hypoxia, electrolyte imbalance, anemia, and hepatic failure. Depression may mimic dementia. Typically, symptoms of depression precede memory loss and depressed patients appear apathetic.

DIAGNOSTIC EVALUATION

There are no definitive tests for diagnosing most of the disorders that cause dementia, including AlzD. The diagnostic evaluation should focus on

recognizing potentially treatable causes of dementia and identifying treatable coexisting illnesses that may be contributing to impaired cognition. History, physical examination, and laboratory testing are indicated to rule out conditions that mimic dementia and to identify reversible causes. Box 78-2 gives a mnemonic, DEMENTIA, to help remember reversible causes of dementia. Appropriate tests include a CBC, sedimentation rate, comprehensive metabolic panel, TSH, vitamin B_{12} and folate levels, and UA. Hearing and vision screening are often useful. A CXR and ECG are commonly done, and HIV testing is indicated for patients with risk factors.

Patients with dementia usually merit some type of neuroimaging procedure such as a CT or MRI of the brain. Testing patients rules out conditions such as a subdural hematoma, normal pressure hydrocephalus, a mass lesion, or vascular dementia. Box 78-3 lists some indications for imaging. A lumbar puncture is useful in evaluating for vasculitis, CNS infection, and MS; it may improve symptoms in those with normal pressure hydrocephalus. Formal neuropsychological testing determines more precisely the extent of cognitive impairment and may be useful in patients with atypical deficits or only a mild cognitive decline.

TREATMENT

Patients found to have reversible causes of dementia should receive prompt and appropriate treatment. For example, those with depression should be started on antidepressants and reevaluated for cognitive improvement. However, because dementia is most often irreversible, the focus in most patients is to maintain quality of life and maximize function. Patients and their caregivers need education about

BOX 78-2. DEMENTIA—Reversible Causes for Dementia

Acronym	Comment
Drugs	Anticholinergics, centrally acting drugs
Emotional disorders	Pseudodementia from depression
Metabolic and endocrine disorders	Thyroid disease common in elderly
Ear and eye impairment	Usually contributes to rather than causes dementia
Nutritional deficiencies	B_{12} and folate deficiency
Trauma or tumor	Subdural hematoma, space-occupying lesion
Infections	Syphilis, HIV
Alcohol and drugs	Can contribute to or cause dementia, easily overlooked

BOX 78-3. Indications for Neuroimaging

Recent onset dementia
Rapid progression
History of head trauma
Younger age
Urinary incontinence and gait disorders
Focal abnormalities on neurologic examination

creating a safe, familiar, and nurturing environment for the patient, managing behavioral problems, and treating comorbid conditions that may exacerbate cognitive decline. Box 78-4 summarizes the management of patients with dementia.

If disruptive behavior persists after optimizing function and using behavioral strategies, the atypical antipsychotics such as quetiapine (Seroquel) are the preferred agents to help control behavior that presents a risk to the patients or others. Phenothiazines (e.g., haloperidol and risperidone) and anticonvulsants are occasionally needed to control disruptive behavior. Because cognitive impairment may be exacerbated by the use of psychoactive medications such as tranquilizers, sleeping pills, anxiolytics, and drugs with anticholinergic activity, they should be used cautiously with careful dosage titration and periodic reassessment of both their indication and dosage. Side effects also include an increased incidence of

BOX 78-4. Managing Patients with Dementia

Optimize Function
Treat medical conditions that impair function
Optimize hearing and vision
Avoid medications that impair cognition
Encourage physical and social activity
Assess nutrition

Identify and Manage Behavioral Complications
Psychosis
Agitation and aggression
Depression
Wandering

Caregiver Education and Support
Discuss prognosis and progression of disease
Discuss advance directives
Discuss community resources
Recommend legal and financial counseling
Review ethical issues
Offer opportunities for new treatments

falls, increased sedation, and—in the case of the phenothiazines—tardive dyskinesia. The dosage and continued use of psychoactive medications should be monitored. Due to their side effect profile and an association with increased mortality these drugs should be considered only when their benefits outweigh their significant risks.

Patients with multiinfarct dementia need to optimize management of blood pressure, diabetes, and hyperlipidemia; if they are smokers, they should stop. If not contraindicated, they should receive an antiplatelet medication such as aspirin or Plavix. Serial lumbar punctures or the placement of a ventricular shunt may benefit patients with normal pressure hydrocephalus. When possible, medications thought to be contributing to or exacerbating the dementia should be changed or discontinued.

Patients with suspected AlzD may benefit from the use of acetylcholinesterase inhibitors such as donepezil (Aricept), rivastigmine (Exelon), or galantamine (Reminyl). These all appear to slow the progression of AlzD, and typically result in a small improvement in symptoms followed by a gradual decline to a level below baseline. An additional medication for moderate to severe AlzD is memantine (Namenda). It is an N-methyl-D-aspartate (NMDA) receptor antagonist and is often combined with the acetylcholinesterase inhibitors. Caregivers of individuals with dementia must be educated regarding home safety, long-term care options, and the importance of a living will. Since caregivers are at high risk for burnout, they may benefit from joining support groups, which can help them to cope with the task of taking care of their loved ones.

Studies examining other therapies for AlzD yield conflicting results. Ginkgo biloba failed to demonstrate a statistically significant and consistent clinical effect over time, except in one small European study. There are also drug–drug interactions to consider, particularly with anticoagulants. Testosterone demonstrated little, if any, long-term effect on memory impairment, but may improve quality of life measures. However, side effects of increased cardiovascular disease limit its usefulness. Selegiline (Eldepryl) showed early improvement in AlzD cognition, but no long-term benefit. It has been used as an adjunct to other AlzD medications.

Medications, herbal products, and supplements show no effect on AlzD including vitamin E, statins, insulin sensitizers, estrogen, and antiinflammatory agents, caprylic acid or coconut oil, Coenzyme Q_{10}, coral calcium, omega-3 fatty acids, and huperzine A.

KEY POINTS

- Dementia is a progressive decline in memory and a loss of intellectual capabilities severe enough to interfere with social or occupational function.

- Multiinfarct dementia because of a series of small-vessel infarctions causes patients to experience discrete episodes of worsening cognition, which occur in a stepwise manner.

- Patients with dementia are diagnosed by history, physical examination, and laboratory testing to rule out conditions that mimic dementia.

- Patients with suspected AlzD may benefit from the use of acetylcholinesterase inhibitors and NMDA receptor antagonists.

79 | Urinary Incontinence

Urinary incontinence (UI) is defined as the involuntary loss of urine severe enough to cause social and hygiene problems. It is a significant cause of disability and caregiver dependency, and can lead to social isolation, depression, skin breakdown, UTIs, and falls. Approximately one-third of community-dwelling elderly women and one-fourth of elderly men experience some degree of incontinence, and the prevalence increases with age. About one-half of patients who are homebound or live in long-term care facilities suffer from incontinence. Despite this prevalence, 50% of incontinent patients have never discussed it with their physicians. Many patients feel incontinence is part of the aging process and are embarrassed to discuss it or believe there is no treatment for it.

PATHOGENESIS

Normal urination is a complex process; knowledge of the pathophysiology is needed to understand the causes of UI.

The lower tract consists of the bladder and urethra. The urethra has two sphincters, an internal one, consisting of smooth muscle, and an external one, with both smooth and striated muscles. The bladder is made up of a smooth muscle called the "detrusor muscle," which is innervated primarily by cholinergic neurons from the parasympathetic system. When these neurons are stimulated, bladder contraction occurs. The sympathetic system innervates both the bladder and the internal sphincter. The beta-adrenergic system in the bladder produces relaxation and the alpha-adrenergic receptors cause sphincter contraction. The striated muscle of the external sphincter allows voluntary interruption of voiding. Additional voluntary control comes from the CNS, which inhibits the autonomic processes described above through the pontine micturition center.

Normal pelvic geometry is important for adequate sphincter function because it allows intra-abdominal pressure to be distributed equally, preventing urine leakage from activities such as coughing, sneezing, laughing, or straining. All of these are associated with increased intra-abdominal pressure.

Three basic mechanisms cause UI: overactivity of the bladder detrusor muscle (urge incontinence), malfunction of the urinary sphincters (stress incontinence), and overflow from the bladder (urinary retention). **Urge incontinence** occurs when uninhibited bladder contractions are sufficient to overcome urethral resistance. **Stress incontinence** is involuntary loss of urine during coughing, sneezing, standing, or exercising. In **overflow incontinence**, either obstruction of urine outflow or ineffective bladder contractions cause urinary retention. As the bladder distention reaches maximum capacity, there is a point at which urethral sphincter pressure is exceeded and overflow leakage from the bladder occurs.

CLINICAL MANIFESTATIONS

HISTORY

Since at least one-half of patients with UI can be helped with relatively simple measures, it is important to identify patients with UI. Incontinence can be classified as transient or chronic. Transient incontinence is urinary leakage that resolves after the underlying cause is treated. Chronic UI does not resolve spontaneously, and is classified into five types: stress, urge, mixed, overflow, or functional. Stress incontinence is caused by urinary sphincter weakness and is the second most common cause in older women. It more common in women who have had vaginal deliveries, and in men risk factors include prostatectomy, transurethral resection of the prostate, and other prostate surgeries. Urge incontinence occurs with detrusor overactivity caused by either local inflammation, infection within the bladder, or neurologic disease that disrupts cerebral inhibition of detrusor contractions. Urge and stress incontinence often occur together and the condition is called "mixed incontinence." Overflow incontinence results from overdistention of the bladder and can be seen in men with obstruction from BPH. Functional incontinence can be caused by mobility problems or cognitive decline.

Patients with incontinence need a complete history, including an obstetric and surgical history, especially about any previous abdominal or pelvic surgery. The medical history should identify problems such as diabetes, CHF, stroke, Parkinson's disease (PD), and UTI. Medication review should include both prescription and OTC medications. Classes of drugs associated with UI include antihypertensives (diuretics, ACEI, calcium channel blockers, alpha-adrenergic antagonists) sedatives, pain medications (narcotics, COX-2 antiinflammatories, muscle relaxants), and anticholinergics. There is often a temporal connection between these drugs and the onset or worsening of incontinence. History can also provide important clues to the type of precipitating factors of UI. Table 79-1 lists important aspects of the history.

PHYSICAL EXAMINATION

The goals of the physical examination are to identify precipitating factors and to establish the underlying pathophysiology. In addition to a general examination, the focus should be on the abdominal, genitourinary, and neurologic examinations. Important findings include a distended bladder, enlarged prostate, uterine prolapse, cystocele, or rectocele. Examining patients for sphincter tone, perineal sensation, and fecal impaction, and for the presence of a rectal mass is important. The neurologic examination should detect evidence of cognitive impairment, spinal cord disease, and CVA.

DIFFERENTIAL DIAGNOSIS

The initial classification can be divided into acute reversible forms and persistent UI. Persistent incontinence occurs over time and is unrelated to an acute event. It can usually be classified by pathophysiology into stress, urge, or overflow incontinence. Stress incontinence, or the involuntary loss of urine when intra-abdominal pressure increases, is most frequently caused by relaxation of the pelvic musculature. It is more common in women who have had vaginal deliveries of children, and also occurs in men whose sphincters may have been damaged by transurethral surgery or radiation therapy. Urge incontinence is usually associated with involuntary detrusor activity. Many neurologic problems such as stroke, dementia, PD, and spinal cord injury are associated with this problem. If no neurologic disease is present, the condition is called "detrusor instability." Patients with urge incontinence typically complain of having the sudden urge to go and being unable to get to the bathroom in time. Occasionally, individuals who have bladder instability can have impaired contractions, creating a combination of urge incontinence and urinary retention. Overflow incontinence, caused by overdistention of the bladder, can be caused by anatomic obstruction (e.g., prostate disease), urethral stricture, or neurologic factors such as diabetes or MS that result in an underactive bladder. Medications such as sympathomimetics, anticholinergics, or narcotics can cause retention. Functional incontinence is the loss of urine from factors outside the urinary tract. In this situation, the urinary system is normal, but the patient cannot reach the toilet in time because of reasons such as decreased awareness, as seen in dementia, poor mobility, or inadequate access to bathroom facilities. Often, UI is a mixture of causes as in the case of someone with urge incontinence whose impaired mobility may cause loss of urine.

Acute reversible UI usually has a sudden onset and is associated with an illness. Acute factors may contribute to worsening of chronic UI. Acute infection is a common cause of UI, along with fecal impaction and inflammatory conditions such as cystitis or urethritis. Any cause that precipitates polyuria, such as uncontrolled diabetes, alcohol ingestion, diuretics, and CHF can cause incontinence, as can the introduction or alteration of medications.

TABLE 79-1. History Taking for Urinary Incontinence
Duration of symptoms
Characteristics of UI—for example, timing and amount of incontinent episodes
Fluid intake
Caffeine and alcohol intake
Other urinary symptoms—for example, nocturia, frequency, hematuria, dysuria
Associated events—for example, surgery
Alteration of bowel function
Use of pads or protective devices

DIAGNOSTIC EVALUATION

Goals of the initial evaluation are to identify correctable causes: UTI, medications, excessive urine output, atrophic vaginitis, fecal impaction, and reduced mobility. The next step is to determine who needs an in-depth evaluation and who can be treated without extensive testing. Generally, this can be accomplished with a clinical assessment and a few simple tests. All incontinent patients need a UA, which can detect infection (a common cause of reversible incontinence), uncontrolled diabetes, and hematuria, which suggests the need for further workup. Postvoid residual (PVR) can be assessed by either US or bladder catheterization. Catheterization is commonly used in women, whereas ultrasound (US) is often preferred in men because catheterization may be more difficult or traumatic. PVRs of <75 mL are considered normal and levels of 75 to 150 mL borderline. A PVR of more than 150 mL requires further investigation.

Laboratory work-up including serum electrolytes, BUN, creatinine, glucose, and calcium should be assessed to determine renal function and identify conditions causing polyuria. An algorithm for the diagnosis of UI is shown in Figure 79-1.

After the initial laboratory and clinical assessment, most potentially reversible causes of UI can be identified and the nature of the incontinence classified. Characteristics suggesting the need for further evaluation and testing include an unclear diagnosis, recent history of pelvic surgery, symptomatic pelvic prolapse, UI with recurrent symptomatic infection, hematuria without infection, PVR >150 mL, prostate nodules, an abnormality suggesting neurologic disease, and failure to respond to adequate treatment. Commonly, when further evaluation and testing are indicated, the patient is referred to a urologist or gynecologist, who may then elect to perform urodynamic testing and/or cystoscopy.

TREATMENT

Treatment of UI includes behavioral, pharmaceutical, and surgical interventions and often a combination of therapies proves beneficial. Generally, the least invasive treatment should be tried first. Behavioral techniques present little risk, but may need to be supplemented with pharmacologic treatment. Bladder retraining involving progressive increases in the intervals between voiding may benefit patients with urge incontinence. Scheduled voiding, where patients are toileted on a regular basis is most successful in patients with functional incontinence. Kegel exercises involving repetitive contraction of the pelvic floor muscles strengthen the pelvic floor, and help improve or control stress incontinence. In addition to behavioral techniques, assessing the environment and improving access to toileting or improving the call system for assistance may resolve incontinence. Simple lifestyle changes such as restricting fluids, decreasing alcohol intake, and eliminating caffeine may resolve or improve mild incontinence. Several medications are available for treatment. These drugs should be started at a low dose and gradually titrated upward to maximize benefits and reduce side effects. Anticholinergic medications (oxybutynin, fesoterodine, imipramine, trospium, and tolterodine) can help control urge incontinence. Drugs such as pseudoephedrine, with alpha-adrenergic properties that stimulate the internal sphincter, may improve stress incontinence, but are not without potential side effects. Topical estrogen may be helpful in patients with atrophic vaginitis and can be used in combination with pseudoephedrine. Effective drugs for overflow incontinence work by stimulating bladder contractions or relaxing the sphincter. Cholinergic agents such as bethanechol stimulate the bladder, and may help patients with an atonic bladder because of neurologic conditions such as diabetic neuropathy; however, medical treatment in overflow incontinence caused by bladder contractility problems is often not very effective. Alpha-adrenergic blockers, such as terazosin, prazosin, or tamsulosin, are often used in men with BPH to relax the internal sphincter. Surgery should be considered in patients with severe stress incontinence. Surgical options for stress incontinence include periurethral bulking agents, transvaginal suspensions, slings, and sphincter prostheses. Patients with an obstructive disease (BPH or urethral stenosis) may also benefit from surgery.

In patients with intractable UI, a variety of absorbent pads, garments, and collection systems are available. The goal of these products is urine containment and prevention of skin breakdown. Pessaries should be tried in women with cystocele and uterine prolapse who will not consider surgery. Although urethral catheters should generally not be used, external collection devices (Texas catheters) are preferable to indwelling catheters in male patients who have not been helped by other measures. External devices are not widely available for women. If internal catheterization is necessary, an intermittent or suprapubic method is recommended to decrease bacteriuria. Indwelling catheters should be reserved for comfort in terminally ill patients, to prevent worsening of pressure ulcers, and for patients with inoperable outflow obstruction.

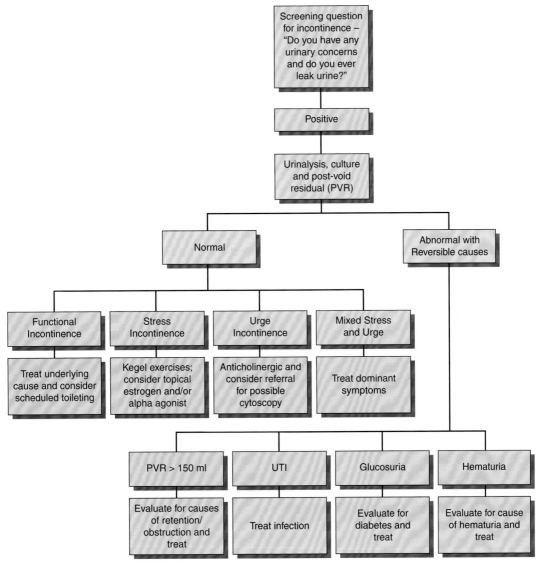

FIGURE 79-1. Evaluation of urinary incontinence. PVR, postvoid residual; UTI, urinary tract infection. (Source: Culligan PJ, Heit M. Urinary incontinence in women: evaluation and management. *Am Fam Physician*. 2000;62[11]:2433–2444.)

KEY POINTS

- Approximately one-third of community-dwelling elderly women and one-fourth of elderly men experience some degree of UI; the prevalence increases with age.

- Three basic mechanisms cause UI: overactivity of the bladder detrusor muscle (urge incontinence), malfunction of the urinary sphincters (stress incontinence), and overflow from the bladder (urinary retention).

- All patients should have a UA, which can detect infection—a common cause of reversible incontinence, uncontrolled diabetes, and hematuria, which suggests the need for further workup.

- PVRs of <75 mL are considered normal and levels of 75 to 150 mL borderline; levels >150 mL require further investigation.

- Treatment of UI consists of behavioral, pharmaceutical, and surgical intervention.

80 | Nursing Home and End-of-Life Care

Nursing homes (NHs) or long-term care (LTC) facilities are institutions that offer around the clock nursing care, as well as medical, social, and personal services to individuals unable to fully care for themselves or those who are in need of skilled rehabilitation to restore function. About one-half of women and one-third of men in the United States will spend some time in a NH before they die. NH admissions rise with age and increase rapidly after age 85.

NH residents are divided nearly evenly between short-term (<6 months) and long-term (>6 months) residents. Short-term residents are divided evenly by those admitted for rehabilitation and those admitted for terminal care. LTC residents typically have physical or cognitive impairments that make them unable to live in the community. Among LTC residents, the prevalence of mental disorders such as dementia, delirium, and mental illness approaches 90%.

COMMON MEDICAL PROBLEMS

Physicians caring for patients in NHs encounter several common problems repeatedly. Some degree of incontinence occurs in more than half of NH admissions and often precipitates admission. More than two-thirds of NH patients fall at least once a year, often with serious injury. Risk factors for falls include psychoactive drugs, overmedication, balance problems, weakness, poor functional status, and nutritional or vitamin D deficiency. Evidence indicates that physical therapy to increase strength and balance and treating vitamin D deficiency reduces the risk of falls.

Nutrition problems are common among NH residents, and weight is an important parameter to follow. Loss of more than 5 lb in 1 month or 10 lb in 6 months is considered significant. Underlying medical conditions common in LTC residents—such

as poor dentition, cancer, and movement disorders, and mechanical problems such as difficulty swallowing—can contribute to malnutrition. Poor nutrition impairs wound healing and the ability to mount an immune response, placing NH patients at greater risk for infection, pressure sores, and other significant problems. Aggressive dietary restrictions should be avoided when weight loss is an issue.

Infections in particular are a serious issue, and up to 15% of NH residents suffer from infection at any given time. Frequently encountered infections include pneumonia, UTI, infected pressure sores, and cellulitis. In addition to fever, infections in the LTC setting present with nonspecific symptoms, such as confusion, change in behavior, loss of appetite, weight loss, weakness, or lethargy. Medications can cause serious side effects. On average, LTC residents take more than eight medications. Medications should be monitored and periodically reviewed for their continued need. Reviewing the diagnosis, symptoms, and severity should be part of evaluating whether a medicine is appropriate, and dosages should be assessed and lowered whenever possible. Psychoactive and antipsychotic medications have a very high side-effect profile and their continued use needs regular reevaluation. Relevant symptoms require documentation, along with evidence that the treatment helps. Attempts to reduce dosages or eliminate psychoactive medications must be considered and documented. As a general rule, NH patients benefit more from reducing the number of medications than adding additional ones.

MONITORING CARE

The goal of the NH is to provide a safe and supportive environment for chronically ill and dependent individuals. Quality of life should be maximized and chronic conditions stabilized, with management directed at delaying the progression of disease and improving function. Each visit merits asking the patient about new complaints and asking the nurse about any changes in status.

A change in status should prompt an assessment for infections such as pneumonia or UTI, fecal impaction, or medication side effects. Symptoms relevant to existing conditions should be sought (e.g., edema and dyspnea in patients with CHF) and addressed when present, along with tests relevant to patients with chronic disease (e.g., blood sugars in patients with diabetes mellitus and electrolytes in patients with CHF). It is important to review nursing notes, to listen to patients, even if they are cognitively impaired, and to make sure patients are examined and touched.

The physical examination should include weight, vital signs, and a targeted examination to evaluate new complaints and to follow active conditions. The assessment should address the stability of active chronic conditions, new complaints, and/or changes in status. The plan should include a medication review, appropriate laboratory screens, testing, consultations, and other therapies that might benefit the patient. Yearly, a more detailed examination and functional assessment, including the MMSE, as well as testing vision and hearing, should be considered.

END OF LIFE

Many cognitively ill patients have lost the capacity for decision making. Advance directives made when the patient is competent allow his or her wishes to be honored and followed in the event the patient is no longer able to communicate these wishes. Despite the recent emphasis on advance directives, only about 15% of the general adult population has completed a directive of this type.

ADVANCE DIRECTIVES

In discussing advance directives, it is important to assure patients their clinical care will be consistent with their preferences. Shared decision making among the patient, his or her proxy, and the physician gives the proxy an opportunity to voice his or her concerns and to be aware of the patient's preferences.

Two common types of advance directives are a living will and health care power of attorney. A living will will contains information about the patient's wishes if the patient were to become incapable of communicating those wishes. The health care power of attorney appoints an individual or surrogate to act as the patient's medical decision maker if the patient should become incapable of making such decisions. Because conflict may develop between family members or the physician about what is in the patient's best interests, discussion in advance about resuscitation, invasive interventions, and enteral nutrition can decrease the stress of making a decision at a time of crisis.

HOSPICE

Hospice care is a type of care provided to patients whose life expectancy is 6 months or less. Hospice care may be provided at home or in an institutional setting such as an NH. Although traditionally associated with cancer care, hospice is appropriate for end-stage patients with conditions such as CHF, COPD, dementia, chronic renal failure, and failure to thrive (sarcopenia). Hospice provides all care related to the patient's terminal diagnosis without cost to the patient. This includes medications, skilled nursing visits, health care aides, counseling, and medical equipment.

Hospice care involves a multidisciplinary team that shifts the emphasis toward palliation, emphasizing symptomatic treatment and comfort measures. The management of pain and relief of symptoms is the primary concern. Special attention is paid to the patient's physical, emotional, and spiritual needs rather than trying to cure his or her illness or prolong life. Referrals to hospice may come from physicians, nurses, social workers, or patients' families. The patient's primary care physician may maintain care of the patient, though most hospices have a medical director who can assume care.

Most hospices use standing orders for the control of common symptoms. Pain is a common symptom in end-of-life care, and medications frequently used for pain control are oxycodone, morphine sulfate, and fentanyl patches. Dyspnea frequently occurs in end-stage CHF, COPD, cancer, and dementia. Opiates are the preferred medication for shortness of breath in end-of-life care. Low-flow oxygen may also be beneficial. Agitation and delirium are common and antipsychotics (risperidone, haloperidol) and anxiolytics (alprazolam) help control symptoms. Antiemetics commonly used include metoclopramide, prochlorperazine, and ondansetron. Many drugs, especially opioids, cause constipation. Useful agents for constipation include senna, docusate, and polyethylene glycol.

Increased secretions can be managed with atropine drops and scopolamine patches. When swallowing becomes an issue, many medications are available in concentrated forms and will be absorbed through the buccal mucosa.

KEY POINTS

- About one-half of women and one-third of men in the United States will spend some time in a NH before they die. NH admissions increase rapidly after age 85.

- Up to 15% of NH residents suffer from infection. Frequently encountered infections include pneumonia, UTI, infected pressure sores, and cellulitis.

- The goal of the NH is to provide a safe and supportive environment for chronically ill and dependent individuals.

- A change in status merits looking for infections such as pneumonia or UTI, fecal impaction, or medication side effects.

- A living will contains information about the patient's wishes if the patient was to become incapable of communicating those wishes; the health care power of attorney appoints an individual or surrogate to act as the patient's medical decision maker if the patient should become incapable of making such decisions.

- Hospice and palliative care are structured around a multidisciplinary team concept to provide end-of-life care for patients and support for caregivers.

CLINICAL VIGNETTES

VIGNETTE 1

An 80-year-old male with advanced dementia is being seen for a regular checkup. He has become nonambulatory and is less verbal than before. The family is challenged in caring for him and is looking at other options for care. He has no active medical issues, but has a history of hypertension for which he is on lisinopril. The family would like to review options in caring for their father with limited financial resources.

1. Which of the following options for living would be potentially covered with government funding?
   a. Nursing home
   b. Assisted living
   c. Staying home with a caregiver
   d. Apartment in a senior living facility
   e. Moving in with a family member

VIGNETTE 2

You are seeing a patient in your office who is asking about receiving hospice services for a family member.

1. Which of the following situations would generally be covered as a hospice patient?
   a. Congestive heart failure, NYHA class 2, edema
   b. Lung cancer, in remission
   c. Dementia, nonverbal, nonambulatory, dysphagia, weight loss
   d. Parkinson disease, slow ambulation, tremor
   e. COPD, chronic cough, O_2 at night, no edema

ANSWERS

VIGNETTE 1 Question 1

1. Answer A:

Funding for long-term care can occur through Medicaid for individuals living in a nursing home or long-term care facility provided the individual qualifies for aid. Assisted living and apartment living in a senior facility do not meet the same criteria as long-term care and are currently paid for by the individual or their family. Likewise, providing a caregiver or moving in with family is not a government-sponsored activity. A hardship often associated with a commitment to long-term care facilities and applying for Medicaid is the need to spend down personal resources before becoming eligible for Medicaid funding. This can lessen resources for surviving family members.

VIGNETTE 2 Question 1

1. Answer C:

Historically, hospice care has been linked as a resource to patients dying from cancer, and the association with other diseases is far more limited. Over time, hospice has been a service that has been expanded to virtually any diagnosis when the disease prognosis predicts a life expectancy of <6 months. This is difficult to predict, so criteria have been developed to define when in the course of various diseases a patient may be expected to have 6 months or less to live. End stage dementia occurs when the patient becomes nonambulatory, nonverbal, struggles to eat, and is losing weight. For the other diseases listed, the stage of the disease is too early for them to qualify for hospice services.

81 | Analgesics: Nonsteroidal Anti-inflammatory and Opioid Medications

NONSTEROIDAL ANTI-INFLAMMATORY DRUGS (NSAIDS)

GENERAL INFORMATION

NSAIDs were first discovered when humans learned that applying plants such as willow bark to their skin decreased pain and swelling. NSAIDs are among the most commonly used drugs in the United States with more than 30 billion OTC tablets sold annually. Over 60 million Americans use NSAIDs regularly, and ~70% of people 65 years or older take NSAIDs at least once per week.

THERAPEUTIC EFFECTS

The three most common indications for NSAIDs are pain, inflammation, and fever. NSAIDs work by blocking COX enzymes and inhibiting the synthesis of prostaglandins that are part of the signaling pathway for pain, inflammation, and fever. Traditional nonselective NSAIDs inhibit two COX enzyme isoforms, COX-1 and COX-2.

Prostaglandins also protect the gastric and duodenal mucosal surface, maintain renal blood flow, and enhance platelet aggregation. By inhibiting both COX-1 and COX-2, nonselective NSAIDs can cause adverse GI and renal effects. Celecoxib (Celebrex), which blocks only the COX-2 enzyme, is less likely to damage the stomach. However, COX-2 inhibitors do not offer a benefit over the traditional NSAIDs for other adverse effects, and one COX-2 inhibitor, rofecoxib, was taken off the market due to cardiovascular (CV) safety concerns.

SIDE EFFECTS

Common side effects from NSAIDs include edema, hypertension, fluid retention, epigastric pain, heartburn, nausea, abdominal pain, dyspepsia, and tinnitus. GI side effects are the most common, and NSAIDs should always be taken with food and a glass of water to help prevent these side effects. Some uncommon but serious side effects include renal failure, bronchospasm, gastric or duodenal ulcer, gastritis, GI hemorrhage, GI perforation, and Stevens–Johnson syndrome.

In the United States, NSAIDs carry black box warnings for adverse cardiac effects and serious adverse GI reactions. NSAIDs increase the risk of cardiovascular thrombotic events, myocardial infarction, and stroke. One strategy to avoid complications is to use the lowest effective dose for the shortest duration and to monitor patients for adverse effects such as increased blood pressure and fluid retention. Both nonselective and COX-2 selective NSAIDs increase the risk of adverse CV events, and while naproxen was once thought to be less likely to cause CV events, a large metaanalysis recently showed that naproxen, celecoxib, and ibuprofen all have similar risks for CV and renal complications. CV risks increase with dose and duration of use, and providers should avoid prescribing celecoxib at doses ≥ 200 mg/day in high-risk CV patients. Because of their risk profile, in diseases such as osteoarthritis where the anti-inflammatory effects of NSAIDs are not considered critical, acetaminophen should be considered as a safer alternative.

NSAIDs also increase the risk of GI bleeding, ulceration, and gastric inflammation, especially in elderly patients or those with a history of peptic ulcer disease, GI bleeding, coagulopathies, smoking, or alcohol use. Providers should use caution when prescribing NSAIDs to patients at increased risk for GI adverse events and consider prescribing a proton pump inhibitor (PPI) in high-risk patients. Concurrent therapy with a PPI is superior to adding either an H_2 blocker or misoprostol. In addition, when NSAIDs and aspirin are combined, gastroprotective therapy should be considered. NSAIDs are contraindicated in patients with active GI bleeding.

Although more expensive, celecoxib, a selective COX-2 inhibitor, is less likely to cause GI side effects. It is not recommended as first-line therapy, but should be considered in patients at high risk for bleeding and for those who fail to tolerate nonselective NSAIDs.

INTERACTIONS

Long-term use of NSAIDs with angiotensin-converting enzyme (ACE) inhibitors can increase the adverse effects of NSAIDs, and may also cause a significant decrease in renal function. Using NSAIDs in conjunction with antihypertensive agents may decrease their effectiveness. NSAIDs reversibly inhibit COX in platelets and may lower the cardioprotective effects of aspirin.

In addition to the black box warning for CV events, NSAIDs also increase the risk of exacerbating heart failure by causing sodium and fluid retention. Patients with an acute kidney injury should not take NSAIDs, and the use of NSAIDs in patients with chronic renal impairment should be monitored closely for adverse effects. The risk for renal injury is greatest in those likely to have poor renal perfusion (e.g., dehydration), liver or cardiac failure, advanced age, or those who take potent diuretics.

SPECIFIC MEDICATIONS

Table 81.1 describes some common NSAIDs available through prescription.

TABLE 81.1. Overview of Nonsteroidal Anti-inflammatory Drugs

Generic (Brand)	OTC/RX	Typical Dose	Renal Dosing[a]	Comments
Diclofenac (Voltaren)	RX	25 mg PO Q 6 hours 50 mg Q 8 hours (max: 150 mg)	• Mild/moderate: no dosage adjustment necessary • Significant or advanced: use is not recommended	• Administer with food to reduce GI upset
Etodolac	RX	IR: 200–400 mg Q 6–8 hours (max: 1000 mg) ER: 400–1000 mg once daily	• CrCl > 88 mL/min: no dosage adjustment necessary • CrCl 37–88 mL/min: no dosage adjustment necessary, however use with caution • CrCl < 37 mL/min: if use must be initiated, use with caution	• COX-2 selective at total daily dose of 600–800 mg • Etodolac 200 mg ≈ Ibuprofen 400 mg
Ibuprofen (Advil, Motrin)	OTC, RX	RX: 400 mg Q 4–6 hours; 800 mg Q 8 hours (max: 3200 mg) OTC: 200–400 mg Q 4–6 hours (max: 1200 mg)	• Mild/moderate: use with caution • Significant or advanced: not recommended	• tid dosing may cause decreased compliance • May have increased risk of renal failure
Indomethacin (Indocin)	RX	IR: 25–50 mg Q 6–8 hours (max: 150 mg) ER: 75 mg once to twice daily	• Mild/moderate: use with caution • Significant or advanced: not recommended	• Daily doses >150–200 mg have increased adverse effects with no increase in clinical benefits • Potent effect on renal prostaglandin synthesis

(continued)

TABLE 81.1. Overview of Nonsteroidal Anti-inflammatory Drugs (*continued*)

Generic (Brand)	OTC/RX	Typical Dose	Renal Dosing[a]	Comments
Ketoprofen	RX	IR: 50 mg Q 6–8 hours ER: 200 mg/day	• Mild: max dose 150 mg/day • Severe (GFR < 25 mL/min/1.73 m^2): max dose 100 mg/day	• Maximum daily dose based on renal impairment and hepatic impairment. • Ketoprofen 25 mg ≈ Ibuprofen 400 mg
Ketorolac	RX	IV/IM: 15–30 mg Q 6 hours (max: 120 mg/day) PO: 10 mg Q 4–6 hours (max: 40 mg/day)	• Mild/moderate: IV/IM: 15 mg Q 6 hours max 60 mg/day • PO: 10 mg Q 6 hours max: 40 mg/day • Advanced renal disease: use is contraindicated	• Total use should not exceed 5 days • Maximum dose based on weight, age, and renal function
Meloxicam (Mobic)	RX	5–7.5 mg PO once daily	• CrCl ≥ 20 mL/min: no dosage adjustment needed • CrCl < 20 mL/min: not studied; not recommended	• Maximum dose based upon indication and age • Long duration of effect, slow onset • COX-2 selective at daily doses of ≤7.5 mg
Naproxen (Aleve, Anaprox)	OTC, RX	*Base:* 250 mg Q 6–8 hours 500 mg Q 12 hours *Sodium:* 275 mg Q 6–8 hours 550 mg Q 12 hours	• CrCl ≥ 30–60 mL/min: use with caution • CrCl < 30 mL/min: not recommended • Advanced renal disease: avoid	• Naproxen base 200 mg, i.e., Naproxen sodium 220 mg • Sodium salt (Anaprox) is more rapidly absorbed and recommended for acute pain • Longer duration of action than ibuprofen
Celecoxib (Celebrex)	RX	100–200 mg once or twice daily	• Mild/moderate: no dosage adjustments provided • Severe: use is not recommended	• Dose adjusted for moderate hepatic impairment (Child-Pugh class B). Reduce dose 50% • COX-2 inhibition only: reduction in GI toxicity compared with a nonselective NSAID

Take NSAIDS with food or milk if GI disturbance occurs or to avoid GI adverse effects.

[a]KDIGO 2012 guidelines provide the following guidance for dosing NSAIDs in renal impairment:

eGFR 30 to <60 mL/min/1.73 m^2: Temporarily discontinue in patients with intercurrent disease that increases risk of acute kidney injury.

eGFR < 30 mL/min/1.73 m^2: Avoid use.

COX-2, cyclooxygenase-2; CrCl, creatine clearance; ER, extended release; IM, intramuscular; IR, immediate release; IV, intravenous; NSAID, nonsteroidal anti-inflammatory drug; OTC, over-the-counter; RX, prescription required.

CLINICAL COMMENTARY

NSAIDs are effective for acute or chronic pain, inflammation, and fever. NSAIDs also decrease opioid requirements in patients on chronic pain management. Although the efficacy of the different NSAIDs is similar at equipotent doses, individual patients exhibit a wide variability in response to an agent. Asking about past response to a specific NSAID can guide the initial choice of an agent. If a patient fails to respond to an NSAID within 2 to 4 weeks, switching to one with a different chemical structure may be effective. Since NSAIDs share the same mechanism of action, there is no therapeutic advantage to combining two different NSAIDs. Although useful for pain, there is no evidence that their anti-inflammatory effects alter the course of musculoskeletal disease.

Chronic NSAID use requires periodically monitoring kidney function, complete blood counts, and liver function tests. In patients with hypertension, NSAIDs may increase blood pressure and decrease the effectiveness of antihypertensive agents. Specifically asking about OTC NSAID use in individuals with poorly controlled hypertension is important, because patients may fail to consider an OTC medicine when asked what medications they are taking.

The widespread use of NSAIDs leads many providers to overlook their hazards. Conservative estimates suggest that each year more than 100,000 patients are hospitalized for NSAID-related GI complications with approximately 16,500 NSAID-related deaths. Providers should carefully monitor patients with comorbid conditions that put them at increased risk for adverse NSAID effects, such as individuals with heart failure, diabetes, alcoholism, renal impairment, and acute myocardial infarction. Patients with a history of GI bleed, ulcer, gastritis, or other GI complication should be educated about the risk of taking any NSAID medication, and consultation with a gastroenterologist should be considered for those at highest risk.

OPIOIDS

GENERAL INFORMATION

Opioids are the most potent analgesics available with the broadest range of efficacy. Thousands of years ago, poppy plants were discovered to have analgesic and psychological effects. Natural, synthetic, and semisynthetic opioids are available for the treatment of acute and chronic nociceptive pain management. Although their effectiveness makes opioids the preferred treatment for moderate to severe cancer pain, their side-effect profile and potential for abuse merit cautious use in the setting of chronic nonmalignant pain.

THERAPEUTIC EFFECTS

Opioids produce their effects by binding to central and peripheral mu, kappa, and delta opioid receptors located in the brain, spinal cord, and smooth muscle cells, respectively. When an agonist binds to these receptors, it decreases nociceptive neurotransmission and thereby decreases the perception of pain. The activity, classification, and side effects of opioid analgesics are based on their relative affinity for these three receptors and where these receptors are located in the body (centrally or peripherally). Opioid analgesics are divided into three types: full agonists, mixed agonist-antagonists, or partial agonists.

Mu receptor activation is the most prominent receptor for producing the effects of opioid medications. Because of genetic variation and expression of these receptors, the potency of opioids and their clinical effectiveness can vary widely between patients.

SIDE EFFECTS

Opioids can cause nausea, vomiting, constipation, drowsiness, sedation, dizziness, dysphoria, euphoria, dry mouth, sweating, pruritus, skin rashes, urinary retention, bradycardia, and hypotension. Patients on opiates should be monitored for level of pain relief, GI side effects, especially constipation, respiratory status, sedation, mental status, blood pressure, and heart rate. Tolerance develops to most side effects except constipation. For patients taking opiates chronically, a bowel regimen including a laxative is recommended to prevent constipation.

Table 81.2 describes some approaches to avoid or limit the adverse effects of opioid analgesics.

Opioids carry a black box warning for their abuse potential and caution is needed when managing pain with opiates. Patients with increased risk of opioid misuse should be monitored closely for signs of misuse, abuse, and addiction. Risk factors for abuse or misuse include the following: personal or family history of substance abuse (e.g., alcohol, drug), mental illness (e.g., depression), history of overdose, multiple prescribers/prescriptions, prolonged use, longer-acting opioids, younger age, high average daily opioid dosages (≥50 mg morphine equivalents per day), and concomitant benzodiazepine or psychotropic medication use.

TABLE 81.2. Management Strategies of Opioid Adverse Effects

Adverse Effect	Preventative or Treatment Measures
Nausea/Vomiting	• Subsides over time • Antiemetic prn (metoclopramide, ondansetron)
Itching	• Switch agent • Diphenhydramine prn
Constipation	• Encourage physical activity and adequate hydration • Bowel regimen: stool softener PLUS stimulant (docusate + senna) • Does not usually decrease over time (no tolerance to this effect)
Sedation	• Monitor sedation and respiratory rate • Avoid concurrent sedative medications (BZD) • Decrease dose, withhold, or change opioid
Respiratory depression	• Avoid with other CNS depressants (alcohol, BZD) • Reverse with opioid reversal agent (naloxone)

BZD, benzodiazepine; CNS, central nervous system; prn, as needed.

INTERACTIONS

When combined with CNS depressants opioids synergistically cause CNS depression, and their concomitant use with benzodiazepines, alcohol, sedative hypnotics, tricyclic antidepressants, and anticonvulsants should be avoided. If combined opioid and CNS depressant therapy is necessary, start at a lower opioid dose and titrate slowly while monitoring for adverse effects such as sedation or respiratory depression.

SPECIFIC MEDICATIONS

Table 81.3 presents an overview of select opioid medications available in the United States.

CLINICAL COMMENTARY

It is not possible to predict the optimal opioid and dosing regimen for a given patient. Therefore, opioid treatment should be individualized, taking into account the type and severity of pain, route of administration, pharmacokinetics, pharmacodynamics, analgesic

TABLE 81.3. Overview of Select Opioid Medications

Generic (Brand)	Equianalgesic (Adults) PO	Equianalgesic (Adults) IV	Onset (minute)	Half Life (hour)	Comments
Codeine	200 mg	NA	10–20	3	• Do not use in children • Metabolized by CYP2D6 to morphine • Do not use in renal or hepatic dysfunction
Fentanyl (Duragesic, Sublimaze, Actiq)	NA	0.1 mg	7–15	3–4	• Metabolized by CYP3A4 • Do not use transdermal in acute pain • Transmucosal, intranasal, sublingual only available via REMS programs
Hydrocodone (Lortab, Vicodin)	30 mg	N/A	30–60	4	• Metabolized CYP2D6, 3A4 • Caution in renal impairment • Caution in hepatic dysfunction
Hydromorphone (Dilaudid)	7.5 mg	1.5 mg	10–20	2–3	• Caution in renal impairment • Caution in hepatic dysfunction

TABLE 81.3. Overview of Select Opioid Medications (*continued*)

Generic (Brand)	Equianalgesic (Adults)		Onset (minute)	Half Life (hour)	Comments
	PO	**IV**			
Methadone (Dolophine)	NA	NA	30–60	8–130	• Metabolized CYP3A4 • Monitor for sedation because of risk for accumulation and long half life • Avoid dose changes <every 2 weeks • Monitor corrected QT interval (QTc) • Not advised in hepatic dysfunction due to variable pharmacokinetics
Morphine	30 mg	10 mg	10–20	2–4	• Metabolized via glucuronidation to active metabolites • Caution in hepatic dysfunction • Active metabolites undergo renal elimination • Caution in renal impairment
Oxycodone (OxyContin, Roxicodone)	20 mg	NA	30–60	2–3	• Metabolized CYP2D6, 3A4 • Metabolized to oxymorphone • Caution in renal impairment • Caution in hepatic dysfunction
Oxymorphone (Opana)	10 mg	1 mg	10–20	2	• Caution in hepatic dysfunction
Tramadol (Ultram)	NA	NA	<60	5–7	• Dose adjust in renal impairment • Binds to mu opiate receptors • Inhibits norepinephrine/serotonin reuptake • Seizure risk: particularly in patients who take antidepressants, neuroleptics, or other drugs that decrease the seizure threshold

IV, intravenous; PO, by mouth; REMS, risk evaluation and mitigation strategy.

effectiveness, side effects, cost, and patient acceptance, other adjuvant analgesic treatments, opioid tolerance (e.g., opioid-naive), comorbid conditions, concurrent medications, and risk of abuse or misuse. Caution should be taken in patients with hepatic or renal impairment because several opioids are metabolized or cleared by each organ respectively. In renal insufficiency, morphine and codeine should be avoided because of the risk of accumulating active metabolites that are renally cleared. Methadone and fentanyl do not have active metabolites and can be used more safely in patients with kidney disease. Meperidine should be avoided because its metabolites can be neurotoxic.

Tramadol is a weak mu agonist and an inhibitor of norepinephrine and serotonin, a quality that gives it a niche in the treatment of neuropathic and radicular pain. Codeine is a prodrug that needs to be converted to morphine to be effective and about 10% of patients lack this enzyme. Doses above 60 mg saturate the enzymes converting codeine, and codeine doses beyond this level do not increase pain relief. Mu agonists have no ceiling effect and doses may be titrated upward until pain is controlled or side effects limit dosing.

Typically, providers should start opioid-naive patients on immediate-release products because extended-release and long-acting opioid medications increase the risk of adverse effects or overdose. Combination products including an opioid and a nonopioid (e.g., hydrocodone/acetaminophen) are of special concern because of the additional risk of overdose with the nonopioid component since many OTC products have similar medications in them (e.g., acetaminophen). Acetaminophen overdose can lead to permanent hepatotoxicity, and the daily dose should not exceed 4 g in healthy adults or more than 3 g in older individuals.

Acute management of pain with opioids should use the lowest effective doses for the shortest duration of treatment. Providers should avoid opioids for treatment of nonmalignant chronic pain due to unknown long-term benefits and an association of serious risks such as overdose and opioid use disorder. When providers prescribe opioids for chronic pain management, they should reevaluate the patient repeatedly for abuse potential, efficacy of therapy, adverse effects, treatment goals, and the need for continued therapy. When discontinuing long-term opioid therapy, the opioid should be discontinued slowly and titrated downward instead of abruptly stopping to avoid withdrawal symptoms.

82 | Antibiotics

PENICILLINS

GENERAL INFORMATION

First discovered in the late 1920s, penicillin remains useful for treating several types of infections encountered in a typical family medicine practice. The penicillins include a broad range of antibiotics characterized by a beta-lactam ring and a shared mechanism of action.

THERAPEUTIC EFFECTS

Penicillins work by binding to penicillin-binding proteins on the bacterial cell wall and inhibiting bacterial wall synthesis. Penicillins can be divided into subclasses: the natural penicillins (penicillin V potassium, penicillin G), the antistaphylococcal penicillins (nafcillin, dicloxacillin), the aminopenicillins (amoxicillin, amoxicillin clavulanate), and the extended-spectrum penicillins (piperacillin/tazobactam, ticarcillin clavulanate). The subclasses differ in their antimicrobial activity and pharmacokinetic properties. Penicillins exhibit bactericidal activity and time-dependent killing with the exception of the Enterococcus species, where penicillins must be combined with an aminoglycoside to demonstrate bactericidal activity. The natural penicillins are mainly active against gram-positive cocci, oral anaerobes, and some spirochetes. They have little gram-negative activity, and, with the exception of the antistaphylococcal penicillins, are not active again most strains of *Staphylococcus aureus*. The antistaphylococcal penicillins (e.g., dicloxacillin) are resistant to staphylococcal penicillinase-mediated resistance and are primarily used to treat methicillin-susceptible staphylococcal infections. The aminopenicillins have a broader spectrum of activity and provide additional gram-negative activity against Haemophilus, Neisseria, *Escherichia coli*, Proteus,

and Klebsiella. The addition of a beta-lactamase inhibitor (clavulanate) increases activity against gram-negative aerobes, gram-negative anaerobes, including *Bacteroides fragilis* and some resistant strains of methicillin-susceptible *S. aureus*. The extended-spectrum penicillins have expanded gram-negative coverage, but are rarely used in outpatient clinic settings. No penicillin subclass is active against atypical organisms.

SIDE EFFECTS

Common side effects include GI disturbances such as nausea, vomiting, and diarrhea. All penicillins have the risk of producing a hypersensitivity reaction that ranges from a mild rash to acute interstitial nephritis or anaphylaxis. The incidence of an IgE-mediated anaphylactic reaction is low (0.01% to 0.05%), but 5% to 10% of those reactions can be fatal. An allergy to any penicillin subclass should be considered as an allergy to all other subclasses. Other class side effects include increased transaminases, myelosuppression with prolonged use, and seizures especially in renal failure where serum levels can accumulate. A nonallergic rash occurs in about 5% to 10% of children taking either amoxicillin or ampicillin and is not a true allergy to penicillin. The rash is characterized by small pink or red flat spots in a symmetrical pattern that usually appear around days 5 to 7 after starting amoxicillin, although it can occur any time while on the medication. Usually, it does not itch and resolves in a few days. The rash reappears in about 5% of children with future doses of amoxicillin.

INTERACTIONS

Penicillins can increase the serum concentrations of methotrexate and decrease the serum concentrations of the active metabolite of mycophenolate, an immunosuppressant. The uricosuric agent probenecid can increase the serum levels of the penicillins by interfering with their renal excretion. Because penicillin works best against actively dividing bacteria, bacteriostatic antimicrobials such as tetracyclines can reduce the effectiveness of penicillin. Most penicillins, with the exception of dicloxacillin, increase the anticoagulant effects of warfarin.

SPECIFIC MEDICATIONS

Table 82-1 provides an overview of select penicillin antibiotics.

TABLE 82-1. Overview of Select Penicillin Antibiotics

Generic	Cost	Formulation	Dosing[a]	Half-Life	Comments
Penicillin VK	$	Tablet, suspension	125–500 mg PO Q 6–12 hours	30 minutes	• Adjust dose for kidney disease • Half-life 10 hours in anuric patients • Indications: upper respiratory tract infections, prophylaxis of rheumatic fever, mild erysipelas, and mild streptococcal infections • Commonly used to treat oropharyngeal infections • Warfarin: increased INR
Penicillin G Benzathine	$$	IM injection	1.2–2.4 million units IM × 1 (frequency varies)	30 minutes	• Do not administer IV; can cause death • Half-life 10 hours in anuric patients • Indications: syphilis, upper respiratory tract infections • STD: drug of choice for syphilis; *Neisseria gonorrheae* resistance common and no longer drug of choice • Warfarin: increased INR
Amoxicillin	$	Tablet, capsule, chewable, suspension	250–500 mg PO Q 8 hours 500–875 mg PO Q 12 hours Amoxicillin XR 775 mg PO daily	0.7–1.4 hours	• Susceptible to penicillinases • Indications: Pharyngitis, otitis media, rhinosinusitis, urinary tract infections, *H. pylori* infections, community-acquired pneumonia, skin and skin structure infections • Drug of choice for acute otitis media depending on local resistance patterns and useful as a component of an *H. pylori* regimen, and as prophylaxis for endocarditis • Active against enterococci, *Listeria monocytogenes*, *E. coli*, *P. mirabilis*, *H. influenza*, and *M. catarrhalis* • Warfarin: increased INR

TABLE 82-1. Overview of Select Penicillin Antibiotics (*continued*)

Generic	Cost	Formulation	Dosing*a*	Half-Life	Comments
Amoxicillin clavulanate	$$–$$$	Tablet, chewable, suspension	500 mg PO tid 875 mg PO bid Amoxicillin clavulanate XR 2000 mg PO bid	0.7–1.4 hours	• Indications: Community-acquired pneumonia, otitis media, rhinosinusitis, skin and skin structure infections, urinary tract infections, diabetic foot, pharyngitis, intra-abdominal infections • Coverage for enterococci, *L. monocytogenes, E. coli, P. mirabilis, H. influenza,* and *M. catarrhalis* • Coverage for beta-lactamase producers and anaerobes • Caution in cholestatic jaundice or hepatic dysfunction with previous use • Warfarin: increased INR
Dicloxacillin	$	Capsule	125–500 mg PO Q 6 hours	0.7 hours	• Treats infections caused by methicillin-sensitive *S. aureus* • No activity against gram-negative organisms • Dicloxacillin can decrease the INR (competition for metabolism) • Skin and soft tissue infections, bite wounds, impetigo

*a*Renal dosage adjustment recommended.

INR, international normalized ratio; IM, intramuscular; IV, intravenous; PO, by mouth; tid, thrice daily; STD, sexually transmitted disease.

CLINICAL COMMENTARY

The penicillins can be used for a broad range of infections ranging from UTIs to meningitis (see Table 82-1). Their low index of side effects often makes them the treatment of choice for sensitive bacterial infections. However, their penicillin susceptibility to beta-lactamases and other forms of resistance make it necessary to examine community resistance patterns when considering empiric antimicrobial therapy. For example, amoxicillin is a drug of choice for nonallergic patients with otitis media. However, if resistance patterns indicate an increased community resistance (>20%) to *Haemophilus influenzae*, then amoxicillin clavulanate may be a better option for empiric therapy. Patients should always be advised to monitor their symptoms for improvement, and if an infection is not responding or worsening, then alternative causative organisms or antibiotic resistance should be considered. Patients should be instructed to take oral penicillins (amoxicillin being an exception) 1 to 2 hours before or after a meal to avoid gastric acid degradation.

CEPHALOSPORINS

GENERAL INFORMATION

Cephalosporins are a member of the class of antibiotics known as beta-lactams and share a mechanism of action and structure similar to penicillin. Generally, organisms sensitive to penicillin are susceptible to cephalosporins. For convenience, cephalosporins are typically grouped by generations with each generation containing drugs with similar characteristics and microbial activity. However, not all experts agree with this classification system because drugs in the same generation may be chemically distinct and differ in spectrum of activity. Cephalosporins, as a class, lack activity against methicillin-resistant *S. aureus* (MRSA), enterococci, Listeria, Mycoplasma, Chlamydia, and Campylobacter. Their safety and broad spectrum of activity make cephalosporins among the most widely prescribed class of antibiotics.

Although there are currently five generations, only the first three generations of cephalosporins are commonly used in the outpatient setting (see Table 82-2). First-generation cephalosporins have good coverage against gram-positive organisms, and as the cephalosporin generations progress, they typically demonstrate increased activity against gram-negative, resistant, and anaerobic organisms but retain less gram-positive activity. In selecting a cephalosporin, the antimicrobial therapy spectrum of activity should be considered along with local resistance patterns. Package inserts for the first three generations of cephalosporins list these medications as pregnancy category B. Providers should also weigh risk versus benefit for nursing mothers because cephalosporins can cross into breast milk. In most cases, both pediatric and adult formulations are readily available.

THERAPEUTIC EFFECTS

Similar to other beta-lactam antibiotics, cephalosporins are bactericidal and exert their antimicrobial effect by attaching to penicillin-binding proteins in the cell wall and interfering with cell wall synthesis. Cephalosporins are less susceptible to beta-lactamase (an enzyme produced by some microbes resulting in resistance to beta-lactam antibiotics) than the penicillins. They are used in a wide variety of infections with good penetration into many tissues.

As noted above, indications for use of cephalosporins vary by generation but generally include the following and are specified, by drug, in Table 82-2:

1. Upper respiratory tract infections
2. Lower respiratory tract infections
3. Skin/skin structure/cellulitis
4. UTIs
5. Joint/bone infections (prosthetic)/prophylaxis
6. Endocarditis prophylaxis
7. Otitis media
8. Sexually transmitted disease
9. CNS infections

SIDE EFFECTS

Cephalosporins are well tolerated with few side effects. GI side effects are the most common and include nausea, vomiting, diarrhea, and dyspepsia. Like other broad-spectrum antibiotics, they can cause an overgrowth of fungus, and it is not uncommon for patients on cephalosporins to develop candida vaginitis or thrush. Less common side effects are anaphylaxis, interstitial nephritis, and rash. Rare but serious dermatologic disorders such as toxic epidermal necrolysis and Stevens–Johnson syndrome have also been reported. Other serious reactions include blood disorders and *Clostridium difficile* diarrhea. Clinical trials data and postmarketing surveillance implicate cephalosporins in seizures, particularly in patients with poor renal function. Providers should adjust the cephalosporin dose based on the patient's estimated creatinine clearance (CrCl). Although an allergy to other beta-lactam antibiotics such as penicillin increases the likelihood of a cephalosporin allergy, the risk of cross-reactivity is often overestimated and may only be about 1%. Unless the patient experienced a life-threatening anaphylactic reaction to penicillin, patients reporting a penicillin allergy can usually be prescribed a cephalosporin when indicated.

INTERACTIONS

Like other antibiotics, cephalosporin administration can potentially lead to *C. difficile* diarrhea, and this risk increases when using it in combination with a PPI. Providers should consider risk versus benefit when these two agents are coadministered. H_2 antagonists and PPIs also may reduce the absorption of oral cephalosporins

Probenecid impairs renal excretion of cephalosporins resulting in increased drug plasma levels. Cephalosporins, can also decrease levels of oral contraceptives by altering intestinal flora. While there is little evidence that antibiotics reduce the effectiveness of oral contraceptive, some providers recommend that women add a backup contraceptive method for that month to reduce the risk of unwanted pregnancy.

CLINICAL COMMENTARY
First-Generation Cephalosporins

First-generation cephalosporins include cephalexin and cefazolin and are effective against sensitive species of *S. aureus* and group A streptococcus. Some species of gram-negative organisms such as *Proteus mirabilis*, *Klebsiella*, and *E. coli* are also covered by

TABLE 82-2. Overview of Select Cephalosporins

Generic (Brand)	Cost	Dose[a], Range, Route, Frequency	Duration (Not specific for all indications)	Dosage Form	Typical Indications (See text listing indications on page 380)	Comments
First Generation						
Cefadroxil (Duricef)	$$	500–2000 mg PO Q 12 or 24 hours	5–10 days	Tablet, capsule, suspension	1, 3, 4, 5	• With or without food • Pediatric doses 30 mg/kg/day • Can decrease effectiveness of birth control • INR may increase when used with warfarin
Cephalexin (Keflex)	$	250–2000 mg PO Q 6–12 hours	5–10 days	Tablet, capsule, suspension	1, 2, 3, 4, 5, 6	• With or without food • Maximum dose 4 g • Pediatric doses 25–50 mg/kg/day • CrCl 30–50 mL/min, daily maximum dose of 1000 mg • Hypoglycemia may occur with metformin use
Second Generation						
Cefaclor (Ceclor, Biocef, Medacef, Keflor, Distaclor, Raniclor)	$$	250–500 mg PO Q 8–12 hours	7–10 days	Tablet, capsule, suspension	1, 2, 3, 4, 7	
Cefprozil (Cefzil)	$$–$$$	250–500 mg PO Q 12–24 hours	7–10 days	Tablet, suspension	1, 2, 3, 7	• With or without food • Pediatric doses range from 7.5 mg/kg/dose to 20 mg/kg/dose • CrCl < 50 mL/min, decrease dose to 50% of the usual dose given every 12 hours • Can decrease effectiveness of birth control, increase renal toxicity with loops, increase INR with warfarin
Cefuroxime (Ceftin, Zinacef)	$$	250–1500 mg IV/IM/PO Q 8–12 hours	7–10 days	Tablet, suspension, injectable	1, 2, 3, 4, 5, 6, 7	• Administer with food • Crosses blood–brain barrier • Pediatric doses range from 20 mg/kg/day to 30 mg/kg/day • Suspension is less bioavailable than the tablet • Can decrease effectiveness of birth control, increase renal toxicity with loops, increase INR with warfarin • Quinapril and antacids containing aluminum hydroxide, calcium, or magnesium, proton pump inhibitors, and H$_2$ antagonists can decrease GI absorption

(continued)

TABLE 82-2. Overview of Select Cephalosporins (*continued*)

Generic (Brand)	Cost	Dose[a], Range, Route, Frequency	Duration (Not specific for all indications)	Dosage Form	Typical Indications (See text listing indications on page 380)	Comments
Third Generation						
Cefdinir (Omnicef)	$$–$$$	300–600 mg PO Q 12–24 hours	5–10 days	Capsule, suspension	1, 2, 3, 7	• With or without food • Administer 2 hours before or 1 hour after antacids or iron products • Pediatric dosing for infants ≥ 6 months of age is 7 mg/kg/dose • Can decrease effectiveness of birth control, increase renal toxicity with loop diuretics, increase INR with warfarin • Vitamins, iron, antacids containing aluminum hydroxide, calcium, or magnesium, proton pump inhibitors, and H_2 antagonists can decrease GI absorption
Cefixime (Suprax)	$$	400 mg PO Q 24–12 hours	7–14 days	Tablet, capsule, suspension	1, 4	
Cefpodoxime (Vantin)	$$–$$$	100–200 mg PO Q 12 hours	5–10 days	Tablet, suspension	1, 2, 3, 4	
Ceftriaxone (Rocephin)	$$–$$$	250–2000 mg IV/IM Q 12–24 hours	7–10 days	Injectable	1, 2, 3, 4, 5, 6, 7, 8, 9	• Reconstitute using sterile water for injection, normal saline, or 1% lidocaine for IM administration • Elimination is extended with renal impairment, no dosage adjustment is necessary • Pediatric dosing 50–75 mg/kg/day • Maximal dose of 4000 mg daily (adult) • Calcium interaction: formation of crystals that can lodge in the lungs and kidneys/fatalities reported in infants. Separate by 48 hours • Can decrease effectiveness of birth control, increase renal toxicity with loops, increase INR with warfarin • May increase effects of some calcium channel blockers • Can cause eosinophilia and changes in LFTs and platelets

[a]Adjustments may be necessary for patients with reduced renal function.

CrCl, creatinine clearance; INR, international normalized ratio; IM, intramuscular; IV, intravenous; LFTs, liver function tests; PO, by mouth.

this generation. First-generation cephalosporins are commonly used for uncomplicated skin and soft-tissue infections, which usually are due to staphylococci and streptococci. They are also effective for uncomplicated urinary infections from susceptible organisms and for streptococcal pharyngitis, but are not indicated for otitis media because of *H. influenza* resistance.

Second-Generation Cephalosporins

Second-generation cephalosporins maintain gram-positive activity, and cefprozil and cefuroxime are active against *Streptococcus pneumoniae*. Coverage for gram-negative organisms is enhanced with added susceptibility for many strains of *H. influenza*, *Moraxella catarrhalis*, and *Neisseria* species; some strains of anaerobic microorganisms are also covered. Their enhanced gram-negative coverage makes these drugs useful for respiratory infections. *B. fragilis* is resistant to oral second-generation cephalosporins. These agents are also clinically effective and considered safe for use to treat UTIs in pregnancy.

Third-Generation Cephalosporins

Most third-generation cephalosporins maintain some gram-positive coverage (product specific), and have enhanced activity against resistant pneumococci compared to first- and second-generation products. They have a wider spectrum of activity against gram-negative organisms, including some *Enterobacter*, *Citrobacter*, *Salmonella*, and *Klebsiella* species. Although more commonly used in the inpatient setting, third-generation cephalosporins can be useful for treating resistant cases of otitis media, UTIs, and uncomplicated gonorrhea. However, their use should be avoided whenever a narrower spectrum antibiotic would be effective.

FLUOROQUINOLONES

GENERAL INFORMATION

Fluoroquinolones are among the most commonly prescribed antibiotics and have a broad spectrum of activity. Commonly prescribed quinolones available in the United States include ciprofloxacin, levofloxacin, ofloxacin, norfloxacin, and moxifloxacin.

THERAPEUTIC EFFECTS

Fluoroquinolones (quinolones) are a class of bactericidal antibiotics unique in their mechanism of action. They target bacterial DNA gyrase (also known as topoisomerase II) as well as topoisomerase IV, which are enzymes involved in the separation of double-stranded DNA required for cellular replication

and DNA damage repair. Most quinolones are available in both oral and IV formulations. However, because the use of broad-spectrum antibiotics encourages the development of resistant bacteria as well as *C. difficile* infections, new guidelines recommend avoiding the use of fluoroquinolones for less severe infections such as acute bacterial sinusitis, acute exacerbation of chronic bronchitis, and uncomplicated UTIs. In addition, prescribing is discouraged for infections where risk factors for multidrug resistance are not present.

SIDE EFFECTS

Although usually well tolerated, quinolones have recently lost favor owing to adverse effects and concerns about resistance. Dizziness and headache occur in about 10% of patients and are the most commonly reported adverse events. Although exceedingly rare, quinolones have a black box warning owing to their association with tendon rupture and tendonitis, most commonly affecting the Achilles tendon. Patients on quinolones should be educated to report any unusual or unexpected pain in their tendons. Quinolones also carry a black box warning for increased muscle weakness in patients with myasthenia gravis. In addition, quinolones have a moderate risk of QTc prolongation, hyperglycemia and can cause a potentially permanent peripheral neuropathy. Other side effects include acute-onset confusion, delirium, or altered mental status, particularly in older adults. Although many broad-spectrum antibiotics increase the risk of developing *C. difficile*-associated diarrhea, after clindamycin, quinolones are associated with the highest risk of *C. difficile* diarrhea. Their risk of *C. difficile* diarrhea, altered mental status, hyperglycemia, and QTc prolongation has led to the recommendation to hold fluoroquinolones in reserve for more serious infections or for when an effective alternative agent is not available.

INTERACTIONS

Although rare, all quinolones carry a risk of QTc prolongation and subsequent arrhythmias. This risk is greatest when used in combination with other agents that prolong QTc such as amiodarone, citalopram, fluoxetine, and quetiapine. Quinolones have chelating properties, meaning they bind to divalent cations such as calcium, magnesium, and aluminum and as such should be separated by at least 2 hours from over-the-counter antacids, calcium-fortified milk, and calcium or mineral supplements. Use during pregnancy should be avoided unless there is no suitable alternative.

SPECIFIC MEDICATIONS

Table 82-3 presents an overview of available quinolones for adult use in an ambulatory setting.

CLINICAL COMMENTARY

The term "respiratory fluoroquinolone" is often used to describe quinolones effective for treating respiratory tract infections and community-acquired pneumonia (CAP). More specifically, this refers to the quinolones that provide adequate activity against streptococcal pneumonia (e.g., levofloxacin and moxifloxacin), the most common pathogen in bacterial respiratory tract infections. Ciprofloxacin can be used to treat bacterial

pneumonia caused by susceptible gram-negative organisms. Due to its broad gram-positive and gram-negative bacterial coverage, levofloxacin is a good choice for moderately severe diabetic foot infections because these are often polymicrobial. However, most skin infections are not polymicrobial and are caused by either staphylococcal or streptococcal infections. Therefore, in uncomplicated cellulitis, levofloxacin is considered unnecessarily broad and could lead to antimicrobial resistance. CAP is an example where levofloxacin provides unnecessarily broad coverage. CAP is predominantly caused by gram-positive organisms, so moxifloxacin may be the preferred agent. Although

TABLE 82-3. Overview of the Most Commonly Used Fluoroquinolone Antibiotics

Generic (Brand)	Cost	Dosing	Comments
Ciprofloxacin (Cipro)	$	Immediate release: 500–750 mg PO Q 12 hours Extended release: 500–1000 mg PO Q 24 hours IV: 400 mg IV Q 8–12 hours	• Strong gram-negative bacterial coverage, including *Pseudomonas*. • Most commonly used for urinary tract infections, intra-abdominal infections (in combination with metronidazole), cat/dog bite-related infections, and other culture and susceptibility confirmed gram-negative infections. • Also available in otic and ophthalmic formulations for otitis externa and bacterial conjunctivitis, respectively. • Requires dose adjustment in renal impairment
Levofloxacin (Levaquin)	$$	250–750 mg IV/PO daily	• Covers gram-positive bacteria as well as gram-negative bacteria, including some *Pseudomonas*. • In addition to the indications for which ciprofloxacin can be used, levofloxacin may also be used to treat sinusitis, community-acquired pneumonia, and skin/skin structure infections. • Also available in an ophthalmic formulation for bacterial conjunctivitis. • Requires dose adjustment in renal impairment.
Moxifloxacin (Avelox)	$$$	400 mg PO/IV daily	• Has the best gram-positive coverage of the class but the weakest gram-negative coverage. Does not provide any coverage of *Pseudomonas* but does cover anaerobic bacteria. • Most commonly used to treat sinusitis, community-acquired pneumonia, and intra-abdominal infections as monotherapy. • Also available in an ophthalmic formulation for bacterial conjunctivitis. • Does NOT require any dose adjustment in renal impairment.

highly effective for UTIs, the quinolones should be considered second-line agents for uncomplicated cystitis to avoid bacterial antimicrobial resistance. However, if a quinolone is used, ciprofloxacin is the preferred agent for UTIs, and in most communities is more than 90% effective. For outpatient treatment of pyelonephritis, fluoroquinolones are considered first-line treatment.

Although moxifloxacin does have some gram-negative coverage, it is the weakest of the class in this respect. Also, moxifloxacin is the only quinolone that is primarily metabolized by the liver and does not require dosage adjustment in renal impairment. However, moxifloxacin does not attain adequate urinary concentrations, making it a poor choice for treating UTIs. Ciprofloxacin and levofloxacin are excreted primarily by the kidney, and therefore require dosage adjustments in renal impairment.

MACROLIDES

GENERAL INFORMATION

Macrolides are one of the most commonly prescribed classes of antibiotics. Erythromycin has been in clinical use since the 1950s, but with the development of newer broader-spectrum macrolides, it is less commonly prescribed now. Providers commonly prescribe macrolides for the treatment of mild to moderate respiratory tract infections, STDs, and infections caused by *Helicobacter pylori* and mycobacteria. The names of the agents in this class end with "thromycin" (erythromycin, clarithromycin, and azithromycin). An exception of note is telithromycin, a relatively new antibiotic, which is not a macrolide but belongs to a closely related antibiotic class known as ketolides. Clindamycin is also a closely related antibiotic but belongs to the class known as lincosamides. Dosing, cost and comments regarding the various macrolides are presented in Table 82-4.

THERAPEUTIC EFFECTS

Macrolides are bacteriostatic antibiotics that inhibit bacterial protein synthesis by reversibly binding to and inhibiting the activity of the 23S ribosomal RNA subunit of the bacterial ribosome. Macrolides are typically active against gram-positive bacteria (e.g., *S. pneumoniae*), campylobacter, atypical bacteria (such as *mycoplasma, chlamydia, ureaplasma,* and *Legionella pneumophila*), *Bordetella pertussis, H. pylori*, and mycobacteria. They have very limited

Brand Name (Generic Name)	Cost	Dosing	Half-life	Comments
TABLE 82-4. Specific Medications Within the Class				
Erythromycin	$	Base: 250–500 mg PO Q 6–12 hours Ethylsuccinate: 400–800 mg PO Q 6–12 hours IV: 250–500 mg IV Q 6 hours	1–2 hours	• Ethylsuccinate formulation has fewer GI adverse effects. • Also available in topical formulation for acne. • Commonly has drug–drug interactions related to CYP3A4 metabolism. • Not commonly used owing to high resistance rates.
Clarithromycin (Biaxin)	$$	Immediate release tablet: 250–500 mg PO Q 8–12 hours Extended release tablet: 1000 mg PO daily	3–7 hours	• Used in treating *H. pylori* and mycobacterial infections. • Commonly has drug–drug interactions related to CYP3A4 metabolism
Azithromycin (Zithromax Z-Pak)	$$	250–500 mg IV/PO daily Other doses are used in treatment of STDs and mycobacterial infections.	50–70 hours	• Part of recommended regimens for community-acquired pneumonia and gonorrhea/chlamydia • Well tolerated, fewer drug interactions than other macrolides

GI, gastrointestinal; IV, intravenous; PO, by mouth; STDs, sexually transmitted diseases.

coverage of gram-negative bacteria. All macrolides are available as oral tablets or capsules and require no dose adjustment in renal impairment. Macrolides are considered first-line agents for empiric outpatient treatment of CAP in patients without significant comorbidities. Their activity against beta hemolytic streptococci and some staphylococci also make then a common substitute for penicillin-allergic patients.

SIDE EFFECTS

Erythromycin commonly causes nausea, vomiting, and diarrhea. The newer agents, clarithromycin and azithromycin, are better tolerated. Although rare, all macrolides carry a risk of QTc prolongation and subsequent arrhythmias. This risk is greatest when used in combination with other agents that prolong QTc. Another rare side effect of macrolides is transaminitis and acute liver injury, which usually occurs with prolonged antibiotic courses. Clarithromycin can cause a troublesome unpleasant taste in about 10% of patients.

INTERACTIONS

The macrolides erythromycin and clarithromycin are metabolized by the CYP3A4 enzyme system. Because the CYP3A4 system is the most common pathway for drugs metabolized by the liver, macrolides have multiple drug interactions. When prescribed with other drugs metabolized by the CYP3A4 system, serum levels increase, resulting in a greater risk of adverse effects. Among the macrolides, azithromycin causes fewer drug interactions. In addition, all three macrolides carry a risk of QTc prolongation and should be used with extreme caution in combination with other high-risk QTc-prolonging agents (e.g., amiodarone, citalopram, fluoxetine, quetiapine).

CLINICAL COMMENTARY

Owing to its high risk of drug interactions, GI intolerance, and bacterial resistance, erythromycin is no longer routinely used in treating bacterial infections. It is most commonly used as a topical agent for acne and in the short-term treatment of diabetic gastroparesis.

Clarithromycin is used clinically in combination regimens for the treatment of peptic ulcer disease due to *H. pylori* and disseminated mycobacterial infections. Otherwise, clarithromycin has limited clinical use owing to its high risk of drug interactions.

Azithromycin is by far the most commonly used macrolide because it is well tolerated with fewer drug interactions. It is a first-line agent for the treatment of CAP and is available as a convenient Z-Pak dosage pack. However, studies indicate that azithromycin is overprescribed and often used inappropriately. Most patients prescribed azithromycin for uncomplicated CAP were found to have simple viral illnesses. This misuse of azithromycin has resulted in increasing bacterial resistance, particularly with *S. pneumoniae*, the most common pathogen in community-acquired bacterial pneumonia. Therefore, providers should cautiously prescribe azithromycin, and guideline recommendations should be closely followed for its use, especially for respiratory infections. Azithromycin is also recommended by the CDC as a single 1 g oral dose in the treatment of gonorrhea and chlamydia in combination with ceftriaxone. Other uses for azithromycin include prophylaxis against *Mycobacterium avium* complex infections in patients with HIV and a CD4 count < 50 cells/μL. In this setting, azithromycin is dosed 1200 mg PO once weekly.

83 | Cardiovascular Medications

ANGIOTENSIN CONVERTING ENZYME INHIBITORS

GENERAL INFORMATION

Researchers developed ACE inhibitors (ACEi) after noting that a peptide in snake venom lowered BP. First formulated in the mid-1970s, ACEi play a crucial role in the management of HTN and CV disease.

THERAPEUTIC EFFECT

ACEi act on the renin-angiotensin-aldosterone system (RAAS), a hormone system that plays a major role in regulating the plasma sodium concentration and arterial BP. ACEi block the conversion of angiotensin I to angiotensin II, a potent vasoconstrictor. Reduction in angiotensin II leads to an increase in plasma renin activity and vasodilation, which decreases BP. Their ability to reduce both preload and afterload make ACEi physiologically beneficial for treating CHF. ACEi also block the breakdown of bradykinin, which not only has a vasodilatory effect but also causes the adverse effect of cough and angioedema.

SIDE EFFECTS

ACEi can cause angioedema (swelling of the face, lips, tongue, or throat), a rare but potentially life-threatening adverse event that may occur at any time during treatment. ACEi should be avoided in patients with previous angioedema caused by ACEi and in those with hereditary angioedema. An angiotensin receptor blocker (ARB) may be used cautiously in patients with a history of angioedema to ACEi.

About 10% of patients on ACEi develop a dry nonproductive cough within the first few months of therapy. If the cough cannot be attributed to another cause, the ACE inhibitor should be discontinued, and if caused by ACEi, the cough should resolve within 1 to 4 weeks after stopping therapy.

Hyperkalemia is a common side effect with ACEi and may require their discontinuation. Risk factors for hyperkalemia include renal impairment, diabetes mellitus, and concomitant use of potassium-sparing diuretics, potassium supplementation, high potassium diets, or using potassium-containing salt substitutes. If there are compelling reasons to use ACEi, lowering potassium intake and stopping potassium supplements or other medications that may contribute to hyperkalemia should be considered before discontinuing therapy.

Providers should monitor kidney function. Increases in serum creatinine of up to 30% may occur after starting an ACE inhibitor but do not require discontinuing treatment. More significant decreases in renal function or hypotension suggest the presence of renal artery stenosis.

Although ACEi rarely cause cholestatic jaundice or hepatitis, they should be discontinued if marked elevation of hepatic transaminases or jaundice occurs. Since fetal death and congenital disabilities can occur, ACEi are contraindicated during pregnancy and should be stopped in women planning a pregnancy, and immediately discontinued if pregnancy is detected. Bone marrow suppression is a rare but serious side effect of ACEi. Treatment should be stopped immediately if this occurs. ACEi can cause dizziness but to a lesser degree than many other antihypertensive agents.

CAUTIONS

Providers should not prescribe ACEi for patients with known renal artery stenosis or aortic stenosis.

INTERACTIONS

The use of ARBs and aliskiren in combination with ACEi increases the risk of renal impairment and hyperkalemia. Combining other antihypertensive agents with ACEi increases the risk of hypotension and syncope. NSAIDs may blunt the effectiveness of an ACE inhibitor and increase the risk of renal impairment. Avoid the use of ACEi with lithium because increased lithium levels may occur.

SPECIFIC MEDICATIONS

Table 83-1 provides an overview of specific ACEi including dosing, cost, and any commentary on the agents' use.

CLINICAL COMMENTARY

ACEi are first-line agents for the treatment of HTN because of their effectiveness and low side effects profile. Although less effective as sole antihypertensive agents in African Americans, they are effective in combination with a diuretic for this population. ACEi are recommended for treating heart failure with reduced ejection fraction and left ventricular dysfunction. Several studies demonstrating reductions in both morbidity and improved survival after MI.

In patients with chronic kidney disease (CKD), ACEi can reduce proteinuria and improve outcomes. They are also indicated for diabetic nephropathy to slow progression of renal insufficiency.

If a cough develops with ACEi, many patients want to switch to another BP agent. If comorbid conditions exist such as diabetes, heart failure, CKD, or post MI, switching to an ARB may confer similar

TABLE 83-1. Overview of ACE Inhibitors

Medication	Dosing	Cost	Comments
Captopril (Capoten)	HTN: 25–100 mg bid HF: 6.25–50 mg tid	$	• May cause neutropenia, myeloid hypoplasia, and agranulocytosis. CBC should be monitored for the first 3 months of therapy. • Take on empty stomach. • Does not require hepatic conversion to active metabolites; may be preferred in patients with severe hepatic impairment • Shortest half-life of the ACE inhibitors (dosed two to three times/day)
Lisinopril (Prinivil, Zestril)	HTN: 10–40 mg daily HF: 2.5–40 mg daily	$	• Does not require hepatic conversion to active metabolites; may be preferred in patients with severe hepatic impairment
Enalapril (Vasotec)	HTN: 2.5–40 mg daily HF: 2.5–20 mg bid	$	
Benazepril (Lotensin)	HTN: 10–80 mg daily	$$	
Fosinopril (Monopril)	HTN: 10–80 mg daily HF: 5–40 mg daily	$$	• May cause less cough than other ACE inhibitors
Moexipril (Univasc)	HTN: 3.75–30 mg daily	$$	• Take on an empty stomach
Perindopril (Aceon)	HTN: 4–16 mg daily HF: 2–16 mg daily	$$$	
Quinapril (Accupril)	HTN: 10–40 mg daily HF: 5–20 mg bid	$$	
Ramipril (Altace)	HTN: 2.5–20 mg daily HF: 1.25–10 mg daily	$	
Trandolapril (Mavik)	HTN: 1–8 mg daily HF: 1–4 mg daily	$$$	

ACE, Angiotensin converting enzyme; CBC, complete blood count; HF, heart failure; HTN, hypertension.

benefits. If the cough does not bother the patient, another option is to continue the ACEi because it is not harmful.

All ACEi seem to be equally effective at equivalent doses, and so the main factors in choosing an agent are cost and convenience. In older patients, hypotension is more common and starting at low doses and lowering concomitant diuretic therapy may reduce the risk of syncope. Using shorter acting agents may also be beneficial.

ANGIOTENSIN RECEPTOR BLOCKERS

GENERAL INFORMATION

The RAAS is an important homeostatic regulator of BP, and an overactive RAAS may elevate BP. ARBs lower BP through modulation of the RAAS system. The names of all medications in this drug class end in "sartan."

THERAPEUTIC EFFECTS

The binding of angiotensin II to its receptors elevates BP via vasoconstriction, increases secretion of aldosterone from the adrenal gland, and activates the sympathetic nervous system. ARBs prevent angiotensin II from binding to the AT_2 receptor, thereby blocking the effects of angiotensin II. In addition to their role in managing HTN, these agents also have indications for type 2 diabetic nephropathy, heart failure, and post MI. ARBs often can be substituted when patients do not tolerate ACEi.

SIDE EFFECTS

ARBs are well tolerated. They are category D for use in pregnancy secondary to the risk of major congenital malformations. ARBs can increase potassium by decreasing aldosterone. Increases in potassium are usually small, but may be clinically significant in patients with CKD and in patients taking potassium supplements or potassium-sparing diuretics. ARBs may decrease glomerular filtration rate by inhibiting ATII vasoconstriction on the efferent arteriole, which reduces pressure within the renal glomerulus and decreases filtration. Increases in serum creatinine are common and an increase of $<30\%$ above baseline serum creatinine or absolute increases <1 mg/dL do not require discontinuing therapy. However, changes above these thresholds should prompt providers to assess for secondary causes. ARBs also precipitate acute kidney failure in approximately 1% of patients, mostly in those with preexisting renal disease such as renal artery stenosis. Modulating the RAAS reduces both preload and afterload, making ARBs useful for treating systolic heart failure.

An increase in bradykinin is the proposed mechanism for the dry cough and angioedema in patients taking ACEi. ARBs do not increase bradykinins, and so cough and angioedema occur far less frequently with ARBs compared to ACEi. However, ARBs should be avoided in patients with a history of angioedema associated with ACEi.

INTERACTIONS

Providers should not combine ARBs with aliskiren because of an increased risk of death. ARBs should not be used concomitantly with ACEi or renin inhibitors, because there is not only no added benefit but there is an increased risk of hypotension, syncope, and hyperkalemia. Providers should avoid potassium supplements in patients taking ARBs because of an increased risk of hyperkalemia, and patients taking medications that can increase serum potassium should be monitored carefully. NSAIDs should be avoided due to the risk of renal dysfunction and decreased antihypertensive efficacy.

SPECIFIC MEDICATIONS

Table 83-2 summarizes details on brand and generic names, cost, dosing, and half-life.

CLINICAL COMMENTARY

ARBs should be initiated at half the maximum dose and titrated upward to the maximum effective dose within 2 to 4 weeks if BP is not at goal. Providers should consider prescribing an ACEi or an ARB to their patients who are ≥ 18 years of age with CKD because these agents appear to slow the progression of disease even in nondiabetics. Although not as effective at lowering BP in blacks, ARBs are considered first-line therapy for black patients with diabetes. Monitoring should include baseline and periodic BP, electrolytes (potassium), and renal function (blood urea nitrogen and serum creatinine).

Although ARBs are used for heart failure and to improve symptoms, the evidence that they are as effective as ACEi in extending survival is not as strong. Most experts recommend initiating therapy with an ACEi and using an ARB in patients who cannot tolerate an ACEi. Current guidelines do not recommend combining an ACE inhibitor and an ARB in patients with heart failure because it increases the risk of side effects with little added benefit.

TABLE 83-2. Overview of Select Angiotensin Receptor Blockers

Generic (Brand)	Cost	Dosing	Half-Life	Comments
Azilsartan (Edarbi)	$$$	40–80 mg daily	11 hours	• No generic available as of 2017
Candesartan (Atacand)	$$$	8–32 mg daily	5–9 hours (>24-hour duration of action)	
Eprosartan (Teveten)	$$$	600–800 mg daily	5–9 hours	• Can be given once daily or divided into two doses
Irbesartan (Avapro)	$$	150–300 mg daily	11–15 hours (>24-hour duration of action)	
Losartan (Cozaar)	$	50–100 mg daily	2 hours	• Most commonly used ARB • Administer without regard to meals; however, administer consistently with respect to food intake at about the same time every day. • Mild to moderate hepatic impairment: initial dose 25 mg once daily • Can be given once daily or divided into two doses
Olmesartan (Benicar)	$$$	20–40 mg daily	13 hours	• May cause symptoms of sprue-like enteropathy (i.e., severe, chronic diarrhea with significant weight loss), which may develop months to years after treatment initiation • If other etiologies have been excluded, discontinue treatment and consider other antihypertensive therapy.
Telmisartan (Micardis)	$$	40–80 mg daily	24 hours (>24-hour duration of action)	
Valsartan (Diovan)	$	80–320 mg daily	6 hours (>24-hour duration of action)	• Food decreases the peak plasma concentration and extent of absorption by 50% and 40%, respectively. • Administer consistently with regard to food.

ARB, angiotensin receptor blocker.

CALCIUM CHANNEL BLOCKERS

GENERAL INFORMATION

Calcium channel blockers (CCBs) inhibit calcium ions from entering the "slow channels" of vascular smooth muscle cells and the myocardium during depolarization, producing relaxation of coronary vascular smooth muscle and coronary vasodilation. There are two categories of CCBs: dihydropyridines and nondihydropyridines. These agents treat a wide variety of conditions including HTN, angina, and Raynaud disease.

THERAPEUTIC EFFECTS

The dihydropyridines vasodilate peripheral arteries and lower vascular resistance and BP. The dihydropyridines decrease afterload but have no direct inotropic or chronotropic effects. All dihydropyridines end in "dipine" (e.g., nifedipine).

Nondihydropyridines (verapamil and diltiazem) inhibit L-type calcium channels of the atrioventricular (AV) node, decreasing heart rate and contractility. They cause coronary vasodilation and increase myocardial oxygen delivery. Both verapamil and diltiazem decrease afterload and have negative inotropic and chronotropic effects.

SIDE EFFECTS

Dihydropyridines cause peripheral edema in about 10% of patients and baroreceptor-mediated reflex tachycardia because of their potent peripheral vasodilatory effects. The peripheral edema is caused by arterial dilation and not left ventricular dysfunction. It is not harmful and may be controlled with support hose and elevation. Reflex tachycardia is more common with short-acting first-generation dihydropyridines, such as nifedipine in its immediate release form. Commonly reported side effects for dihydropyridines include stomach pain, nausea, dizziness, flushing, headache, and lethargy. Dihydropyridines may also cause gingival hyperplasia.

Because of their effects on the AV node, nondihydropyridines may cause bradycardia and AV block. Other class adverse effects include dizziness, constipation, nausea, headache, and lethargy. Both verapamil and diltiazem can worsen systolic heart failure and should be avoided in this patient population.

INTERACTIONS

Grapefruit and grapefruit juice can inhibit hepatic metabolism of CCBs. In general, medications and herbals that inhibit CYP3A4, such as St. John's Wort, should be avoided or used with caution when taken concomitantly with dihydropyridines. Other medicines to avoid or to modify the dose when prescribed with dihydropyridines include carbamazepine, phenobarbital, rifampin, phenytoin, macrolides, and the antifungal "azoles."

Both nondihydropyridines, especially verapamil, inhibit CYP3A4. Medications with contraindications for simultaneous use with nondihydropyridines include lomitapide, flibanserin, aprepitant, domperidone, and ivabradine. Nondihydropyridines also have major interactions with colchicine, clozapine, clarithromycin, erythromycin, digoxin, simvastatin, and dronedarone. Concomitant use with BBs increases the risk of heart block.

SPECIFIC MEDICATIONS

Table 83-3 summarizes the brand/generic, cost, dosing, half-life, and comments specific to CCBs available in the United States.

CAUTIONS

Patients with sick sinus syndrome or second- or third-degree AV block should not take diltiazem unless they have a functioning artificial pacemaker. Diltiazem should also be avoided in cases of acute MI or pulmonary congestion. Patients may experience transient dermatologic reactions with diltiazem use, but if the reaction persists, it should be discontinued.

Short-acting CCBs have been associated with an increased incidence of MI and sudden death, possibly due to their rapid onset of action and shorter half-lives which cause wide swings in BP. As a result, amlodipine and the long-acting formulation of nifedipine are preferred agents in patients with chronic angina.

Verapamil is contraindicated in patients with severe left ventricular dysfunction, hypotension (SBP < 90 mmHg), or cardiogenic shock. Patients with sick sinus syndrome or second- or third-degree AV block (except those with a functioning artificial ventricular pacemaker) should not take verapamil.

CLINICAL COMMENTARY

Dihydropyridines reduce the risk of strokes and CV events. Amlodipine is among the most widely prescribed CCBs because it is well tolerated and causes less reflex tachycardia. It is available in combination with several other antihypertensive medications to reduce the pill burden for patients and to improve medication adherence. Peripheral edema is most common with nifedipine, but does occur with other dihydropyridine CCBs. Nondihydropyridines are used primarily for rate control (e.g., atrial fibrillation) and are not preferred for managing HTN or angina. Nondihydropyridines should not be combined with BBs because of the risk of bradycardia and AV node block. Verapamil is more effective at slowing AV conduction than diltiazem, but is also more negatively inotropic. Caution is indicated with these agents in the setting of heart failure or conduction abnormalities. Both agents are contraindicated in Wolff–Parkinson–White (WPW) syndrome.

CCBs are equally effective in all racial and ethnic groups, and dihydropyridines are effective in older patients with isolated systolic HTN. All CCBs are pregnancy category C and are not recommended for use during pregnancy. No laboratory monitoring is required, but BP and heart rate monitoring are recommended. Although verapamil and diltiazem are metabolized in the liver and may cause increases in liver function tests, providers do not need to routinely monitor liver function tests.

ALPHA BLOCKERS

GENERAL INFORMATION

Alpha blockers were first introduced for treating BP, but are now more widely used to provide symptomatic relief for BPH. Although previously considered

TABLE 83-3. Overview of Calcium Channel Blockers

Generic (Brand)	Cost	Dosing	Half-life	Comments
Dihydropyridines				
Amlodipine (Norvasc)	$	5–10 mg daily	30–50 hours	• Most commonly used dihydropyridine CCB • Pulmonary edema (in HF patients: 7%–15%) • Caution with simvastatin, lomitapide, and other CYP3A4 inhibitors • Do not exceed 20 mg of simvastatin with amlodipine.
Felodipine (Plendil)	$$	5–10 mg daily	11–16 hours (>24-hour duration of action)	• Swallow tablet whole; do not divide, crush, or chew. • High fat or high carbohydrate meals may increase concentration. • Pills may contain lactose; so avoid in patients intolerant to lactose. • Caution with cimetidine
Cardene (Nicardipine)	$$	20–40 mg tid	8 hours (≤8 hours duration of action)	• Avoid use with silodosin and use caution with amiodarone and celecoxib.
Nifedipine IR (Procardia)	$	10–20 mg tid; max 60 mg tid.	2 hours	• Avoid use for acute angina and 1–2 weeks after MI or ACS • Not used for HTN; used for chronic stable angina • Administration with low-fat meals may decrease flushing but will decrease absorption.
Nifedipine ER (Adalat CC, Afeditab CR, Procardia XL)	$	30–90 mg daily	7 hours	• Take on an empty stomach. • Swallow whole; do not crush, split, or chew. • Procardia XL: Active drug release from nonabsorbable shell. Patients may notice "ghost" tablet in their stool.
Nondihydropyridines				
Diltiazem IR (Cardizem)	$	Depends on indication	3–4.5 hours	• Take before meals and at bedtime. • Swallow whole; do not split, crush, or chew. • Caution with rifampin, lovastatin, cyclosporine, and atorvastatin (all diltiazem formulations). • Do not exceed 10 mg simvastatin, 20 mg lovastatin, and limit atorvastatin use (all diltiazem formulations).
Diltiazem ER (Taztia XT, Tiazac)	$	Depends on indication	5–10 hours	• Capsules may be opened and sprinkled on a spoonful of applesauce. • Swallow without chewing, followed by drinking a glass of water.
Diltiazem ER (Cardizem SR)	$	Depends on indication	5–10 hours	• Do not open, chew, or crush; swallow whole. • Administer at same time of day, either morning or evening. • Cardizem CD, Cardizem LA, Cartia XT: Administer without regard to meals. • Dilacor XR and Dilt XR: Administer on an empty stomach.

TABLE 83-3. Overview of Calcium Channel Blockers (*continued*)				
Generic (Brand)	**Cost**	**Dosing**	**Half-life**	**Comments**
Verapamil IR (Calan)	$	Depends on indication	4.5–12 hours	• Caution with dofetilide and silodosin (all verapamil formulations) • No evidence of additional benefit beyond 360 mg • May cause gingival hyperplasia • Do not exceed 10 mg simvastatin, 20 mg lovastatin, and limit atorvastatin use (all verapamil formulations).
Verapamil SR (Verelan, Calan SR)	$	Depends on indication	4.5–12 hours	• May administer capsule contents sprinkled on one tablespoon of applesauce and swallow immediately without chewing. • Do not subdivide contents of capsules. • Follow by a glass of cool water. • When switching from IR to ER/SR, the total daily dose remains the same unless formulation strength does not allow for equal conversion. • May cause gingival hyperplasia

ACS, American Cancer Society; CCB, calcium channel blockers; HF, heart failure; HTN, hypertension; MI, myocardial infarction.

first-line antihypertensives, since the ALLHAT trial showed more favorable results for thiazide diuretics, alpha blockers are prescribed less often for BP control.

THERAPEUTIC EFFECTS

Alpha blockers bind to alpha 1 receptors in the prostate, blocking the action of norepinephrine and leading to smooth muscle relaxation of the bladder neck and prostate. Alpha blockers also bind to alpha 1 receptors on vascular smooth muscle, causing vasodilation and lowering BP. Selectivity for alpha 1A receptors (prevalent in the prostate) and alpha 1B receptors (predominant in vasculature) varies among the agents in this class, causing differences in side-effect profiles. Tamsulosin, alfuzosin, and silodosin are selected more often for relaxing the smooth muscle in the prostate and have little effect on BP.

SIDE EFFECTS

The vasodilation causes orthostatic hypotension, which is the principle side effect of alpha blockers and is more common with doxazosin, prazosin, and terazosin. Orthostatic hypotension is least common with silodosin and tamsulosin because of their selectivity for the alpha 1A receptors. Vasodilation can also cause headache. Alpha blockers can cause abnormal ejaculation, impotence, and priapism. Sexual dysfunction occurs more frequently with tamsulosin and silodosin. Alpha blockers may also rarely cause QT prolongation, more commonly with alfuzosin than the other alpha blockers. Floppy iris

syndrome is reported with tamsulosin and may complicate cataract surgery. Although most closely linked to tamsulosin, other alpha blockers may also increase the risk of floppy iris syndrome.

INTERACTIONS

When using alpha blockers with other antihypertensive medications, there is an increased risk of hypotensive effects. Phosphodiesterase inhibitors also increase the risk for hypotension and should be used cautiously in combination with an alpha blocker, starting at lower doses with close BP monitoring.

SPECIFIC MEDICATIONS

Table 83-4 outlines the cost, dosing, pharmacokinetic profile, and drug interactions within the class.

CLINICAL COMMENTARY

Alpha blockers are first-line agents for the treatment of BPH and improve symptoms in about 70% of patients. Since the doxazosin arm of the ALLHAT study ended prematurely because of increased risk of the secondary outcomes of stroke, heart failure, and CV events compared to chlorthalidone, alpha blockers are infrequently used for treating HTN. However, in patients with high BP and prostate disease, many clinicians use an alpha blocker such as doxazosin to attempt treating both conditions with a single medication. Starting patients with a low initial dose and titrating up slowly helps prevent hypotension. BP should be monitored with the

TABLE 83-4. Overview of Alpha Blockers

Medication	Cost	Dosing	Comments	Drug Interactions
Alfuzosin (Uroxatral)	$$$	BPH: 10 mg daily	• Long acting • Nonselective • Contraindicated in hepatic disease	CYP450 inhibitors
Doxazosin (Cardura)	$	BPH: 1–8 mg daily HTN: 1–16 mg daily	• Long acting • Nonselective	CYP450 inhibitors
Prazosin (Minipress)	$	HTN: 1–15 mg/day divided two to three times per day	• Short acting • Nonselective	
Silodosin (Rapaflo)	$$$	BPH: 8 mg daily	• Long acting • Selective for alpha 1A receptors • Needs dose adjustment in patients with CrCl <50 mL/min; do not use if CrCl <30 mL/min. • Contraindicated in hepatic disease	CYP450 inhibitors and P-glycoprotein inhibitors
Tamsulosin (Flomax)	$$	BPH: 0.4–0.8 mg daily	• Long acting • Selective for alpha 1A receptors	CYP450 inhibitors
Terazosin (Hytrin)	$	HTN: 1–20 mg daily BPH: 1–20 mg daily	• Long acting • Nonselective	

BPH, benign prostatic hyperplasia; CrCl, creatinine clearance; HTN, hypertension.

first dose and with each dose increase thereafter. Because of their vasodilating effects, these agents can help improve vasospastic symptoms from Raynaud disease.

BETA ADRENERGIC AGONISTS

GENERAL INFORMATION

Beta adrenergic antagonists or beta blockers (BBs) have several therapeutic indications including CAD, control of heart rate with supraventricular arrhythmias, and as part of the therapeutic regimen for CHF. Although used for HTN, they are no longer considered first-line agents unless there is another compelling indication for their use. BBs affect the heart by decreasing myocardial oxygen demand and by their negative chronotropic and inotropic effects on the heart. BBs also reduce AV conduction that slows the heart rate, and their negative chronotropic effects counteract the reflex tachycardia when added to regimens that include vasodilators. Their ability to decrease renin secretion and inhibit sympathetic nervous system activity reduces cardiac remodeling and dysfunctional neurohumoral responses in patients with systolic dysfunction. These effects create compelling indications for the use of BBs in heart failure (HF), recent MI, nonvasospastic stable angina, atrial fibrillation or atrial flutter, and tachycardia.

BBs are also useful in reducing tremor, preventing migraines, and treating symptoms associated with thyrotoxicosis. The preferred BBs for these conditions tend to be nonselective and lipophilic because of their ability to block beta receptors in noncardiac tissue and to cross the blood–brain barrier. Their ability to block sympathetic activity also makes BBs useful for catecholamine-mediated symptoms such as tremor or tachycardia associated with panic disorder, social phobias, and other anxiety disorders.

THERAPEUTIC EFFECTS

BBs affect both beta 1 and beta 2 receptors. Beta 1 receptors concentrate in the heart and kidney, and blocking this receptors account for the CV benefits of BBs. Cardioselective agents preferentially block the beta 1 receptors and are less likely to cause side effects associated with beta 2 blockade. Beta 2 receptors concentrate in the lungs, liver, pancreas, and arteriolar smooth muscle. When blocked, they contribute to side effects such as bronchospasm, vasoconstriction, and inhibition of glycogenolysis.

Although properties vary among individual BBs, all BBs inhibit renin release and have negative chronotropic and inotropic effects because of beta 1 receptor blockade. These negative effects can reduce cardiac output. The exception is BBs with intrinsic sympathetic activity (ISA), because they partially agonize cardiac beta receptors that minimize the reduction in cardiac output at low doses.

Nonselective BBs inhibit both beta 1 and beta 2 receptors and have a higher risk of exacerbating bronchospastic lung disease. Cardioselective BBs selectively inhibit beta 1 receptors at low and moderate doses, but with higher dosages, cardioselectivity decreases. The exact dose when the cardioselectivity of a beta receptor blockade disappears varies among patients. Table 83-5 outlines the cardioselectivity of commonly used BBs.

Some BBs also block alpha receptors. Alpha receptor antagonism increases vasodilation, which can add to BP lowering and increase the risk of orthostatic hypotension. The alpha blocking activity of labetalol and carvedilol make these agents useful in individuals with both HTN and CHF. BBs with ISA partially stimulate beta receptors while antagonizing overstimulation (partial-agonist) and tend to have less impact on heart rate, contractility, and conduction. These agents can be useful in patients with bradycardia who might benefit from a BB, because resting heart rate, cardiac output, and peripheral blood flow are less effected by BBs with ISA. At higher doses, the agonist effects of BBs with ISA tend to be overcome by their beta-blocking activity. Providers should avoid using a BB with ISA post MI.

SIDE EFFECTS

Bronchoconstriction is the most common serious side effect of BBs. However, although they need to be monitored carefully, most patients with a history of asthma can tolerate low to moderate doses of cardioselective agents. Beta 2 receptor blockade can also cause peripheral vasoconstriction and ischemia, or exacerbate peripheral arterial disease and Raynaud phenomenon.

Monitoring heart rate is necessary because bradycardia may limit dose titration. Patients taking a BB can experience exercise intolerance or pronounced orthostatic hypotension owing to delayed compensatory heart rate elevation. BBs may mask adrenergic symptoms associated with hypoglycemia such as tachycardia, anxiety, and tremor.

Beta receptor blockade in peripheral tissues decreases insulin secretion, decreases glycogenolysis,

and stimulates lipolysis. These effects can elevate blood sugars, increase very-low-density lipoproteins (VLDL), and lower HDL.

BBs with increased lipophilicity are absorbed more rapidly, have shorter half-lives, and may have greater CNS effects owing to their ability to cross the blood–brain barrier. Common side effects include fatigue and drowsiness; there is also an association of depression with BB use. Sexual dysfunction is commonly reported by male patients but may be lower with less lipophilic BBs.

INTERACTIONS

In general, providers should not combine BBs with nondihydropyridine CCBs (verapamil and diltiazem) owing to the potential to synergistically block AV node conduction. In addition, combining a BB with other antihypertensive medications increases the risk of hypotension. Peripheral beta 2 receptor blockade can cause vasoconstriction, which when combined with alpha adrenergic agonists can exaggerate hypertensive reactions. Finally, BBs reduce the effectiveness of sympathomimetic agents.

CAUTIONS

Providers should avoid BBs in patients with severe bradycardia, sinoatrial or AV node dysfunction, and should not combine agents that block AV conduction with BBs because this could result in heart block. Providers should not prescribe BBs in patients with decompensated HF or use BBs at higher than recommended doses because the reduction in cardiac output can exacerbate HF. Providers should use caution in patients with low heart rate, low BP, vascular disease, bronchospastic disease, and insulin dependence with frequent hypoglycemia.

SPECIFIC MEDICATIONS

Table 83-5 compares BBs and their relative cardioselectivity, lipid solubility, partial agonist effect, and alpha-blocking activity. Table 83-6 compares dosing, costs, and significant differences between medications within the class.

CLINICAL COMMENTARY

In general, the choice of BB is based on cost, need for cardioselectivity, and duration of action. Other factors to consider are ISA activity, lipid solubility, and the benefit of having added alpha agonist activity. Low cost, cardioselectivity, and once-to-twice daily

TABLE 83-5. Comparison of Beta Blocker Properties

Beta Blocker	Acebutolol (Sectral)	Atenolol (Tenormin)	Bisoprolol (Zebeta)	Carvedilol (Coreg)	Labetalol (Trandate)	Metoprolol (Toprol XL or Lopressor)	Nebivolol (Bystolic)	Propranolol (Hemangeol or Inderal LA or XL)
Cardio-selective (beta 1) at low dose[a]	Yes <800 mg	Yes ≤100 mg	Yes <20 mg			Yes <100 mg	Yes <10 mg	
Nonselective				Yes	Yes			Yes
Mixed alpha and beta blockers				Yes (1:10)	Yes (1:3)			
Intrinsic sympathomimetic activity	Yes				Yes (beta 2)			
Pharmacokinetics								
Lipophilicity	Low	Lowest	Moderate	High	Moderate	Moderate to high	High	Highest
Half-life (hours)	3–12	6–9	9–12	7–10	6–8	3–7	10–12	3–10
Time to peak On HR On BP	1–1.5 hours 2–8 hours	2–4 hours	2–4 hours	1–2 hours	1–4 hours	1–2 hours	1.5–4 hours	1–14 hours Days to weeks
Bioavailability	30%–50%	50%–60%	80%	IR 25%–35% ER 85%	25%	40%–77%	12%–96%	25%
First-pass metabolism	Extensive	50%	Approx. 20%	Extensive	Extensive	Approx. 50%	Extensive	Extensive
Hepatic elimination	1° 50%–60%	Limited	Yes 50%	Yes—biliary 98%	Yes—100%	Yes—100%	Yes—100%	Yes—100%
CYP substrate	No	No	3A4, 2D6	2D6, 2C9, 3A4, 2C19, 1A2, 2E1	No	2D6	2D6	2D6, 1A2
Renal elimination	2° 10%–50%	Yes 40%–50%	Yes 50%	No	Metabolites only	95% as metabolites	Yes, active metabolites	96%–99% as metabolites
Removed by dialysis	Hemo	Hemo 1–12%	No	No	No	No	Not studied	No

[a]Total daily dose.

BP, blood pressure; CYP, cytochrome P450; ER, extended release; HR, heart rate; IR, immediate release.

TABLE 83-6. Overview of Select Beta Blockers

Generic Name	Initial Dose	Renal (R) or Hepatic (H) Dose Adjustment	Typical Maintenance Dose	Maximum Daily Dose	Cost	Comments
Acebutolol	200–400 mg/day	Yes—R	400–800 mg/day	1.2 g/day 800 mg in elderly	$$	• Usually dose is divided into bid. • Higher doses used in ventricular arrhythmias (600–1200 mg daily) • Not recommended for CVD; may cause tachyarrhythmias and little impact on CO
Atenolol	25–50 mg daily	Yes—R	100 mg daily	200 mg daily	$	• Can increase to 200 mg daily for angina; unlikely added benefit in HTN • Low lipophilicity; does not cross BBB
Bisoprolol	2.5–5 mg daily	Yes—R, H	2.5–10 mg daily	20 mg daily	$$	• HF: start with 1.25 mg daily and target 10 mg daily • Crosses BBB
Carvedilol	6.25 mg bid	Yes—H	6.25–25 mg bid	50 mg bid	$	• 3.125 mg bid of IR can be converted to 10 mg daily of CR • HF: Start with carvedilol 3.125 mg bid or CR 10 mg daily • HF: Target carvedilol 25 mg bid (50 mg bid if weight >85 kg) or CR 80 mg daily • Take IR form with food to slow absorption and reduce risk of orthostasis. • Can take CR with food to increase absorption
Carvedilol CR	20 mg daily	Yes—H	20–80 mg daily	80 mg daily	$$	
Labetolol	100 mg bid	Yes—H	200–400 mg bid	2400 mg daily (in divided doses)	$$	• Do not titrate more than increments of 200 mg bid • Best evidence of safety in pregnancy • Can take with food to increase absorption
Metoprolol tartrate/ Metoprolol succinate ER	25–50 mg/day	No	100–200 mg/day	450 mg daily (tartrate) 400 mg daily (succinate)	$ $$	• Convert between formulations using total daily dose. • Tartrate is dosed bid and ER is dosed once daily. • HF: (succinate only) Start with 12.5–25 mg daily and target 200 mg daily. • Migraines: 200 mg per day • Crosses BBB • Can take with food to increase absorption
Nebivolol	5 mg daily	Yes—R, H	5–10 mg daily	40 mg daily	$$$	• Most beta 1 selective agent • Additional vasodilatory effect: stimulates endothelial release of NO

(continued)

TABLE 83-6. Overview of Select Beta Blockers (*continued*)

Generic Name	Initial Dose	Renal (R) or Hepatic (H) Dose Adjustment	Typical Maintenance Dose	Maximum Daily Dose	Cost	Comments
Propranolol	40 mg bid	No	120–240 mg/day	640 mg/day	$	• IR formulation divided into bid to tid dosing
Propranolol LA	80 mg/day	No	120–240 mg/day	640 mg/day	$$$	• FDA approval for several noncardiac conditions: essential tremor, migraines, pheochromocytoma
Propranolol XL	80 mg/day	No	120 mg daily	120 mg daily	$$$	• Highest lipophilicity; easily crosses BBB
						• Take IR formulation before meals and bedtime. Take LA/XL consistently with or without food.
						• Also available as an oral solution that should be diluted when taken

BBB, blood–brain barrier; CAD, coronary artery disease; CR, extended release; CO, cardiac output; CVD, cardiovascular disease; ER, extended release; FDA, Food and Drug Administration; HF, heart failure; HTN, hypertension; IR, immediate release; La/XL, long acting; NO, nitrous oxide; SE, side effects.

administration make generic metoprolol and atenolol the most commonly prescribed BBs for patients with CAD. Heart rate should be monitored to assess the adequacy of therapy, with the goal being a resting heart rate of 50 to 60 beats/minute indicating beta blockade.

Although BBs are no longer first-line agents for BP management, combining a BB with a diuretic can create synergy and more effective BP lowering. BBs with relative beta 1 selectivity are preferred by clinicians in patients with asthma, type 1 diabetes, or peripheral vascular disease.

Providers should counsel patients that abruptly discontinuing a BB can result in rebound HTN and tachycardia because of beta receptor upregulation. To avoid rebound effects, BBs should be tapered over 1 to 2 weeks by decreasing the dose in half for 1 week, then every other day for 1 week before stopping the drug. Rebound effects are less common with long-acting agents and BBs with longer half-lives. Patients with HF should be stable and relatively euvolemic before starting a BB. Therapy should be started at the lowest dose and doubled no more often than every 2 weeks to avoid exacerbation

of HF. Patients with HF should be advised that symptoms may worsen slightly before a positive effect is seen.

ANTIPLATELET MEDICATIONS

GENERAL INFORMATION

Platelets are an important part of a complex pathway used to preserve hemostasis in the arterial system. Under some pathologic conditions, such as atherosclerosis, platelets may aggregate and cause thrombosis or arterial occlusion leading to ischemia or necrosis of tissue in the affected region. Antiplatelet therapy is used to limit or prevent this arterial thrombosis in the management of CAD and peripheral artery disease (PAD), and for noncardioembolic stroke prevention.

THERAPEUTIC EFFECTS

Antiplatelet medications inhibit the activation of platelets through multiple mechanisms resulting in reduced platelet aggregation. This process is irreversible for the lifespan of the platelet (~7 to 10 days).

SIDE EFFECTS

In general, antiplatelet therapy is well tolerated, and the main adverse effect is an increased risk of bleeding. This risk is greater in older patients (≥75 years old), those with a recent surgery, a history of GI bleeding or active peptic ulcer disease, severe hepatic impairment, heavy ethanol use (>3 drinks/day), or weight less than 60 kg.

Ulcers and upper GI bleeding are serious adverse events related to aspirin therapy. In those patients at high risk for a GI bleed, taking a PPI with aspirin reduces the risk of bleeding. Because clopidogrel does not inhibit prostaglandin synthesis, the risk of a GI bleed is lower than with aspirin. Aside from GI bleeding, the risk of other adverse bleeding events is similar for clopidogrel and aspirin. Combination therapy increases the risk of bleeding and often adds little benefit.

If a patient does experience significant active bleeding associated with antiplatelet use, platelet transfusions can help restore hemostasis.

INTERACTIONS

In addition to antiplatelet medications, other classes of medications can increase bleeding risk. Combining these medications with antiplatelet medications further increases the bleeding risk. In cases where the following medications are used concomitantly with an antiplatelet agent, patients should be monitored closely for signs and symptoms of bleeding:

• Anticoagulants: warfarin, dabigatran, apixaban, rivaroxaban, edoxaban
• SSRIs: citalopram, escitalopram, fluoxetine, paroxetine, sertraline, vilazodone
• NSAIDs: diclofenac, ibuprofen, indomethacin, ketorolac, nabumetone, naproxen
• Herbal products: Ginkgo biloba, omega-3-fatty acids, vitamin E

SPECIFIC MEDICATIONS

There are currently several antiplatelet medications on the market. Although they all inhibit platelets, each has different properties that may cause it to be favored over another agent. Table 83-7 outlines the properties of the available agents.

CLINICAL COMMENTARY

The primary indications for antiplatelet therapy include noncardioembolic stroke prevention, primary and secondary prevention of CV disease, treatment of PAD, and following percutaneous coronary intervention with stent placement.

Following coronary stent placement, current guidelines recommend dual antiplatelet therapy for at least 1 month with a bare metal stent, and at least 12 months following a drug-eluting stent placement to prevent restenosis. Dual antiplatelet therapy is defined as a P2Y12 inhibitor (clopidogrel, prasugrel, or ticagrelor) plus aspirin. After receiving antiplatelet therapy for the specified period, discontinuing the P2Y12 inhibitor may be considered, though aspirin should be continued indefinitely.

Antiplatelet therapy is also indicated for the prevention of noncardioembolic stroke. Aspirin, clopidogrel, and a combination of aspirin and dipyridamole are all options for preventing noncardioembolic ischemic stroke or TIA. However, there is some evidence to suggest that clopidogrel or a combination of aspirin and dipyridamole may be superior to aspirin in the secondary prevention of noncardioembolic stroke or TIA. The combination of aspirin and clopidogrel offers a modest increase in efficacy, but these benefits are offset by increased cost and risk of bleeding. Typically, dual therapy is reserved for those at highest risk.

Aspirin reduces the risk of heart attack in patients with chronic angina. In PAD, antiplatelet therapy is indicated because of the increased risk of future CV events. Aspirin, clopidogrel, and cilostazol have all been studied in the treatment of PAD. Cilostazol has vasodilating properties in addition to its antiplatelet effect, and is approved for the symptomatic treatment of intermittent claudication. Side effects include headache, tachycardia, and cardiac arrhythmias. It has a black box warning because of the risk of sudden death in patients with CHF, and this risk along with only a modest benefit in increased walking distance limits its use.

Because of the increased risk of bleeding associated with antiplatelet use, these medications should be stopped for 5 to 7 days before surgery, with the exception of minor procedures such as dental surgery. Special consideration should be given to patients with cardiac stents who have not completed their full course of dual antiplatelet therapy, and delaying surgery should be considered when possible.

TABLE 83-7. Overview of Antiplatelet Medications

Generic (Brand)	Dosing	Significant Drug Interactions	Cost	Comments
Aspirin	81 mg, PO, Q day		$	• Most studies indicate that higher doses of aspirin are not more effective than 81 mg daily. Increased doses are associated with increased bleeding risk. • Avoid use in children and adolescents due to risk of Reye syndrome.
Clopidogrel (Plavix)	75 mg, PO, Q day	• PPIs ($\downarrow$clopidogrel active metabolites) • Grapefruit juice ($\downarrow$clopidogrel active metabolites)	$$	• Prodrug metabolized to the active drug by the liver. • Clopidogrel should not be used in patients who are CYP2C19 poor metabolizers, because they cannot metabolize clopidogrel to its active form. Genetic testing may be considered prior to using clopidogrel in high-risk patients.
Prasugrel (Effient)	10 mg, PO, Q day <50 kg: 5 mg, PO, Q day		$$$	• Prodrug metabolized to the active drug by the liver. • Does not interact with PPIs. • Generally not recommended in patients ≥75 years owing to increased risk of bleeding. • Superior to clopidogrel in reducing cardiovascular events, but with a slight increase in bleeding complications
Ticagrelor (Brilinta)	90 mg, PO, bid	• Colchicine ($\uparrow$ colchicine) • CYP3A4 Inducers ($\downarrow$ticagrelor) • CYP3A4 Inhibitors ($\uparrow$ticagrelor) • Lovastatin ($\uparrow$ lovastatin) • Simvastatin ($\uparrow$simvastatin)	$$$	• Superior to clopidogrel in reducing cardiovascular events with a slight increase in bleeding complications • Aspirin >100 mg/day reduces the efficacy of ticagrelor and should be avoided. • Dyspnea is a common side effect. • Avoid use in patients with gout.
Cilostazol (Pletal)	100 mg, PO, bid on an empty stomach	• Grapefruit juice ($\uparrow$cilostazol) • CYP3A4 inhibitors ($\uparrow$cilostazol) • CYP3A4 inducers ($\downarrow$cilostazol) • CYP2C19 inhibitors ($\uparrow$cilostazol)	$$	• Should be avoided in patients with congestive heart failure • Use with caution in patients with moderate to severe hepatic impairment. • Use with caution in patients with severe renal impairment. • Most common side effects are headache, diarrhea, and rhinitis.
Aspirin/ Dipyridamole (Aggrenox)	25 mg/200 mg, PO bid	• Colchicine ($\uparrow$colchicine)	$$	• Avoid use in patients with severe hepatic and renal impairment. • Avoid use in children and adolescents due to risk of Reye syndrome. • Most common side effect is headache.

PPIs: omeprazole, esomeprazole, lansoprazole, rabeprazole, pantoprazole.

CYP3A4 inducers: carbamazepine, phenytoin, oxcarbazepine, phenobarbital, St. John's Wort, pioglitazone.

CYP3A4 inhibitors: clarithromycin, verapamil, diltiazem, erythromycin, fluconazole, ketoconazole.

CYP2C19 inhibitors: fluconazole, omeprazole, ticlopidine.

PO, by mouth; PPIs, proton pump inhibitors.

STATINS (3-HYDROXY-3-METHYLGLUTARYLCOENZYME A REDUCTASE INHIBITORS)

GENERAL INFORMATION

The 3-hydroxy-3-methylglutarylcoenzyme A (HMG-CoA) reductase inhibitors or statins are the mainstay of cholesterol treatment and are among the most commonly prescribed class of medications in the United States. Nearly a quarter of adults in the United States take a statin, and, based on the most recent guidelines, another 12.8 million are considered candidates for statin therapy.

THERAPEUTIC EFFECTS

By inhibiting HMG-CoA reductase, the rate-limiting step in cholesterol synthesis, statins lower cholesterol. In addition to lowering LDL levels, statins also upregulate LDL receptors on hepatocytes, modestly increase HDL, decrease triglycerides, and appear to have other beneficial effects such as inhibiting platelets and reducing inflammation. Statins reduce all-cause mortality both in patients with known CV disease (secondary prevention) as well as in those with risk factors for developing CV disease (primary prevention). Among lipid-lowering agents, statins lower LDL by the highest percentage, and their effectiveness makes them the primary drug intervention in lipid management. Moderate-dose therapy lowers LDL cholesterol by 30% to 50% and high-dose therapy by 50% or more.

SIDE EFFECTS

In general, statin therapy is well tolerated. The most common complaint resulting in statin discontinuation is myalgia. The reported frequency of statin-associated myalgia varies depending on the source and has been reported to be anywhere from 1% to 29%. Rhabdomyolysis, the most severe myopathy associated with statins, is very rare (approximately 0.1%) and is most commonly associated with simvastatin 80 mg daily, a dose no longer recommended by the FDA. The risk of myopathy increases with renal insufficiency or when statins are combined with medications that impair their metabolism.

In addition to myalgia, statins increase the incidence of type 2 diabetes mellitus by about 10%. The increased risk of developing diabetes occurs mostly with high-intensity statin use and in patients already at risk of developing diabetes. When considering the risk of developing diabetes associated with statin use, it is important to consider that the CV risk reduction with statins in patients with diabetes is similar to that in nondiabetics. Given the high risk of CV disease associated with diabetes, the benefits of arteriosclerotic cardiovascular disease (ASCVD) risk reduction generally outweigh the risk.

Statins are associated with increases in LFTs, especially during the first 12 weeks of therapy. However, the risk of hepatotoxicity is <1%, and current guidelines do not recommend routine monitoring of LFTs. Other side effects include indigestion, constipation or diarrhea, fatigue, headache, and runny or bloody nose. Despite a few small studies suggesting cognitive impairment, the burden of evidence indicates that statins most likely do not cause cognitive decline.

INTERACTIONS

Drug–drug interactions with statins primarily occur through three mechanisms: CYP3A4/5 inhibition (amiodarone, macrolides, CCBs, protease inhibitors, azole antifungals, grapefruit juice, rifampin, carbamazepine); drugs that interfere with transport proteins (cyclosporine); and drugs that affect glucuronidation (gemfibrozil).

SPECIFIC MEDICATIONS

There are currently seven statins available on the US market. The statins vary in potency and drug interactions as shown in Table 83-8.

CLINICAL COMMENTARY

Because statins reduce all-cause mortality, the 2013 ACC/AHA guidelines identified four groups of patients who benefit from moderate- or high-intensity statin therapy: (1) those older than 21 years of age who already have established clinical ASCVD; (2) those older than 21 years of age with LDL-C levels of ≥190 mg/dL; (3) those 40 to 75 years of age with diabetes without known ASCVD and LDL-C of 70 to 189 mg/dL; and (4) those who do not meet any of the above criteria, but have an estimated 10-year risk of developing ASCVD of 7.5% or greater. Patients in any of these four groups should receive statin therapy unless contraindications, such as pregnancy, exist.

Many patients fail to remain on long-term statin therapy and myopathy is the most common reason for their lack of adherence. Because statins markedly reduce CV risk, poor adherence is an important clinical issue. If a statin myopathy is suspected, the statin should be discontinued for 2 to 3 weeks and the patient rechallenged with the initial statin. If the patient still cannot tolerate the statin, a different statin, a lower dose, or less than daily dosing may

TABLE 83-8. Overview of Statin Medications

Generic (Brand)	Dosing			Important Interacting Agents				
	Low Intensity	Moderate Intensity	High Intensity	Amiodarone	Carbamazepine	Clarithromycin	Cyclosporine	Diltiazem
Atorvastatin (Lipitor)		10–20 mg daily	40–80 mg daily	X	X	X	X	X
Fluvastatin (Lescol)	20–40 mg QHS	80 mg QHS or 40 mg bid					X	
Lovastatin (Mevacor, Altoprev)	20 mg QHS	40 mg QHS		X	X	X	X	X
Pitavastatin (Livalo)	1 mg daily	2–4 mg daily						
Pravastatin (Pravachol)	10–20 mg QHS	40–80 mg QHS					X	
Rosuvastatin (Crestor)		5–10 mg daily	20–40 mg daily				X	
Simvastatin (Zocor)	10 mg QHS	20–40 mg QHS		X	X	X	X	X

bid, twice daily; PO, by mouth; QHS, every night at bedtime.

be tried. Studies show that many statin-intolerant patients do well when they are challenged with a different statin or by reducing dosage.

DIURETICS

GENERAL INFORMATION

In outpatient practice, diuretics are most often prescribed for HTN, HF, and other fluid-retaining conditions. Diuretics consist of a diverse group of medications that act on the kidney to increase urine output. The mechanism and site of action of a diuretic affects its typical side effects. Understanding the pharmacologic differences among these medications assists providers in choosing the most appropriate medication for their patient.

THERAPEUTIC EFFECTS

A diuretic is any substance that promotes urine excretion. The kidneys filter blood to excrete waste and to help maintain the proper balance of electrolytes, water, and pH. The filtration byproduct, urine, contains metabolic waste products such as urea and nonwaste products such as water, electrolytes, and glucose. Most diuretics promote excretion of waste and nonwaste products by inhibiting the reabsorption of electrolytes (primarily sodium) through the renal tubules. Sodium and other unabsorbed components create an osmotic gradient that draws water along with them, increasing urine output.

Prescription diuretics vary in their site of action in the kidney, potency, and proclivity to cause electrolyte imbalances. Diuretics can be divided into five categories: thiazide/thiazide-like, loop, potassium-sparing, osmotic, and carbonic anhydrase inhibitors. Figure 83-1 shows the site of action for thiazide and thiazide-like, loop, and potassium-sparing diuretics. Agents that cause a greater diuresis are typically used for edematous disorders (HF, nephrotic syndrome, refractory ascites), whereas those causing less diuresis are used for HTN. Loop diuretics are the most potent, whereas thiazide/thiazide-like diuretics

Fluconazole	Gemfibrozil	Grapefruit juice	Itraconazole	Ketoconazole	Protease inhibitors	Rifampin	Cost	Comments
	X	X	X	X	X	X	$$	Long half-life, decrease frequency with myopathy; low doses for HIV
X						X	$	Well tolerated, less myopathy
	X	X	X	X	X	X	$	
							$$$	Less risk of developing diabetes
	X					X	$$	Safest statin for HIV (less drug interactions)
X	X					X	$$$	Long half-life, decrease frequency with myopathy
	X	X	X	X	X	X	$	FDA warning against 80 mg/day—higher rates of rhabdomyolysis

are less potent and have a longer duration of action. Potassium-sparing diuretics are the least potent with a duration of action similar to that of thiazides. The thiazide/thiazide-like diuretics, often in combination with potassium-sparing diuretics, are most commonly used for BP control and less often for edema.

SIDE EFFECTS

The most common side effects of diuretics are fluid and electrolyte imbalances. Loop and thiazide/thiazide-like diuretics can cause hyponatremia, hypokalemia, and hypomagnesemia. Potassium-sparing diuretics inhibit reabsorption of potassium and can cause hyperkalemia. Of note, thiazide/thiazide-like diuretics can cause hypercalcemia, whereas loop diuretics can cause hypocalcemia. Thiazide-induced hypercalcemia usually resolves in 7 to 10 days, and persistent hypercalcemia suggests the possibility of undiagnosed hyperparathyroidism. Common symptoms include dizziness, dry mouth, thirst, weakness, headaches, muscle cramps, nausea and vomiting,

and drowsiness. In more severe cases seizures, confusion, hypotension, inability to urinate, kidney damage, and arrhythmias can occur. Monitoring fluid and electrolyte status prevents many of these side effects from occurring.

Other side effects include impotence, gout, and hyperglycemia. Hyperglycemia is usually mild, and the degree of both the hyperglycemia and hyperuricemia are usually clinically insignificant. Impotence is often overlooked, and asking patients taking diuretics about their sexual function is important. Although textbooks often mention a cross-reactivity of thiazide to sulfonamide antibiotics, the sulfur-containing components differ in the two molecules and cross-reactivity is rare. Most patients tolerate diuretics well and report few or no significant side effects.

GENERAL DRUG INTERACTIONS

There are many drug interactions with diuretics and providers should evaluate a patient's medications for potential drug–drug and drug–disease state

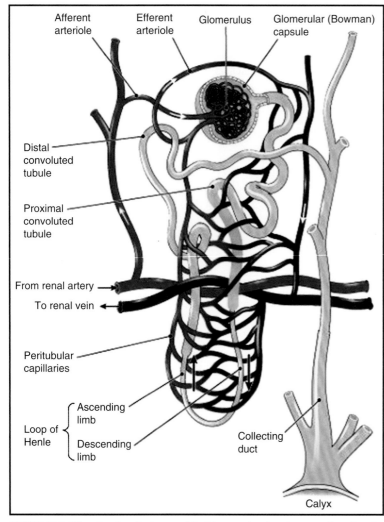

Afferent arteriole
Efferent arteriole
Glomerulus
Glomerular (Bowman) capsule

Distal convoluted tubule

Proximal convoluted tubule

From renal artery
To renal vein

Peritubular capillaries

Ascending limb
Loop of Henle
Descending limb

Collecting duct

Calyx

> Loop diuretics act at the proximal convoluted tubule, Loop of Henle, and distal convoluted tubule

> Thiazide and thiazide like diuretics act at the Loop of Henle and distal convoluted tubule

> Potassium Sparing diuretics act at the proximal convoluted tubule and Loop of Henle

FIGURE 83-1. Site of action for loops, thiazides, and potassium-sparing diuretics. (From Cohen BJ, ed. *Memmler's The Human Body in Health and Disease*. 12th ed. Philadelphia, PA: Lippincott Williams & Wilkins; 2012.)

interactions. Common interactions include the following: nonsteroidal anti-inflammatory agents that can blunt the effectiveness of diuretic agents; reduced lithium clearance and an increased risk of lithium toxicity; diuretic-induced hypokalemia causing digoxin toxicity; and worsened glycemic control that, on occasion, may merit medication adjustment. Patients taking antiarrhythmic medications require careful monitoring of their fluid and electrolyte status because imbalances can induce or worsen electrophysiologic changes.

SPECIFIC MEDICATIONS

Table 83-9 shows typical indications, dosing, potency, half-life, cautions/contraindications, typical costs, and suggested monitoring of select thiazide/thiazide-like, loop, and potassium-sparing diuretics.

CLINICAL COMMENTARY

Thiazide and Thiazide-like Diuretics

Recent research regarding the clinical equivalency between hydrochlorothiazide and chlorthalidone stirred debate about the preferred drug for HTN. The half-life of chlorthalidone is longer than that of hydrochlorothiazide, spurring speculation that chlorthalidone could affect CV morbidity and mortality to a greater extent. A recent metaanalysis showed that chlorthalidone decreased CV events by 12% and heart failure by 21% compared to hydrochlorothiazide. However, since chlorthalidone costs more than hydrochlorothiazide, affordability should be considered when determining which product may be best for an individual patient. Both thiazide and thiazide-like diuretics lose effectiveness at CrCl of <30 mL/min, and providers should discontinue thiazides in these cases and use a loop diuretic instead. Thiazides also

TABLE 83-9. Overview on Select Diuretics

Medications	Typical Indications	Typical Dosing	Diuretic Potency	Half-Life	Cautions/ Contraindications	Costs	Monitoring
Thiazide or Thiazide-like Diuretics							
Hydrochloro-thiazide	Hypertension	12.5–25 mg once daily	Moderate	4–15 hours	Anuria, pregnancy, hepatic dysfunction	$	• Sodium, potassium (higher doses), blood urea nitrogen and creatinine
Chlorthalidone	Hypertension	25–50 mg once daily	Moderate	30–60 hours	Anuria, pregnancy, hepatic dysfunction	$$	• Sodium, potassium (higher doses), blood urea nitrogen and creatinine
Loop Diuretics							
Furosemide	Heart failure or edema	20–80 mg once daily	High	2 hours	Anuria, hepatic dysfunction	$	• Sodium, potassium, blood urea nitrogen and creatinine; magnesium and phosphate if indicated
Bumetanide	Heart failure or edema	0.5–2 mg once daily	High	4–6 hours	Anuria, hepatic dysfunction, sulfa allergy	$$	• Sodium, potassium, blood urea nitrogen and creatinine; magnesium and phosphate if indicated
Potassium Sparing Diuretics							
Amiloride	Combined with loop or thiazide for heart failure or edema	5–10 mg once daily	Low	6–9 hours	Hyperkalemia, anuria, hepatic dysfunction	$–$$	• Potassium, blood urea nitrogen and creatinine
Triamterene	Combined with thiazide for hypertension	37.5–50 mg once daily	Low	1–3 hours	Hyperkalemia, anuria, hepatic dysfunction	$	• Potassium, blood urea nitrogen and creatinine

reduce peripheral resistance, probably by lowering intracellular sodium in the vascular smooth muscle cells and relaxing the arterial wall smooth muscle.

Metalozone, a sulfonamide similar to thiazide diuretics, is more effective in patients with renal impairment. It can be combined with a loop diuretic for refractory cases of edema.

Loop Diuretics

Manufacturing shortages over the last 10 to 15 years have affected the availably of furosemide, making a knowledge of alternatives necessary in the event of future shortages. Alternatives include torsemide and bumetanide, which are more potent than furosemide. Ethacrynic acid is another loop diuretic; however, its use is limited because of a higher incidence of ototoxicity. Although loop diuretics are not traditionally used for BP control, they do lower BP and may be a better choice in patients with renal impairment (CrCl < 30 mL/min). When prescribing a loop diuretic for BP control, providers can consider twice-daily dosing with the last dose early in the afternoon to avoid nocturia.

Because of their potency, loop diuretics should be used cautiously. Postural hypotension, prerenal azotemia (BUN to creatinine ratio > 20:1), lightheadedness, and fatigue are clues to hypovolemia and overdiuresis. Hypokalemia is the most serious metabolic consequence, and potassium supplementation is indicated if levels fall below 3.5 mg/dL. In cases of heart failure, loop diuretics help control congestive symptoms and edema, but do not extend longevity.

Potassium-Sparing Diuretics

Potassium-sparing diuretics should be used cautiously with other agents that can raise serum potassium levels such as potassium supplements, ACEi, and ARBs. These patients need frequent serum potassium monitoring. Potassium-sparing diuretics are weak diuretics when used alone, but are often used in fixed-dose combinations in conjunction with thiazides to avoid hypokalemia.

In patients with HF due to systolic dysfunction with an ejection fraction <30%, adding either spironolactone or eplerenone improves outcomes. Spironolactone is the diuretic of first choice in fluid retention related to liver failure, but is also more likely to cause gynecomastia or breast pain (up to 10%) than eplerenone (up to 0.5%).

Carbonic Anhydrase Inhibitors

These agents do not have a potent diuretic effect, and their main use in the ambulatory care setting is for the prophylaxis of altitude sickness and as a topical preparation in glaucoma patients.

Osmotic diuretics are rarely used in the outpatient family medicine setting.

84 | Endocrine Medications

CORTICOSTEROIDS

GENERAL INFORMATION

Family practice providers use corticosteroids for a wide variety of conditions. They are very effective anti-inflammatory and immune-modulating agents, but are limited in use by their long-term side effects. This section focuses on corticosteroids and their indications, general use, side effects, dosing, relative potency, and clinical pearls (Table 84-1). Anabolic steroids differ from corticosteroids and are most commonly used to treat male hypogonadism. They are often abused by athletes seeking to enhance performance.

THERAPEUTIC EFFECTS

Cortisol release from the adrenal glands is stimulated by adrenocorticotropic hormone (ACTH) which is released by the pituitary in response to corticotropin-releasing hormone (CRH) secreted by the hypothalamus. A negative feedback loop controls the release of CRH and ACTH based on circulating levels of cortisol. There is a diurnal pattern of cortisol release with higher blood levels in the early morning and late afternoon. Additionally, cortisol levels increase during times of stress. Corticosteroids are often referred to as glucocorticoids because cortisol increases gluconeogenesis making glucose more available during stressful times. They also have very potent anti-inflammatory and immune response properties. Some corticosteroids also have mineralocorticoid properties that cause sodium and water retention. Many of the therapeutic uses and side effects of the corticosteroids are due to the glucose, immune-modulating, and mineralocorticoid properties. Corticosteroids can be taken orally, inhaled, applied topically, and injected intravenously, intramuscularly, and into joints for arthritis.

Another type of steroid is the anabolic steroids related to testosterone. Anabolic refers to the muscle-building effect of these steroids, and androgenic means they increase male sex characteristics.

INDICATIONS

In family practice, providers most often prescribe corticosteroids by mouth for short-term treatment of inflamed and painful joints, allergic reactions, and acute respiratory illness. Long-term oral uses include rheumatoid arthritis (or other autoimmune disorders), adrenal insufficiency, and solid organ transplant. For asthma and more advanced cases of COPD, providers usually prescribe inhaled corticosteroids (ICS). In addition, corticosteroids can be applied topically to treat many skin disorders such as atopic dermatitis and eczema.

SIDE EFFECTS

Side effects of corticosteroids are diverse and can be severe. Generally, clinicians should not be concerned about long-term effects when prescribing corticosteroids for 2 weeks or less (unless prescribed frequently), or when delivered as an inhaled or topical preparation. When used acutely, the corticosteroids can cause dyspepsia, mild euphoria, and mild hyperglycemia. When used long term, corticosteroids can cause weight gain with fat redistribution, skin thinning, osteoporosis, increased risk of infections, hyperlipidemia, hypertension, hyperglycemia, cataracts, glaucoma, gastritis, euphoria, and psychosis. The extent to which these side effects occur is related to the dose, duration, and route of administration. Therefore, to avoid long-term effects, prescribers should use the smallest effective dose for the shortest period possible. Also, clinicians should promote exercise and appropriate vitamin D and calcium intake to help prevent osteoporosis.

ICS are not absorbed extensively from the lungs exerting their effects primarily in the lungs. Side effects of ICS include an increased risk of thrush, hoarse voice, and lower respiratory infections.

TABLE 84-1. Overview of Selected Corticosteroids

Generic (Brand)	Cost	Dosage Forms	Relative Potency
Oral			
Prednisone (Deltasone)	$	• Solution 5 mg/5 mL • Concentrated solution 5 mg/mL • Tablet 1, 2.5, 5, 10, 20, and 50 mg	Medium
Methylprednisolone (Medrol)	$	• Tablet 4, 8, 16, and 32 mg	Medium
Dexamethasone (Decadron)	$	• Solution 0.5 mg/5 mL • Concentrated solution 1 mg/mL • Tablet 0.5, 0.75, 1, 1.5, 2, 4, and 6 mg	High
Prednisolone (Prelone, Orapred)	$	• Suspension 15 mg/5 mL • Syrup 15 mg/5 mL • Tablet 5, 10, 15, and 30 mg	Medium
Topical			
Hydrocortisone (Cortisone 10 OTC, Hytone)	$	• Cream 0.5%, 1%, 2.5% • Ointment 0.5%, 1%, 2.5% • Spray 1% • Lotion 1%	Low
Triamcinolone acetonide (Kenolog, Aristocort)	$	• Cream 0.025%, 0.1%, 0.5% • Ointment 0.025%, 0.1%, 0.5% • Lotion 0.025%, 0.1%	Low (0.025%) Medium (0.1%) High (0.5%)
Mometasone furoate (Elocon)	$$	• Cream 0.1% • Ointment 0.1% • Lotion 0.1%	Medium
Betamethasone dipropionate (Diprosone, Diprolene)	$	• Cream 0.05% • Ointment 0.05% • Lotion 0.05%	High
Clobetasol propionate (Temovate, Clobex, Olux)	$$–$$$	• Cream 0.05% • Ointment 0.05% • Gel 0.05% • Lotion 0.05% • Foam 0.05% • Shampoo 0.05%	Very high
Inhaled			
Fluticasone (Flovent)	$$$	• 44–220 µg/inhalation	Medium
Mometasone (Asmanex)	$$$	• 110–220 µg/inhalation	Medium
Beclomethasone (Qvar)	$$$	• 40–80 µg/inhalation	High
Nasal Spray			
Fluticasone (Flonase OTC)	$	• 50 µg/spray	Medium
Triamcinololone (Nasacort OTC)	$	• 55 µg/spray	Medium

OTC, over-the-counter.

Although controversial, patients who use long-term, high-dose ICS may be at an increased risk for osteoporosis. Similarly, use of long-term, high-dose ICS in pediatric and adolescent patients carries a small risk of decreased overall growth. Rinsing the mouth with water after use of an ICS is an effective method to avoid oral thrush.

Nasal steroid sprays are very effective for allergic rhinitis and can be used safely long term. Recently, two products (Flonase and Nasacort) became available as over-the-counter medications. Systemic absorption is low, and side effects include an increase in bloody nose and taste disturbances.

Topical corticosteroids also have limited systemic absorption, but the absorption can increase with the use of high-strength topical steroids. Side effects of topical use include skin atrophy, acneiform eruptions, purpura, and hypopigmentation. High-potency corticosteroids can suppress the HPA axis, and can lead to glaucoma and other systemic side effects especially when used for longer than 2 weeks. In addition, tachyphylaxis may occur with prolonged use. Guidelines suggest using topical corticosteroids for no longer than 2 weeks at a time with at least 1-week drug-free intervals between uses. Also, avoid applying high-potency agents to the face, especially in the skin surrounding the eyes and mouth, to avoid acneiform eruptions and skin thinning.

Anabolic steroids also have significant side effects, and although useful for patients with testosterone deficiency and for patients who lose muscle mass from AIDS or cancer, their nonmedical use should be discouraged. Short-term side effects include paranoia, irritability, impaired judgment, swelling, acne, and hypertension. Long-term use can cause kidney and liver disease, high BP, high cholesterol, cardiac hypertrophy, and an increased risk of heart attack and stroke. Their androgenic effect in men can cause decreases in sperm count, baldness, gynecomastia, and testicular atrophy. Women can experience masculinization with male pattern baldness, hirsutism, enlarged clitoris, and deepened voice.

CLINICAL COMMENTARY

Clinically, steroid use is complicated by suppression of the HPA-axis. Recommendations for those needing to be tapered off steroids include the following:

- Patients taking 20 mg or more of daily prednisone for more than 3 weeks;
- Patients taking an evening dose of prednisone greater than 5 mg for more than 2 weeks;
- Anyone with a Cushing-type appearance.

Any dose of corticosteroids for less than 3 weeks does not usually warrant a steroid taper to prevent HPA-axis suppression; however, owing to the serious nature of HPA-axis suppression, many clinicians suggest tapering steroids in frail or seriously ill patients. Although there is no set way to taper steroids, one general rule is to decrease the dose by 10% to 20% each week. The patient should be monitored for any

recurrence of the baseline disease and for symptoms of adrenal insufficiency. Commercial "dose packs" are available for short-term use and have a taper built into the dosing regimen. Although tapering is not necessary for short-term steroid use, dose packs are easy to prescribe and easy for patients to use. Adrenal suppression is usually not a concern with topical or inhaled corticosteroids.

Patients should be counseled to take their oral corticosteroids with food and to take them first thing in the morning to coincide with the peak of endogenous adrenal activity. For topical administration, it is important to counsel the patient to apply a small amount and to limit use to 2 weeks. Ointments tend to deliver more medication than creams or lotions. For ICS, patients should rinse their mouths after each inhalation.

SULFONYLUREAS

GENERAL INFORMATION

Sulfonylureas (SUs) were one of the first oral agents discovered for the management of type 2 diabetes and have been in use for more than 50 years. They can be used as monotherapy or in conjunction with other oral antihyperglycemic medications. Although still one of the most widely used agents, their use as a first-line agent is decreasing as data emerge associating metformin with better CV outcomes. SUs lower HbA_{1C} by approximately 1.5% to 2%, and are useful in treating mild to moderately severe disease. As with other antihyperglycemic agents, HbA_{1C} and blood glucose readings should be monitored to assess effectiveness.

THERAPEUTIC EFFECTS

Insulin is released by the pancreas, and the SUs stimulate endogenous insulin secretion by binding to receptors on the beta cells and stimulating potassium channels sensitive to ATP. SUs are ineffective when there is an absolute deficiency in insulin production as in type 1 diabetes or in those with pancreatic insufficiency. SUs may also reduce serum glucagon and increase insulin sensitivity, but the mechanisms of action for these effects remain uncertain.

About 25% of patients with type 2 diabetes are controlled long term with a SU alone. The natural history of the disease and the gradual, progressive loss of beta cell function results in decreased efficacy and worsened glycemic control despite an initial response to a SU and increasing to maximal doses. In these patients, a second agent is required to meet treatment targets. Providers occasionally combine SUs with insulin.

SIDE EFFECTS

SUs can cause hypoglycemia and weight gain of approximately 5 to 10 lbs. Their hypoglycemic effect makes it important to discuss the management of hypoglycemia when prescribing or increasing the dose of a SU. Weight gain can be troublesome because most patients with type 2 diabetes are overweight or obese, and gaining weight heightens insulin resistance and the risk of CVD. Other class side effects include nausea and rarely elevated liver transaminases that require discontinuing the drug.

INTERACTIONS

Any medication that alters blood glucose levels can interact with SUs; when combined with SUs, other oral antihyperglycemic agents enhance the risk of hypoglycemia. Medications that increase blood glucose, like BBs or thiazide diuretics, can decrease the efficacy of SUs, but this is typically not clinically relevant. BBs can also mask symptoms of hypoglycemia for a SU. Since meglitinide and SUs share the same mechanism of action, they should not be combined.

SUs are cytochrome P (CYP) 2C9 substrates and lower SU concentrations may occur when used in patients treated with CYP2C9 inducers such as carbamazepine, phenytoin, phenobarbital, primidone, and rifampin. Higher concentrations of SUs can occur in patients treated with CYP2C9 inhibitors, such as gemfibrozil, fluorouracil, nicardipine, cimetidine, and fluconazole. SUs like glipizide and glyburide may be displaced from albumin when taken with highly protein-bound drugs such as oral anticoagulants, salicylate, NSAIDs, protein-bound anticonvulsants, and sulfonamides.

SUs should be taken at least 4 hours before colesevelam to avoid problems with absorption. On rare occasions, patients taking a SU experience disulfiram reactions with alcohol.

CAUTIONS

SUs are structurally related to sulfonamides and should be avoided in patients with a severe sulfa allergy. They are also contraindicated for use in type 1 diabetes because these patients do not have functioning beta cells.

SUs should be used with caution in patients with hepatic or renal dysfunction and the elderly. The elderly are at greater risk for hypoglycemia and may be less likely to display symptoms of hypoglycemia.

SPECIFIC MEDICATIONS

The three most commonly used SUs in the United States are glipizide, glimepiride, and glyburide, all of which are available in generic forms. Table 84-2 compares the pharmacokinetic properties and dosing of these agents. When patients switch from one SU to another, they should be started at the initial dose of the new SU because there are no clear dose conversions between agents.

CLINICAL COMMENTARY

SUs can cause hypoglycemia at any dose. Fasting and postprandial sugars should be monitored with doses adjusted upward every 1 to 2 weeks as needed. If a patient is elderly or has decreased renal function, providers should start at lower doses and titrate up more slowly. Glipizide is preferred in older adults because of a shorter half-life and a lower incidence of hypoglycemia. Over time, SUs lose effectiveness as beta cell function declines; typically adding other medications to a SU are needed to control a patient's blood glucose levels.

METFORMIN

GENERAL INFORMATION

First approved in 1994 for the treatment of type 2 diabetes, metformin is the only approved drug among a class of agents called biguanides. Prior to metformin, phenformin was an FDA-approved biguanide but was withdrawn from the market owing to an increased risk of lactic acidosis and excess CV mortality. Based on its effectiveness and risk–benefit ratio, the American Diabetes Association recommends metformin as initial therapy for most individuals with type 2 diabetes, especially those who are obese. Metformin is available as a low-cost generic drug and lowers HbA_{1C} by about 1.5% to 2.0%.

THERAPEUTIC EFFECTS

Metformin improves glycemic control primarily by decreasing hepatic gluconeogenesis, and also reduces intestinal glucose absorption and improves

TABLE 84-2. Overview on Sulfonylureas

Generic (Brand)	Cost	Dose	Half-Life	Comments
Glipizide (Glucotrol) Glipizide ER (Glucotrol XL)	$	5 mg daily to start; 40 mg maximum (glipizide); 20 mg maximum (glipizide ER)	2–5 hours	• Split dose if it exceeds 15 mg daily • Maximum therapeutic effect is 20 mg daily. • 30 minutes before meals (preferred breakfast) • When switching between drug formulations, switch to same daily dose. • Not recommended in pregnancy; stop 1 month prior to delivery if used in pregnancy. • Lactation—case reports suggest it does not cross into breastmilk. • Renal impairment: may be less likely to cause hypoglycemia; recommended to avoid extended release formulation. • May cause vomiting, diarrhea, or constipation.
Glimepiride (Amaryl)	$–$$	1–2 mg daily to start; 8 mg maximum	5–9 hours	• Take before first meal of the day. • Not recommended in pregnancy • Renal impairment: use cautiously • Hepatic impairment: has not been studied
Glyburide (Diabeta) Micronized glyburide (Glynase PresTab)	$	2.5–5 mg daily (glyburide) to start; 20 mg maximum (glyburide) 1.5–3 mg daily (micronized) to start; 12 mg maximum (micronized)	4 hours (glyburide) 10 hours (micronized)	• Split dose if it exceeds 10 mg daily (glyburide) or 6 mg daily (micronized). When switching between drug formulations, start from initial dose and retitrate. • 30 minutes before meals, ideally first main meal • Crosses placenta; however, most common SU used in pregnancy. Stop 2 weeks before anticipated delivery. • Lactation—does not cross into breastmilk. • Renal impairment: not recommended if eGFR <60 mL/min • Do not use in elderly if possible; can cause extended hypoglycemia • Rarely can cause epigastric fullness, diarrhea, or heartburn • Increased serum aminotransferase concentrations can occur with bosentan; do not use concomitantly.

eGFR, estimate glomerular filtration rate; SU, sulfonylureas

insulin sensitivity which increases glucose utilization. Because it does not stimulate insulin release, metformin does not cause hypoglycemia when used alone; however, it increases the risk of hypoglycemia when used with insulin or drugs that stimulate insulin secretion.

Although similar in overall effectiveness to the second-generation SUs, metformin is an insulin-sensitizing agent rather than a secretagogue and in contrast to a SU, it may be effective when an initial fasting blood level (>300 mg/dL) indicates poor beta cell responsiveness. The ability to enhance insulin sensitivity also makes metformin a logical choice to combine with insulin or a secretagogue such as a SU.

SIDE EFFECTS

The most common side effects associated with metformin are dose related, and are predominantly GI including diarrhea, bloating, flatulence, abdominal discomfort, and nausea. These side effects occur more frequently with the immediate release form than the sustained release products. Taking metformin with meals may reduce the incidence of GI upset.

Lactic acidosis is a rare (<0.03%) but potentially fatal adverse effect. The risk is greatest in patients who are hypovolemic, hypoxic, or have renal insufficiency. Because the drug is excreted by the kidney, serum levels can rise in patients with poor kidney function and cause impaired hepatic metabolism of lactate. Symptoms of lactic acidosis include respiratory distress, lethargy, abdominal discomfort, malaise, and myalgia. In these situations, metformin should be discontinued immediately and supportive measures initiated.

Patients receiving intravenous (IV) contrast for a radiologic procedure are also at increased risk for developing lactic acidosis. Although there is disagreement about exactly when to stop and restart metformin for patients scheduled to receive an IV contrast dye, many physicians recommend withholding metformin for 48 hours before administering contrast to patients with an eGFR <60 mL/min and waiting 48 hours before restarting metformin. Others feel that the risk is minimal for patients with normal renal function or for those receiving only a small amount of contrast and that no dose adjustment is needed.

INTERACTIONS

Metformin interactions are primarily due to competition for proximal renal tubular secretion. Potential interactions include trimethoprim, triamterene, vancomycin, procainamide, ranitidine, digoxin, and amiloride. However, these interactions usually are clinically insignificant. Other drug interactions that could potentially decrease glycemic control include thiazide diuretics, corticosteroids, thyroid products, estrogens, and isoniazid.

PHARMACODYNAMICS/PHARMACOKINETICS

Metformin is excreted in the urine unchanged and does not undergo liver metabolism. However, the half-life varies depending upon the extended release versus immediate release formulations. The extended release formulation allows for once-daily dosing whereas the immediate release formulation is typically prescribed twice daily.

PRECAUTIONS AND CONTRAINDICATIONS

Caution should be used when prescribing metformin to elderly patients owing to decreased renal function.

Reduced renal function prolongs the half-life, increasing metformin plasma concentration. Previously, contraindications for metformin use included SCr ≥1.5 mg/dL (males), SCr ≥1.4 mg/dL (females), or in patients over the age of 80 unless renal function was found to be normal. However, in 2016, the FDA required manufacturers to change the assessment of renal function to the eGFR because eGFR takes into account other patient-specific factors such as age, gender, weight, and race. The FDA recommended a baseline eGFR before starting metformin, and if the eGFR is ≤30 mL/min/1.73 m^2, metformin is contraindicated. If the eGFR is between 30 and 45 mL/min/1.73 m^2, it is not recommended. For patients taking metformin, monitoring kidney function annually is sufficient unless a patient is elderly or has renal insufficiency. Providers should avoid metformin in patients with HF, active alcoholism, or liver disease. Metformin should not be used in patients with diabetic ketoacidosis or any metabolic acidosis.

COST

Metformin is inexpensive compared to many other antihyperglycemic agents, and can cost as little as $ 4/month for the immediate release formulation, making it a good alternative for self-pay patients. Extended release formulations are more expensive but are covered by most insurance companies.

CLINICAL COMMENTARY

Metformin is considered first-line therapy for patients with newly diagnosed diabetes unless renal function is impaired. If the A$_{1C}$ is ≥ 10%, temporary initiation of long-acting insulin (no >10 units/day) in addition to the metformin is advised. Initial metformin doses should not exceed 500 mg by mouth twice daily (primarily owing to GI side effects). If the patient tolerates this dose but is not adequately controlled, the dose can be increased to a maximum of 2500 mg daily. Extended release formulations are more costly, but should be prescribed for patients with intolerable side effects or those with adherence issues.

In some cases, metformin may suppress appetite and induce a mild weight loss, making it exceptionally useful in obese patients.

85 | Gastrointestinal Medications

PROTON PUMP INHIBITORS

GENERAL INFORMATION

Proton pump inhibitors (PPIs) are the most effective and potent class of acid inhibitors available to treat gastric and esophageal disorders related to gastric acid production. Common indications include dyspepsia, gastric and duodenal ulcers, gastro-esophageal reflux disease, erosive esophagitis, and Barrett esophagus. They are considered the drug of choice for Zollinger–Ellison syndrome, and when used with NSAIDs reduce the risk of GI bleeding. PPIs also appear to have an antibacterial effect on Helicobacter and are incorporated in treatments to eradicate *Helicobacter pylori*.

Because they effectively treat common stomach disorders with relatively few side effects, several PPIs can be purchased over the counter although at lower dosages than pills available by prescription. Omeprazole, released in 1988, represents the first PPI and is now one of many in the class that includes lansoprazole, esomeprazole, dexlansoprazole, pantoprazole, and rabeprazole. Despite extensive marketing, there is no documented therapeutic advantage between generic and brand-named PPIs.

THERAPEUTIC EFFECTS

As a class, PPIs irreversibly bind to the H+/K+/ATPase (proton pump) located in gastric parietal cells and decrease acid production in the stomach, which increases the gastric pH to levels associated with mucosal healing (pH > 4).

SIDE EFFECTS

Adverse effects associated with short-term use of PPIs are infrequent and usually mild. These include nausea, vomiting, diarrhea, flatulence, and headache. However, more severe adverse effects have been implicated in long-term use including an increased risk of fractures secondary to osteoporosis, reduced calcium absorption, and hypomagnesemia secondary to reduced magnesium absorption. To minimize the risk of osteoporosis associated with a PPI, some physicians recommend supplemental calcium and vitamin D to enhance calcium absorption.

Stomach acid also helps protect against infection, and long-term acid suppression modestly increases the risk of *Clostridium difficile*-associated diarrhea, community acquired pneumonia (CAP), and gastric cancer from an *H. pylori* infection. Individuals on long-term high-dose therapy should be tested for *H. pylori* and treated if positive.

INTERACTIONS

PPIs are metabolized by the cytochrome P450 metabolic pathway in the liver and can cause drug interactions with other agents metabolized by this pathway. Monitoring and possible dose adjustments may be needed. Other common interactions center on the need for an acid environment for some drugs to be absorbed. For example, protease inhibitors used in the treatment of HIV need a low gastric pH to achieve peak drug levels, and acid suppression may render some protease inhibitors ineffective. Long-term PPI use is also associated with atrophic gastritis and poor B_{12} absorption, requiring B_{12} levels be monitored annually.

SPECIFIC MEDICATIONS

Tables 85-1 and 85-2 summarize the doses and indications of PPIs.

CLINICAL COMMENTARY

Since the release of omeprazole, PPIs have become the mainstay of therapy related to stomach acid production. Judicious use can alleviate and treat many acid-related GI disorders. However, because of their

TABLE 85-1. Doses and Indications for Proton Pump Inhibitors

Drug	Equivalent Dose	Clinical Dose Range	Dose/ Duration GERD	Dose/Duration Duodenal Ulcer	Dose/ Duration Gastric Ulcer	Dose/ Duration Erosive Esophagitis	[b]Dose/ Duration for *Helicobacter pylori*
Omeprazole	[a]20 mg	20–40 mg daily	20 mg 4 weeks	20 mg 4–8 weeks	40 mg 4–8 weeks	20 mg 4–12 weeks	20 mg bid 14 days
Esomeprazole	[a]20 mg	20–40 mg daily	20 mg 4–8 weeks		20–40 mg 6 months	20–40 mg 4–8 weeks	20 mg bid 10 days
Lansoprazole	[a]15 mg	15–30 mg daily	15 mg 4–8 weeks	15 mg 4 weeks	30 mg 4–8 weeks	30 mg 8–16 weeks	30 mg bid 14 days
Dexlansoprazole	30 mg	30–60 mg daily	30 mg 4 weeks			60 mg 4–8 weeks	
Pantoprazole	20 mg	20–40 mg daily				40 mg 4–8 weeks	
Rabeprazole	20 mg	Daily	20 mg 4 weeks	20 mg 4 weeks		20 mg 4–16 weeks	20 mg 7 days

[a]Available in this strength OTC.
[b]In combination with amoxicillin, clarithromycin, or metronidazole.
bid, twice daily; GERD, gastroesophageal reflux disease; OTC, over-the-counter.

TABLE 85-2. Overview of Proton Pump Inhibitors

Generic (Brand)	Cost	Dosage Forms	Half-Life	Comments
Omeprazole (Prilosec)	$	• Delayed release capsules • Enteric coated tablets • Oral packet and suspension (Rx only)	0.5–1 hour; effect lasts up to 72 hours	• Best on empty stomach 30–60 minutes before a meal • Zollinger–Ellison may require significantly higher doses; 60 mg daily or 40 mg twice daily up to 120 mg three times daily • Metabolized in the liver; inhibitor of CYP2C19 and lesser extent CYP3A4 • Clopidogrel ineffective when combined with omeprazole • Cross-reactivity with other PPIs (allergic hypersensitivity) • Hepatic impairment (Child–Pugh class A, B, or C), and those of Asian descent may require dose reduction
Esomeprazole (Nexium)	$$–$$$	• Delayed release capsule • Delayed release tablet • Oral packet, and injectable (Rx only)	1–1.5 hours; effect lasts up to 72 hours	• Best on empty stomach 30–60 minutes before a meal • Zollinger–Ellison syndrome require significantly higher doses; 40 mg twice daily with upward ranges of 240 mg twice daily • Metabolized in the liver; inhibitor of CYP2C19 and lesser extent CYP3A4 • Potential to render clopidogrel ineffective • Linked to cutaneous and systemic lupus • Severe liver impairment (Child–Pugh class C): no more than 20 mg daily

TABLE 85-2. Overview of Proton Pump Inhibitors (*continued*)

Generic (Brand)	Cost	Dosage Forms	Half-Life	Comments
Lansoprazole (Prevacid)	$$	• Delayed release capsule • Oral dispersal tablet, and suspension (Rx only)	1–1.5 hours; effect lasts up to 72 hours	• Best on empty stomach 30–60 minutes before a meal • Half-life extended in the elderly and in those with hepatic impairment • Zollinger–Ellison syndrome requires significantly higher doses; 60 mg daily with upward ranges of 90 mg twice daily • Metabolized in the liver; inhibitor of CYP2C19 and lesser extent CYP3A4 • May interact with clopidogrel; manufacturer does not recommend dosage adjustment; consider alternative agents if possible.
Dexlansoprazole (Dexilant)	$$$	• Delayed release capsule	1–2 hours; effect lasts up to 72 hours	• Less potent than lansoprazole • Food increases absorption (can take with or without food) • A 30 mg maximum dose is recommended for patients with Child–Pugh class B and use in patients with Child–Pugh class C is not recommended. • Same precautions and interactions as lansoprazole
Pantoprazole (Protonix)	$$$	• Delayed release tablet • Oral packet • Injectable	3.5 hours	• Doses should be taken 30 minutes before a meal • Half-life extended in hepatic impairment • 40 mg maximum dose is recommended for patient's hepatic insufficiency • Weak inhibitor of CYP2C19 and lesser extent CYP3A4 • May interact with clopidogrel; manufacturer does not recommend dosage adjustment; consider alternative agents if possible. • Linked to systemic lupus erythematosus
Rabeprazole (Aciphex)	$$$	• Delayed release tablet • Sprinkle capsule	2–5 hours; effect lasts up to 24 hours	• Doses should be taken 30 minutes before a meal • Half-life is extended in those with hepatic impairment; avoid in Child–Pugh class C. • Zollinger–Ellison syndrome requires significantly higher doses; 60 mg once daily with dose adjustments up to 100 mg daily or 60 mg twice daily • Metabolized by CYP2C19 and CYP3A4 • May render clopidogrel ineffective; consider alternative agents if possible

CYP, cytochrome; PPIs, proton pump inhibitors

low side-effect profile, they tend to be used in patients who do not need chronic acid suppression. Clinicians should not only know when to initiate therapy, but also when to stop therapy to avoid side effects associated with chronic use. As PPIs are costly, patient insurance or prescription plan should be considered when making a decision on product selection.

For patients with mild symptoms, an H_2 blocker may suffice and may be preferred over a PPI because of lower cost and the potential risks of chronic PPI therapy. However, for those who do not respond to an H_2 blocker, a PPI is indicated.

ANTIEMETICS

GENERAL INFORMATION

Patients take antiemetic agents for a wide variety of circumstances including motion sickness, prevention of nausea and vomiting associated with chemotherapy, diabetic gastroparesis, hyperemesis gravidarum, idiosyncratic drug reactions, and surgery or illnesses associated with nausea and vomiting. The antihistamines are a group of antiemetics commonly used for motion sickness. These include diphenhydramine, dimenhydrinate, and meclizine (see Antihistamine section, Chapter 87). Scopolamine, an anticholinergic medication, available as a patch placed behind the ear, is commonly prescribed for motion sickness. The patch should be applied at least 4 hours before its effects are needed, and lasts up to 3 days. Doxylamine and pyridoxine (vitamin B_6) are first-line medications for treating hyperemesis gravidarum. Dopamine receptor antagonists are helpful for nausea and vomiting associated with chemotherapy or diabetic gastroparesis. Agents include prochlorperazine, promethazine, and metoclopramide. Because metoclopramide also has a prokinetic effect on the GI tract, it is commonly prescribed for diabetic gastroparesis. Currently, the most widely used antiemetic agents in the community setting are the 5-HT_3 receptor antagonists. These agents include palonosetron, dolasetron, granisetron, and ondansetron. Ondansetron is the most frequently prescribed and is well tolerated, with fewer reported side effects than antihistamines and dopamine receptor antagonists.

Cannabinoids may be useful for refractory nausea and vomiting in patients undergoing chemotherapy.

THERAPEUTIC EFFECTS

As noted, several classes of drugs are used as antiemetic agents and include anticholinergics, antihistamines, cannabinoids, 5-HT receptor antagonists,

and phenothiazines. The anticholinergic medication, scopolamine, appears to block cholinergic transmission from the CNS to the vomiting center, whereas the dopamine receptor antagonists block dopamine receptors in the chemotherapy trigger zone. The 5-HT_3 receptor antagonists block the action of serotonin at the 5-HT_3 receptors located in the GI and CNS. Phenothiazines (e.g., promethazine) inhibit dopamine, muscarinic, and histamine receptors in the vomiting center and chemoreceptor zone. Metoclopramide blocks both dopaminergic and serotonergic receptors, which account for both its antiemetic action and extrapyramidal side effects. It accelerates gastric emptying by enhancing the effect of acetylcholine on the upper GI tract.

SIDE EFFECTS

Common side effects of the dopamine receptor antagonists include sedation, lethargy, and rash. Less common but more worrisome side effects include Parkinsonian-like symptoms, neuroleptic malignant syndrome (NMS), seizures (lowers seizure threshold), QT prolongation, cholestatic jaundice, hyperprolactinemia, galactorrhea, and extrapyramidal symptoms.

Although the 5-HT_3 receptor antagonists are generally well tolerated, their side effects include constipation or diarrhea, malaise, fatigue, dizziness, and headache. These agents can also prolong the QTc and PR interval; however, this is more common with IV formulations.

INTERACTIONS

Avoid concomitant use of other dopamine antagonists with prochlorperazine, promethazine, and metoclopramide.

Using 5-HT_3 receptor antagonists with other serotonergic agents (SSRIs, SNRIs, MAOIs, fentanyl, lithium, tramadol, mirtazapine, and IV methylene blue) increases the risk of serotonin syndrome, a group of symptoms associated with too much serotonin. Serotonin syndrome symptoms can range from mild, such as shivering, sweatiness, headache, restlessness, and diarrhea, to more severe symptoms including confusion, muscle rigidity, fever, and seizures. Mild symptoms usually respond to supportive care and stopping the medication, whereas severe serotonin syndrome requires hospitalization and can be fatal.

PRECAUTIONS AND CONTRAINDICATIONS

Dopamine receptor antagonists are contraindicated in individuals with Parkinson disease. All patients taking dopamine receptor antagonists should be monitored for Parkinsonian and extrapyramidal symptoms. High fever, muscle rigidity, and mental status changes can be indicative of NMS, a rare but life-threatening idiosyncratic reaction. For patients with suspected NMS, the medication should be discontinued immediately and emergency services provided. Providers should avoid the use of dopamine receptor antagonists in patients with a history of seizures, or in combination with medications or illicit drugs that lower the seizure threshold (bupropion, TCAs, some antibiotics, cocaine, etc.). Because QT prolongation can occur, providers should weigh the risks and benefits of using these agents in patients at risk for arrhythmias.

Providers should also monitor for rhythm changes when using 5-HT_3 receptor antagonists in patients with electrolyte abnormalities, HF, history of arrhythmias, or other agents that prolong the QTc interval. Cases of torsade de pointes have been reported in postmarketing surveillance. These agents can also cause constipation, lethargy, tremor, fever, dizziness, nervousness, asthenia, thirst, and muscle pain.

SPECIFIC MEDICATIONS

See Table 85-3 for an overview of dopamine receptor antagonists and 5-HT_3 receptor antagonists including dosing, costs, indications, precautions, and contraindications.

TABLE 85-3. Overview of Dopamine Receptor Antagonists and 5-HT_3 Receptor Antagonists

Brand/Generic Name	Cost	Typical Dose	Indications	Comments
Dopamine Receptor Antagonists				
Prochlorperazine (Compazine)	Oral tablets $ Rectal suppositories $$	Oral tablets 10 mg PO Q 6 hours Rectal suppositories 25 mg rectally Q 12 hours May be taken as needed or scheduled	Nausea and vomiting associated with chemotherapy, migraine, and surgery	• Increased mortality in elderly with dementia-related psychosis • Significant anticholinergic effects • Leukopenia and agranulocytosis • Cholestatic jaundice • Parkinson-like symptoms • Sedation and lethargy • Neuroleptic malignant syndrome • Lowers seizure threshold • QT interval prolongation • EPS • Avoid concomitant use of other dopamine antagonists • Not recommended for use in pregnancy (Category C)
Promethazine	Oral tablets and syrup $ Rectal suppositories $$	Oral tablets, syrup 12.5–25 mg PO Q 4 hours prn Rectal suppositories 12.5–25 mg rectally Q 4 hours prn May be taken as needed or scheduled	Nausea and vomiting associated with surgery or anesthesia and motion sickness	• Fatal respiratory depression seen in children <2 years of age (do not use in children <2 years) • Do not use in comatose patients • Significant anticholinergic effects (caution with other anticholinergics) • Leukopenia and agranulocytosis • Cholestatic jaundice • Parkinson-like symptoms • Sedation and lethargy (do not use with other CNS depressants) • Neuroleptic malignant syndrome • Lowers seizure threshold • QT prolongation • EPS • Avoid concomitant use of other dopamine antagonists • May reverse epinephrine effectiveness • Pregnancy category C

(continued)

TABLE 85-3. Overview of Dopamine Receptor Antagonists and 5-HT$_3$ Receptor Antagonists (*continued*)

Brand/Generic Name	Cost	Typical Dose	Indications	Comments
Metoclopramide (Reglan)	Oral tablet $ Oral solution $$ Oral disintegrating tablet $$$	Oral tablet, disintegrating tablet, or solution 10–40 mg PO Q 6 hours	Prevention of nausea and vomiting after surgery and chemotherapy	• Irreversible tardive dyskinesia can occur. Avoid use longer than 12 weeks. • Do not use if patient has GI hemorrhage, mechanical obstruction, or perforation. • Contraindicated in pheochromocytoma • Patients with NADH-cytochrome b5 reductase deficiency may develop methemoglobinemia and sulfhemoglobinemia • Lowers seizure threshold • EPS • Neuroleptic malignant syndrome • Parkinson-like symptoms • Depression • Hypertension • If fluid retention develops, discontinue • Do not use with anticholinergics (slowed GI motility) • Absorption of drugs from the stomach may be decreased; small bowel absorption may be increased. • Pregnancy category B and excreted in breast milk (consult with OB before use) • Hypotension • Restlessness and agitation

5-HT$_3$ Receptor Antagonist

Brand/Generic Name	Cost	Typical Dose	Indications	Comments
Zofran Ondansetron	Oral tablet $$$ Oral soluble film $$$ Oral solution $$$ Oral disintegrating tablet $$$	8–24 mg PO Q 8 hours	Treatment of chemotherapy-induced and postoperative nausea and vomiting	• Avoid concomitant use of apomorphine owing to enhanced hypotensive effects • Reduce dose in hepatic insufficiency • Less drowsiness or lethargy than dopamine receptor antagonists • In Child–Pugh score of ≥10, do not exceed 8 mg/day

CNS, central nervous system; EPS, extrapyramidal side effects; GI, gastrointestinal; NADH, nicotinamide adenine dinucleotide; OB, obstetrician; PO, by mouth.

CLINICAL COMMENTARY

For pediatric patients, antiemetic use is discouraged in cases of mild to moderate vomiting owing to the side-effect profiles of these agents. Most antiemetic agents can cause drowsiness, and patients should be cautioned about driving while taking these agents. Anticholinergic agents such as meclizine seem to be most effective for nausea and vomiting related to motion sickness or vertigo.

86 | Psychiatric Medications

BENZODIAZEPINES

GENERAL INFORMATION

Benzodiazepines (BZDs) are a class of medications often referred to as sedatives or hypnotics. There are many medications in this class, and their indications are broad. In the outpatient setting, providers prescribe BZDs for the short-term treatment of anxiety, panic attacks, and alcohol withdrawal. Other indications for BZDs include seizure disorders, muscle spasms, preprocedure anxiety, and insomnia. Although widely used in the past, most recent clinical guidelines no longer recommend BZDs as first-line treatment for anxiety.

THERAPEUTIC EFFECTS

BZDs exert their sedative and anxiolytic effects by enhancing the actions of gamma-aminobutyric acid (GABA) in the brain, which results in increased neuronal inhibition and CNS depression. Over time, patients can develop tolerance and physical dependence because of receptor adaptation.

SIDE EFFECTS

General side effects of BZDs include sedation, next-day fatigue, dizziness, depression, confusion, anterograde amnesia, increased fall risk, and disinhibition. BZDs can be addictive, and providers should consider their abuse potential when prescribing BZDs and be on the alert for concurrent alcohol or other substance use. Patients on BZDs need regular followup, and these medicines should not be prescribed by phone.

Physical dependence can occur and withdrawal symptoms can develop when stopping BZDs. Withdrawal symptoms are generally mild, and can include rebound anxiety, insomnia, and restlessness. However, seizures or a delirium tremens-like syndrome can occur after abruptly stopping a BZD. To prevent seizures and withdrawal, BZDs should be slowly tapered.

INTERACTIONS

BZDs in combination with other CNS depressants increase the risk of oversedation, falls, and respiratory depression. Even at therapeutic doses, the effects of a BZD can become life threatening when used in combination with other CNS agents or taken with opioids and alcohol. Although BZD overdoses alone are rarely fatal, an overdose in combination with alcohol or other CNS depressants can be life threatening. BZDs are pregnancy category D or X, with the greatest risk occurring in weeks 2 to 8 of pregnancy.

SPECIFIC MEDICATIONS

Several BZDs are on the market, and most are available in relatively inexpensive generic forms. All agents in this class are similar in their sedative, hypnotic, anxiolytic, muscle relaxant, and anticonvulsant activity, but differ in their time of onset, active metabolites, and duration of action. BZDs with a rapid onset and shorter half-life, such as alprazolam, are considered more habit forming than others in the class. Longer-acting agents are preferred for alcohol withdrawal.

BZDs are metabolized by the liver, and hepatic function and age play a role in the choice of agent. For elderly patients and those with hepatic dysfunction, lorazepam, oxazepam, and temazepam are preferred because they lack active metabolites. Table 86-1 provides information on the most commonly prescribed BZDs.

CLINICAL COMMENTARY

It is best to use caution when prescribing BZDs, starting with low doses and only prescribing them for the minimum duration necessary. Evidence indicates that long-term BZD use can have negative outcomes, including memory impairment and dependence. Older adults are more sensitive to their effects and should be started at half the usual starting dose and limit the dose to half the usual maximum

TABLE 86-1. Commonly Prescribed Benzodiazepines

Generic Name (Brand Name)	Typical Dosing	Half-Life and Onset	Important Drug Interactions	Pricing	Clinical Commentary
Alprazolam (Xanax)	0.25–0.5 mg tid	$T_{1/2}$ 12–15 hours Rapid onset	• CNS depressants • Alcohol • Opioids • Fluvoxamine can increase alprazolam levels	$	• Rapid onset and short duration of action • Can be difficult to taper off after long-term use • One of the more widely abused benzodiazepines
Clonazepam (Klonopin)	0.25–1 mg bid	$T_{1/2}$ 18–50 hours Intermediate onset	• CNS depressants • Alcohol • Opioids	$	• Intermediate onset and long duration of action
Diazepam (Valium)	2–5 mg tid	$T_{1/2}$ 100 hours Rapid onset	• CNS depressants • Alcohol • Opioids	$	• Rapid onset and long duration of action
Lorazepam (Ativan)	1–2 mg tid	$T_{1/2}$ 10–20 hours Intermediate onset	• CNS depressants • Alcohol • Opioids	$	• Intermediate onset and short duration of action • A preferred choice for elderly patients or those with hepatic dysfunction
Temazepam (Restoril)	15–30 mg qhs	$T_{1/2}$ 1.5–5 hours Slow onset	• CNS depressants • Alcohol • Opioids	$	• Slow onset and short duration of action • Typically prescribed for insomnia

CNS, central nervous system; qhs, every night at bedtime; tid, thrice daily.

dose. Delirium can occasionally develop with the use of BZDs. If this occurs, consider switching to an alternative agent, such as phenobarbital, to mitigate this side effect. Physical dependence can develop in as little as 14 days of BZD use. If used for anxiety or insomnia, a short course of 5 to 10 days is typically recommended. For alprazolam, withdrawal seizures can occur with as short as 1 to 2 months of therapy.

SELECTIVE SEROTONIN REUPTAKE INHIBITORS

GENERAL INFORMATION

SSRIs are considered a first-line option for treating depression, anxiety disorders, obsessive compulsive disorder (OCD), and post-traumatic stress disorder (PTSD). Although SSRIs do not exhibit superior efficacy compared with other antidepressants, these agents typically have better tolerability and side-effect profiles.

THERAPEUTIC EFFECTS

SSRIs selectively inhibit the reuptake of serotonin into the presynaptic neuron by blocking the serotonin transporter. This increases the serotonin in the synaptic cleft available to bind to the postsynaptic receptor, causing an increase in neurotransmission. It may take several weeks for postsynaptic serotonin receptors to begin to downregulate and for peak neurotransmitter response. As a result, a full clinical response may take 4 to 6 weeks and sometimes up to 12 weeks. However, most patients begin to see improvement in the physical symptoms of depression (sleep difficulties, lack of energy, appetite) within 1 to 2 weeks. Table 86-2 summarizes SSRI treatment timeline and typical symptom response.

SIDE EFFECTS

Most patients tolerate SSRIs without significant problems. Common side effects include anorexia, insomnia, headache, sweating, nausea, diarrhea, sexual dysfunction, and hyponatremia. Hyponatremia is more common in older patients. Nausea, vomiting, and diarrhea are more closely associated with sertraline. Most side effects tend to dissipate with time, particularly the GI side effects. Sexual dysfunction with SSRIs most commonly manifests as delayed ejaculation for men and anorgasmia for women. If sexual dysfunction occurs with an SSRI, it rarely improves with continued SSRI treatment (sexual dysfunction symptoms abate in 1 in 10 patients). As such, alternative therapy may be needed. There is an increased risk of GI bleeding

TABLE 86-2. Treatment Timeline for SSRIs

Treatment Timeline	Response
First few days	Decreased agitation, decreased anxiety
First week	Improved sleep and appetite
2–3 weeks	Increased activity, improved sex drive, self-care, concentration, memory, thinking, and movements
2–4 weeks (may take up to 12 weeks)	Relief of depressed mood, return of experiencing pleasure, less hopelessness, subsiding of suicidal thoughts

SSRIs, selective serotonin reuptake inhibitors.

with SSRIs, especially when combined with NSAIDs. All antidepressants, including SSRIs, carry a black box warning for suicidal thinking and behavior, with the highest risk seen in children, adolescents, and young adults up to age 24. The risk is greatest during the first 2 weeks of initiating therapy, but patients should be monitored closely for the first 1 to 2 months of therapy for any suicidal thoughts or behavior.

INTERACTIONS

Serotonin syndrome is a rare and potentially fatal adverse event associated with SSRIs. SSRIs alone rarely precipitate serotonin syndrome; the syndrome primarily occurs when an SSRI is taken in combination with other serotonergic medications. Signs and symptoms of serotonin syndrome include hyperreflexia, altered mental status, hyperthermia, and autonomic dysregulation.

SSRIs are predominantly metabolized by the liver and can cause drug–drug interactions, although most of these interactions are not clinically significant. Table 86-3 summarizes specific drug interactions. SSRIs usually do not need dose adjustments for kidney dysfunction.

TABLE 86-3. SSRI Dosing, Interactions, and Clinical Commentary

Generic Name (Brand Name)	Typical Dosing	Half-Life	Important Drug Interactions	Pricing	Clinical Commentary
Citalopram (Celexa)	10–40 mg once daily	35 hours	• Avoid with other QT-prolonging medications • Maximum of 20 mg with (es)omeprazole	$	• Possibly more risk of QT prolongation than other SSRIs
Escitalopram (Lexapro)	5–20 mg once daily	35 hours		$	• Considered to be better tolerated with fewer drug interactions • More likely to cause hyponatremia than others
Fluoxetine (Prozac)	10–80 mg once daily	4–6 days		$	• More activating than most
Fluvoxamine (Luvox)	50–300 mg once daily	16 hours	• Could increase effect of metoprolol and propranolol • Could increase levels of alprazolam and triazolam • Could increase warfarin effects • Could increase clozapine levels • Cigarette smoke could decrease levels.	$$	• Only FDA-approved drug for OCD in pediatric patients • Can be sedating (dose in the evening to reduce daytime sedation)
Paroxetine (Paxil)	10–50 mg once daily	21 hours	• Use caution with other anticholinergic medications	$	• Anticholinergic; avoid in elderly • More side effects reported • Worst discontinuation syndrome/slow tapering required
Sertraline (Zoloft)	25–200 mg once daily	26 hours		$	• Typically more GI side effects; one of the more activating SSRIs

GI, gastrointestinal; OCD, obsessive-compulsive disorder; SSRI, selective serotonin reuptake inhibitor.

Contraindications to SSRIs include allergy, taking an monamine oxidase inhibitors (MAOIs) which if used concurrently or within the past 14 days can cause a life-threatening interaction. SSRIs lower the seizure threshold and should be used with caution in patients with a history of a seizure disorder. In addition, they may trigger a manic episode in patients with an unrecognized or untreated bipolar disorder.

SPECIFIC MEDICATIONS

Table 86-3 lists currently available SSRIs. All are available as generic medications. No SSRI has been proven to have superior efficacy, and so providers should weigh side-effect profile, patient comorbidities, and drug interaction potential when choosing an SSRI.

CLINICAL COMMENTARY

SSRIs are the most commonly used medications to treat depression and anxiety. The choice of antidepressant depends on comorbidities, symptoms, and side effects. SSRIs tend to be "activating," and an SSRI with more energizing effects may be a better choice for patients exhibiting apathy, excessive sleepiness, or psychomotor retardation. However, although SSRIs are generally energizing, up to 20% of patients may experience sedation as a side effect. In patients who experience sleepiness, taking the pill at night may allow them to "sleep" through the sedation. Although considered equally effective as TCAs for treating mild to moderate depression, some experts believe that TCAs may be more effective for treating severe depression. Although all SSRIs appear equally effective in trials, individual patients may respond differently to one SSRI, and it may take trial and error to determine the best agent and dose for a particular patient.

It is important to note that patients should not abruptly discontinue therapy with an SSRI because this can lead to a withdrawal syndrome, characterized by flulike symptoms, insomnia, irritability, nausea, sensory disturbances, and a reemergence of symptoms such as anxiety. Although usually mild, withdrawal symptoms can be severe. To avoid withdrawal, patients should be slowly tapered off their medication rather than stopping it abruptly. The only exception is fluoxetine, which has a long half-life and tends to self-taper upon discontinuation. Among the SSRIs, paroxetine has the strongest anticholinergic effect and should be avoided in older patients.

Some recent literature suggests that SSRIs may also be an effective nonhormonal treatment for hot flashes and premenstrual dysphoric disorder (PMDD).

ANTIPSYCHOTICS

GENERAL INFORMATION

Antipsychotics, also referred to as neuroleptics or major tranquilizers, were the first medications developed to treat schizophrenia and to manage positive psychotic symptoms such as delusions, hallucination, disordered thinking, and paranoia. Two classes of antipsychotics exist, first-generation (FG) or "typical" antipsychotics and second-generation (SG) or "atypical" antipsychotics. Presently, SG antipsychotics are more widely used owing to more favorable side-effect profiles and superiority in treating negative symptoms such as anhedonia, impoverished thought, blunted affect, and a lack of initiative or motivation (avolition).

THERAPEUTIC EFFECTS

FG antipsychotics act by blocking dopamine-2 (D_2) receptor in the brain. Blocking D_2 receptors is thought to be the mechanism for ameliorating positive symptoms, such as the delusions and hallucinations of schizophrenia. FG antipsychotics also have anticholinergic and antihistaminic properties. SG antipsychotics have a similar mechanism of action as FG antipsychotics, and also partially antagonize the serotonin 5-HT$_{2A}$ receptor. Aripiprazole, brexpiprazole, and cariprazine have a slightly different mechanism of action because they are also partial D_2 agonists. Both FG and SG antipsychotics have similar efficacy except clozapine, an SG antipsychotic with greater efficacy, but its use is limited by its side-effect profile to patients who fail other drugs. Clozapine causes agranulocytosis in about 4% of patients and requires careful monitoring including frequent CBCs. Usually, clozapine therapy is comanaged with a specialist with experience using the drug.

SIDE EFFECTS

General class side effects for FG antipsychotics include sedation, weight gain, anticholinergic side effects, elevated prolactin levels, orthostatic hypotension, QT prolongation, extrapyramidal side effects (EPS), and neuroleptic malignant syndrome (NMS). Of these side effects, NMS and EPS are considered the most worrisome. Although rare, NMS is an idiosyncratic life-threatening reaction that presents with autonomic instability (e.g., tachycardia, sweatiness), lead-pipe rigidity, hyperthermia, and mental status changes. Patients with NMS require hospitalization and aggressive treatment in the ICU. EPS include akathisia (restlessness, a compelling need to move, and agitation), pseudoparkinsonism, dystonia, and tardive dyskinesia (TD). Parkinsonian symptoms are more common in elderly patients, and are reported more frequently with higher potency antipsychotics. Symptoms include masked facies, tremor, bradykinesia, rigidity, cogwheeling, and drooling. TD, characterized by slow, repetitive, involuntary movements of the lips, face, or arms is a feared complication. It is resistant to treatment and may be progressive and irreversible despite discontinuing the drug. SG antipsychotics have a similar side-effect profile as FG antipsychotics, but tend to have a lower risk of both EPS and hyperprolactinemia. SG antipsychotics have a higher incidence of metabolic side effects, including weight gain, lipid abnormalities, and hyperglycemia. Despite the widespread belief that SG antipsychotics are safer than FG antipsychotics, research has failed to demonstrate a clear advantage of the newer "atypical drugs." Their touted advantages must be weighed against their increased cost.

All antipsychotics contain a boxed warning cautioning about use in elderly patients with dementia-related psychosis, owing to an increased risk of sudden death. All antipsychotics should be used with caution in patients with Parkinson disease, because their extrapyramidal effects may exacerbate parkinsonian symptoms.

INTERACTIONS

Metabolized by the liver, these drugs should be used cautiously in patients with liver disease or when combined with other drugs cleared by the liver. Providers should avoid using FG and SG antipsychotics in combination with medications that cause QT prolongation because further widening of the QT complex and arrhythmias can occur. Other interactions depend on the specific agent and Tables 86-4 and 86-5 provide additional information about specific agents.

SPECIFIC MEDICATIONS

The literature differentiates FG antipsychotics by potency, which correlates to their affinity for blocking the D_2 receptor. The higher the affinity of an agent for the D_2 receptor, the greater its potency and the greater its risk for EPS. Among these, haloperidol and fluphenazine are the two most potent FG antipsychotics (see Table 86-4). Guidelines commonly recommend SG antipsychotics over FG antipsychotics, although FG agents such as chlorpromazine, haloperidol, and fluphenazine are still widely used. Providers prescribe chlorpromazine primarily for its anticholinergic properties rather than its antipsychotic properties.

There are currently 12 SG antipsychotics on the market, and not all of them are available as generic medications, making cost a factor when selecting

TABLE 86-4. Select First-Generation Antipsychotics

Generic/Brand	Typical Dosing	Contraindications	Pricing	Clinical Commentary
Chlorpromazine (Thorazine)	25–800 mg divided twice to four times daily	• Hypersensitivity • Concomitant use with other CNS depressants • Comatose	$$	• More commonly used for nausea, vomiting, and intractable hiccups • Use with caution with other QT-prolonging medications
Haloperidol (Haldol)	2–5 mg given twice to three times daily (maximum 100 mg daily)	• Hypersensitivity • Parkinson disease • Severe CNS depression • Comatose	$	• Available as a long-acting injectable every 4 weeks • Short-acting injection often used for acute agitation • Use with caution with other QT-prolonging medications
Fluphenazine (Prolixin)	2.5–10 mg divided three to four times daily	• Hypersensitivity • Severe CNS depression • Comatose • Subcortical brain damage • Blood dyscrasias • Hepatic impairment	$$	• Most potent FG antipsychotic • Highest risk for EPS • Available as a long-acting injectable every 4 weeks

CNS, central nervous system; EPS, extrapyramidal side effects; FG, first generation.

TABLE 86-5. Select Second-Generation Antipsychotics

Generic/Brand	Typical Dosing	Contraindications	Pricing	Clinical Commentary
Aripiprazole (Abilify)	5–15 mg once daily	• Hypersensitivity	$$$	• Slightly different mechanism of action: partial D_2 agonist and partial 5-HT_{1A} agonist • Lower metabolic risks • Less sedating • No risk of prolactin elevation • May worsen/cause pathologic gambling
Olanzapine (Zyprexa)	5–20 mg at bedtime	• Hypersensitivity	$$$	• Very sedating • High metabolic risk • Increased incidence of cerebrovascular events • Cigarette smoke can decrease olanzapine concentrations.
Quetiapine (Seroquel)	300–600 mg at bedtime	• Hypersensitivity	$$	• Most sedating • Moderate metabolic risk • Thyroid dysfunction
Risperidone (Risperdal)	2–6 mg daily (can be divided twice daily)	• Hypersensitivity	$-$$	• High risk of prolactin elevation • Highest risk of SG antipsychotics for EPS • Increased incidence of cerebrovascular events • Floppy iris syndrome in patients undergoing cataract surgery
Ziprasidone (Geodon)	20–80 mg twice daily	• Hypersensitivity • History or current prolonged QT or congenital long QT syndrome • Concurrent use with other QT-prolonging agents • Recent MI • Uncompensated heart failure	$$$	• Use with caution with other QT-prolonging medications • Lower metabolic risks • Greatest potential for QT prolongation • Must be taken with a (minimum) 500-calorie meal • Dermatologic reactions • Electrolyte imbalances (especially hypomagnesemia and hypokalemia)

EPS, extrapyramidal side effects; MI, myocardial infarction; SG, second generation.

an agent. It is also important to consider patient comorbidities, other drug therapy, and side effects when selecting an SG antipsychotic. For example, a patient with difficulty sleeping in addition to symptoms of psychosis may benefit from a more sedating SG antipsychotic, such as quetiapine or olanzapine. A patient who has diabetes and is already overweight may be better suited for ziprasidone, an SG antipsychotic with a lower risk of metabolic side effects. Table 86-5 provides information about the most commonly used SG antipsychotics.

CLINICAL COMMENTARY

When starting a patient on an antipsychotic, it is important to follow the patient closely in the initial months of therapy to assess efficacy and side effects. Patients started on antipsychotics, especially SG antipsychotics, should have their weight, abdominal circumference, hemoglobin A_{1C} or fasting blood glucose, lipids, and BP monitored routinely. TD is a feared complication and requires early recognition and discontinuing the drug. Recently, some providers prescribe antipsychotics for sleep with no other indication (such as bipolar disorder or schizophrenia), a practice that should be discouraged owing to the high-risk side-effect profile associated with these medications.

Atypical antipsychotics are also used in conjunction with mood stabilizers, such as lithium, to treat bipolar disorder or psychosis associated with major depressive disorder.

87 | Other Medications

BRONCHODILATORS

GENERAL INFORMATION

Inhaled bronchodilators are a cornerstone of treatment for asthma and COPD. There are two classes of inhaled bronchodilators: beta 2 agonists and antimuscarinic (anticholinergic) agents, both of which are available as short- or long-acting formulations. The third class of bronchodilators, the methylxanthines (e.g., theophylline) are available in oral or intravenous formulations. The methylxanthines are used less frequently because of their side-effect profile, and because they are less effective when compared to inhaled bronchodilators. However, they still play a role in a limited number of patients whose symptoms remain uncontrolled despite optimal inhaled therapy and who suffer from troubling nighttime symptoms. Because of their low cost, they can be an alternative for those patients who cannot afford inhalers. Beta agonists are also available in oral formulations (tablets or capsules) but are rarely prescribed because they are less effective and have more side effects.

THERAPEUTIC EFFECTS

Beta 2 agonists relax bronchial smooth muscles, increasing airflow, decreasing dyspnea, improving pulmonary function, and increasing exercise tolerance. Short-acting beta 2 agonists (SABAs) and long-acting beta 2 agonists (LABAs) are currently approved by the FDA for the treatment of asthma and COPD. Antimuscarinic agents reduce airway constriction by blocking the acetylcholine (ACh) parasympathetic receptors on bronchial smooth muscle. These agents are available as both short-acting antimuscarinic agents (SAMAs) and long-acting antimuscarinic agents (LAMAs) for the treatment of COPD. Tiotropium is approved as add-on maintenance therapy for asthma patients experiencing exacerbations while taking a high-dose inhaled corticosteroids (ICS) and LABA concurrently.

SIDE EFFECTS

Beta 2 agonists can cause heart palpitations, tachycardia, and tremor. These effects are dose related and dose increases the incidence of side effects increases. Antimuscarinic agents can cause dry mouth, and some patients report a bad taste immediately after use. Because these agents act on the anticholinergic muscarinic receptors, they can cause urinary retention, especially in those with obstructive bladder disease such as men with preexisting BPH.

INTERACTIONS

Beta 2 agonists can potentially interact with nonselective beta blockers (BBs) such as propranolol, sotalol, pindolol, carvedilol, and labetalol.

With any inhaled antimuscarinic agent, there is a small potential for additive anticholinergic adverse effects if given concurrently with other anticholinergics. However, this is more likely to occur with tiotropium than aclidinium owing to its higher bioavailability. Anticholinergic effects include constipation, urinary retention, blurred vision, dry mouth, an increase in ocular pressure, and worsening of narrow-angle glaucoma.

PRECAUTIONS AND CONTRAINDICATIONS

In 2017, the FDA rescinded its black box warning about LABAs combined with ICS. However, they should always be used in conjunction with an ICS and never as monotherapy. If a patient is adequately controlled on dual LABA-ICS therapy, clinicians should consider stepping down therapy by first discontinuing the LABA. Avoid antimuscarinic bronchodilators in patients with prostatic hypertrophy, obstructive bladder, or those who are taking other anticholinergic agents. Patients should be informed to limit their use of SABAs to acute exacerbations and not for regular maintenance.

SPECIFIC MEDICATIONS

Table 87-1 provides an overview of bronchodilators.

CLINICAL COMMENTARY

When selecting a bronchodilator, it is important to take into account a patient's comorbidities and concomitant medications.

Short-acting bronchodilators work rapidly to relieve acute symptoms and are rescue medications that provide temporary relief from flare-ups. They take 15 to 20 minutes to work and last 4 to 6 hours. When taken 20 minutes before exercise, they can prevent exercise-induced bronchospasm. Individuals with controlled asthma should not use their rescue inhalers more than twice per week. More frequent use suggests uncontrolled asthma and should prompt a review of the patient's medication with goals of optimizing anti-inflammatory therapy, such as ICS and perhaps adding a LABA. LABAs should not be used as monotherapy in asthma but in combination with an ICS. LABAs have a longer onset of action and should not be used as a rescue medication.

Long-acting anticholinergics such as tiotropium are first-line agents for patients with COPD.

TABLE 87-1. Overview of Bronchodilators

Brand/Generic	Cost	Half-Life	Dosing	Comments
Inhaled SABAs				
Albuterol (Proair, Proventil, Ventolin)	$–$$	3.8–5 hours	1–2 inhalations every 4–6 hours as needed	• May cause tremor, tachycardia • Used primarily as a rescue medication
Inhaled LABAs				
Salmeterol (Serevent)	$$$	5.5 hours	1 inhalation twice daily	• Not to be used as monotherapy • Should be used in combination with inhaled corticosteroid • Not for acute bronchospasm
Formoterol (Foradil Aerolizer)	$$$	10–14 hours	Inhale 1 puff (12 µg) every 12 hours	• Not for acute bronchospasm
Indacaterol (Arcapta Neohaler)	$$$	40–56 hours	Inhale contents of 1 capsule (75 µg) once daily using neohaler	• Not for acute bronchospasm • Contains lactose; avoid use in patients with milk allergy
Inhaled SAMAs				
Ipratropium bromide (Atrovent)	$–$$	2 hours	2 inhalations 4 times daily; maximum dose: 12 inhalations in 24 hours	• Avoid contact with eyes • Better tolerated in some patients than beta agonists
Inhaled LAMAs				
Aclidinium bromide (Tudorza Pressair)	$$$	5–8 hours	Inhale 1 puff (400 µg) twice daily	• Contains lactose: avoid use in patients with milk allergy
Tiotropium bromide (Spiriva, Spiriva Respimat)	$$$	Asthma: 44 hours COPD: 25 hours	Max: Respimat 2.5 µg inhaled daily for asthma Max: Respimat 5 µg inhaled once daily for COPD HandiHaler: inhale contents of 1 capsule (18 µg) once daily	• Capsule contains lactose: avoid in patients with milk allergy • Do not swallow capsules • Avoid contact with eyes, which could lead to blurred vision. • Can take 2–8 days to reach maximal bronchodilation • Indicated for prevention of bronchospasm for COPD

COPD, chronic obstructive pulmonary disease; LABAs, long-acting beta 2 agonists; LAMAs, long-acting antimuscarinic agents; SABAs, short-acting beta 2 agonists; SAMAs, short-acting antimuscarinic agents.

Although they do not extend life, they reduce exacerbations and improve the quality of life for many patients. They need to be used with caution in patients with preexisting prostatic hypertrophy, bladder obstruction, or those taking other anticholinergic agents. For these patients, a LABA might be a better therapeutic choice. BBs may worsen asthma and COPD symptoms secondary to bronchoconstriction. Avoid using nonselective BBs in this population.

BISPHOSPHONATES

GENERAL INFORMATION

Bisphosphonates are the most commonly prescribed therapy for osteoporosis in the United States. This drug class treats bone loss and reduces the fracture risk in postmenopausal women. The literature classifies bisphosphonates as either first generation (FG) or second generation (SG). SG bisphosphonates are more potent and less toxic than FG bisphosphonates making them preferred over the FG bisphosphonates.

THERAPEUTIC EFFECTS

Bone is a metabolically active tissue and is maintained by cells that build bone (osteoblasts) and cells that break bone down (osteoclasts). Bisphosphonates work by inhibiting osteoclastic activity, which prevents bone loss as evidenced by improvement or stabilization of BMD. Bisphosphonate therapy reduces both vertebral and nonverterbral fractures. A feature of bisphosphonates is that their effect can continue for years after stopping the drug, and is believed to result from the tight bonding of the bisphosphonate to the bone mineral.

In addition to prevention and treatment of osteoporosis, bisphosphonates are the drug of choice for treating Paget disease and are approved for the treatment of primary hyperparathyroidism, hypercalcemia, multiple myeloma, metastatic bone cancer, and other diseases that cause bone fragility. Alendronate and risedronate are also approved for the prevention of bone loss associated with steroid therapy and for treating osteoporosis in men.

SIDE EFFECTS

GI side effects such as abdominal pain, constipation, and diarrhea are common with bisphosphonate therapy. Weekly and monthly drug formulations have fewer GI side effects than daily formulations. Oral formulations may cause esophageal irritation/ulceration if taken incorrectly. IV formulations may cause injection site reactions and musculoskeletal pain.

Although uncommon, osteonecrosis of the jaw (ONJ) and atypical femur fractures can occur with bisphosphonate use. ONJ occurs more commonly in cancer patients receiving chemotherapy and/or radiation, and in patients on glucocorticoid therapy receiving higher-dose IV bisphosphonate therapy. Patients with significant dental disease should be advised to have major dental work completed before starting bisphosphonate therapy. If the patient is already on therapy and needs major dental work, the provider should carefully weigh the risks and benefits of withholding bisphosphonate therapy while the dental work is completed. A link between atypical femur fractures and bisphosphonate treatment is less clear, but studies suggest that patients on long-term (>3 to 5 years) therapy may be at an increased risk. Rarely, bisphosphonates cause severe musculoskeletal pain, which usually improves with discontinuing therapy.

INTERACTIONS

The manufacturer recommends administering oral bisphosphonates apart from other oral medications and supplements secondary to poor bioavailability. Medications or OTC products that contain a cation (calcium, magnesium, etc.,) can bind to the oral bisphosphonate and prevent absorption of both agents. Providers should avoid any medication known to irritate the esophageal or stomach lining when prescribing bisphosphonates.

PRECAUTIONS AND CONTRAINDICATIONS

Oral bisphosphonates should be avoided in pregnant women and patients who have esophageal strictures, esophageal varices, hypocalcemia, an inability to stand or sit upright, and people at increased risk of aspiration.

SPECIFIC MEDICATIONS

Table 87-2 provides an overview of the brand and generic names, cost, dosing, and any additional commentary specific to each medication.

CLINICAL COMMENTARY

Oral tablets must be taken with at least 6 oz of plain water and at least 30 (60 for ibandronate) minutes before consuming any food, supplements (including calcium and vitamin D), or medications. Tablets should be swallowed whole, without any crushing, chewing, or sucking. Delayed-release risedronate

TABLE 87-2. Overview of Bisphosphonates

Generic (Brand)	Cost	Dosing	Comments
First Generation			
Etidronate (Didronel)	$$$	• 5–10 mg/kg/day (not to exceed 6 months) • 11–20 mg/kg/day (not to exceed 3 months)	• Oral and IV formulation • Ensure adequate calcium and vitamin D intake
Tiludronate (Skelid)	$$$	• 400 mg daily for 3 months	• Oral and IV formulation • Use: PD • CrCl < 30 mL/min: not recommended
Second Generation			
Risedronate (Actonel or Atelvia)	$$$	• 5 mg once daily • 35 mg once weekly • 150 mg once monthly	• Oral formulation only • Use: OP and PD • CrCl < 30 mL/min: not recommended
Ibandronate (Boniva)	$$$	• 3 mg every 3 months • 150 mg once monthly • 6 mg every 3–4 weeks	• Oral and IV formulation • Use: PM OP, HM, metastatic bone disease due to breast cancer • CrCl < 30 mL/min: not recommended
Alendronate (Fosamax, Binosto)	$$–$$$	• 5 mg or 10 mg once daily • 35 mg once weekly • 70 mg once weekly	• Oral formulation only • Use: PM OP, OP, PD • CrCl < 30 mL/min: not recommended
Pamidronate (Aredia)	$$	• 30–90 mg over 2–24 hours	• IV formulation only • Use: androgen deprivation-induced OP, PD, HM, MM
Zoledronic acid (Reclast or Zometa)	$$$	• 5 mg once or every 2 years • 4 mg once every 3–4 weeks	• IV formulation only • Use: OP, PD, HM, MM • Nononcology: CrCl < 35 mL/min: not recommended • Oncology: CrCl < 30 mL/min: not recommended

CrCl, creatinine clearance; HM, hypercalcemia of malignancy; IV, intravenous, MM, multiple myeloma; OP, osteoporosis; PD, Paget's disease; PM, postmenopausal.

is administered immediately following breakfast with at least 4 oz of plain water. Patients must remain upright (either sitting or standing) for at least 30 minutes after alendronate and risedronate and 1 hour after ibandronate administration. Patients who forget to take a weekly dose can take it the next day. If more than 1 day has elapsed, the patient should skip the dose. If a patient misses a monthly dose, it can be taken up to 7 days before the next administration. The choice of bisphosphonate is based on preference, convenience, cost, and adherence to the dosing schedule.

For patients who cannot tolerate oral therapy, IV therapy with either ibandronate (infused every 3 months) or zoledronic acid (infused once a year) are alternatives. The optimal duration of therapy remains controversial, but many experts recommend treating for 3 to 5 years for those at lower risk for fracture and beyond 5 years for those at high risk (e.g., history of hip or vertebral fracture, hip BMD <2.5 after treatment). Lower doses are used to prevent osteoporosis in patients with osteopenia or for those on long-term steroid therapy.

Assuring adequate calcium and vitamin D intake for patients taking bisphosphonates is also important and is a commonly overlooked part of optimizing bone health.

ANTIHISTAMINES

GENERAL INFORMATION

Histamine 1 (H_1) receptor antagonists, or antihistamines, are used to treat allergic disorders including rhinitis, pruritus, urticaria, and allergic reactions.

Selection of an antihistamine is based on multiple factors including the type of allergy, severity, patient age, and presenting symptoms. Diphenhydramine, chlorpheniramine, brompheniramine, and hydroxyzine are FG antihistamines; newer agents such as loratadine, fexofenadine, and cetirizine, desloratadine, and levocetirizine are SG antihistamines. SG agents are usually more expensive but have fewer side effects. Many antihistamines are available OTC either alone or in combined formulation with cough and cold medications (Table 87-3).

THERAPEUTIC EFFECTS

Antihistamines competitively bind to the H_1 receptor and suppress the effects of histamine such as itching, redness, sneezing, and rhinorrhea. FG antihistamines also have anticholinergic and antimuscarinic effects resulting in antiemetic, antidyskinetic, and sedative properties. SG antihistamines exhibit no muscarinic blocking effects and little to no anticholinergic effects at recommended doses. SG agents inhibit mast cell and basophil inflammatory mediator release resulting in antiallergic and anti-inflammatory effects in addition to H_1 antagonism.

SIDE EFFECTS

Side effects of antihistamines result primarily from their anticholinergic properties. These are more pronounced in the FG lipophilic agents that cross the blood–brain barrier and may limit their use due to sedation. Impaired performance in driving, work, and academics are associated with FG antihistamines even in patients who do not report drowsiness. Although uncommon, paradoxical CNS stimulation has been reported with antihistamine use, particularly in children. Other common side effects include dry mouth, urinary retention, constipation, weight gain, and cognitive impairment, especially in older adults. SG antihistamines are lipophobic and more selective for the H_1 receptor, resulting in fewer side effects. Loratadine, fexofenadine, and desloratadine do not usually cause sedation at recommended doses, although higher than recommended doses of loratadine or desloratadine may cause some sedation. Sedation can occur with the use of cetirizine at recommended doses.

INTERACTIONS

FG antihistamines are more likely to cause clinically relevant drug interactions, including the risk of QT prolongation when used with other QT-prolonging agents and augmented CNS depression when used with other sedating agents. Agents that irritate the gastric mucosa, such as oral potassium salts, should be avoided when giving FG antihistamines due to decreased gastric emptying and an increased risk of ulceration.

SPECIFIC MEDICATIONS

First-Generation Antihistamines

There is no demonstrated difference in efficacy among the FG antihistamines. Onset is rapid, generally between 1 and 4 hours, with peak serum concentrations occurring within 2 to 3 hours. Their short half-life necessitates multiple doses per day. However, these agents are associated with prolonged sedation beyond the elimination half-life. FG agents are all available generically and are inexpensive.

Second-Generation Antihistamines

Among SG agents, cetirizine and levocetirizine are thought to be the most potent, albeit with an increased likelihood of causing sedation. Longer half-lives allow for once-daily dosing. These agents are slightly more expensive than FG agents.

CLINICAL COMMENTARY

Antihistamines are not only useful for allergic conditions, but are also sometimes used for anxiety, nausea, motion sickness, vertigo, and insomnia. Many of these indications are off label. Providers should avoid the use of FG antihistamines in elderly patients because side effects are often more pronounced. FG agents may be more effective for pruritus because sedation may contribute to their effectiveness for this indication. For allergic symptoms, prescribing a nonsedating agent for daytime use and a less costly sedating agent at night is a common strategy. Topical antihistamines may be useful for allergic conjunctivitis. Azelastine is available as a nasal spray, but its side effects (somnolence, bitter taste) and high cost make it less desirable than oral agents and nasal steroids for allergic rhinitis. Hydroxyzine is contraindicated in early pregnancy. However, other antihistamines have relatively good safety profiles in pregnancy. These agents are widely available in combinations with decongestants, antitussives, antipyretics, and expectorants.

Many antihistamines are found in OTC cold remedies. However, their benefit in treating URIs remains controversial. Typically, they dry secretions and may be helpful in reducing rhinorrhea, sneezing, and watery eyes. Decongestants appear to be more effective than antihistamines for nasal congestion.

TABLE 87-3. Overview of Antihistamines

Brand/Generic	Cost/Availability	Adult Dosing	Comments
First Generation			
Diphenhydramine (Benadryl)	$/OTC	25–50 mg every 4–6 hours	• Typically used for severe allergic reactions and for acute dystonic reactions • Often in OTC sleep preparations
Chlorpheniramine (ChlorTrimeton)	$/OTC	4 mg every 6 hours (maximum 16 mg/day)	• Tolerance to sedation may develop with continued use.
Hydoxyzine (Atarax)	$/Rx only	Every 4–6 hours	• Most significant QT-prolongation risk; avoid in early pregnancy • Often used as an anxiolytic
Meclizine (Antivert)	$/OTC	12.5–25 mg every 6–8 hours	• Often used for dizziness and nausea associated with vestibular dysfunction • Should not be used until diagnosis is established.
Second Generation			
Loratadine (Claritin)	$/OTC	10 mg once daily or 5 mg bid	
Desloratadine (Clarinex)	$$$/Rx only	5 mg once daily	
Fexofenadine (Allegra)	$/OTC	60 mg bid or 180 mg daily	• Least likely to cause sedation • Can be chelated by magnesium salts and lanthanum. Administration should be separated by several hours. • Often used for urticaria at higher than recommended doses
Cetirizine (Zyrtec)	$/OTC	10 mg once daily	• Most likely second-generation agent to cause sedation
Levocetirizine (Xyzal)	$$/Rx only	5 mg once daily	• Cut dose in half in renal impairment

OTC, over-the-counter.

Questions

1. A 7-year-old child moved to the United States 6 months ago. His past medical history and physical examination are unremarkable. You review his immunization records and note that he has missed a few immunizations. When providing "catch-up" shots, which of the following immunizations can you safely omit at this age?
   a. Mumps, measles, rubella (MMR)
   b. Influenza
   c. *Haemophilus influenzae*
   d. Pertussis
   e. Hepatitis B

2. A 23-year-old female presents for a colposcopy and cervical biopsy. Which of the following is a true statement about obtaining informed consent on this patient?
   a. Informed consent is not needed.
   b. Informed consent is implied by the patient allowing the procedure to be performed.
   c. Risks and benefits of the procedures must be included in the discussion.
   d. Alternative forms of treatment do not need to be reviewed.
   e. Patient can be told that there are possible side effects, but specific side effects do not need to be reviewed.

3. Mr. Jones presents to your office with a desire to quit smoking. He would like to set a date to quit, but first wants to get nicotine replacement or other therapy to help with his attempt. You determine that he is in which of the following "stages of readiness" to quit smoking?
   a. Precontemplation
   b. Contemplation
   c. Preparation
   d. Action

4. Which of the following is important in deciding that a test is appropriate for screening?
   a. A low prevalence of disease being tested
   b. Lack of effective therapies for the disease
   c. High specificity of the test
   d. High sensitivity of the test
   e. Both c and d

5. A 40-year-old male presents for an annual physical examination. He has no significant family history and a normal physical examination. Which of the following tests will you recommend for screening this patient?
   a. Cholesterol
   b. Prostate-specific antigen (PSA)
   c. Colonoscopy
   d. Stress treadmill
   e. Glucose

6. A 2-month old presents for a well-child examination and is noted to have bruising on the torso and extremities. The mother seems unconcerned and states that she thinks he fell. An appropriate course of action would now include which of the following:
   a. Observation
   b. Notification of Child Protective Services
   c. Referral for hematology consultation
   d. Supplementation with vitamin with iron
   e. Psychiatric evaluation of the mother

7. An 86-year-old male presents with the following skin lesion. Treatment options for this would include

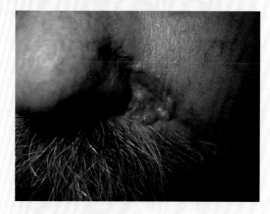

   a. Topical clindamycin
   b. Salicylic acid topically
   c. Retinoic acid topically
   d. No therapy
   e. Surgical excision

8. A 74-year-old female presents with a flat affect, poor eye contact, and limited interaction during the interview. Upon physical examination, there is no rigidity, bradykinesia, or tremors noted and

the neurologic examination appears to be normal. During the Mini-Mental State Examination (MMSE) questions, she responds to many of the questions with "I don't know." A likely diagnosis in this patient is:
a. Parkinson disease
b. Dementia
c. Delirium
d. Stroke
e. Depression

9. An 85-year-old male presents with his daughter, who notes that he has had a gradually progressive loss of function resulting in forgetfulness and inability to live alone because of loss of IADLs. He scores a 22/30 on his MMSE and otherwise has a nonfocal neurologic examination. Which of the following is the most likely cause for his findings?
a. Multiinfarct dementia
b. Lewy body dementia
c. Parkinson disease
d. Alzheimer disease
e. Huntington disease

10. When assessing a patient to distinguish dementia from delirium, which of the following is true?
a. Both have a gradual onset and are progressive.
b. Delirium is only associated with alcohol withdrawal.
c. Sleep is unaffected by delirium.
d. Patients with dementia rarely develop delirium.
e. Medication reactions and infections commonly cause delirium.

11. A 70-year-old male presents with a rhythmic tremor in his right hand while sitting and talking to you. Upon testing his neurologic function in that hand, the tremor disappears. Although the man moves about very slowly, his examination is otherwise normal. Which of the following are true regarding his diagnosis and treatment?
a. He has an essential tremor and needs no treatment.
b. Urgent therapy is needed utilizing levodopa.
c. Parkinson disease is unlikely because it is asymmetric.
d. He has suffered a stroke and requires hospitalization.
e. Metoclopramide (Reglan) may induce or aggravate his condition.

12. A 75-year-old female presents with history of urinary incontinence. She notes that she cannot get to the bathroom in time when she feels the sensation to urinate. She has no pain or fever. She takes sertraline for anxiety but otherwise is healthy. Initial steps in management of this patient include:
a. Discontinuing the sertraline
b. Urine culture
c. Cystoscopy
d. Use of anticholinergic medication such as oxybutynin
e. Advising her to curtail her liquid intake

13. When performing a geriatric assessment, which of the following tests should be considered routine?
a. PSA
b. Rheumatoid factor
c. Gait evaluation
d. Liver function tests
e. Serum iron

14. When considering involuntary weight loss in the geriatric population, which of the following is true?
a. More than 4% loss is predictive of death within 2 years.
b. Only about 5% have no identifiable cause.
c. Hyperthyroidism is the most common cause.
d. Functional impairments rarely cause weight loss.

15. The family of an 85-year-old patient with advanced dementia is inquiring about hospice care. When counseling this family, which of the following considerations will be important to advise?
a. Hospice care can only be provided in a hospital setting.
b. Hospice is not appropriate for dementia patients.
c. Over 90% of patients enrolled in hospice have cancer as their diagnosis.
d. Patients enrolled in hospice should not be told because it will demoralize them.
e. An important criteria for hospice is life expectancy <6 months.

16. A 75-year-old male presents with increasing difficulty reading and has loss of central vision. He reports no additional problems related to bright lights. You make a referral for him to see an ophthalmologist because you are concerned about which of the following?
a. Presbyopia
b. Glaucoma
c. Cataracts
d. Macular degeneration
e. Strabismus

17. You are seeing a patient in your office with elevated liver enzymes on recent blood testing and suspect alcohol abuse as a potential cause. You administer

the "CAGE" questionnaire. When utilizing this test, which of the following must you consider?
a. Results provide a conclusive diagnosis.
b. Sensitivity of the test is >95%.
c. Specificity of the test is around 90%.
d. The test requires referral for accurate interpretation.
e. Over half of adults meet criteria for substance abuse.

18. Somatic symptom disorders are characterized by which of the following?
a. Onset after age 50 years
b. More common in men
c. Extreme loyalty to one physician
d. Symptoms in an isolated organ/system
e. Exaggeration of patient complaints

19. You are seeing a 14-month-old male for a well-child visit. Which of the following are recommended at this age as screening or preventive care measures?
a. Blood lead level
b. Serum glucose
c. Serum bilirubin
d. Human papillomavirus vaccine
e. Serum cholesterol

20. Which of the following medical conditions may present as an anxiety disorder?
a. Posttraumatic stress syndrome
b. Obsessive–compulsive disorder
c. Postconcussion syndrome
d. Panic disorder
e. Phobias

21. You are implementing a smoking cessation program within your office and in setting up the program will be providing education to the staff. Important considerations to emphasize include:
a. You should wait for patients to show interest in quitting before discussing smoking with them.
b. Older patients will derive no health benefit from quitting.
c. Teenagers are a low-risk subgroup for smoking.
d. Lung cancer risk is never reduced by quitting.
e. Risk of a second heart attack drops by 50% in 1 to 2 years.

22. A 65-year-old male presents with his wife, who notes that he is getting up every 2 hours to urinate. He denies any pain or fever. Physical examination is unremarkable other than a slightly enlarged prostate with a firm nodule. Urinalysis by dipstick in the office is negative. His PSA value is 8 ng/mL. To evaluate this patient further, which of the following is indicated?

a. CT scan of the abdomen and pelvic
b. Ultrasound of the renal system
c. No further testing
d. Serum glucose
e. Needle biopsy of the prostate

23. A 50-year-old male presents with a painful red eye and notes that, in the affected eye, he sees halos around lights. Upon eliciting the history and performing the examination, which of the following confirms the need for urgent referral?
a. Unilateral involvement
b. Purulent discharge
c. Severe itching
d. Dilation of the pupil
e. A nodular lesion on the lid margin

24. You are seeing a 45-year-old male who noted onset of back pain 1 week ago after working in his yard and doing heavy lifting. When considering the causes for his back pain, which of the following would be most common?
a. Muscle strain
b. Malignancy
c. Infection
d. Herniated disc
e. Nephrolithiasis

25. A 40-year-old female presents with asymptomatic hematuria with 8 RBCs/hpf. This is confirmed by a repeat urine examination on another occasion. At this point, which of the following would you recommend?
a. Renal biopsy
b. MRI
c. Antinuclear antibody test
d. Urine culture
e. Cystoscopy

26. You are seeing a 76-year-old male with constant leaking of urine and a PVR of 210 mL of urine. Appropriate initial treatment of this patient would include which of the following?
a. Pseudoephedrine
b. Oxybutynin
c. Urecholine
d. Foley catheterization
e. Finasteride

27. Which of the following represents age-related hearing loss?
a. Meniere disease
b. Otosclerosis
c. Acoustic neuroma
d. Presbycusis
e. Labyrinthitis

28. A 21-year-old female presents with a history of a breast lump on her right side. She initially noted the

lump about 18 months ago. It is not painful. She believed it had begun after being hit in the chest during a basketball game. It initially grew for 2 to 3 months but has been stable in size since then. The presentation of this mass is most consistent with which of the following?
a. Breast cancer
b. Fibroadenoma
c. Fibrocystic breast disease
d. Mastitis
e. Intraductal papilloma

29. A 42-year-old male has painful joints in the hands, especially the metacarpophalangeal joints. On examination, there is soft-tissue swelling about the joints and x-ray reveals bony erosion in the periarticular bone. Which of the following would be the most likely cause for these joint pains?
a. Systemic lupus erythematosis
b. Wegener granulomatosis
c. Osteoarthritis
d. Rheumatoid arthritis
e. Scleroderma

30. A 65-year-old male presents for follow-up on his congestive heart failure and hypertension. His last echocardiogram revealed an ejection fraction of 65% with diastolic dysfunction. He has been very stable on his current medical regimen that includes aspirin, carvedilol, lisinopril, furosemide, and digoxin. He has not been hospitalized or symptomatic in over 3 years, and his current examination reveals clear lungs, regular heart rate and rhythm with an S_4, but no murmurs, and no edema. He would like to discontinue some of his medications. Which of the following medications should be discontinued initially?
a. Carvedilol
b. Lisinopril
c. Digoxin
d. Furosemide
e. Aspirin

31. A mother brings in her 12-year-old daughter with concerns about weight. The daughter is obese with a BMI of 31. The mother wants an evaluation to find out why she is overweight and you proceed to educate the mother with the following information:
a. Secondary causes are common and treatable.
b. Therapy for obesity in children involves taking a daily diet pill.
c. The causes for obesity are multifactorial.
d. Thyroid replacement cures most cases.
e. To lose 1 lb of fat, the patient must have a 2000-calorie deficit.

32. A phlebotomist in your office is drawing blood from a patient who is HIV positive. She accidentally is stuck by the needle after drawing his blood. She comes to see you immediately and you advise which of the following:
a. Check HIV titers in 2 weeks.
b. Wait and see if she becomes ill, then draw laboratory tests and consider treatment.
c. Because no blood was injected into her, she is not at risk.
d. Begin pneumocystis, toxoplasmosis, and mycobacteria prophylaxis now.
e. Begin antiviral prophylactic therapy for HIV now.

33. You are evaluating an 18-year-old male for a preparticipation sports examination. He was noted to have proteinuria and a 24-hour sample was collected with separate daytime and nighttime samples. He has daytime proteinuria but virtually no protein is excreted into the urine at night. Further evaluation or counseling of the patient should include which of the following:
a. He may not participate in sports until the proteinuria resolves.
b. Strict bedrest with reevaluation of his urine in 2 weeks
c. Referral for renal biopsy
d. Reassurance that his condition is benign and does not need treatment
e. Four weeks of a steroid burst and reevaluation of his urine

34. A 35-year-old female has been treated for *Helicobacter pylori*, and now has recurrence of epigastric discomfort. Her diagnosis was initially made by testing for serum *H. pylori* antibodies. In order to determine whether her exposure to *H. pylori* currently represents an active disease state, which of the following would you recommend?
a. Repeat serology
b. Barium swallow
c. Ambulatory esophageal pH monitoring
d. Abdominal CT scan
e. Stool for *H. pylori* fecal antigen

35. A 46-year-old patient presents for follow-up care for his hypertension, elevated lipids, and diabetes. His current medications include glipizide, simvastatin, enalapril, and verapamil. He notes increasing problems with constipation since his last visit. Appropriate management of his symptoms would include which of the following?
a. Referral for colonoscopy
b. Initiation of laxative therapy
c. Metoclopramide 10 mg orally four times daily
d. Changing his verapamil to alternative therapy
e. Recommending a low fat diet

36. You are evaluating a 60-year-old male for new onset of jaundice. He is experiencing no pain and minimal symptoms. His skin has a yellowish hue and his sclera are icteric. You plan to order laboratory tests and perform additional testing to determine the etiology. Match the following laboratory test with the disease that it can assist with diagnosis:

1. Antismooth muscle antibodies   a. Hemochromatosis

2. Ferritin   b. Hemolytic anemia

3. Ceruloplasmin   c. Autoimmune hepatitis

4. Antimitochondrial antibody   d. Wilson disease

5. Haptoglobin   e. Primary biliary cirrhosis

37. A 32-year-old male presents with an enlargement in his axilla that he believes has been there and unchanged for the past 2 weeks. There has been no injury, pain, or drainage from the lesion. He notes no other arm problems or injuries. On examination, you note a 2 cm, enlarged, soft, mobile lymph node in the patient's left axilla. There is no redness and the remainder of the upper extremity examination is normal. There are no other areas of lymphadenopathy noted. Which of the following would you recommend for your patient at this time?
   a. Observation for 4 weeks
   b. Surgical removal
   c. Fine needle aspiration
   d. Empiric cephalexin for 10 days
   e. PET scan imaging

38. A 58-year-old male presents with complaints of vomiting <1 hour after eating, and, often, nearly immediately after eating. This has been present for the past 4 months and he believes he has lost some weight as a result. After vomiting, he feels fine until this recurs the next time he eats. It occurs nearly every time he eats, and is not associated with nausea, fever, diarrhea, or other abdominal symptoms. He has tried over-the-counter antiemetics, such as Dramamine, with no change in symptoms. He takes no other medications, does not drink, occasionally smokes, and is physically very active. In addition to ordering laboratory tests, which of the following would you recommend?
   a. Colonoscopy
   b. Abdominal ultrasound
   c. Barium esophagogram
   d. Abdominal CT scan
   e. Chest x-ray

39. A 10-year-old male presents with a red, warm patch on his left arm that you believe is consistent with cellulitis. In prescribing an antibiotic for this patient, which of the following organisms should be included in the coverage?
   a. *Pseudomonas aeruginosa*
   b. *Staphylococcus aureus*
   c. *H. influenzae*
   d. *Clostridium difficile*
   e. *Streptococcus pneumoniae*

40. A 5-month-old girl presents with fever of 103.8°F. Besides a slight increase in crying and a slight decrease in appetite, there are no other obvious symptoms. Specifically, there is no cough, congestion, emesis, diarrhea, or rash. On examination, the ears, mouth, lungs, and skin are all clear and the child has a soft fontanelle and normal neurologic examination for age. Laboratory tests include a WBC count of 16,000 and urinalysis with 5 to 10 WBCs/hpf. Appropriate management would include which of the following?
   a. Admit and obtain urine and blood cultures along with empiric antibiotic coverage.
   b. Counsel about medications for fever and follow up with phone call the next day.
   c. Start oral amoxicillin for a 10-day course.
   d. Obtain chest x-ray.
   e. Reassure the parents and follow up prn.

41. A 2-year-old male presents with an upper respiratory infection and his mother is concerned about his breathing. He has laryngitis and a harsh barking cough along with some obvious dyspnea. On auscultation, he has good air entry, minimal inspiratory and expiratory stridor, but no retractions or cyanosis. His oxygen saturation is 99% on room air. Appropriate management of this patient would include which of the following?
   a. Albuterol by nebulizer every 4 hours as needed
   b. Albuterol syrup orally three times per day
   c. Prednisone 1 mg/kg daily for 7 days
   d. Inhaled racemic epinephrine
   e. Oral dexamethasone for one dose

42. A 4-year-old male presents after a seizure described as generalized and lasting 5 minutes. He is currently somnolent but without any focal deficits. His temperature is 102°F. He has nasal congestion and an erythematous pharynx. Management of this patient should include which of the following?
   a. Lumbar puncture
   b. CT scan of the brain
   c. Initiate therapy with phenytoin
   d. Administer antipyretic medications
   e. Empiric therapy with IV ceftriaxone

43. An 18-year-old female presents for physical examination before heading off to college. She has had regular care throughout childhood.

She currently has no complaints. She has no significant past medical history. Her parents and siblings are healthy. She has been sexually active for 1 year. She has a boyfriend, is currently on contraception, and states that she regularly uses condoms. In providing her preventive health care, which of the following are recommended at this time?

a. Pap smear screening
b. Cholesterol screen
c. STD screening
d. Urinalysis
e. ECG

44. A mother brings in her 7-year-old male child for evaluation for possible attention deficit disorder. His teacher has noted inattentiveness, impulsivity, and that he forgets to take home or bring back necessary books or assignments. He has a calm demeanor and does not seem fidgety in the office. He is quiet during your examination, which is otherwise normal. To diagnose attention deficit disorder, which of the following is true?

a. CT scan of the brain is part of the evaluation.
b. Ages and Stages questionnaire can accurately diagnose ADHD.
c. TSH should be obtained in all patients.
d. ADHD is a clinical diagnosis.
e. Hyperactivity is a universal element of this disorder.

45. A 14-year-old girl presents for evaluation of amenorrhea. She has never had a menstrual period, and is of normal weight and body build. Upon physical examination, you note that she is lacking both breast development and pubic hair, but otherwise appears to have normal genital anatomy. Next steps in the evaluation and management of this patient should include:

a. Karyotype
b. MRI of brain
c. Serum gonadotropin levels
d. Medroxyprogesterone challenge test
e. Serum testosterone

46. A 35-year-old female presents at her 6-week postpartum visit with complaints of feeling down. She notes frequent crying spells and fatigue. Most days, she is so tired that she does not shower or change out of her pajamas until her husband gets home from work in the evening. She denies any suicidal or homicidal thoughts. She has a past medical history of depression for which she took medication. Her husband has returned to work, but is extremely supportive and helps with all childcare and housework. Her family is out of town but call frequently and offer support. Which

of the following are important considerations in caring for this patient?

a. Depression is unlikely after a happy event such as childbirth.
b. Her prior history of depression puts her at increased risk for postpartum depression.
c. Her supportive family puts her at low risk for postpartum depression.
d. She cannot take antidepressant medication during the postpartum period.
e. This degree of fatigue and "postpartum blues" is normal in the postpartum period.

47. A 35-year-old female presents for contraceptive care and advice. She has four children and is currently married in a monogamous relationship. They are still unsure if they want additional children. Her last two children were conceived unintentionally in association with first condoms and then oral contraceptive use. The patient admits to having an irregular schedule and to not being reliable with the use of these contraceptive choices. Which form of contraception would be most appropriate in meeting her current needs?

a. Intrauterine device
b. Hormonal contraceptive patch
c. Postcoital contraception
d. Female condoms
e. Tubal ligation

48. A 24-year-old female with a history of one lifetime sexual partner undergoes an annual gynecologic examination and is found to have atypical cells of undetermined significance on her Pap smear. Reflex testing for HPV is negative. Follow-up for this patient should include which of the following?

a. Loop electroexcision procedure (LEEP)
b. Repeat Pap smear in 4 months
c. Repeat Pap smear in 12 months
d. Colposcopy
e. Conization

49. You are caring for a 21-year-old G1P0, who, on initial screen, is found to have a positive urine culture for *Escherichia coli*. The *E. coli* is sensitive to all antibiotics tested. She is afebrile, asymptomatic, and has no allergies. Appropriate follow-up care for this patient would include which of the following?

a. Repeat culture to confirm true infection
b. Treatment with amoxicillin
c. Treatment with ciprofloxacin
d. Ultrasound of her kidneys
e. No treatment is necessary

50. A 25-year-old G2P1 female presents for routine glucose testing during her pregnancy. When

counseling her about gestational diabetes and its treatment, which of the following is true?

a. Intrauterine growth retardation occurs with inadequate treatment.
b. Goals of therapy are to prevent maternal retinopathy and neuropathy.
c. Dietary treatment is the only option during pregnancy.
d. The maternal risks associated with diabetes resolve upon delivery.
e. Oral diabetic medications are now a common part of treatment.

51. A 20-year-old waitress complains of cough and a low-grade fever. She feels tired and has shortness of breath on exertion. She denies any pleuritic pain or night sweats. Her temperature is 100.6°F (38.1°C), heart rate 100, and respiratory rate 22. Examination of the ears, nose, and throat is normal. Auscultation of the lungs reveals a few fine crackles at the right lung base. The heart rate is regular with no murmurs. The next step in the management of this patient is which of the following:

a. Treatment with antibiotics for sinusitis
b. Treatment with a cough suppressant for postviral syndrome
c. A chest x-ray for suspected pneumonia
d. Sputum for Gram stain and culture
e. Initiate incentive spirometry to treat atelectasis

52. A 25-year-old woman complains of vaginal itching and burning. The pH of the vaginal discharge is 4. The most likely diagnosis is:

a. Atrophic vaginitis
b. Candidal vaginitis
c. Trichomoniasis
d. Bacterial vaginosis
e. Human papillomavirus

53. A 52-year-old man presents with a complaint of dyspnea, which has troubled him for the preceding 8 months. He has had minimal prior medical care, notes no prior medical problems, and denies any medication use. He admits to having smoked a pack of cigarettes daily for the past 30 years. He is currently stable, and his physical examination is remarkable for a prolonged expiratory phase and diminished breath sounds bilaterally. In evaluating this patient, which of the following is the most likely cause for his chronic dyspnea?

a. Pulmonary embolus
b. Chronic obstructive pulmonary disease
c. Diabetes mellitus
d. Myocardial infarction
e. Pneumonia

54. An asymptomatic 15-year-old youth presents for a preparticipation sports examination and is found to have a systolic ejection murmur at the left sternal border that decreases with squatting and increases on standing. With regard to hypertrophic cardiomyopathy, which of the following is true?

a. Most patients with hypertrophic cardiomyopathy have symptoms.
b. It is the most common cause of sudden cardiac death in those over the age of 50.
c. It is an autosomal recessive trait.
d. Diagnosis is made via echocardiogram.
e. Squatting decreases venous return and thus decreases the intensity of the murmur.

55. A 40-year-old man presents with a painful, swollen right knee and a low-grade temperature. The most useful test for this individual is:

a. CBC
b. Uric acid level
c. ESR
d. Rheumatoid factor
e. Joint fluid analysis

56. A previously healthy 26-year-old man presents with abdominal cramping and fever that has lasted for 2 days. He has had 10 stools in the last 24 hours. A stool specimen reveals the presence of blood and WBCs. The most likely diagnosis is:

a. Staphylococcal food poisoning
b. Rotavirus
c. Crohn disease
d. Shigellosis
e. Irritable bowel syndrome

57. A 22-year-old woman complains of a severe unilateral throbbing headache accompanied by emesis and photophobia. She has a history of "bad headaches" and states that her mother and sister also have "headache problems." The patient takes no medications, is afebrile, and other than being moderately uncomfortable, has a normal physical examination. The most likely diagnosis is:

a. Tension headache
b. Sinusitis
c. Meningitis
d. Temporal arteritis
e. Migraine headache

58. A 30-year-old obese woman presents with right upper quadrant pain and low-grade fever. Her symptoms started 2 weeks earlier with myalgias, fatigue, and anorexia. They are worsening progressively; now she also has nausea and vomiting. Her physical examination reveals mild jaundice and right upper quadrant pain.

The CBC shows mild elevation of WBC count. Hemoglobin, hematocrit, and platelet levels are within normal limits. The liver function test shows elevated AST, ALT, and total bilirubin with a high conjugated fraction. Which of the following is the best management option?

a. Because the patient has abdominal pain with nausea and vomiting, admit her for possible appendicitis.

b. Because she has three risk factors for gallstone disease as well as right upper quadrant pain, she needs a cholecystectomy.

c. Her jaundice is secondary to hemolysis and should be evaluated and treated accordingly.

d. Advise the patient to continue oral fluids and bed rest, and order a hepatitis profile to determine the type of hepatitis.

e. Endoscopic retrograde cholangiopancreatography should be performed to assess for a pancreatic mass.

59. A 21-year-old sexually active woman comes in with complaints of pain in the genital area, mild vaginal discharge, and painful urination. On examination, painful vesicles and ulcers are noted on the cervix. You tell the patient the most likely diagnosis is:

a. Syphilis
b. Urinary tract infection
c. Yeast vaginitis
d. Herpes simplex
e. Cervicitis

60. A 41-year-old obese woman presents with an acute onset of sharp, intermittent right upper quadrant pain associated with eating. She denies any fever or chills. On examination, there is no abdominal mass or tenderness. The CBC is normal. Liver function tests show elevated total and conjugated bilirubin levels as well as alkaline phosphatase. The next step in management is:

a. Ultrasound of the right upper quadrant
b. MRI of the abdomen
c. Esophagogastroduodenoscopy (EGD)
d. Empiric PPI therapy
e. Liver biopsy

61. A 76-year-old man complains of progressively worsening fatigue over the preceding 6 months. He has difficulty walking two blocks because of this. He has a poor appetite and has lost 15 lb. Physical examination reveals pale conjunctivae. The lungs are clear to auscultation bilaterally. The heart rhythm is regular and the rate is 96 beats/minute. There are no heart murmurs. The CBC shows hemoglobin of 7 with decreased mean corpuscular volume (MCV). The total iron-binding

capacity is increased and the ferritin level is low. This patient's anemia is most likely secondary to:

a. Thalassemia
b. Anemia of chronic disease
c. Folate deficiency
d. B_{12} deficiency
e. Iron deficiency anemia

62. A 15-year-old white adolescent girl complains of "bad skin." On examination, the patient is noted to have whiteheads and blackheads, as well as some papules and pustules, on her face and upper back. Treatment options are many for this patient. The medication reserved for severe acne is:

a. Tretinoin (Retin A)
b. Sulfur preparations
c. Isotretinoin (Accutane)
d. Topical clindamycin
e. Benzoyl peroxide

63. A 55-year-old black man complains of pain and some swelling in his right great toe. He has also noticed some "bumps" on his skin. On examination, his toe is swollen, red, and very painful. There are scattered tophi on his skin. Many causes of arthritis have systemic manifestations. A common association is:

a. Nail pitting and psoriatic arthritis
b. Tophi and rheumatoid arthritis
c. Malar rash and scleroderma
d. Fingertip atrophy and telangiectasias with systemic lupus erythematosus (SLE)
e. Erythema migrans and dermatomyositis

64. A 60-year-old woman presents with complaints of fatigue for the past 6 months. Her condition has been worsening progressively. Now, she is beginning to notice weakness and unsteadiness in her gait. Physical examination shows pale conjunctivae. Her lung and heart examinations are unremarkable, but neurologic examination shows a decreased vibration sense. Hemoglobin level is 8 and MCV is high. The most common cause of her condition is:

a. Iron deficiency anemia
b. Folate deficiency
c. Pernicious anemia
d. Anemia of chronic disease
e. Thalassemia

65. A 32-year-old gravida 3, para 2–0–0–2 presents for her prenatal visit. Based on her last menstrual period, the current gestational age is 10 weeks and 4 days. The patient states that she is sure of her dates. She denies any problems. Her BP is 125/80. On physical examination, the uterus is barely palpable above the pubis. Fetal heart

sounds are heard at a rate of 140 beats/minute. Management of this patient should include:

a. Laboratory evaluation for preeclampsia
b. Routine care with follow-up in 4 weeks
c. Ultrasound to confirm gestational age
d. Amniocentesis to evaluate chromosomes
e. Abdominal x-ray to rule out any pelvic masses

66. A 32-year-old woman presents with palpitations, tachycardia, and exophthalmos. You are concerned she may have Graves disease. With regard to that disease, which of the following statements is true?

a. Serum TSH is decreased whereas free T4 is elevated.
b. Thyroid scan shows a "hot" nodule.
c. Tests for thyroid antibodies are negative.
d. Both serum TSH and free T4 are elevated.
e. Fine needle aspiration is required for diagnosis.

67. A 20-year-old man with no past medical problems complains of a runny nose, which he has had for several months. The nasal discharge is watery and clear. He also has a nonproductive chronic cough, for which he has tried several over-the-counter medications, with no relief. His symptoms are worse at night. On physical examination, the patient has a pale nasal mucosa. The bridge of the nose also has a nasal crease. The most likely diagnosis is:

a. Vasomotor rhinitis
b. Allergic rhinitis
c. Sinusitis
d. Rhinitis medicamentosa
e. Nasal foreign body

68. A 40-year-old man with no past medical problems complains of left-sided chest pain with no radiation. He denies any nausea or diaphoresis. His pain is located at midclavicular line at the fourth intercostal space. The pain becomes worse with inspiration. His vital signs are stable. Physical examination shows a tender spot at the fourth intercostal space. The remainder of the physical examination is unremarkable. The ECG shows a normal sinus rhythm at 70 beats/minute. The most likely diagnosis is:

a. Myocardial infarction
b. Pneumonia
c. Costochondritis
d. Esophageal spasm
e. Pericarditis

69. A 55-year-old man with a history of hemorrhoids complains of weakness and dizziness. Over the last 2 days, he has had two episodes of painless rectal bleeding. He denies any fever or chills. Vital signs are BP 100/60, temperature 98.4°F (36.8°C), respiratory rate 22, and heart rate 98. The conjunctiva is pale. His lung and heart examinations are unremarkable. The abdomen is not distended. The bowel sounds are active. There is no abdominal tenderness. Rectal examination shows bright red blood per rectum (BRBPR). His hemoglobin level is 7 with microcytic and hypochromic RBCs, and the WBC count is 8000. Which of the following is the most likely diagnosis with this presentation?

a. Diverticulosis
b. Colon cancer
c. Ulcerative colitis
d. Irritable bowel syndrome
e. *Clostridium difficile* colitis

70. A 30-year-old woman, gravida 1, para 0, comes in for her second trimester prenatal visit at 16 weeks' gestation. She has had prenatal care since her pregnancy diagnosis at 8 weeks' gestation, and has had all routine prenatal testing performed according to schedule. In continuing to provide routine care, which one of the following tests should now be offered?

a. A CBC to rule out anemia
b. Atypical antibody screen
c. Hepatitis B surface antigen
d. Quadruple marker screen
e. Glucose screening for diabetes

71. A 68-year-old white woman comes in to discuss the results of her dual energy x-ray absorptiometry (DEXA) scan. Her T score is −2.7. You explain that she has osteoporosis and requires treatment. Management of osteoporosis includes:

a. Daily intake of 500 mg of calcium
b. Avoidance of weightbearing exercise
c. Taking bisphosphonates on a full stomach
d. Smoking cessation
e. Estrogen replacement therapy

72. A 60-year-old man complains of left lower quadrant abdominal pain, fever, and chills, which he has had for the past 2 days. His appetite is poor and he feels nauseous. Vital signs are as follows: blood pressure 140/90, temperature 101°F (38.3°C), respiratory rate 22, and heart rate 90. The patient looks sick and appears to be in pain. The lung and heart examinations are unremarkable. His abdomen is distended, with decreased bowel sounds. The left lower quadrant is tender to palpation. Rectal examination is normal. The CBC shows leukocytosis of 15,000 and hemoglobin of 12. The test of choice to diagnose this patient's condition is:

a. Ultrasound
b. CT of the abdomen
c. Barium enema
d. Bleeding scan
e. Colonoscopy

73. A 20-year-old man with no prior medical problems complains of a dry cough, which he has had for the past month. He denies any fever, chills, or night sweats. The cough started with a runny nose and low-grade fever. All the other symptoms resolved within a week, but the cough has been persistent. His vital signs are stable, and physical examination is unremarkable. The most likely diagnosis is:
   a. Sinusitis
   b. Postviral syndrome
   c. Pneumonia
   d. Psychogenic cough
   e. Asthma

74. A 9-month-old Native American boy is brought in by his mother; with a one day history of a fever of 101°F (38.3°C). She denies any diarrhea, nausea, or vomiting. This morning he began pulling on his right ear. His symptoms began after he developed a cold, couple of days ago. He has had four other similar episodes in the past 6 months. The mother is very concerned and states that antibiotics usually take care of the problem. His vital signs show a temperature of 100°F (37.7°C). The child is irritable but consolable. Examination of the ear shows an erythematous tympanic membrane with decreased mobility. The remainder of the physical examination is unremarkable. The best management option for this child should include:
   a. Observation; this is most likely a viral URI.
   b. Treatment for acute otitis media with antibiotics
   c. Antibiotics for acute otitis and then prophylaxis for 6 months
   d. Antibiotics for acute otitis and then daily oral decongestants
   e. Referral to ENT specialist for myringotomy and tympanostomy tube placement

75. A 62-year-old black man complains of fever, cough, and chest pain. On examination, the patient has a temperature of 102°F (39.8°C), obvious chills, and rales at the left lung base. The patient should be admitted if he has:
   a. Pulse >120
   b. O$_2$ saturation <95%
   c. Age >50
   d. Systolic BP <110
   e. Pleural effusion

76. A 60-year-old woman presents with chronic dyspnea and a long history of smoking. Based on the history and physical examination, you diagnose COPD and initiate treatment to relieve the patient's symptoms. In addition to this therapy, additional recommendations should include:
   a. V/Q scan of the chest
   b. Exercise avoidance
   c. Smoking cessation
   d. *H. influenzae* b vaccination
   e. Referral for bronchoscopy

77. A 40-year-old woman complains of intermittent palpitations, which began 3 weeks earlier and occur daily. The symptoms are not associated with any medication use, activity, or other symptoms. The physical examination, including heart rate, is within normal limits. CBC, FSH, and TSH testing is within normal limits, and event monitor testing shows sinus rhythm during the occurrence of symptoms. Which of the following is most likely in this patient?
   a. Menopause
   b. Cardiac arrhythmias
   c. Anemia
   d. Panic attacks
   e. Hyperthyroidism

78. A 70-year-old man has been treated for a gastric ulcer—positive for *H. pylori*—diagnosed 6 weeks earlier. He presents for follow-up and is asymptomatic. Current recommendations should include which of the following?
   a. Lifetime use of a PPI
   b. Rotating antibiotic use every 6 weeks
   c. EGD
   d. Observation for recurrence of symptoms
   e. *H. pylori* antibody testing

79. A 23-year-old woman complains of dizziness. On questioning, she says that she sometimes feels the room spinning. She has no significant past medical history, is on no medications, and has not been ill recently. On physical examination, she is noted to have vertical nystagmus unaffected by position. Her physical examinations, including vital signs, orthostatic BP, and pulse readings, are normal. A hearing evaluation is performed and is within normal limits. Which of the following diagnoses should be considered in the further evaluation of this patient?
   a. Multiple sclerosis
   b. Ménière disease
   c. Benign positional vertigo
   d. Vestibular neuronitis
   e. Psychiatric disease

80. A 65-year-old man presents for preoperative medical evaluation for a vascular procedure to treat symptoms of claudication. He has a past medical history of hypertension that has been well controlled the past 2 years with ACEi. He is on no

other medications except for 1 aspirin per day. He has had two prior uncomplicated surgeries for an inguinal hernia and a herniated lumbar disc. He quit smoking 10 years ago. Other than decreased peripheral pulses, his physical examination is within normal limits. The surgeon has requested that the patient have a CBC, basic metabolic profile, ECG, and chest x-ray performed. What other testing is indicated in this patient before proceeding with surgery?

a. Prothrombin time
b. Cardiac stress test
c. Pulmonary function tests
d. Holter moniter
e. Venous duplex scan

81. The parents of a 4-year-old and a newborn child present for wellness care and seek counseling with regard to vaccinations for their children. Which of the following is a true statement that may be part of the counseling you provide to encourage appropriate vaccination?

a. Hepatitis A vaccine is recommended for all children.
b. Inactivated poliovirus vaccine (IPV) has been associated with vaccine-related polio infection.
c. Pneumococcal vaccine is recommended only for high-risk adults.
d. Chronic hepatitis B infection develops in 90% of infected teens and adults.
e. Children receiving aspirin therapy should not receive influenza or varicella vaccines.

82. A mother brings in her 12-year-old son for a routine health care visit. She expresses concern about their family's history of elevated cholesterol and heart disease. She would like her son to have his cholesterol evaluated. A true statement regarding cholesterol and cholesterol screening in children is:

a. Normal cholesterol in children is ≤ 240 mg/dL.
b. Childhood cholesterol levels are predictive of adult levels.
c. Screening is recommended for children with a parental history of hypercholesterolemia.
d. Cholesterol values in children are unaffected by diet and physical activity.
e. Screening is recommended for children beginning at 12 months of age.

83. A 35-year-old man presents for an initial physical examination. He has had no significant past medical history, and reports that both of his parents are alive and well, as are his siblings. He does not smoke or drink, and exercises regularly. He received his last tetanus shot 5 years ago. His physical examination, including vital signs and

weight, is normal. You now recommend which of the following:

a. ECG
b. Chest x-ray
c. Lipid profile
d. Exercise stress test
e. Occult blood testing of stool

84. You are seeing a 15-month-old boy for follow-up of a pruritic skin rash that you diagnosed as atopic dermatitis. The child has erythema, scaling, and lichenification of the flexural creases of the arms and legs. There is a family history of eczema and allergies. No identifiable triggers have been identified for the child's atopic dermatitis, and he is otherwise well. The mother is concerned about the long-term implications of this condition. You advise her that:

a. Atopic dermatitis is a rare condition.
b. Resolution of the atopic dermatitis by age 2 is common.
c. Affected children rarely develop allergic rhinitis or asthma.
d. Most cases are diagnosed after age 2.
e. In teenagers, the face and cheeks are more commonly affected.

85. A 15-year-old adolescent girl presents with recurrent episodes of wheezing, which she experiences three or four times per year in association with URIs. During the episodes, medical evaluation has documented a peak expiratory flow of 70% predicted. She has no nocturnal symptoms and no other significant past medical history. You diagnose asthma and now recommend which of the following therapies?

a. Oral steroids daily
b. Short-acting beta agonists as needed
c. Inhaled steroids daily
d. Inhaled nedocromil daily
e. Antibiotics to be used with exacerbations

86. A 40-year-old, overweight, Hispanic woman complains that she has feelings of hopelessness, insomnia, recent weight gain, constipation, and no energy. On examination, the patient cries, makes little eye contact, has a somber affect, and shows psychomotor retardation. Depression is diagnosed. Possible treatment strategies would include:

a. Use of buproprion because of the insomnia
b. Use of antidepressants for 6 to 12 months for the first episode of depression
c. Use of an SSRI if agitation is a complaint
d. Use of mirtazapine because of weight gain
e. Use of TCAs to relieve constipation

87. A 30-year-old white woman complains of fatigue, sore throat, and low-grade fever. On examination,

her throat is mildly erythematous and there are shotty cervical nodes. The heterophile test is negative. The most common cause of a heterophile-negative, mononucleosis-like syndrome is:
a. Cytomegalovirus
b. Toxoplasmosis
c. Rubella
d. HIV
e. Hepatitis A

88. A 10-year-old male presents for evaluation of his asthma. He reports daily symptoms and wakes from sleep about once a week because of symptoms. He is currently using albuterol as needed for his symptoms. Current therapeutic recommendations should include:
a. Oral steroids daily
b. Antibiotics for 10 days
c. Nedocromil daily
d. Inhaled steroids and long-acting beta agonists
e. No change in therapy

89. A 45-year-old previously healthy male presents for a physical examination. His last physical examination was performed 10 years earlier and was normal. He has no significant past medical history and is on no medications. He does not smoke, and consumes two to three alcoholic drinks weekly. His family history is significant for hypertension in his mother. He denies any physical complaints. His physical examination is normal with the exception of a BP of 148/98. You recommend a recheck on his BP in 1 month; the repeat measurement is then found to be 150/100. Further evaluation of this patient should include which of the following:
a. Serum and urine catecholamines
b. Cardiac stress testing
c. ECG
d. No testing
e. Renal scan

90. An 18-year-old man presents for a preparticipation sports examination. He has no significant past medical or family history and a normal physical examination. His mother asks whether he should have any cardiac screening performed. Which of the following statements are true and helpful in addressing her concerns?
a. Routine screening with an ECG or echocardiogram has been shown to be cost effective.
b. History taking is used to identify those at risk for sudden cardiac death.
c. In those below age 40, CAD is the most common cause of sudden cardiac death.
d. Aortic stenosis is the most common cause of sudden death in those over age 40.
e. Stress testing is recommended routinely for preparticipation sports examinations.

91. A 20-year-old woman presents with concerns that her thyroid gland is overactive, because she has not been feeling well and her mother had a similar condition. In the evaluation of this patient, which of the following would be a symptom of hyperthyroidism?
a. Palpitations
b. Weight gain
c. Constipation
d. Depression
e. Fatigue

92. A 30-year-old woman complains of fatigue, cold intolerance, and dry skin. She has no other medical problems and takes birth control pills. Her physical examination is normal. Laboratory evaluation reveals TSH, at 8.9, to be elevated. The next step in evaluating her thyroid function would be to:
a. Arrange for a thyroid scan
b. Start her on thyroxine and recheck her TSH in 3 months
c. Administer TRH
d. Order a thyroid ultrasound
e. Test free T4

93. A 26-year-old man presents to the emergency department with complaints of the acute onset of the "worst headache of my life." Appropriate diagnostic evaluation/treatment would include which of the following?
a. Sumatriptan 6 mg subcutaneously (SC)
b. CT scan of the head, which if negative, should be followed by lumbar puncture.
c. CT scan of the head
d. Ibuprofen 600 mg by mouth every 6 hours
e. ESR and, while awaiting results, corticosteroid therapy

94. A 56-year-old white man expresses concerns regarding diabetes. His mother has diabetes, which is controlled with glipizide, and his brother was just diagnosed with the disease, controlled by diet. Appropriate screening is guided by the following criteria:
a. Hemoglobin A_{1C} cannot be used for screening for diabetes.
b. All patients over 55 years of age should be screened with a fasting blood sugar every 4 years.
c. Random blood glucose >200 with polyuria, polydipsia, and polyphagia establishes a diagnosis of diabetes.
d. A single fasting blood sugar >126 signifies diabetes.
e. For patients over age 30 with diabetes, screening for microalbuminemia should be done every 6 months.

95. An otherwise healthy 18-year-old, sexually active, white man complains of a persistent watery discharge in both eyes. On examination, both conjunctivae are slightly erythematous with a watery discharge. The likely diagnosis for this patient's red eye is:
  a. Blepharitis
  b. Bacterial conjunctivitis
  c. Viral conjunctivitis
  d. Iritis
  e. Inclusion (chlamydial) conjunctivitis

96. A 39-year-old gravida 5, para 2, comes in for a prenatal visit. She is 20 weeks pregnant and, at her last visit, a maternal serum alpha fetoprotein was ordered; it is decreased. The most probable cause is:
  a. Twin pregnancy
  b. Neural tube defects
  c. Pregnancy-induced HTN
  d. Trisomy 21
  e. Trisomy 18

97. A 5-year-old child is brought in by her mother for follow-up. She was diagnosed with acute otitis media 2 weeks earlier and given an antibiotic. The child's fever and ear pain have resolved. On examination, you note that the effusion behind the ear is still present. The tympanic membrane is normal. Management of this child should include:
  a. Antibiotics
  b. A tympanostomy tube
  c. Observation
  d. Referral to an ear, nose, and throat (ENT) specialist
  e. Hearing evaluation

98. A 68-year-old man presents for routine physical examination. In addition to obtaining a complete history and examination, which of the following would you routinely recommend?
  a. Chest x-ray
  b. Hepatitis B vaccine
  c. DEXA scan
  d. Pneumococcal vaccine
  e. Electrocardiography

99. A 42-year-old woman returns from a business trip and notes the sudden onset of dyspnea along with a pleuritic right-sided chest pain. Her past medical history is unremarkable. She is currently on birth control pills. Her vital signs are BP 120/70, heart rate 100, regular respiratory rate 24, and temperature 98.6°F (37.0°C). Cardiac and lung examinations are unremarkable. There is no chest wall tenderness. Examination of her extremities reveals no cyanosis or clubbing, but there is pitting edema in her right leg. Testing should be done promptly to exclude the following:
  a. Fibromyalgia
  b. Costochondritis
  c. Pulmonary embolus
  d. Lymphedema
  e. Varicose veins

100. A 50-year-old man complains of recurrent chest pain that radiates down his left arm and has been occurring over the past 9 months. The pain is described as a retrosternal pressure. It is brought on by walking or other strenuous exercise and is relieved by 2 minutes of rest. His vital signs are stable and the physical examination is unremarkable. The most likely diagnosis is:
  a. Myocardial infarction
  b. Stable angina
  c. Unstable angina
  d. Pericarditis
  e. Pleurisy

Answers

1.   c (Chapter 4 [Table 4-1])

c is correct because *H. influenzae* flu type B (Hib) vaccine is not administered after the age of 5, because children over age 5 generally achieve a natural immunity and are less affected by the disease. Hib should be administered at 2 months, 4 months, 6 months, and a fourth dose scheduled between 12 and 15 months of age. Not administering this vaccine to young children can be harmful, because *H. influenzae* type B can cause devastating illnesses such as meningitis and epiglottitis.

a is incorrect because the first MMR vaccine is due when the child is 12 months old and the second MMR when the child is between 4 and 6 years old. Omitting these can lead to harmful consequences regardless of the age group. Mumps is associated with parotitis, orchitis, oophoritis, pancreatitis, myocarditis, and encephalitis. One to three out of 1000 inflicted with measles die owing to neurologic and respiratory complications. Rubella is one of the TORCH infections and is associated with ophthalmologic, cardiac, and neurologic defects, including mental retardation in those children born to mothers with this infection during pregnancy.

b is incorrect because the CDC recommends influenza vaccine for all children over 6 months of age, replacing the previous recommendations restricting vaccine use under 24 months to high-risk children. This new recommendation is because this age range being at highest risk for hospitalizations secondary to influenza. Although universally recommended, the influenza IM vaccine is especially important for children 6 months of age or older with risk factors such as asthma, HIV, cardiac disease, sickle cell disease, and diabetes and if the child is in close contact with a high-risk group. Healthy people ages 5 to 49 years are eligible to receive the intranasal live attenuated influenza vaccine. Because of the vaccine's live attenuated virus, viral shedding can occur for up to 7 days; the live vaccine is not recommended for health care workers, asthmatics, immunocompromised individuals, or those within close contact to them.

d is incorrect because pertussis, along with diphtheria and tetanus (TDaP), should be administered in four doses at 2 months, 4 months, 6 months, and with a booster shot recommended at 15 to 18 months. The fifth and final dose of the series should be given at age 4 to 6 years. Furthermore, TDaP should be repeated at age 11 and 12 years if at least 5 years have elapsed since the last dose of tetanus and diphtheria toxoid-containing vaccine. Subsequent routine TDaP boosters are recommended every 10 years thereafter provided one booster of pertussis was given during the teen years. In individuals with potentially contaminated wounds and more than a 5-year lapse since their last TDaP, a booster is recommended. In individuals with high-risk wounds and no previous tetanus immunization, passive immunization with tetanus immunoglobulin (TIg) is indicated in addition to starting the primary series at initial presentation for wound care.

e is incorrect because the hepatitis B vaccine should either be administered at birth (before hospital discharge) or before 2 months of age. The second dose is given between 1 and 4 months of age (at least 4 weeks after the first dose), and the third dose given between 6 and 18 months of age (at least 16 weeks after the first dose and 8 weeks after the second). The third dose should not be given before 24 weeks of age. Infants born to hepatitis B vaccine surface antigen (HBsAg) positive mothers should receive hep B vaccine and 0.5 mL of hep B immunoglobulin (HBIg) at separate sites within 12 hours of birth. The second dose is recommended between age 1 and 2 months, and the final dose of the immunization series administered after 24 weeks of age (same as in normal mothers). HBsAg and anti-HBs antibody testing should be performed on these infants between 9 and 15 months of age.

2.   c (Chapter 2)

Patients undergoing surgical or other invasive procedures need to give informed consent. Describing the nature of the patient's condition and its consequences, including whether it is disabling or life threatening, are essential components of informed consent. Recommended treatment and alternatives should also be reviewed, including proposed benefits, risks, costs, discomfort, and specific side effects.

3.   c (Chapter 2 [Table 2-1])

The patient is ready to make a change by setting a specific quit date; at this stage, nicotine replacement and further therapy should be offered to help the patient achieve this goal.

a is incorrect because in the precontemplation stage the patient is not considering quitting, may not believe he/she is able to quit, and/or may not believe he/she is susceptible to severe illness owing to the habit. At this stage, it is appropriate to ask the patient about their knowledge of the health consequences of smoking.

b is incorrect because at the contemplation stage the patient is merely considering cessation. He/she also recognizes the dangers of smoking and may still be upset by previous failed attempts. At this stage, it is appropriate to encourage the patient to quit and provide educational materials.

d is incorrect because the patient is not in the process of cessation. At this point, support and positive reinforcement are most appropriate, as well as discussing strategies if relapse were to occur. Maintenance occurs when a patient has successfully quit smoking and is continuing to live tobacco free. Continuing support of this and aiding if relapse occurs are most appropriate at this stage.

4.   e (Chapter 3)
Both high sensitivity and high specificity are desirable characteristics of a screening test. Sensitivity (or the true positive rate) is the percentage of cases that a test may detect. Specificity (also called the true negative rate) measures the proportion of negatives that are correctly identified as such (i.e., the percentage of healthy people who are correctly identified as not having the condition).

A low prevalence of disease being tested (**a**) would increase the cost/benefit ratio of the disease being screened in a population. A lack of effective therapies for the disease (**b**) would not warrant a screening test because it would not decrease the morbidity or mortality associated with early detection of a disease. As a review, positive predictive value is the likelihood percentage that a person with a positive test has the disease. A negative predictive value is the likelihood percentage that a person who tests negative for the disease does not truly have it. Below are examples of how to calculate each of the quantities in variable as well as numerical forms.

	Disease Present	Disease Absent
Positive test	A	B
Negative test	C	D
Sensitivity	A/(A + C)	
Specificity	B/(B + D)	
Positive predictive value	A/(A + B)	
Negative predictive value	D/(C + D)	

	Disease Present	Disease Absent
Positive test	80	40
Negative test	20	60
Sensitivity	[80/(80 + 20)] × 100% = 80%	
Specificity	[60/(40 + 60)] × 100% = 60%	
Positive predictive value	[80/(80 + 40)] × 100% = 66%	
Negative predictive value	[60/(20 + 60)] × 100% = 75%	

5.   a (Chapter 5)
A cholesterol screening is warranted for this patient, as he is over the age of 35. Routine cholesterol screening is recommended every 5 years starting at age 35.

Yearly prostate cancer screening, including a PSA and a digital rectal examination, is no longer recommended for screening purposes.

The patient is below the age of 50 and has no high risk factors for colon cancer or prostate cancer based on family history and medical history; therefore, he is not at increased risk for these cancers. The USPSTF recommends a colonoscopy for all average risk patients at and above the age of 50 years, and if that initial screening test is normal recommends repeat colonoscopy every 10 years. Annual occult blood testing along with flexible sigmoidoscopy every 5 years is an alternative method for colon cancer screening for low-risk patients; for example, those with no family history of colon cancer before age 50. However, a full colonoscopy is warranted for those with signs or symptoms such as anemia, weight loss, and/or heme-positive stools

Stress testing is warranted if there is a suspicion of cardiac disease such as those with anginal symptoms but is not indicated for an asymptomatic 40-year-old male.

Glucose testing in the form of fasting glucose and subsequent glucose tolerance testing is only warranted in individuals younger than age 45 if family history or personal history causes suspicion for diabetes mellitus. Beginning at age 45, fasting blood glucose levels should be checked every 3 years.

Additional recommended screening tests in this age group for women include mammography every 1 to 2 years (by ACS whose recommendation differs from USPSTF) starting at age 40 and Pap smears every 3 years in low-risk women.

6.   b (Chapter 7)
In any case of suspected child abuse or neglect, local child protective service agencies must be contacted. The explanation for why the child is bruised appears

vague, and more importantly the lack of concern for the child's injuries suggests abuse or at the very minimum neglect. Observing (a) the situation may expose the child to further neglect or abuse. Referral for a hematology consultation (c) might be considered if there are no obvious causes for bruising and/or other symptoms or signs to suggest a clotting defect, and concerns about child abuse have been eliminated. Supplementation with iron (d) is appropriate therapy for iron deficiency anemia; however, there is currently no evidence to suggest the child has this condition. A psychiatric evaluation (e) may be appropriate in the future, but the immediate concern is for the safety and well-being of the child.

7. e (Chapter 77)

The pink nodular, pearly white translucent appearance with inverted edges and telangiectatic vessels are typical of a basal cell carcinoma (BCE). Biopsy is diagnostic and the most common therapies include surgical excision or curettage and electrodesiccation. This malignancy rarely metastasizes but can become locally invasive and destructive over the course of years. This lesion occurs more commonly on sun-exposed areas (80% on the head and neck). Other risk factors include fair skin, family history of skin cancer, history of sunburns, and outdoor occupations. Squamous cell carcinoma is another common skin malignancy that more readily metastasizes than a BCE and can have a prior premalignant lesion called actinic keratosis. These premalignant lesions are primarily seen in older individuals, induced by UV light, common in fair-skinned individuals, and appear as asymptomatic, rough, scaly lesions on sun-exposed sites. Actinic keratoses have a 1% yearly risk of developing into squamous cell carcinoma. Actinic keratoses can be treated by cryotherapy or curettage. Extensive lesions can be treated with a topical agent such as 5-fluorouracil. Malignant melanoma is one of the few potentially fatal skin diseases. It readily metastasizes, and risk factors include fair complexion, light hair and eyes, and those with excessive sun exposure. An excisional biopsy is required of suspicious lesions. Survival is most closely related to depth of tumor invasion.

8. e (Chapter 42)

This patient demonstrates a lack of interest in the interviewer's questions and possibly poor concentration. She also demonstrates a flat affect. Depression presents as a 2-week or greater history of depressed mood and/or disinterest (anhedonia) accompanied by impaired function along with at least four of the following: weight changes, sleep disturbance, loss of energy, feelings of worthlessness or guilt, poor concentration, psychomotor retardation or agitation, thoughts of death, or recurrent suicidal ideations.

The patient does not have Parkinson disease (PD) (a) because of an absence of the cardinal symptoms of PD rigidity, bradykinesia, and tremors. Dementia (b) would be suspected if the patient had difficulty recalling objects or recent events, experienced marked forgetfulness or a history of getting lost, neglected personal hygiene, was socially withdrawn, had frustrating emotional outbursts, or difficulty driving. Delirium (c) is an acute state of confusion that affects memory and cognition. It usually occurs suddenly over hours to days and is associated with a clouding of consciousness and disruption of the sleep cycle. None of these appears to be the case with this patient. Stroke (d) could present as an acute confused state, a sudden loss in motor function, or loss of vision. No such acute events are depicted in this scenario.

9. d (Chapter 78)

Progressive memory loss accompanied by loss of IADLs is consistent with a diagnosis of AlzD. AlzD patients usually develop social withdrawal over time. It is the most common cause of dementia, accounting for over half of the cases of dementia in the United States. Histologic findings include intracellular neurofibrillary tangles comprised of tau proteins and extracellular beta amyloid proteins plaques. These changes lead to neuronal loss and subsequent disturbance in the cholinergic system, resulting in cognitive decline. Most AlzD cases are sporadic, but an autosomal dominant form involving the amyloid protein has been described. Risk factors include advanced age, female gender, and family history of the disease. APO-E4 apolipoprotein on chromosome 19 is associated with increased risk for AlzD.

Multiinfarct dementia is a type of vascular dementia. It presents in discrete episodes of stepwise worsening cognition. Multiinfarct dementia is usually due to a series of lacunar strokes (owing to small vessel hyaline arteriolosclerosis). Risk factors for all types of vascular dementias include HTN, diabetes, history of smoking, and known arterial disease.

Lewy body dementia patients have a rapid clinical decline, visual hallucinations, episodic delirium, and extrapyramidal motor signs. This patient does not have these signs. Lewy body dementia is characterized by the presence of Lewy bodies (intracytoplasmic inclusions) and by decreased neuronal density in the amygdala, hippocampus, cortex, and other portions of the brain.

Parkinson disease is characterized by bradykinesia (slowing of voluntary muscle movements), a resting tremor, described as "pill-rolling," micrographia, blunting of affect, a shuffling gait, and cogwheel rigidity. Dementia occurs in some cases, but it is not a consistent or diagnostic finding. The pathophysiology of Parkinson disease is degeneration of dopaminergic neurons in the substantia nigra. This patient lacks the motor symptoms mentioned earlier.

Huntington chorea is an autosomal dominant disease associated with chorea (spasmodic movements of body and limbs) and muscle rigidity or dystonia which are not present in this patient. The pathophysiology involves atrophy/loss of neurons of the globus pallidus, putamen, and caudate. This patient does not possess these motor symptoms.

10.   e (Chapter 78)
Delirium, or an acute confusional state, affects memory and cognition, typically occurs over hours to days, and is most commonly caused by medications, infection, dehydration, hypoxia, electrolyte imbalance, anemia, and hepatic failure. It is associated with a clouding of consciousness and disruption of the sleep cycle, and commonly occurs in patients with dementia.

Dementia is a progressive decline in memory and intellectual capabilities severe enough to interfere with social or occupational functioning. It can encompass impairment in language, judgment, cognition, visuospatial skills, and personality with the functional decline occurring over years. One percent of the population is affected by age 60 and almost 50% by age 85. Dementia is usually subcategorized into either the Lewy body type, Alzheimer type, frontotemporal (Pick's disease), or multiinfarct dementia.

11.   e (Chapter 77)
This patient likely has parkinson's disease (PD). Metoclopramide (Reglan), which stimulates GI tract motility, does so by blocking the gastric dopamine receptor. This can cause dystonic reactions, restlessness, drowsiness, and can exacerbate Parkinsonian symptoms in patients with PD.

The treatment of choice for PD is levodopa with carbidopa. Levodopa is a dopamine precursor that can cross the blood–brain barrier and helps replenish the loss of dopamine owing to the degeneration of neurons in the substantia nigra seen in PD. Carbidopa, a peripheral dopa decarboxylase inhibitor, increases the bioavailability of levodopa in the brain and inhibits its peripheral conversion to dopamine, thus limiting peripheral side effects. This also helps decrease the daily requirements of levodopa by approximately 75%.

a is incorrect because an essential tremor is a tremor associated with voluntary movements, not a resting tremor as seen in PD.

c is incorrect because Parkinsonian tremor usually begins as a "pill-rolling tremor" (as though a pill were being rolled between the thumb and fingers with mild external and internal rotation of the wrist) unilaterally, and progresses to include both hands. The tremor may also include the chin, lips, legs, and trunk, and may be exacerbated by stress. The tremor typically has a unilateral onset.

d is incorrect because the patient has no history significant for a stroke, such as a focal or hemi deficit. This patient has the bradykinesia and resting tremor associated with PD.

12.   d (Chapter 79)
This patient has detrusor instability. Her symptoms of urgency and incontinence suggest urge incontinence owing to contractions of the bladder with filling. It is idiopathic in most cases but can be neurogenic. Cystometry (electronic measure of pressure changes as water fills and is expelled from the bladder), not cystoscopy (**c**) is diagnostic. It shows bladder contraction on filling. Anticholinergic medications such as oxybutynin (Ditropan), tolterodine tartrate (Detrol LA), propantheline bromide (Pro-Banthine), or imipramine (Tofranil) are the medications of choice to treat detrusor instability. Additionally, behavior modification such as timed voiding and not inhibiting liquid intake (**e**) can also be beneficial.

a is incorrect because sertraline, an SSRI, does not usually cause urinary symptoms, but may cause GI upset, insomnia, somnolence, sexual dysfunction (anorgasmia), dry mouth, weight loss, and exacerbation of mania.

b is incorrect because a urinalysis would be appropriate initially but a culture is appropriate in the workup for UTI, which would typically present with dysuria. If a urinalysis suggests infection, then a culture is warranted.

13.   c (Chapter 76)
Gait evaluation is particularly important because geriatric patients are at increased risk for falls and this examination may uncover correctable gait disturbances such as peripheral neuropathy secondary to vitamin B_{12} deficiency. PD may present with a shuffling gait.

a is incorrect because PSA is often elevated owing to benign prostatic hypertrophy, but marked elevations or increasing values are suggestive of prostate cancer. Further evaluation of patients with possible prostate cancer should be undertaken only if the diagnosis would result in a change in management.

Both rheumatoid factor and ANA tests are commonly positive in low titers and rarely indicate disease in the elderly.

d is incorrect because LFTs are unchanged with aging. However, abnormal liver tests may indicate necessity for further evaluation for hepatitis, cirrhosis, or hepatocellular carcinoma.

e is incorrect and is not a recommended part of an assessment in an asymptomatic adult. However, serum iron is important in the evaluation of microcytic anemia, as in iron deficiency anemia, which may be secondary to oncologic causes, such as cancers of the GI tract.

14. a (Chapter 77)

Unintended weight loss of 4% over 1 year is the single best predictor of death within 2 years in the geriatric population. The causes of weight loss in the geriatric population are similar to those in middle-age adults. The most common causes are depression and cancer, especially GI and pulmonary malignancies. Although hyperthyroidism does cause weight loss, it is not one of the most common causes; so **c** is incorrect. Both CHF and COPD can cause weight loss in later stages. Other causes of weight loss in this population include renal failure (anorexia and weight loss as early symptoms), infection (such as tuberculosis), endocrine disorders such as diabetes, and medication-induced decrease in appetite. Alteration in taste and nausea is also associated with weight loss in this population. Functional impairments, such as from poorly fitted dentures, secondary to stroke or arthritis, or from difficulty swallowing, can also cause weight loss in this population. In about 25% (not 5%) of cases, weight loss remains unexplained and no identified cause is found.

15. e (Chapter 80)

Hospice care is a type of palliative care provided to patients whose life expectancy is 6 months or less. It emphasizes symptomatic treatment and comfort measures. The management of pain and relief of symptoms is the primary concern. Special attention is paid to the patient's physical, emotional, and spiritual needs rather than trying to cure his or her illness or prolong life. It is important for the patient and family members to understand hospice care because it will help them fulfill the needs mentioned above.

a is incorrect. Hospice care can be provided at the patient's place of residence (home, nursing home).

b is incorrect. Hospice care is appropriate for end-stage patients with conditions such as cancer, CHF, COPD, chronic renal failure, and dementia.

c is incorrect. Although traditionally associated with cancer care, other end-stage diseases make up more than 10% of enrolled patients in hospice care (only 41.3% had cancer as a primary diagnosis, not 90%). National Hospice and Palliative Care Organization reported in October 2008 that the previous year's non–cancer-related admissions were at 58.7%.

d is incorrect. Although this is not always possible due to dementia and/or severe prolonged bouts of delirium, an attempt to explain hospice care is important and provides a way for the patient to take control of how he or she is affected by disease as life comes to an end.

16. d (Chapter 77)

Macular degeneration is atrophy of the cells in the central macula. It is associated with a loss of central vision and blurring of vision. It is the most common cause of visual impairment in elderly Caucasians. There are two types of macular degeneration. Wet macular degeneration involves formation of new, abnormally weak blood vessels under the macula. These vessels rupture and leak blood and fluid, which can lead to central vision loss. Photocoagulation can be helpful in this type of macular degeneration. Dry macular degeneration is more common than wet and progresses more slowly than the wet form. It involves formation of deposits, drusen, which form under the retina and damage the macula. Patients with macular degeneration should be monitored for visual changes with an Amsler grid (grid with black dot in the middle used to monitor changes in central vision). Antioxidant therapy (including using Ocuvite) helps reduce progression.

Presbyopia is an age-associated loss of the ability of the eye to accommodate. It is not associated with a loss of central vision. Most individuals need glasses for reading by their 50s.

Untreated glaucoma leads to loss of peripheral vision (not central) and eventual blindness. Glaucoma is characterized by an elevated intraocular pressure (measured by tonometry) and increased optic cup-to-disc ratio. There is an increase in pressure of the aqueous humor (produced by ciliary bodies) while it flows from the posterior chamber to the anterior chamber of the eye past the trabecular meshwork into the canal of Schlemm. Open-angle glaucoma is a slowly progressive blockage of outflow of aqueous humor, whereas closed-angle glaucoma (acute blockage of the canal of Schlemm) presents as an acute emergency. Treatment to lower pressures is indicated when intraocular pressures exceed 25 mmHg or in the presence of optic nerve atrophy or visual field loss. Pharmacologic treatment includes drops that either decrease the aqueous production (BBs, adrenergic agents) or increase aqueous drainage (mitotic) and thus lower the pressure. Surgical intervention is only indicated when pressures are poorly controlled by topical agents or when visual loss progresses. Glaucoma is the most common cause of blindness in African Americans.

Cataract is a loss of transparency of the crystalline lens (cloudy appearance). Risk factors for cataracts include sun exposure, smoking, steroid use, and diabetes mellitus. Treatment consists of surgical removal of the lens and is indicated if the visual acuity is 20/50 or worse and/or if there is functional impairment from the cataract. Cataracts usually cause a generalized clouding of vision and do not usually begin as a loss of central vision.

Strabismus is a misalignment of one of both eyes and is not a defect in central vision of the eyes (like macular degeneration). It involves inability of the eyes to coordinate focus on an object and is usually due to problem with the muscles of the eyes. It generally presents in childhood and if a child has unilateral strabismus, the eye without the defect is covered for a significant amount of time to allow the defected eye's muscles to strengthen. There are different types of strabismus including esotropia (crossed eyes) and exotropia ("wall-eyes," or eyes directed laterally).

17. c (Chapter 35)
The specificity ranges between 85% and 95%. The CAGE questionnaire is a screening tool and is not diagnostic of abuse because many factors go into diagnosing substance abuse. The CAGE questionnaire is an acronym for the following questions.

Have you ever felt the need to "Cut down" on your drinking?

Are you "Annoyed" by people criticizing your drinking?
Have you ever felt "Guilty" about your drinking?

Do you ever need a drink in the morning to steady your nerves or hangover? ("Eye-opener")

The test is a screening test and does not diagnose substance abuse; the diagnosis of abuse depends on a constellation of medical, social, and psychological clues.

When using the CAGE test and given two "yes" answers, the sensitivity ranges from 70% to 85% and the specificity ranges from 85% to 95%.

d is incorrect because interpretation of the CAGE questionnaire is straightforward. However, the CAGE questionnaire is a screening test and is not diagnostic; therefore, further questioning, testing, or referral is indicated to arrive at a diagnosis of substance abuse in those instances of a positive screen.

13% of the adult population meets the diagnostic criteria for substance abuse and 20% of adults in the United States are at risk for substance abuse.

18. e (Chapter 31)
Somatic symptom disorders are defined as emotional or psychological distress that is experienced and expressed as physical complaints. It is characterized by multiple, unexplained symptoms in multiple organs (**d** is incorrect) before the age of 30 (**a** is incorrect). Most patients with these disorders will "doctor shop" (search for the answers to their health concerns from multiple doctors) (**c** is incorrect). Women who have this disorder outnumber men by 6:1 (**b** is incorrect).

19. a (Chapter 67)
Blood lead and hemoglobin levels are generally obtained between 9 and 15 months of age. Serum glucose and bilirubin levels are obtained shortly after birth (**b** and **c** are incorrect). Patients born to diabetic mothers may have hypoglycemia owing to increased insulin because of the mother's elevated blood sugar. Bilirubin levels can be high in the immediate neonatal period because of immaturity of the newborn's hepatobiliary system. This may result in clinical jaundice that may require therapy.

The HPV vaccine was developed as a preventive tool for preventing cervical cancer. It is active against the strains of virus most commonly associated with cervical cancer. It is recommended for girls beginning at 11 years of age. Pap smears are recommended beginning at age 21. Repeat smears are initially recommended every year and can be spaced out to every 3 years for women in a monogamous relationship (or not sexually active) with three previously normal Pap smears. HPV DNA testing is recommended for sexually active females with abnormal Pap smears.

Serum cholesterol measurements are recommended for men age 35 and older and women age 45 without significant risk factors for cardiac disease. For men and women with an increased risk for CHD, however, screening should begin at age 20. In children with a family history of CHD at a young age, cholesterol screening is recommended beginning at age 2 years.

20. c (Chapter 37)
PTSD, OCD, panic disorder, and phobias are all types of anxiety disorders. Postconcussion syndrome refers to a neurologic disorder following mild or moderate head injury. The main features are dizziness, headache, fatigue, and difficulty in concentration. An uneasy or anxious feeling is also a commonly reported symptom.

PTSD is a psychiatric disease with anxiety symptoms that develop and last at least 1 month after an individual experiences a distressing event outside the normal human response. There may be delayed onset after the inciting event and the patient may experience flashbacks.

OCD also is a psychiatric disease and a type of anxiety disorder. OCD involves intrusive, unwanted thoughts and repetitive behaviors performed in a ritualistic manner.

Panic disorder is a specific form of anxiety disorder that involves episodes of intense fear or apprehension accompanied by at least four somatic complaints, such as diaphoresis, dyspnea, dizziness, or flushing, accompanied by behavior changes because of unrealistic and persistent worry.

Phobias are anxiety disorders characterized by persistent or irrational fear of a specific object, activity, or situation.

21. e (Chapter 55)
Smoking reduces the risk of a second MI by 50% within 1 to 2 years of smoking cessation. Even older individuals benefit from stopping tobacco use after years of smoking or after quitting subsequent to a smoking-related illness. Lung cancer risk drops significantly 10 years after a smoker quits. Adolescent smoking has fallen less than in other age groups since its peak in the 1970s, and in teenage girls it has increased in recent years. This is despite the fact that the overall adult population smoking in the United States has declined to about 15%.

The National Cancer Institution lists four As for office-based intervention:

1. *A*sk about smoking at every opportunity possible. Ask those who smoke whether they are interested in cessation.

2. *A*dvise every smoker with a clear, direct message. Tailor the advice to the patient's individual situation.

3. *A*ssist patients in their efforts to stop. If a smoker is ready to quit, ask him or her to set a date. Offer self-help material and pharmacologic therapy, such as nicotine replacement. Consider a referral to a formal smoking cessation program. If the individual is ready to quit, discuss the benefits and barriers to smoking cessation. Make the information as relevant to the individual as possible. Advise the smoker to avoid exposing family members to secondhand smoke. Indicate a willingness to help in the future when the smoker is ready, and continue to ask about quitting in follow-up visits.

4. *A*rrange and negotiate a follow-up appointment generally within 1 to 2 weeks after the quit date. Make sure to congratulate those who have successfully quit and reinforce the benefits of giving up smoking. Discuss high-risk situations for relapse and review coping mechanisms. For those who fail to quit, provide positive reinforcement for taking the first step toward quitting. Ask about what obstacles the patient encountered and discuss strategies to overcome these in the future. Encourage the patient to set another quit date.

22. e (Chapter 52)

Any firm nodule in the prostate should be biopsied. Ultrasound-guided needle biopsy from 6 to 12 sites to improve sampling is the usual procedure. The patient's PSA is in an abnormal range, but in a range often due to benign conditions. Values under 4 are considered normal, whereas those above 10 are considered suspicious for carcinoma. For the value of 8 (between 4 and 10), additional PSA measures such as the percent of free PSA or the ratio of free PSA: total PSA can help determine the need for biopsy. Using a cutoff of 25% free PSA in patients with values of 4 to 10 may eliminate many unnecessary biopsies without significant loss in sensitivity. Urinalysis helps rule out transitional cell carcinoma of the bladder (blood in urine is often present) as well as nonmalignant diseases such as cystitis or renal lithiasis.

CT scan of the abdomen and pelvis is not indicated for patients with prostatic symptoms or physical findings. CT scan does not show the prostate well. In patients with prostate cancer and suspected metastases, CT scan can be beneficial in assessing the spread of prostate cancer.

Renal ultrasound is the imaging method of choice for urinary obstruction, renal tumors, renal vein thrombosis, and is part of the evaluation of renal failure. While a prostate ultrasound might be useful, a renal ultrasound would not be helpful for assessing a prostate nodule or elevated PSA.

Evaluation of prostate cancer, which while usually lower mortality rate than most other cancers, can cause significant morbidity in a symptomatic patient. In elderly males with significant comorbidities, one option may be to manage symptoms and not pursue invasive procedures. Screening PSA testing is no longer routinely recommended.

Generally, glucose testing would be indicated to evaluate polyuria such as is present in this patient. However, this patient is advanced in age, has no glucosuria, and an enlarged prostate with a suspicious nodule. Glucose testing could be performed to be thorough but is not the test of choice to evaluate this patient's findings.

23. d (Chapter 77)

The patient is likely suffering from closed-angle glaucoma. It typically presents with blurred vision, halos around lights, pain, redness in the eye, and a moderately dilated pupil that does not respond to light. Dilation of the pupil helps distinguish closed-angle glaucoma from other causes of a painful red eye (e.g., iritis). Emergent treatment is needed to prevent permanent loss of vision.

As depicted in the answer explanation for question 16, glaucoma. Glaucoma left untreated leads to a loss of peripheral vision (not central) and eventual blindness. Glaucoma is the most common cause of blindness in African Americans. Many diseases (such as those mentioned below) can present with unilateral involvement. Unilateral involvement alone does not indicate a need for emergent treatment.

b is incorrect because purulent discharge suggests an infectious etiology such as conjunctivitis or dacryocystitis, neither of which usually affects vision. Bacterial conjunctivitis is usually due to *S. aureus* or beta hemolytic *Streptococci*. They usually start as a unilateral condition, but often become bilateral from cross contamination.

Itching of the eye is not typical of acute angle glaucoma. It is more consistent with allergic conjunctivitis.

A nodular lesion is usually either a chalazion (a chronic granulomatous lesion of the meibomian gland, which is hard and painless) or a hordeolum, which is an abscess over the upper or lower eyelid also known as a stye. Neither of these eye nodules presents with halos around lights.

24. a (Chapter 9)

The onset of pain following heavy lifting in an adult under 50 years of age suggests a muscular cause for this patient's pain.

b and **c** are incorrect as tumor, infection, or inflammation can cause nighttime awakenings owing to pain that does not improve with rest.

d is incorrect as disc herniations usually occur after a very trivial stress (may just be a cough or sneeze). The most common levels for these to occur are L5–S1 (nerve root for S1) and L4–L5 (nerve root for L5). The L5 nerve root includes motor function for extension of the great toe, as well as sensory for the dorsum of the foot/base of the first great toe. The nerve root for S1 includes the ankle jerk reflex, plantar flexion (motor), and sensory for the buttock, posterior thigh, calf, lateral ankle, and foot.

Although nephrolithiasis can cause back pain, the pain usually radiates to the groin unilaterally. In cases of suspected nephrolithiasis, a UA is necessary. If a stone is detected on CT scan and it is <4 mm, the patient would probably be able to pass it with adequate hydration within 1 to 2 weeks. The urine must be strained during this time, and a follow-up x-ray in 1 to 2 weeks recommended. If the stone is not passed in 2 weeks or if the stone is larger than 4 mm, then extracorporeal shockwave lithotripsy or surgical intervention would be necessary.

25. d (Chapter 18)
In asymptomatic individuals, the initial test for evaluating hematuria is a urine culture. An entirely normal repeat study after treatment of an infection in healthy individuals under 35 to 40 years of age usually requires no further evaluation other than repeating the UA in 1 to 2 months. Although there are many causes of hematuria, including SLE (+ANA), Henoch–Schonlein purpura (presents with purpura on lower extremities and buttock), various other forms of nephritis, renal vein/artery embolus, tuberculosis, polycystic kidney disease, bladder carcinoma (if suspected, diagnostic modality of choice is cystoscopy), medullary sponge kidney, renal cell carcinoma (warrants CT scan or MRI), exercise, trauma, renal stones, Foley placement, prostatitis, and BPH. The key to this question is making sure to rule out more benign and easily treatable causes such as infection before putting the patient through unnecessary treatments or diagnostic imaging studies making **a**, **b**, **c**, and **e** incorrect.

26. e (Chapter 79)
This 76-year-old man is most likely suffering from overflow incontinence secondary to BPH. Finasteride is a 5-alpha-reductase blocker used to reduce prostatic hypertrophy and therefore help alleviate obstruction to voiding. Overflow incontinence usually presents with constant leakage of urine and a PVR >200 mL. It can be caused by anatomic obstruction (prostate disease, urethral stricture) or neurologic factors such as diabetes or multiple sclerosis, or can be caused by medications such as narcotics, anticholinergics

(disinhibits beta relaxation of bladder), or sympathomimetics (increases beta relaxation).

Oxybutynin is an anticholinergic used to control urge incontinence, which is usually due to detrusor muscle instability, or secondary to stroke, dementia, PD, or spinal cord injury. Patients often complain of having the sudden urge to go to the bathroom but are unable to get to the bathroom before micturition occurs. Because oxybutynin can relax the bladder detrusor muscle, it can worsen overflow incontinence.

Urecholine is a cholinergic that is used to stimulate bladder contractions in an atonic bladder owing to conditions such diabetes mellitus or MS. It is not hydrolyzed by cholinesterase and therefore has a longer duration of action than similar parasympathomimetics like bethanechol, which is also used in overflow incontinence in diabetics. However, medical treatments of overflow incontinence owing to bladder contractility problems are generally not very efficacious. Also, if obstruction contributes to overflow incontinence, it should be reversed if possible.

d is incorrect because catheterization usually predisposes the patient to infection. If necessary, a suprapubic catheter is inserted or intermittent catheterization is preferred to indwelling catheters. Indwelling catheters should be reserved for comfort in terminally ill patients, to prevent worsening of pressure ulcers, or for patients with inoperable outflow obstruction.

27. d (Chapter 77)
Presbycusis is a bilateral loss of hearing related to aging. It is a sensorineural hearing loss, which affects hearing at higher frequencies more than at lower frequencies. It is associated with age-related degeneration of the hair cells of the cochlea and is thought to result from cumulative noise-induced damage over time.

Meniere disease is an acquired, idiopathic condition, not age related, that affects the inner ear and can affect balance and hearing. It is characterized by episodes of tinnitus and progressive hearing loss. The hearing loss associated with Meniere disease is low pitched in nature and is usually unilateral and caused by endolymphatic hydrops, resulting in increased pressure within the semicircular canals and damage to the sensory hair cells. Hyperacusis and nystagmus may also be present. It usually develops between 30 and 60 years of age. Chronic therapy includes diuretics (acetazolamide or hydrochlorothiazide) and salt restriction.

Otosclerosis is a hereditary disorder, not age related, in which ossification of the labyrinth of the inner ear occurs, resulting in tinnitus and eventual conductive hearing loss. The ossification can lead to fusion of the ossicles causing conductive hearing loss. Treatment is generally surgical. An acoustic neuroma is a schwannoma of the eighth cranial nerve that gradually grows to compress the eighth cranial nerve and eventually the brainstem. This can occur sporadically or can be found in neurofibromatosis type 2 syndrome (MISME syndrome, multiple inherited schwannomas, meningiomas, and ependymomas). Acoustic neuromas are treated surgically.

Labyrinthitis is an inflammation of the labyrinth and often follows a viral upper respiratory tract infection. It can cause vomiting and severe vertigo. Recovery is generally within 1 to 6 weeks. Meclizine, dimenhydrinate, antiemetics, and BZDs are used for symptomatic treatment. Long-term sequelae can include dysequilibrium and dizziness, which can last for months to years.

28.   b (Chapter 61)

Fibroadenomas commonly present in younger women as discrete, painless, rubbery masses. After an initial several month period of growth, fibroadenomas generally stabilize in size, remain mobile, and do not spread to adjacent lymph nodes. They can be observed but are often surgically removed because of their associated anxiety and discomfort.

Breast cancer typically presents in a postmenopausal woman as an isolated painless mass discovered on self-examination or as part of routine screening. The mass usually does not have discrete borders, and often fixed. Over time, cancerous masses enlarge, and may be associated with palpable lymph nodes. Other signs of breast cancer include skin dimpling, nipple inversion, nipple discharge in a nonlactating woman (especially bloody discharge), and skin edema or inflammation. Although this woman's mass is painless, the age and stability in growth over 18 months make a diagnosis of breast cancer highly unlikely in her case.

Fibrocystic breast disease usually presents as diffusely lumpy tender breasts. Fibrocystic changes vary with the menstrual cycle and are most commonly found in young women. Cysts that persist through the menstrual cycle, fail to resolve with aspiration, or those with bloody aspirate may be malignant. This woman's mass is not painful, is discrete, and does not vary with her menstrual cycle. Fibrocystic change is not likely the cause for the mass in this case.

Mastitis usually presents in a lactating woman as an erythematous, painful area on the breast. Purulent discharge may be present. *S. aureus* is usually the implicated pathogen. It is recommended to continue breastfeeding or pumping of the affected breast. Antibiotics with appropriate MRSA coverage should be prescribed for 2 to 4 weeks. Heat or ice packs may be used for 24 hours for symptom relief. If an abscess is present and can be percutaneously drained with complete resolution, antibiotic therapy can be withheld with the patient monitored closely. If the patient is not lactating, inflammatory carcinoma must be ruled out, and referral for possible biopsy would be warranted. Intraductal papillomas usually present with nipple discharge (bloody or serous). Grossly, they appear as pink to tan, friable, lesions within the duct and are attached to the involved duct by a stalk. They are generally not palpable on clinical breast examination. They are rarely malignant, but if multiple lesions are present (usually in younger women), they may undergo malignant transformation.

29.   d (Chapter 23)

RA is a chronic multisystem disease of unknown cause. The characteristic feature of established RA is persistent inflammatory synovitis of the peripheral joints, including metacarpophalangeal, wrist, knee, and joints of the feet, in a symmetric distribution. Two-thirds of patients present with an insidious onset of fatigue, anorexia, generalized weakness, and vague musculoskeletal symptoms until appearance of synovitis. Stiffness is frequent following periods of inactivity. Morning stiffness is common, as in many other inflammatory joint diseases. X-rays show bony erosions in the periarticular bone of the wrists or hands. The earliest changes, however, occur in the wrists or feet and consist of soft tissue swelling and juxtaarticular demineralization. Treatment may include NSAIDs or COX-2 inhibitors, but disease-modifying antirheumatic drugs (DMARDs), such as methotrexate, should be started as soon as the diagnosis is certain to prevent long-term disfigurement and to preserve function. SLE may present with arthritis of the hands and wrist, but x-rays do not show bony erosions. The diagnosis of SLE is based on having at least four of the following at any point in the patient's history: malar rash, discoid rash, photosensitivity, oral ulcers, arthritis, serositis, renal disease, seizures or psychosis with no other known cause, hemolytic anemia or leukopenia, antidouble-stranded DNA, anti-Smith antigen or antiphospholipid, and antinuclear antibodies. Severe systemic illness can occur with fever, anemia, prostration, and weight loss and require glucocorticoid therapy.

Wegener granulomatosis is a small vessel vasculitis that affects both the upper and lower respiratory tracts and glomerulonephritis. Presenting symptoms not only include upper respiratory symptoms (nasal congestion, sinusitis, otitis media, mastoiditis, inflammation of the gums, or stridor) but can also include migratory oligoarthritis specifically in the large joints, ocular disease, and dysesthesia secondary to neuropathy, purpura, fever, and weight loss. Three-fourths of patients have renal involvement, which may be subclinical until renal insufficiency is advanced. Induction treatment includes prednisone and cyclophosphamide (or prednisone and methotrexate).

Osteoarthritis usually presents in the cervical, or lower lumbar vertebrae, first metacarpal phalangeal, hip, knee, and first metatarsal phalangeal, and distal and proximal interphalangeal joints. There is usually joint space narrowing on x-ray along with osteophytes, but erosions do not occur. Osteoarthritis is uncommon in adults under age 40 and highly prevalent in those over age 60. Scleroderma is a multisystem disease that frequently presents with Raynaud phenomenon, GERD with or without dysmotility, skin changes, swollen fingers, and arthralgias. The American College of Rheumatology diagnostic criteria include thickened skin changes proximal to the metacarpophalangeal joints or at least two of the following: sclerodactyly, digital pitting (loss of tissue on finger pads secondary to ischemia), and bibasilar pulmonary fibrosis. A diagnosis can also be made if the patient has three out of five features of CREST syndrome (calcinosis, Raynaud phenomenon, esophageal dysmotility, sclerodactyly, and telangiectasis). A positive ANA is usually present in patients with scleroderma. This patient does not satisfy either criterion for a diagnosis of scleroderma.

30. c (Chapter 41)

Digoxin can improve left ventricular contractility in patients with systolic CHF and also helps control heart rate in patients with atrial fibrillation. There is no data to suggest benefit for patients in sinus rhythm with diastolic CHF. Initial management could include discontinuing the digoxin. Patients with diastolic HF generally benefit from reduction in heart rate and increased left ventricular relaxation and filling time. BBs, such as carvedilol, are useful therapeutic agents in achieving these goals and are a cornerstone of therapy for diastolic HF. In addition, carvedilol was associated with significant (65%) reduction in all-cause mortality, during the U.S. Carvedilol trial. This effect was independent of sex, age, etiology of HF, or ejection fraction.

Lisinopril should be maintained to provide afterload reduction and adequate BP control. ACEi are beneficial in HF, particularly in those with diabetes mellitus, HTN, or additional CV risk factors.

Acutely, patients with diastolic CHF will benefit from aggressive diuresis. Once fluid retention is no longer a concern, the diuretic dose may be reduced to the minimal level necessary to maintain euvolemia. In many cases, diuretics may ultimately be discontinued. In this patient, discontinuing furosemide may be a logical next step after discontinuing the digoxin.

Aspirin continues to be recommended as a preventive medication for MI and ischemia in those patients with CVD or risk factors.

31. c (Chapter 49)

The exact causes for obesity are not known, but appear to be multifactorial. Important factors most likely include a genetic disposition and psychosocial factors such as socioeconomic status.

Many patients present wanting to find an underlying medical condition that would account for their being overweight or obese. Secondary causes for obesity are unusual, and the medical examination and laboratory workup for obesity generally does not uncover a cause. Very often patients want to take a pill to lose weight. The current state of knowledge and treatment for obesity does not lend itself to this approach. Even in the cases where hypothyroidism is incidentally discovered, treatment of the hypothyroidism results in a euthyroid overweight or obese patient. Hypothyroidism may cause symptoms but it is generally not the cause for obesity. Treatment efforts focus on diet and exercise with the goal of increasing caloric expenditure and limiting intake to healthy, less-calorie dense choices. Expenditure of 3500 more calories than are taken in can result in weight loss of 1 lb.

32. e (Chapter 45)

Antiviral prophylaxis should be instituted as soon as possible after a health care provider is exposed to HIV-infected material. Early chemoprophylaxis may destroy the virus and prevent infection. Waiting to check titers or to see if the patient becomes ill puts her at unnecessary risk of developing infection that may then become a long-term health problem. Even though she did not "inject" blood into herself, the accidental stick with a needle that contained blood from an HIV-positive patient potentially exposes her to the HIV virus from any residual blood on or in the needle. Prophylaxis for pneumocystis, toxoplasmosis, or mycobacteria would not be appropriate until active HIV infection is established. Initiating such therapies is determined based on the patient's CD4 counts. Pneumocystis prophylaxis with TMP-SFX begins at a CD4 count of 200. Toxoplasmosis begins with a CD4 count of <100. *M. avium* complex prophylaxis with clarithromycin begins with a CD4 count of 50.

33. d (Chapter 26)

Orthostatic proteinuria is a benign condition of unknown etiology. Proteinuria is often discovered incidentally during a school or sports examination. Causes for proteinuria include intrinsic renal diseases such as minimal change disease, glomerulosclerosis, polycystic kidney disease, or Alport syndrome. Other conditions associated with proteinuria include diabetes, immunologic or connective tissue diseases, medications, and cancers such as multiple myeloma. These conditions are associated with a continuous proteinuria that does not depend on the upright or supine position. In contrast, orthostatic proteinuria is associated with protein leakage into the urine in significant quantities only upon assuming the upright posture and diminishes in the supine position. The exact cause for this condition is unknown, but patients have been followed for years and uniformly follow a benign course with no additional follow-up or treatment being required. Thus, no additional workup or restrictions are needed for this patient.

34. e (Chapter 17)

Testing the stool for *H. pylori* antigen would determine if the infection is active. Other means to test for active disease would include the Campylobacter-like organism (CLO) test performed on samples obtained via endoscopy, pathologic examination of biopsy specimens, and urea breath testing. The use of the fecal antigen testing is a good means to detect disease activity because it is more readily available than urea breath testing and it is not invasive.

Serologic testing is highly sensitive and specific and would be more convenient than fecal antigen testing. Unfortunately, this test remains positive indefinitely in patients who have had a history of *H. pylori* infection, even posttreatment. Barium swallow is a useful test for detecting anatomic abnormalities such as esophageal cancers, achalasia, or esophageal pouches, but is not sensitive for detecting the surface inflammatory changes associated with the *H. pylori* gastritis. Ambulatory pH monitoring is useful in correlating heartburn symptoms with gastroesophageal reflux in patients with symptoms but no visible changes detected on EGD. This test would not be helpful in detecting *H. pylori*–related disease. Abdominal CT would play no role in diagnosing heartburn-related symptoms. CT scans do play a role in the evaluation of acute and chronic abdominal pain to help define the anatomy and to detect associated abnormalities that can identify the cause for pain. CT scans are especially helpful in acute abdominal pain when nephrolithiasis, pancreatitis, appendicitis, or diverticulitis are suspected. CT scans are also obtained in cases of bowel obstruction to help identify the level of the obstruction and the possible cause for obstruction.

35. d (Chapter 11)

Verapamil, a calcium channel blocker, can cause constipation. Changing Verapamil to an alternative medication may relieve this patient's symptoms. Other medications that may cause constipation include opiates, anticholinergics, TCAs, diuretics, antacids, clonidine, levodopa, and laxative abuse. Other causes of constipation include insufficient dietary fiber, inactivity, hypokalemia, hypercalcemia, hypothyroidism, scleroderma, amyloidosis, pregnancy, neurologic disorders such as PD, paraplegia, prior pelvic surgery, diabetes mellitus, IBS, colonic mass, Hirschsprung disease, perianal pathology such as fissure(s), hemorrhoids, rectoceles, rectal prolapse, and diverticular disease. If the patient had no other potential causes for his change in bowel habits, then consideration should be given to the possibility of a lesion such as colon cancer. Because there is an identifiable potential cause for his symptoms, this should be addressed first. If his symptoms resolve with a change in medication, then he should undergo routine colonoscopy screening at age 50 or age 40 in those with a first-degree relative with colon cancer.

Laxative medication or preferably an increase in activity level and fiber and fluid intake are helpful measures for relieving the symptoms of constipation and tried first before additional medications are prescribed. In addition, long-term use of motility agents is thought to damage the myenteric nerves, thus negatively impacting GI motility. Metoclopramide is a promotility agent used for nausea and vomiting. It has its primary effect on the esophagus and gastroesophageal sphincter and does not have a role in treating constipation.

Recommending a low-fat, high-fiber diet is part of constipation management, and may be beneficial for individuals prone to constipation. This step could be taken along with modification of the patient's medication regimen. Other important steps in evaluating constipation include treating underlying disorders causing constipation, such as hypothyroidism, bowel obstruction, or anal fissure (or any of the above-mentioned causes). For functional constipation, increasing fluid and fiber intake is the first step. Patients should drink eight 8-oz glasses of water per day and consume large amounts of bran, fresh fruit, vegetables, beans, and whole grains. Other means to increase dietary fiber in those who have difficulty ingesting sufficient quantities in the diet include over-the-counter products, such as psyllium (Metamucil), methylcellulose (Citrucel), and polycarbophil (FiberCon). Patients may also benefit from bowel retraining, which involves devoting 10 to 15 minutes each day for quiet and unhurried time on the commode. This should take place at the same time each day and occur following a meal, to take advantage of the gastrocolic reflex. Bowel retraining often requires 2 to 3 weeks before becoming effective. Other medications include osmotic laxatives such as lactulose, magnesium salts, and sorbitol, which are nonabsorbable solutes that draw water fluid into the intestinal lumen by creating an osmotic gradient. Stimulants such as phenolphthalein (Ex-Lax) and bisacodyl (Dulcolax) stimulate intestinal smooth muscle activity. Stool softeners like docusate sodium (Colace), which is used for hard stools that are difficult to pass, decrease surface tension, and allow water and fat to mix in the stool. Stool softeners must be taken with plenty of water to work optimally. Enemas and suppositories work by distension and stimulation of the rectum, which leads to evacuation, and is especially useful in bedridden patients and those with stool impaction.

36. (Chapter 19)

1. **c.** Antismooth muscle antibodies can be found in type 1 and type 2 autoimmune hepatitis. ANAs are usually also elevated in autoimmune hepatitis.

2. **a.** Ferritin is used to diagnose hemochromatosis. Elevated ferritin, decreased transferrin, and increased transferrin saturation suggest hemochromatosis,

an iron storage disease affecting the liver, joints, pancreas, and other organs.

3. **d.** Decreased ceruloplasmin levels are found in 90% of Wilson disease patients; however, 20% of carriers also have reduced serum ceruloplasmin levels. Kayser-Fleischer rings are present in 99% of patients with the neurologic form of the disease; however, only 30% to 50% of patients present with the purely hepatic or presymptomatic states of Wilson disease. These rings are diagnosed definitively using an ophthalmologist's slit-lamp examination. Definitive diagnosis of the disease is made by liver biopsy and with quantitative copper assays. Wilson disease involves abnormal excretion of copper with subsequent buildup in the liver, the iris, and the brain causing parkinsonism. Trientine is the chelator being used more often in treatment, because it is less toxic than penicillamine.

4. **e.** Antimitochondrial antibodies are used to screen for primary biliary cirrhosis. Primary biliary cirrhosis is a disease with insidious onset characterized by autoimmune destruction of the intrahepatic bile ducts and cholestasis.

5. **b.** Haptoglobin is a glycoprotein synthesized in the liver that binds free hemoglobin. It is increased in obstructive liver disease or diseases associated with increased ESR. It is decreased in any type of hemolysis, liver disease, anemia, mildly with oral contraceptives, or in childhood and infancy.

37.   a (Chapter 21)

Deciding when to aggressively work up a patient with lymphadenopathy can be difficult. Important considerations include assessing for inciting causes and associated symptoms that may indicate increased risk for serious diseases such as metastatic cancer or lymphoma. Fever, weight loss, and generalized lymphadenopathy are examples of symptoms that suggest infection or malignancy as the potential etiology. Frequently, localized adenopathy can result from a viral infection or local inflammatory condition (e.g., tinea pedis, onychomycosis).When there are no worrisome signs or symptoms, then observation for up to 4 weeks is one option. Nodes that are unchanged or larger after 4 weeks should be biopsied. Nodes that have not resolved in 12 weeks should also be evaluated for possible biopsy.

Fine needle aspiration is one method for obtaining tissue. However, fine needle aspirates often obtain inadequate samples and therefore surgical excision is generally the preferred method for evaluating undiagnosed lymphadenopathy.

If there were signs of infection, such as redness, tenderness, fever, or an identified lesion, then empiric cephalexin would be reasonable during the observation period for resolution of the node. PET scanning has no role in evaluating this type of patient and is generally reserved for evaluating patients with known malignancies for metastases.

38.   c (Chapter 22)

The symptoms this patient is experiencing suggest an esophageal obstruction. Lesions that could cause obstruction of this nature include cancer, stricture, and achalasia. A barium esophagogram and upper endoscopy are tests that would help identify the type of lesions that may cause obstruction. A colonoscopy may be indicated as a routine screening tool in patients this age but would not be warranted as part of the evaluation for these symptoms. Other indications for colonoscopy would include change in bowel habits and melena or hematochezia.

Abdominal ultrasound is not a useful tool for examining the esophagus, the stomach, or the intestines. The only exception to this is that ultrasound has been used to assess for appendicitis, particularly in children. Ultrasound is useful in examining the organs both intraabdominally and in the pelvis. This would include the liver, kidneys, pancreas, uterus, and ovaries.

Abdominal CT is useful for assessing the organs and for inflammatory conditions such as pancreatitis, diverticulitis, and appendicitis. CT, like ultrasound, is not as useful for evaluating the esophagus, stomach, or intestines except for more advanced disease where there may be significant wall thickening or mass effect. Chest x-ray would not be expected to show any significant findings. Without contrast material, the esophagus is generally not apparent on chest x-rays, although on occasion, lesions such as a hiatal hernia are apparent due to the associated "gas bubble" that can be seen.

39.   b (Chapter 54)

S. aureus is the most common cause of cellulitis. *Streptococcus pyogenes* is also a common offending agent. With *S. pyogenes,* a golden crust is often present. Oral or IV beta-lactams, including dicloxacillin, cefazolin, and cephalexin are commonly prescribed.

Pseudomonas aeruginosa is a common respiratory pathogen in patients with cystic fibrosis or those that are immunocompromised. *Pseudomonas* is also associated with osteomyelitis in sickle cell patients and is a cause of foot infections because it grows well in tennis shoes.

H. influenzae type B is a common cause of epiglottitis. Nontypeable H. flu is the second most common cause of otitis media infections and sinusitis and is implicated in many acute pneumonias in COPD patients.

C. difficile is the cause of pseudomembranous colitis. These infections can occur after eradication of normal gut flora from a course of antibiotics that then leads to an overgrowth of enteric *C. difficile*. The change in gut flora is generally associated with use of antibiotics that kill off the normal flora but not *C. difficile*.

S. pneumoniae is the most common cause of bacterial otitis media, sinusitis, and a common cause of pneumonia, as well as of bronchitis, bacteremia, meningitis, and other infectious processes.

40.   a (Chapter 72)
Children between the age of 3 months and 3 years, with a temperature over 102°F, are at increased risk of occult bacteremia and an underlying bacterial infection. One approach to these children is to first obtain a CBC. Those with WBCs >15,000 need urine and blood cultures ordered. A chest x-ray in these children is indicated when respiratory symptoms or signs are present. Children in whom cultures are obtained should generally receive empiric antibiotic coverage until culture results are available. Many experts recommend admitting these children and starting antibiotics. The risk of bacteremia is higher in younger children, in those with a temperature over 102°F, and in those with WBCs >15,000. Children, in this age category, with temperatures above 102°F who are not admitted, should have follow-up the next day.

For neonates (birth to 1 month of age) and ill-appearing infants (age 1 to 3 months), a fever workup involves a full septic workup that entails a CBC, blood cultures, chest x-ray, UA, urine culture, and lumbar puncture. Hospitalization and empiric antibiotic coverage to cover the most common pathogens is indicated until culture results are available. Infants 1 to 3 months of age who appear well with normal laboratory studies, reliable parents, and a WBC between 5000 and 15,000 may be discharged with a follow-up in 24 hours. Empiric coverage (such as ceftriaxone IM) is usually given pending follow-up and culture results. In children older than age 3, occult bacteremia is less common and clinical evaluation by history and physical examination can usually distinguish the source of fever. Laboratory evaluation in these older children is dictated by clinical findings.

41.   e (Chapter 70)
This patient has mild croup and no signs of respiratory distress. Dexamethasone as a single dose lessens the need for reevaluation and hospitalization in children with croup. Croup is a respiratory infection or laryngotracheobronchitis generally caused by the parainfluenza virus. Children may appear nontoxic at rest, but with crying or activity experience respiratory distress. Because the lungs are not affected, oxygen saturation is generally within normal limits, except in very severe cases. Anterior–posterior soft tissue neck x-rays may demonstrate steeple sign of upper tracheal narrowing; if present, this helps to confirm the diagnosis.

Inhaled racemic epinephrine is used in patients with moderate-to-severe croup. Following therapy with racemic epinephrine, the child should be observed for 2 to 3 hours to assure that rebound symptoms do not occur. This may entail an extended emergency room stay or admission to observe the child. Dexamethasone is generally prescribed along with any racemic epinephrine treatments. Nebulized or oral albuterol (beta 2 agonist) is indicated for treatment of asthma or COPD. Albuterol is not indicated in treatment of croup.

Oral prednisone at a dose of 1 to 2 mg/kg for asthma for 3 to 10 days or until peak expiratory flow returns to above 80% can be used for an acute exacerbation. This is not indicated in the treatment of croup.

42.   d (Chapter 70)
Febrile seizures occur with fever, and the rate of rise of temperature is more closely associated with a seizure than the absolute temperature. With this in mind, treatment attempts should be made to control or reduce the fever with antipyretics. Therapy with antiepileptics is not indicated for simple febrile seizures. After trying to control the temperature, the next step should be to assess and treat the underlying cause of the fever. Lumbar puncture or CT scan is indicated if based on the history or physical examination: for example, if there are signs or symptoms suggesting meningitis, encephalitis, or other CNS lesions might be present. The presence of a febrile seizure alone, particularly when there is an identifiable cause for the fever, is not an indication for these tests. Likewise, antibiotics are not routinely recommended because of the seizure, but need an indication based on the evaluation of the patient.

43.   c (Chapter 53)
STDs (infections) should be tested for at this time, because the patient is sexually active and is in a high-risk age group for sexually transmitted infections.

Pap smear screening begins at age 21 years, and, if normal for 3 years, is repeated every 3 years in low-risk individuals.

Cholesterol screening is indicated in male patients beginning at 35 years of age and female patients at 45 years of age. Screening may start earlier in high-risk individuals.

Routine UA is not indicated as part of adolescent care. ECGs are indicated in specific disease conditions, such as HTN and heart disease, but are not a part of routine health screening at this age.

44.   d (Chapter 71)
ADHD is a clinical diagnosis based on the following DSM-IV criteria for ADHD:

I: Either **a** or **b** or combined type.

a. Six or more of the following symptoms of inattention have been present for at least 6 months to a point that is disruptive and inappropriate for developmental level. Inattention: (1) Often does not give close attention to details or makes careless mistakes in schoolwork, work, or other activities. (2) Often has trouble keeping attention on tasks or play activities. (3) Often does not seem to listen when spoken to directly. (4) Often does not follow instructions and fails to finish schoolwork, chores, or duties in the workplace (not due to oppositional behavior or failure to understand instructions). (5) Often has trouble organizing activities. (6) Often avoids, dislikes, or does not want to do things that take a lot of mental effort for a long period of time (such as schoolwork or homework). (7) Often loses things needed for tasks and activities (e.g., toys, school assignments, pencils, books, or tools). (8) Is often easily distracted. (9) Is often forgetful in daily activities.

    b. Six or more of the following symptoms of hyperactivity–impulsivity have been present for at least 6 months to an extent that is disruptive and inappropriate for developmental level. Hyperactivity: (1) Often fidgets with hands or feet or squirms in seat. (2) Often gets up from seat when remaining in seat is expected. (3) Often runs about or climbs when and where it is not appropriate (adolescents or adults may feel very restless). (4) Often has trouble playing or enjoying leisure activities quietly. (5) Is often "on the go" or often acts as if "driven by a motor." (6) Often talks excessively. Impulsivity: (1) Often blurts out answers before questions have been finished. (2) Often has trouble waiting one's turn. (3) Often interrupts or intrudes on others (e.g., butts into conversations or games).

    II: Some symptoms that cause impairment were present before age 7 years.

    III: Some impairment from the symptoms is present in two or more settings (e.g., at school/work and at home).

    IV: There must be clear evidence of significant impairment in social, school, or work functioning.

    V: The symptoms do not happen only during the course of a pervasive developmental disorder, schizophrenia, or other psychotic disorder. The symptoms are not better accounted for by another mental disorder.

    CT scanning and TSH testing are not indicated as part of the evaluation. The Ages and Stages questionnaire is an evaluation used to screen for developmental problems in children in four domains: cognitive, motor, self-help, and language. It is used for ages 3 months to 5 years.

45. c (Chapter 60)

Because this patient has primary amenorrhea and is also lacking secondary sex characteristics, her hypothalamic/pituitary function needs assessment. If the FSH and LH are within normal limits, then an ultrasound is indicated to determine if the uterus and ovaries are present or absent. If the FSH and LH are abnormally elevated, or if on ultrasound there is no evidence of

a uterus or ovaries, then genetic testing is needed to determine the karyotype. If the FSH and LH are abnormally low, then the patient should be evaluated for hypogonadotropic hypogonadism including an assessment for medical illnesses and an MRI of the brain. The medroxyprogesterone challenge test would be performed if there were evidence of both a uterus and presence of estrogen (e.g., breast development). This test evaluates the presence of estrogenic action on the uterus and the presence of an intact outflow tract. Testosterone would be useful if there were virilization or clitoral hypertrophy.

46. b (Chapter 66)

History of major depression puts this patient at increased risk for developing postpartum depression. Postpartum depression is relatively common after childbirth. Although this patient has a supportive family, the strongest predictors of postpartum depression include prior psychopathology (such as depression), low levels of social support, stressful life events, and poor marital status. This patient, despite having strong family support, is still at significant risk due to her previous personal history of depression. Postpartum depression should be treated immediately to minimize the impairment to caregiving mothers. SSRIs are usually first-line agents. Cognitive behavioral therapy and group therapy can also help. Postpartum blues have an onset of 2 to 14 days after childbirth with a duration of <2 weeks. This heightened emotional reactivity can develop in 50% of women. The key element to this question is both duration and severity of symptoms.

47. a (Chapter 62)

An intrauterine device (IUD) is a good choice for a woman in a monogamous relationship, who may still want to have children in the future. Further, the patient's irregular schedule would not be of concern if using an IUD. IUDs such as Progestasert have theoretical and actual failure rates of 2.0%. This device works by interfering with sperm mobility and fertilization. IUDs are highly effective, inexpensive, and reversible. Complications include pregnancy, undiagnosed vaginal bleeding, and PID. Relative contraindications include nulliparity, prior ectopic pregnancy, history of multiple partners, as well as history of STDs or an abnormal Pap smear. Complications include PID, ectopic pregnancy, spontaneous abortions, increased menstrual flow and pain, and uterine perforation during insertion.

    Hormonal contraceptive patches still require weekly changes and may not be ideal for this woman with an irregular schedule and failure of prior hormonal contraception. Postcoital contraception requires taking the equivalent of two oral contraceptive pills within 72 hours of coitus as well as 12 hours later. One form of postcoital contraception utilizes ethinyl estradiol 50 μg with 0.5 mg norgestrel given in a regimen of two tablets initially followed by two tablets 12 hours later. This method has nausea as potential adverse effect. Emergency postcoital contraception prevents at least three of four pregnancies that would have occurred. These methods should not be relied upon as a means of contraception.

Female condoms have an actual failure rate of 21.0% to 26.0% (although the theoretical failure rate is as low as 6%), and require use every time coitus occurs. This patient's history suggests poor use of such contraception. This patient is not sure if she desires more children. A tubal ligation should be considered permanent and would be inappropriate in this case.

48. c (Chapter 58)

The patient has atypical squamous cells of undetermined significance (ASCUS), but has no history of previously abnormal Pap smears and, most importantly, a negative HPV test. This patient should have a repeat Pap smear in 12 months. A subsequent abnormal Pap smear is an indication for colposcopy. If the patient is at risk for not adhering to this regimen, then immediate colposcopy is the preferred option.

Higher grade lesions, positive endocervical curettage, or an inadequate colposcopy may require conization or loop electroexcision procedure (LEEP). Lower grade lesions may be treated with observation, laser, cryotherapy, or by LEEP depending on size and location of the lesion.

49. b (Chapter 65)

The patient should be treated with amoxicillin, nitrofurantoin, or cephalexin for 7 to 10 days. Although most patients are not treated for asymptomatic bacteriuria, pregnant women are an exception. All pregnant women should be screened and, if positive, treated for asymptomatic bacteriuria to reduce the risk of acute pyelonephritis of pregnancy requiring hospitalization and parenteral antibiotic therapy. After treatment, a culture to document clearing of the infection is indicated, and cultures should be repeated monthly thereafter until delivery. If infections are recurrent, continuous low-dose prophylaxis with nitrofurantoin is indicated. All asymptomatic bacteriuria in pregnancy are treated to avoid pyelonephritis because the physiologic hydronephrosis of pregnancy predisposes to development of pyelonephritis.

Ciprofloxacin, other fluoroquinolones, and tetracyclines should be avoided in pregnancy for risk of teratogenicity in the fetus.

Ultrasound of the kidneys of a pregnant woman is likely to show mild hydronephrosis that is a physiologic change of pregnancy and not secondary to a disease process. Ultrasound would be useful in cases of pyelonephritis to evaluate for obstruction.

50. e (Chapter 65)

Oral medications such as metformin are now commonly used in the management of gestational diabetes. Although dietary management is part of all treatment, medications are often required, in the form of either an oral agent or insulin.

Macrosomia is a complication of gestational diabetes, not intrauterine growth retardation (IUGR). IUGR is a potential complication for women with preexisting type 1 diabetes, who become pregnant. Macrosomic babies are at greater risk of complications, such as shoulder dystocia, cephalopelvic disproportion, and hypoglycemia in the neonatal period (secondary to fetal increase in insulin due to maternal hyperglycemia). Goals of therapy are to prevent complications and to maintain the mother's blood sugar levels in a normal range. Retinopathy and nephropathy are not generally concerns associated with gestational diabetes.

Concerns about gestational diabetes do not vanish after delivery and women should be followed up and tested postpartum. A woman who has had gestational diabetes is at a much higher risk for developing T2DM later on in life.

51. c (Chapter 12)

With symptoms of fever, dyspnea, and abnormal findings on lung examination, this patient most likely has pneumonia, which can be documented by obtaining a chest x-ray. Sinusitis is not likely, given the absence of nasal symptoms or headaches and a normal ear, nose, and throat examination. Symptomatic treatment with cough suppressants or incentive spirometry may be appropriate; however, evaluation and treatment of the underlying condition is the first priority in a patient with these signs and symptoms. Sputum cultures are generally not very helpful in the outpatient setting. However, if the patient does not respond to antibiotics, a sputum culture may be considered.

52. b (Chapter 63)

Atrophic vaginitis is usually seen in postmenopausal women. HPV infections are generally asymptomatic and discovered by palpation or visualization of a wart-like lesion or by Pap smear testing. In menstruating women, *Trichomonas*, bacterial vaginosis, and *Candida* cause 90% of vaginitis symptoms. All three may cause itching, but the discharge seen in bacterial vaginosis and trichomoniasis usually has a pH > 4.5. The diagnosis can be confirmed by examining a wet mount and then adding KOH to the slide, which will dissolve epithelial cells but not the spores and hyphae seen in candidal infections.

53. b (Chapter 29)

The most common cause of chronic dyspnea in a smoker without other significant prior medical problems is COPD. In evaluating this patient, other causes for chronic dyspnea must also be considered. A chest x-ray and laboratory work can help to exclude causes such as pleural effusion, CHF, and anemia. When the diagnosis is in doubt, additional testing, including pulmonary function testing, may help arrive at the diagnosis. Diabetes mellitus does not generally cause dyspnea except in association with ketoacidosis, which would present acutely in a patient younger than this. Patients with pneumonia, pulmonary embolus, and MI present with acute dyspnea.

54.   d (Chapter 74)

Hypertrophic cardiomyopathy is inherited as an autosomal dominant trait with variable expression. It is the most common cause of sudden death in those younger than 35 years. Most patients with this condition are asymptomatic, and, unfortunately, sudden cardiac death may be the initial presentation. Definitive diagnosis is made via echocardiogram, which shows asymmetric septal hypertrophy and left ventricular outflow obstruction. In this condition, decreased venous return increases the obstruction and the intensity of the murmur. Squatting increases venous return, whereas standing increases venous pooling and limits venous return.

55.   e (Chapter 20)

Although a CBC, uric acid level, rheumatoid factor, and ESR are useful tests, a joint fluid analysis is the most critical test to determine whether this patient has a septic joint and to detect uric acid crystals (gout) or calcium pyrophosphate crystals (pseudogout). Prompt diagnosis of a septic joint is important because delays in treatment can lead to permanent joint damage.

56.   d (Chapter 13)

The presence of WBCs and blood in the stool is consistent with an inflammatory process. Food poisoning, rotavirus, and irritable bowel are noninflammatory processes. Although Crohn disease can cause bloody stools with WBCs, there is no previous history of GI complaints. The most likely cause is diarrhea from a bacterial infection, such as shigellosis.

57.   e (Chapter 16)

Migraine headaches are characterized by severe unilateral, throbbing pain, which are often accompanied by photophobia, nausea, and emesis. Migraines preceded by auras (transient neurologic abnormalities such as the sensation of flashing lights or strange odors) are called classic migraines, whereas those not associated with auras are called common migraines. A family history of migraines occurs in most cases and can be an important diagnostic clue.

58.   d (Chapter 19)

The subacute course, myalgias, fatigue, and elevated liver function tests suggest hepatitis. Patients with appendicitis have nausea and vomiting along with right lower quadrant pain but usually do not have elevated liver enzymes. Although this patient does have risk factors for gallstones, patients with cholelithiasis typically present more acutely and have intermittent pain that is aggravated with food. Although hemolysis can cause jaundice, it is unlikely to be the cause of her problems because the CBC is normal and the unconjugated fraction of bilirubin is elevated in hemolytic disease. Painless jaundice is the classic presentation for pancreatic cancer involving the head of the pancreas.

Supportive care is generally recommended for patients with hepatitis. Determining the specific viral cause may help determine the need for follow-up testing, the likelihood of developing chronic hepatitis, and guide how to counsel family members regarding testing.

59.   d (Chapter 54)

Herpes simplex virus causes painful genital ulcers, often with fever and dysuria. Syphilis ulcers are painless. UTIs do not cause genital ulcers. Although women with cervicitis may note vaginal discharge, dysuria, or spotting, most are asymptomatic. Petechial or pustular skin lesions are sometimes seen on the dorsal aspect on the distal extremity, ankles, or wrist joints with gonorrheal infections, but ulcers are not seen on the cervix.

60.   a (Chapter 19)

This patient most likely has cholelithiasis. She has risk factors for gallstone disease and her total and conjugated bilirubin levels are elevated, indicating that the stone may be obstructing the common bile duct. She may ultimately need endoscopy and endoscopic retrograde cholangiopancreatography (ERCP), but an ultrasound or CT scan is generally done prior to the ERCP to confirm the diagnosis. MRI and liver biopsy are not indicated in this situation. Peptic ulcers can sometimes present with right upper quadrant pain; however, they do not cause liver enzyme abnormalities.

61.   e (Chapter 36)

This patient has an iron deficiency anemia, indicated by low ferritin levels and increased total iron-binding capacity. The most probable cause of his anemia is chronic GI blood loss, possibly from a colon cancer. Patients with thalassemia can have microcytic anemia; however, the iron-binding capacity and ferritin levels would be normal. Similarly, the serum ferritin levels are normal or increased in anemia of chronic disease. Vitamin B_{12} or folate deficiency causes megaloblastic anemias.

62.   c (Chapter 34)

Most cases of acne are pleomorphic and include comedones, papules, pustules, and nodules. Topical agents such as tretinoin are often the first line of therapy. Other milder comedolytics include salicylic acid, sulfur preparations, and azelaic acid. To reduce the follicular bacterial population, topical antibiotics such as erythromycin and clindamycin may be tried. Benzoyl peroxide also has bacteriostatic properties, which makes it effective for mild acne. Isotretinoin (Accutane) is reserved for severe acne and should not be used as the first line of treatment for this patient. It is teratogenic and in females should only be used patients with a secure means of birth control; its use should be restricted to dermatologists or those providers who are experienced with its use.

63. a (Chapter 23)
Nail pitting is commonly seen in psoriatic arthritis. Other skin lesions and associated diseases include tophi and gout, malar rash and mouth ulcers with lupus erythematosus, and erythema migrans with Lyme disease. Fingertip atrophy or ulcers along with calcinosis and telangiectasias are signs of scleroderma. Keratoderma blennorrhagicum, a hyperkeratotic lesion on the palms and soles, and balanitis circinata, a shallow painless ulcer on the penis, are signs of Reiter syndrome.

64. c (Chapter 36)
The patient has a macrocytic anemia, indicated by the high MCV. Thalassemia, iron deficiency, and anemia of chronic disease typically cause microcytic anemia. Both vitamin B_{12} and folate deficiencies may cause megaloblastic anemia; however, only B_{12} deficiency causes neurologic symptoms. The most common cause of B_{12} deficiency is pernicious anemia.

65. c (Chapter 64)
Although this patient is sure of her last menstrual period (LMP), the physical findings do not correlate with the gestational age by LMP. At 10 weeks, the uterus is not palpable above the pubis, and it is unlikely that fetal heart tones would be detected by Doppler. Therefore, an ultrasound is needed to confirm the gestational age as well as to document a single fetus and normal uterus. The incidence of chromosomal abnormalities does not exceed the risk of amniocentesis until after a maternal age of 35 years. Preeclampsia does not occur before 20 weeks of gestation. Abdominal x-rays should be avoided in pregnancy because the radiation may adversely affect the fetus.

66. a (Chapter 47)
Graves disease is a common cause of hyperthyroidism and is the result of serum thyroid-stimulating antibodies. These antibodies act on the TSH receptors of the thyroid, causing an excessive release of thyroid hormone. As a result, TSH is low and free T4 levels are high. Thyroid scan shows diffuse uptake and thus helps differentiate between Graves disease and a nodular disorder. Fine-needle aspiration is performed to assess for cancer in patients with nodular lesions, but it would not be helpful in those with Graves disease.

67. b (Chapter 8)
This patient has the typical symptoms and signs of allergic rhinitis. The nasal crease is a sign of chronic nasal itching, a common symptom associated with allergic rhinitis. Vasomotor rhinitis is characterized by chronic nasal congestion with pink nasal mucosa that is brought on by sudden changes in temperature, humidity, or odor. Although rhinitis occurs with sinusitis, it is unlikely that the patient has sinusitis. The nasal discharge in sinusitis is purulent rather than watery. Rhinitis medicamentosa is a condition caused by chronic use of cocaine or nasal decongestants. There is nothing in the history to suggest that the rhinorrhea may be secondary to rhinitis medicamentosa. Foreign body is associated with purulent, malodorous discharge and is unlikely in a patient this age.

68. c (Chapter 10)
This patient has the classic signs and symptoms of costochondritis without any other symptoms to suggest cardiac or pulmonary problems. This history and the fact that his pain is reproducible with palpation suggest that it is not cardiac but rather musculoskeletal. A normal ECG while having discomfort also argues against a cardiac cause. In pneumonia, patients can have chest pain worsened with inspiration, but they also have other symptoms, such as cough and fever, along with physical examination findings such as inspiratory rales. Esophageal spasm is often associated with eating or drinking but is not affected by breathing.

69. b (Chapter 44)
Patients with diverticular disease, colon cancer, or colon polyps can present with painless GI bleeding, as in this patient. Diverticular bleeding is generally an acute episode and although the hemoglobin may drop significantly, RBC indices are generally normal with acute blood loss. Colitis associated with rectal bleeding is generally not painless but associated with cramps and diarrhea. Although hemorrhoids can cause rectal bleeding, the bleeding is generally not severe enough to cause a significant anemia. Before assuming that rectal bleeding and anemia are because of hemorrhoids, the patient should undergo diagnostic testing to eliminate other causes for his anemia. Colon cancer commonly presents with hypochromic microcytic anemia, and an acute bleeding episode may lead to laboratory testing that suggests chronic blood loss. Irritable bowel syndrome is a benign condition—where people feel cramping abdominal pain, relieved with a bowel movement—and is not associated with GI bleeding.

70.   d (Chapter 64)

Quadruple marker screening should be offered to the patient in the second trimester. It includes the maternal serum AFP (MSAFP), estriol, inhibin A, and HCG. This is a screening test for neural tube defects and Down syndrome. High levels of MSAFP are associated with neural tube defects. Low levels of MSAFP and estriol are associated with trisomy 21. Inhibin A and HCG levels are increased in trisomy 21. However, dating errors and multiple fetuses should be ruled out before ordering further testing for neural tube defects or trisomy 21. Not all women choose to have the quadruple screen performed. Counseling about the tests, possible test results, additional testing for abnormal results, and options available to the woman faced with an abnormal fetus should be provided to assist in her making the decision to be tested. All other listed tests are done in the first trimester except glucose screening, which is generally performed around 28 weeks' gestation.

71.   d (Chapter 51)

The first line of prevention for osteoporosis is lifestyle changes, but pharmaceutical agents along with preventive measures are important for treatment of the disease. Smoking cessation, modest alcohol consumption, weightbearing exercises, and good dietary habits should be stressed. Calcium intake should be 1000 mg/day for premenopausal women and 1200 mg/day for postmenopausal women. As patients age, the risk for falls increases and measures to decrease falls—such as correcting visual problems, decreasing sedative medications, and initiating balance exercises—are beneficial. Medical management is indicated for women with a T score below −2.0 without risk factors and for those with a T score below −1.5 and risk factors, such as women above age 70 or those on long-term corticosteroids. The bisphosphonates must be taken on an empty stomach with at least an 8-oz glass of water while the patient remains upright, without eating, for at least 30 minutes. Although useful in treating menopausal symptoms, estrogen replacement therapy is no longer considered first-line therapy for osteoporosis.

72.   b (Chapter 44)

This patient has diverticulitis. Although a barium enema or colonoscopy can help diagnose diverticular disease, these tests should not be done in acute diverticulitis because of the risk of perforation. In the acute setting, the test of choice is an abdominal CT scan. Ultrasound is useful in diagnosing appendicitis and other abdominal disorders but has not been shown to be a useful test for diagnosing diverticulitis.

73.   b (Chapter 12)

This patient had a viral illness prior to the onset of the cough, and a postviral syndrome can cause coughing for up to 8 weeks. It is unlikely that the patient has sinusitis without nasal congestion, headaches, or any other symptoms of sinusitis. Pneumonia is unlikely in the absence of fever, dyspnea, or sputum production. Psychogenic cough is a possibility, but the viral prodrome and the short duration of symptoms make it unlikely. Asthma is a chronic condition characterized by repetitive episodes of cough associated with wheezing on physical examination.

74.   c (Chapter 73)

This child has recurrent otitis media. Acute otitis media is often associated with a URI. Treatment should be initiated with antibiotics that cover *S. pneumoniae*, *H. influenzae*, and *Moraxella catarrhalis,* the bacterial organisms most likely to cause otitis media. Children with recurrent otitis media should be started on prophylactic antibiotics for 6 months to suppress recurrent infections and allow fluid resolution. Otitis media tends to occur less frequently as children advance in age, and the prophylactic antibiotics may allow the child to grow and develop further while also suppressing recurrent infections. Myringotomy and tympanostomy tube placement is an option for those who fail suppressive therapy and for children with persistent otitis media with effusion, particularly when associated with hearing loss. Decongestant therapy has not been shown to be effective prophylactic treatment for otitis media.

75.   e (Chapter 29)

In patients with pneumonia, it is important to determine the best locus of care. Indications for hospitalization are (a) systolic BP <90; (b) pulse rate >140; (c) O_2 saturation <90% or PO_2 <60 mmHg; (d) presence of abscess or pleural effusion; (e) marked metabolic abnormality; (f) age >65; and (g) unreliable social situation. Underlying disease states such as CHF, renal failure, malignancy, diabetes, or severe COPD are also important factors in considering whether to hospitalize an individual with pneumonia.

76.   c (Chapter 40)

Patients with COPD are commonly treated with bronchodilators, anticholinergics, and inhaled steroids. During acute exacerbations, antibiotics and oral steroids are often prescribed. Nonmedication recommendations include smoking cessation and pulmonary rehabilitation, which includes exercise. Spiral CT scanning and bronchoscopy are not recommended routinely in patients with COPD except to assist in the diagnosis of suspected pulmonary embolus, lung cancer, or other structural lung lesions that may complicate or contribute to a patient's symptoms. Routine vaccinations recommended for patients with COPD include pneumococcal vaccine and an annual influenza vaccine. Hib vaccine is not recommended for patients with COPD.

77. d (Chapter 24)

All of these conditions are diagnoses with palpitations as significant symptoms. Diagnostic testing is often warranted to evaluate patients presenting with a complaint of palpitations. Cardiac evaluation may include an echocardiogram, 24-hour Holter monitor, or event monitor. The echocardiogram evaluates cardiac structure. A 24-hour Holter monitor may detect arrhythmias occurring on a daily basis, whereas an event monitor is more useful to detect those that occur more sporadically. A CBC, TSH, and FSH may help diagnose the other listed causes of palpitations. Panic disorder is diagnosed clinically; thus, although diagnostic testing is useful for excluding other potential causes, no test diagnoses panic disorder.

78. c (Chapter 17)

Following therapy for gastric ulcers, ulcer healing must be documented to help ensure that the ulcer did not represent a gastric carcinoma. Once ulcer healing has been documented, observation for recurrence of symptoms is appropriate. Repeated therapy with antibiotics or extended use of PPIs is not necessary in an asymptomatic patient provided the EGD results are normal. If the ulcer persists and remains *H. pylori*–positive, a repeat course of antibiotics and PPIs may be warranted. *H. pylori* antibody testing is not useful as a test of cure, because antibody levels remain abnormal for an indefinite time.

79. a (Chapter 14)

A central cause is likely in this patient with vertigo in light of the physical finding of vertical nystagmus. Vertical nystagmus does not occur with peripheral etiologies. The lack of association of the patient's symptoms with positional changes and the normal findings on hearing evaluation also help localize the process to a central etiology. Evaluation for possible MS should be performed with MRI of the brain and possibly with brainstem auditory evoked responses. A psychiatric cause is unlikely and would not cause the finding of vertical nystagmus.

80. b (Chapter 6)

The patient presented is undergoing vascular surgery, which is a high-risk surgery for concomitant CAD. Thus, a cardiac stress test should be ordered. Several studies indicate that a prothrombin is not indicated as a routine test, but is indicated for those requiring warfarin therapy and for those with suspected liver disease. Pulmonary function testing may help define the severity of lung disease, but is not recommended as a screening test and does not define a prohibitive level of lung function for surgeries other than lung resection. An echocardiogram may help in assessing patients with known or suspected CHF or valvular heart disease. Venous duplex imaging is helpful in those suspected of having DVT but is not recommended as a screening test.

81. a (Chapter 4)

Hepatitis A is generally a mild, self-limited infection in children. Vaccination for hepatitis A is currently recommended for all children. Hepatitis B is associated with chronic infection and can cause lifelong liver disease. Whereas most teens and adults develop immunity after infection with hepatitis B, up to 90% of infants who are infected will develop chronic hepatitis B infection. Oral poliovirus has been associated with vaccine-related infection and has led to recommendations for universal use of IPV, which does not use live virus and does not cause vaccine-related infection. Pneumococcal vaccine is recommended for all children as well as high-risk adults, although the vaccine for children is different than the one for adults. Individuals who require chronic aspirin therapy should receive influenza and varicella vaccines to limit the risk for developing Reye syndrome.

82. c (Chapter 3)

Some controversy surrounds the issue of cholesterol screening in children, because childhood values are not always predictive of future adult values. Cholesterol values tend to be variable and are affected by diet and level of physical activity; if they are elevated, therefore, they must be confirmed on one or more occasions. Elevated levels are those >200 mg/dL, with values of 170 to 199 mg/dL considered borderline and those below 170 mg/dL normal. Screening is currently recommended for children above 2 years of age with a family history of premature CVD (before age 55) in the parents or grandparents or with a parental history of hypercholesterolemia.

83. c (Chapter 5)

Routine health care of a healthy 35-year old with no medical disease, no significant family or social history, and a normal physical examination including BP will involve minimal laboratory work. The primary focus of the examination is a review of risk factors, including those for accidents, injury, and exposures to STDs, cigarettes, and drugs. Routine ECG, chest x-ray, and stress testing are not supported by the literature in any age group. Occult blood testing of the stool generally commences at age 50 but earlier at age 40 in those with a family history of colon cancer. Lipid profile evaluation is recommended beginning at age 35 in men and at age 45 in women.

84. b (Chapter 39)

Atopic dermatitis is a common disease affecting infants, with over 60% of cases diagnosed by 1 year of age and an additional 30% diagnosed by age 5.

The lifetime incidence for atopic dermatitis is over 20%; however, many cases spontaneously resolve by age 2, and most of the remaining cases resolve during the teen years. In infancy, the face and cheeks are commonly affected, along with the trunk and extremities. In children and teens, atopic dermatitis spares the face and most commonly localizes to the flexural creases of the extremities. Atopic dermatitis is associated with other allergic diseases, and children who develop atopic dermatitis may go on to develop allergic rhinitis or asthma.

85. b (Chapter 38)
The patient described has mild intermittent asthma, for which short-acting beta agonists are recommended as needed for the acute exacerbations. Oral steroids may be used for acute exacerbations but are generally reserved for those with severe symptoms. Daily medication use is reserved for those with mild, moderate, or severe persistent asthma. Patients with persistent asthma have symptoms more than twice per week and/or nocturnal symptoms more than twice per month. Chronic oral steroids are reserved for those with chronic persistent asthma that is refractory to other therapies. Antibiotic therapy is not recommended for the treatment of uncomplicated asthma.

86. b (Chapter 42)
Different classes of antidepressants are equally effective. The choice of medication depends on the patient's symptoms, current medications, and side-effect profile. In a patient with insomnia, a TCA, trazodone, or mirtazapine is a good choice. Bupropion is a good choice in patients with somnolence. If anxiety or agitation is a complaint, SSRIs should be avoided because they can be energizing. The key to successful treatment is duration. For the first episode, depression should be treated for 6 to 12 months.

87. a (Chapter 25)
The classic symptoms of infectious mononucleosis caused by heterophile-positive Epstein-Barr virus (EBV) are fever, sore throat, malaise, lymphadenopathy, and splenomegaly. In adolescence, these symptoms are seen in 75% of the patients, whereas EBV infections in infants and young children may be asymptomatic or have a mild pharyngitis. The heterophile test is used for diagnosis in children and adults; however, the mononucleosis spot test (Monospot) is more sensitive and more commonly used than the heterophile. All the above infections can produce a mononucleosis-like syndrome, but CMV is the most common. Patients with CMV mononucleosis are usually older and have fever and malaise as the major manifestations. Pharyngitis and lymphadenopathy are less common than with EBV mononucleosis.

88. d (Chapter 38)
The patient described has moderate persistent asthma, for which daily therapy with inhaled steroids and long-acting beta agonists are recommended. The presence of daily symptoms requires daily medications to suppress the inflammation and reactivity of the airways of asthmatic patients. Oral steroids are reserved for severe persistent asthma and those with severe acute exacerbations. Nedocromil is useful for mild persistent asthma and may be used in combination with other therapies for more severe disease.

89. c (Chapter 46)
Ninety-five percent of patients with a diagnosis of HTN have primary or essential HTN. Evaluation for secondary causes is generally reserved for those refractory to medical therapy or those presenting with hypertensive crisis. Although this patient may be at increased risk for cardiac disease in the future, a screening cardiac stress test is not routinely recommended for any patient. Testing is recommended to detect the secondary effects of HTN, evaluate other CV risk factors, and help choose medical therapy. Recommended testing includes an ECG, chest x-ray, CBC, glucose, cholesterol, electrolytes, creatinine, calcium, uric acid, and UA.

90. b (Chapter 74)
An important part of the preparticipation evaluation (PPE) is to identify those at risk for sudden cardiac death. Although ECG, echocardiogram, or stress testing may be appropriate in those at risk for sudden cardiac death, these tests have not been shown to be effective in mass screening of those with a normal history and physical examination. Because the incidence of CAD increases with age, it is the most common cause of sudden cardiac death in athletes over the age of 40. Hypertrophic cardiomyopathy is the most common cause for death in athletes under age 40.

91. a (Chapter 47)
Constipation, weight gain, depression, and fatigue are common in those with hypothyroidism and uncommon in those with hyperthyroidism. Geriatric patients may present with "apathetic hyperthyroidism" and appear clinically depressed because of the underlying hyperthyroidism. Younger patients do not generally present in this manner. Patients who complain of palpitations, unintended weight loss, loose stools, heat intolerance, nervousness, or have goiter, exophthalmos, or atrial fibrillation on physical examination should be evaluated for hyperthyroidism.

92. e (Chapter 48)
The most appropriate next step is to determine the levels of free T4. TSH levels are useful to screen for thyroid dysfunction, whereas free T4 levels provide information

about the amount of thyroid hormone being produced by the thyroid gland. If the free T4 levels are normal, this patient most likely has subclinical hypothyroidism, although if the levels of free T4 are low, she has overt hypothyroidism and requires medication.

93. b (Chapter 16)

Sudden onset of a severe headache, especially the "worst headache of my life" should elicit concern about subarachnoid hemorrhage (SAH). Diagnostic steps include an emergent CT scan of the head. Because the CT scan will identify only 90% of all SAH, a negative scan should be followed up by a lumbar puncture to avoid missing 1 of every 10 SAHs. Empiric therapy without these tests would be inappropriate. Temporal arteritis is a consideration in the evaluation of headaches, particularly in patients over age 50. ESRs are significantly elevated. If temporal arteritis is seriously suspected, steroid therapy should be started prior to results and arrangements made for temporal artery biopsy.

94. c (Chapter 43)

The American Diabetes Association recommends screening high-risk individuals for diabetes with a fasting blood sugar and screening all patients over age 45 with a fasting blood sugar every 3 years. Hemoglobin A_{1C} is another means to screen for diabetes. Fasting blood sugars >126 on two or more separate occasions signify diabetes. Classic symptoms along with a random glucose over 200 mg/dL are also diagnostic of diabetes. Diabetic patients over age 30 need to be checked yearly for microalbuminuria.

95. e (Chapter 27)

Inclusion conjunctivitis is seen in neonates and young adults with STDs. It is associated with a persistent watery discharge of the eye. With blepharitis, one sees chronic lid margin erythema, scaling, and loss of eyelashes. Bacterial conjunctivitis presents with a purulent discharge, whereas iritis is associated with pain, photophobia, pupillary constriction, and a cloudy cornea. Viral conjunctivitis would be self-limited and not persistent.

96. d (Chapter 64)

In the second trimester, between 15 and 20 weeks, an MSAFP level should be offered as a screening test. Causes of an elevated MSAFP include an incorrectly dated pregnancy, twin pregnancy, and neural tube defects. Decreased levels are associated with pregnancy date errors or trisomy 21. Many physicians order an ultrasound to confirm the expected date of delivery (EDD) established by the LMP to help interpret the MSAFP results.

97. c (Chapter 73)

Middle ear effusions may persist for several weeks following an episode of acute otitis media. At 2 weeks, 60% of children will still have effusions. Further therapy may be indicated if the effusions persist and are associated with hearing loss. Although antibiotics and systemic corticosteroids have been studied and may be helpful as medical therapy, most effusions resolve spontaneously within 2 to 3 months. Thus, follow-up examination should be performed in 2 months to reassess for persistence of effusion. If the effusion is persistent, hearing evaluation should be considered. Bilateral effusions that persist for more than 4 to 6 months and are associated with bilateral hearing deficits of 20 decibels or more are indications for tympanostomy tube placement.

98. d (Chapter 75)

Of the tests and vaccines listed, only pneumococcal vaccine is a part of the routine recommendations for health care in a 68-year-old man. The heptavalent pneumococcal vaccine is currently recommended for children. The 23-valent pneumococcal vaccine is recommended for all patients over age 65 and for high-risk individuals of other ages (e.g., those with asplenia, diabetes, asthma, or COPD). Chest x-rays are not routinely recommended in any age group. Hepatitis vaccine is recommended for children and for adults who are at risk. DEXA scanning is not routinely suggested for men under age 70. ECGs, although often routinely performed during physical examinations, are not recommended for routine screening.

99. c (Chapter 29)

PE is high on the list of possible diagnoses in the patient presented. She has two significant risk factors for developing PE: history of recent travel and use of oral contraceptives. Fibromyalgia is a chronic non–life-threatening disease that may present with chest pains but will be associated with trigger points elsewhere on physical examination. In addition, peripheral edema is not a characteristic of fibromyalgia. Costochondritis may cause chest pain and on occasion may be associated with dyspnea. The chest pain is typically reproduced by palpation of the costochondral margin. Both costochondritis and fibromyalgia are clinical diagnoses and no diagnostic tests exist for either. Varicose veins may be associated with the development of edema and are a risk factor for developing DVT and PE; however, varicose veins themselves are not life threatening and do not cause dyspnea or chest pain. Lymphedema can cause swelling in the lower extremity but would not typically cause dyspnea.

100.   b (Chapter 10)

This patient has the classic presentation of stable angina. Typical cardiac pain is a substernal pressure with radiation to left arm, shoulder, or jaw. A distinguishing feature in this case is the duration of the pain. In MI, the pain usually lasts longer than 20 minutes. The pain associated with stable angina lasts <10 minutes.

Unstable angina by definition occurs at rest or with increasing frequency or less strenuous activity. The pain of pericarditis and pleurisy is sharp and worsened with breathing. Both of these conditions are acute in nature and generally do not present with chronic symptoms, as described in this patient.

Appendix
Evidence-Based Resources

CHAPTER 1

Haggerty JL, Reid RJ, Freeman GK, et al. Continuity of care: a multidisciplinary review. *BMJ*. 2003;327(7425):1219–1221.

CHAPTER 2

Bourgeut C, Gilchrist V, McCord G. The consultation and referral process: a report from NEON. Northeastern Ohio Network Research Group. *J Fam Pract*. 1998;46:47–53.

Bull SA, Hu XH, Hunkeler EM, et al. Discontinuation of use and switching of antidepressants: influence of patient-physician communication. *JAMA*. 2002;288:1403–1409.

Emanuel EJ, Emanuel LL. Four models of the physician-patient relationship. *JAMA*. 1992;267(16):2221–2226.

CHAPTER 3

American Heart Association. Prevention guidelines. 2013 Prevention guidelines tools: CV risk calculator. http://my.americanheart.org/cvriskcalculator. Accessed December 29, 2016.

Stone NJ, Robinson JG, Lichtenstein AH, et al. 2013 ACC/AHA guideline on the treatment of blood cholesterol to reduce atherosclerotic cardiovascular risk in adults: a report of the American College of Cardiology/American Heart Association Task Force on Practice Guidelines. *Circulation*. 2014;129(25 suppl 2):S13.

U.S. Preventive Services Task Force. https://www.uspreventiveservicestaskforce.org.

CHAPTER 4

Centers for Disease Control and Prevention. Diphtheria: clinicians. 2016. https://www.cdc.gov/diphtheria/clinicians.html. Accessed December 29, 2016.

Centers for Disease Control and Prevention. Vaccines and preventable diseases: about diphtheria, tetanus and pertussis vaccines. 2016. https://www.cdc.gov/vaccines/vpd/dtap-tdap-td/hcp/about-vaccine.html. Accessed December 29, 2016.

Centers for Disease Control and Prevention. Viral hepatitis: hepatitis B FAQs for health professionals. 2016. https://www.cdc.gov/hepatitis/hbv/hbvfaq.htm. Accessed December 29, 2016.

Centers for Disease Control and Prevention. Recommended immunization schedule for children and adolescents aged 18 years or younger, UNITED STATES, 2017. Birth-18 years and "Catch-up" and Birth-18 years recommended immunization schedules. 2017. https://www.cdc.gov/vaccines/schedules/hcp/child-adolescent.html. Accessed December 29, 2016.

Schweitzer A, Horn J, Mikolajczyk RT, et al. Estimations of worldwide prevalence of chronic hepatitis B virus infection: a systematic review of data published between 1965 and 2013. *Lancet*. 2015;386:1546.

CHAPTER 5

Iglar K, Katyal S, Matthew R, et al. Complete health checkup for adults. *Can Fam Physician*. 2008;54:84–88.

CHAPTER 6

Arnold MJ, Beer J. Preoperative evaluation: a time-saving algorithm. *J Fam Pract*. 2016;65(10):702–704, 706–710.

Fleisher LA, Fleischmann KE, Auerbach AD, et al. 2014 ACC/AHA guideline on perioperative cardiovascular evaluation and management of patients undergoing noncardiac surgery: executive summary: a report of the American College of Cardiology/American Heart Association Task Force on Practice Guidelines. *Circulation*. 2014;130:2215–2245.

CHAPTER 7

American College of Obstetricians and Gynecologists. Committee opinion: intimate partner violence. 2012. http://www.acog.org/Resources-And-Publications/Committee-Opinions/Committee-on-Health-Care-for-Underserved-Women/Intimate-Partner-Violence. Accessed April 16, 2017.

Centers for Disease Control and Prevention. Violence prevention. 2016. https://www.cdc.gov/violenceprevention/. Accessed April 16, 2017.

Klevens J, Kee R, Trick W, et al. Effect of screening for partner violence on women's quality of life: a randomized controlled trial. *JAMA*. 2012;308(7):681–689. doi:10.1001/jama.2012.6434.

National Institute of Justice. Extent of elder abuse victimization. 2017. https://nij.gov/topics/crime/elder-abuse/Pages/extent.aspx. Accessed April 16, 2017.

Wilkins N, Tsao B, Hertz M, et al. Connecting the dots. https://www.cdc.gov/violenceprevention/pdf/connecting_the_dots-a.pdf. Accessed April 16, 2017.

CHAPTER 8

Bousquet J, Khaltaev N, Cruz AA, et al. Algorithm for allergic rhinitis diagnosis and management. *Allergy*. 2008;63(suppl 86):8–160.

Seidman MD, Gurgel RK, Lin SY, et al; Guideline Otolaryngology Development Group. AAO-HNSF. Clinical practice guideline: allergic rhinitis. *Otolaryngol Head Neck Surg*. 2015;152(1 suppl):S1–S43. Also available at http://oto.sagepub.com/content/152/1_suppl/S1.full. Accessed November 03, 2016.

Yawn BP, Fenton MJ. Summary of the NIAID-sponsored food allergy guidelines. *Am Fam Physician*. 2012;86(1):43–50.

CHAPTER 9

Chou R, Qaseem A, Snow V, et al. Diagnosis and treatment of low back pain: a joint clinical practice guideline from the American College of Physicians and the American Pain Society. *Ann Intern Med*. 2007;147:478–491.

Metzger RL. Evidenced-based practice guidelines for the diagnosis and treatment of lumbar spinal conditions. *Nurse Pract*. 2016;41:30–37.

Speed C. Low back pain. *BMJ*. 2004;328(7448):1119–1121.

van Tulder MW, Touray T, Furlan AD, et al; Cochrane Back Review Group. Muscle relaxants for nonspecific low back pain: a systematic review within the framework of the Cochrane collaboration. *Spine*. 2003;28(17):1978–1992.

CHAPTER 10

Amsterdam EA, Wenger NK, Brindis RG, et al. 2014 AHA/ACC guideline for the management of patients with non–ST-elevation acute coronary syndromes: executive summary. *J Am Col Cardiol*. 2014;64(24):2645–2687. doi:10.1016/j.jacc.2014.09.016.

Pulivarthi S, Gurram MK. Effectiveness of D-dimer as a screening test for venous thromboembolism: an update. *N Am J Med Sci*. 2014;6(10):491–499. doi:10.4103/1947-2714.143278.

Stone NJ, Robinson JG, Lichtenstein AH, et al. 2013 ACC/AHA guideline on the treatment of blood cholesterol to reduce atherosclerotic cardiovascular risk in adults: a report of the American College of Cardiology/American Heart Association Task Force on Practice Guidelines. *Circulation*. 2014;129(25 suppl 2):S9.

van Belle A, Büller HR, Huisman MV, et al; Writing Group for the Christopher Study Investigators. Effectiveness of managing suspected pulmonary embolism using an algorithm combining clinical probability, D-dimer testing, and computed tomography. *JAMA*. 2006;295:172–179.

CHAPTER 11

Bharucha AE, Dorn SD, Lembo A, et al. American Gastroenterological Association medical position statement on constipation. *Gastroenterology*. 2013;144:211–217.

Foxx-Orenstein AE, McNally MA, Odunsi ST. Update on constipation: one treatment does not fit all. *Cleve Clin J Med*. 2008;75(11):813–824.

Horwitz BJ, Fisher RS. The irritable bowel syndrome. *N Engl J Med*. 2001;344:1846–1850.

Jamshed N, Lee ZE, Olden KW. Diagnostic approach to chronic constipation in adults. *Am Fam Physician*. 2011;84(3):299–306.

Nurko S, Zimmerman LA. Evaluation and treatment of constipation in children and adolescents. *Am Fam Physician*. 2014;90(2):82–90.

CHAPTER 12

Currie GP, Gray RD, McKay J. Chronic cough. *BMJ*. 2003;326(7383):261.

Gibson P, Wang G, McGarvey L, et al. Treatment of unexplained chronic cough: CHEST Guideline and Expert Panel Report. *Chest*. 2016;149(1):27–44.

Morice AH, Kastelik JA. Chronic cough in adults. *Thorax*. 2003;58(10):901–907.

Pratter MR, Brightling CE, Boulet LP, et al. An empiric integrative approach to the management of cough: ACCP evidence-based clinical practice guidelines. *Chest*. 2006;129(1 suppl):222S–231S.

CHAPTER 13

DuPont HL. Persistent diarrhea: a clinical review. *JAMA*. 2016;315:2712–2723. Also available at http://jamanetwork.com/journals/jama/fullarticle/2530542. Accessed March 07, 2017.

Riddle MS, DuPont HL, Conner BA. ACG guideline: diagnosis, treatment, and prevention of acute diarrheal infections in adults. *Am J Gastroenterol*. 2016;111:602–622.

Thomas PD, Forbes A, Green J, et al. Guidelines for the investigation of chronic diarrhea, 2nd edition. *Gut*. 2003;52 (suppl 5):v1–v15.

CHAPTER 14

Baloh RW. Vestibular neuritis. *N Engl J Med*. 2003;348:1027–1032.

Chawla N, Olshaker JS. Diagnosis and management of dizziness/vertigo. *Med Clin North Am*. 2006;90(2):291–304.

Labuguen RH. Initial evaluation of vertigo. *Am Fam Physician*. 2006;73(2):244–251.

Walther LE. Current diagnostic procedures for diagnosing vertigo and dizziness. *GMS Curr Top Otorhinolaryngol Head Neck Surg*. 2017;16:Doc02. doi:10.3205/cto000141.

CHAPTER 15

Mohandas H, Jaganathan SK, Mani MP, et al. Cancer-related fatigue treatment: an overview. *J Cancer Res Ther*. 2017;13(6):916–929. doi:10.4103/jcrt.JCRT_50_17.

Rosenthal TC, Majeroni BA, Pretorius R, et al. Fatigue: an overview. *Am Fam Physician*. 2008;78(10):1173–1179.

Whiting P, Bagnall AM, Sowden AJ, et al. Interventions for the treatment and management of chronic fatigue syndrome: a systematic review. *JAMA*. 2001;286(11):1360–1368.

CHAPTER 16

Becker WJ, Findley T, Moga C, et al. Guideline for primary care management of headache in adults. *Can Fam Physician*. 2015;61:670–679.

Cady R, Dodick DW. Diagnosis and treatment of migraine. *Mayo Clin Proc*. 2002;77:255–256.

Evans RW. Diagnostic testing for migraine and other primary headaches. *Neurol Clin*. 2009;27(2):393–415.

Trainor A, Miner J. Pain treatment and relief with primary headaches subtypes in the ED. *Am J Emerg Med*. 2008;26(9):1029–1034.

CHAPTER 17

Kahrilas PJ, Shaheen NJ, Vaezi MF, et al; American Gastroenterological Association. American Gastroenterological Association medical position statement on the management of gastroesophageal reflux disease. *Gastroenterology*. 2008;135:1383–1391.

Richter JE. The many manifestations of GERD: presentation, evaluation and treatment. *Gastroenterol Clin North Am*. 2007;36(3):577–599.

Talley NJ, Goodsall T, Potter M. Functional dyspepsia. *Aust Prescr*. 2017;40(6):209–213. doi:10.18773/austprescr.2017.066.

CHAPTER 18

Davis R, Jones S, Barocas DA, et al. Diagnosis, evaluation and follow-up of asymptomatic microhematuria (AMH) in adults: AUA guideline. Linthicum, MD: American Urological Association (AUA). 2012. http://www.auanet.org/education/guidelines/asymptomatic-microhematuria.cfm. Accessed February 19, 2017.

Jimbo M. Evaluation and management of hematuria. *Prim Care*. 2010;37(3):461–472. doi:10.1016/j.pop.2010.04.006.

Sharp VJ, Barnes KT, Erickson BA. Assessment of asymptomatic microscopic hematuria in adults. *Am Fam Physician*. 2013;88(11):747–754. Also available at: http://www.aafp.org/afp/2013/1201/p747.html. Accessed February 19, 2017.

CHAPTER 19

Kruger D. The assessment of jaundice in adults: tests, imaging, differential diagnosis. *JAAPA*. 2011;24(6):44–49.

Taylor A, Stapley S, Hamilton W. Jaundice in primary care: a cohort study of adults age >45 years using electronic medical records. *Fam Pract*. 2012;29:416–420.

CHAPTER 20

Hunter DJ, McDougall JJ, Koefer FJ. The symptoms of osteoarthritis and the genesis of pain. *Rheum Dis Clin North Am*. 2008;34(3):623–643.

Jones BQ, Covey CJ, Sineath MH Jr. Nonsurgical management of knee pain in adults. *Am Fam Physician*. 2015;92(10):875–883.

Solomon DH, Simel DL, Bates DW, et al. Does this patient have a torn meniscus or ligament of the knee? Value of the physical examination. *JAMA*. 2001;286:1610–1620.

CHAPTER 21

Bozemore AW, Smucker DR. Lymphadenopathy and malignancy. *Am Fam Physician*. 2002;66:2103–2110.

Gaddey HL, Riegel AM. Unexplained lymphadenopathy: evaluation and differential diagnosis. *Am Fam Physician*. 2016;94(11):896–903.

Nield LS, Kamat D. Lymphadenopathy in children: when and how to evaluate. *Clin Pediatr*. 2004;43(1):25–33.

CHAPTER 22

Anderson WD III, Strayer SM. Evaluation of nausea and vomiting in adults: a case-based approach. *Am Fam Physician*. 2013;88(6):371–379.

Magee LA, Mazzotta P, Koren G. Evidence-based view of safety and effectiveness of pharmacologic therapy for nausea and vomiting of pregnancy. *Am J Obstet Gynecol*. 2002;186(5 suppl):S256–S261.

Scarza K, Williams A, Phillips JD, et al. Evaluation of nausea and vomiting. *Am Fam Physician*. 2007;76(1):76–84.

Spiller RC. ABC of the upper gastrointestinal tract: anorexia, nausea, vomiting, and pain. *BMJ*. 2001;323(7325):1354–1357.

CHAPTER 23

Becker JA, Daily JP, Pohlgeers KM. Acute monoarthritis: diagnosis in adults. *Am Fam Physician*. 2016;94(10):810–816.

Kim PS. Role of injection therapy: review of indications for trigger point injections, regional blocks, facet joint injections, and intra-articular injections. *Curr Opin Rheumatol*. 2002;14:52–57.

Manek NJ. Medical management of osteoarthritis. *Mayo Clin Proc*. 2001;76:533–539.

CHAPTER 24

Hood RE, Shorofsky JR. Management of arrhythmias in the emergency department. *Cardiol Clin*. 2006;24(1):125–133.

Snow V, Weiss KB, LeFevre M, et al. Management of newly detected atrial fibrillation: a clinical practice guideline from the American Academy of Family Physicians and the American College of Physicians. *Ann Intern Med*. 2003;139:1009–1017.

Wexler RK, Pleister A, Raman S. Outpatient approach to palpitations. *Am Fam Physician*. 2011;84(1):63–69.

CHAPTER 25

Alcaide ML, Bisno AL. Pharyngitis and epiglottis. *Infect Dis Clin North Am*. 2007;21(2):449–469.

Choby BA. Diagnosis and treatment of streptococcal pharyngitis. *Am Fam Physician*. 2009;79(5):383–390.

Kalra MG, Higgins KE, Perez ED. Common questions about streptococcal pharyngitis. *Am Fam Physician.* 2016;94(1):24–31.

CHAPTER 26

Snyder S, Jones SJ. Workup for proteinuria. *Prim Care Clin Office Pract.* 2014;41:719–735.

Stevens LA, Levey AS. Current status and future perspectives for CKD. *Am J Kidney Dis.* 2009;53(3 suppl 3):517–526.

Toblli JE, Bevione P, DiGennaro F, et al. Understanding the mechanisms of proteinuria: therapeutic implications. *Int J Nephrol.* 2012;2012:546039. doi:10.1155/2012/546039.

CHAPTER 27

Cronau HL, Kankanala RR. Diagnosis and management of the red eye in primary care. *Am Fam Physician.* 2010;81(2):137–144.

Wirbelauer C. Management of the red eye for the primary care physician. *Am J Med.* 2006;119(4):302–306.

CHAPTER 28

File TM Jr, Garau J, Blasi F, et al. Guidelines for empiric antimicrobial prescribing in community-acquired pneumonia. *Chest.* 2004;125(5):1888–1901.

Moran GJ, Talan DA, Abrahamian FM. Diagnosis and management of pneumonia in the emergency department. *Infect Dis Clin North Am.* 2008;22(1):53–72.

Yoon YK, Park CS, Kim JW, et al. Guidelines for the antibiotic use in adults with acute upper respiratory tract infections. Infect Chemother. 2017;49(4):326–352. doi:10.3947/ic.2017.49.4.326.

Zoorob R, Sidani MA, Fremont RD, et al. Antibiotic use in acute upper respiratory tract infections. *Am Fam Physician.* 2012;86(9):817–822.

CHAPTER 29

Chunilal SD, Eikelboom JW, Attia J, et al. Does this patient have pulmonary embolism? *JAMA.* 2003;290(21):2849–2858.

Gehlbach BK, Geppert E. The pulmonary manifestations of left heart failure. *Chest.* 2004;125(2):669–682.

Shiber JR, Santana J. Dyspnea. *Med Clin North Am.* 2006;90(3):453–479.

Stokes NR, Dietz BW, Liang JJ. Cardiopulmonary laboratory biomarkers in the evaluation of acute dyspnea. *Open Access Emerg Med.* 2016;8:35–45.

Torres M, Maayedi S. Evaluation of acutely dyspneic elderly patients. *Clin Geriatr Med.* 2007;23(2):307–325.

CHAPTER 30

Burbank KM, Stevenson JH, Czarnecki GR, et al. Chronic shoulder pain: part 1 evaluation and diagnosis. *Am Fam Physician.* 2008;77(4):453–460.

Burbank KM, Stevenson JH, Czarnecki GR, et al. Chronic shoulder pain: part 2 treatment. *Am Fam Physician.* 2008;77(4):493–497.

Monica J, Vredenburgh Z, Korsh J, et al. Acute shoulder injuries in adults. Am Fam Physician. 2016;94(2):119–127.

Stevenson JH, Trojian T. Evaluation of shoulder pain. *J Fam Pract.* 2002;51(7):605–611.

CHAPTER 31

Ballas CA, Staab JP. Medically unexplained physical symptoms: toward an alternative paradigm for diagnosis and treatment. *CNS Spectr.* 2003;8(12 suppl 3):20–26.

Kroenke K, Rosmalen JG. Symptoms, syndromes, and the value of psychiatric diagnostics in patients who have functional somatic disorders. *Med Clin North Am.* 2006;90(4):603–626.

Oyama O, Paltoo C, Greengold J. Somatoform disorders. *Am Fam Physician.* 2007;76(9):1333–1338.

CHAPTER 32

Trayes KP, Pickle S, Tully AS. Edema: diagnosis and management. *Am Fam Physician.* 2013;88(2):102–110.

O'Brien JG, Chennubhotla SA, Chennubhotla RV. Treatment of edema. *Am Fam Physician.* 2005;71(11):2111–2117.

CHAPTER 33

DeLegge MH, Drake LM. Nutritional assessment. *Gastroenterol Clin North Am.* 2007;36(1):1–22.

Gaddey HL, Holder K. Unintentional weight loss in older adults. *Am Fam Physician.* 2014;89(9):718–722.

Rolland Y, Kim MJ, Gammack JK, et al. Office management of weight loss in older persons. *Am J Med.* 2006;119(12):1019–1026.

CHAPTER 34

Haider A, Shaw JC. Treatment of acne vulgaris. *JAMA.* 2004;292(6):726–735.

Tan HH. Topical antibacterial treatments for acne vulgaris comparative review and guide to selection. *Am J Clin Dermatol.* 2004;5(2):79–84.

Titus S, Hodge J. Diagnosis and treatment of acne. *Am Fam Physician.* 2012;86(8):734–740.

CHAPTER 35

Asplund CA, Aronson JA, Hadassah EA. Three regimens for alcohol withdrawal and detoxification. *J Fam Pract.* 2004;53(7):545–554.

Muncie HL, Yasinian Y, Oge L. Outpatient management of alcohol withdrawal syndrome. *Am Fam Physician.* 2013;88(9):589–595.

CHAPTER 36

DeRossi SS, Raghavendra S. Anemia. *Oral Surg Oral Med Oral Pathol Oral Radiol Endod.* 2003;95(2):131–141.

Short MW, Domagalski JE. Iron deficiency anemia: evaluation and management. *Am Fam Physician.* 2013;87(2):989–104.

Tefferi A. Anemia in adults: a contemporary approach to diagnosis. *Mayo Clin Proc.* 2003;78(10):1274–1280.

CHAPTER 37

Kroenke K, Spitzer RL, Williams JB, et al. Anxiety disorders in primary care: prevalence, impairment, comorbidity, and detection. *Ann Intern Med.* 2007;146(5):317–325.

Locke AB, Kirst N, Shultz CG. Diagnosis and management of generalized anxiety disorder and panic disorder in adults. *Am Fam Physician.* 2015;91(9):617–624. Also available at http://www.aafp.org/afp/2015/0501/p617.html. Accessed December 29, 2016.

Solvason HB, Ernst H, Roth W. Predictors of response in anxiety disorders. *Psychiatr Clin North Am.* 2003;26(2):411–433.

CHAPTER 38

National Heart, Lung, and Blood Institute. National Asthma Education and Prevention Program. Guidelines for the diagnosis and management of asthma (EPR-3). Summary report 2007:343. http://www.nhlbi.nih.gov/guidelines/asthma/asthgdln.htm. Accessed December 31, 2016.

Centers for Disease Control and Prevention. Most recent asthma data. http://www.cdc.gov/asthma/most_recent_data.htm. Updated June 2017. Accessed December 31, 2016.

Falk NP, Hughes SW, Rodgers BC. Medications for chronic asthma. *Am Fam Physician.* 2016;94(6):454–462. Also available at http://www.aafp.org/afp/2016/0915/p454.html. Accessed December 31, 2016.

CHAPTER 39

American Family Physician. Practice guidelines. Management of atopic dermatitis: guideline from the American academy of dermatology. *Am Fam Physician.* 2014;90. Also available at http://www.aafp.org/afp/2014/1201/p798.pdf. Accessed January 02, 2017.

Pongdee T. Skin Care Tips for Individuals with Atopic Dermatitis (Eczema). Milwaukee, WI: American Academy of Allergy Asthma & Immunology. https://www.aaaai.org/conditions-and-treatments/library/allergy-library/skin-care-tips-atopic-dermatits. Accessed January 02, 2017.

U.S. Food & Drug Administration. Press announcements. http://www.fda.gov/bbs/topics/news/2006/NEW01299.html. Accessed December 14, 2009.

CHAPTER 40

Evensen AE. Management of COPD exacerbations. *Am Fam Physician.* 2010;81(5):607–613.

Lee H, Kim J, Tagmazyan K. Treatment of stable chronic obstructive pulmonary disease: the GOLD guidelines. *Am Fam Physician.* 2013;88(10):655–663.

Yawn BP, Thomashaw B, Mannino DM, et al. The 2017 Update to the COPD Foundation COPD Pocket Consultant Guide. *Chronic Obstr Pulm Dis.* 2017;4(3):177–185. doi:10.15326/jcopdf.4.3.2017.0136.

CHAPTER 41

Francis GS, Felker GM, Tang WH. A test in context: critical evaluation of natriuretic peptide testing in heart failure. *J Am Coll Cardiol.* 2016;67(3):330–337.

Okwuosa IS, Princewill O, Nwabueze C, et al. The ABCs of managing systolic heart failure: past, present, future. *Cleve Clin J Med.* 2016;83(10):753–765.

Yancy CW, Jessup M, Bozkurt B, et al. 2013 ACCF/AHA guideline for the management of heart failure: a report of the American College of Cardiology Foundation/American Heart Association Task Force on Practice Guidelines. *Circulation.* 2013;128:e240–e327.

Yancy CW, Jessup M, Bozkurt B, et al. 2016 ACC/AHA/HFSA focused update on new pharmacological therapy for heart failure: an update of the 2013 ACCF/AHA guideline for the management of heart failure: a report of the American College of Cardiology/American Heart Association Task Force on clinical practice guidelines and the heart failure society of America. *Circulation.* 2016;134:e282–e293. Also available at http://circ.ahajournals.org/content/134/13/e282. Accessed June 18, 2017.

CHAPTER 42

Kessler RC, Berglund P, Demler O, et al. The epidemiology of major depressive disorder: results from the National Comorbidity Survey Replication. *JAMA.* 2003;289:3095–3105.

McIntyre RS, Suppes T, Tandon R, et al. Florida best practice psychotherapeutic medication guidelines for adults with major depressive disorder. *J Clin Psychiatry.* 2017;78(6):703–713. doi:10.4088/JCP.16cs10885.

National Institute of Mental Health (n.d.). Major depression among adults. https://www.nimh.nih.gov/health/statistics/prevalence/major-depression-among-adults.shtml. Accessed July 21, 2017.

Sharp LK, Lipsky, MS. Screening for depression across the lifespan: a review of measures for use in primary care settings. *Am Fam Physician.* 2002;66:1001–1008, 1045–1046, 1048, 1051–1052.

CHAPTER 43

American Diabetes Association. Type 2 diabetes practice guidelines. www.guideline.gov and www.diabetes.org.

Field S. The American Association of Clinical Endocrinologists. Medical guidelines for the management of diabetes mellitus: the AACE system of intensive diabetes self-management: 2002 update. *Endocr Pract.* 2002;8(suppl 1):40–86.

George CM, Brujin LL, Will K, et al. Management of blood glucose with noninsulin therapies in type 2 diabetes. *Am Fam Physician.* 2015;92(1):27–34.

Institute for Clinical Systems Improvement (ICSI). Diagnosis and management of type 2 diabetes mellitus in adults. National Guideline Clearinghouse; 2008:12693. Also availbalbe at https://www.icsi.org/guidelines__more/catalog_guidelines_and_more/catalog_guidelines/catalog_endocrine_guidelines/diabetes/. Accessed April 16, 2017.

CHAPTER 44

Martel J, Raskin JB. History, incidence and epidemiology of diverticulosis. *J Clin Gastroenterol.* 2008;42(10):1125–1127.

Stollman N, Smalley W, Hirano I, et al. American Gastroenterological Association Institute Guideline on the management of acute diverticulitis. *Gastroenterology.* 2015;149:1944–1949.

CHAPTER 45

Centers for Disease Control and Prevention. HIV/AIDS. https://www.cdc.gov/hiv/default.html/.

Chobanian AV, Bakris GL, Black HR, et al. The seventh report of the Joint National Committee on Prevention, Detection, Evaluation, and Treatment of High Blood Pressure: the JNC 7 report. *JAMA.* 2003;289:2560–2572. Also available at http://www.nhlbi.nih.gov/guidelines/hypertension/express.pdf. Accessed August 2, 2003.

Goldschmidt RH, Chu C, Dong BJ. Initial management of patients with HIV infection. *Am Fam Physician.* 2016;94(9):708–716.

CHAPTER 46

The ALLHAT Officers and Coordinators for the ALLHAT Collaborative Research Group. Major outcomes in high-risk hypertensive patients randomized to angiotensin-converting enzyme inhibitor or calcium channel blocker vs. diuretic: the Antihypertensive and Lipid-Lowering Treatment to Prevent Heart Attack Trial (ALL-HAT). *JAMA.* 2002;288:2981–2997. Also available at http://www.acc.org/latest-in-cardiology/ten-points-to-remember/2017/11/09/11/41/2017-guideline-for-high-blood-pressure-in-adults.

CHAPTER 47

Cooper DS. Antithyroid drugs in the management of patient with Graves disease: an evidence-based approach to therapeutic controversies. *J Clin Endocrinol Metab.* 2003;88(8):3474–3481.

CHAPTER 48

Fatourechi V. Subclinical hypothyroidism: an update for primary care. *Mayo Clin Proc.* 2009;84:65–71.

Gaitonde DY, Rowley KD, Sweeney LB. Hypothyroidism: an update. *Am Fam Physician.* 2012;86(3):244–251.

Nygaard B. Primary hypothyroidism. *Am Fam Physician.* 2015;91(6):359–360.

Stathatos N, Wartofsky L. Perioperative management of patients with hypothyroidism. *Endocrinol Metab Clin.* 2003;32(2):503–518.

CHAPTER 49

Bray GA. Medical consequences of obesity. *J Clin Endocrinol Metab.* 2004;89(6):2583–2589.

Erlandson M, Ivey LC, Seikel K. Update on office-based strategies for the management of obesity. *Am Fam Physician.* 2016;94(5):361–368.

Greenwood JL, Stanford JB. Preventing or improving obesity by addressing specific eating patterns. *J Am Board Fam Med.* 2008;21(2):135–140.

Slentz CA, Duscha BD, Johnson JL, et al. Effects of the amount of exercise on body weight, body composition, and measures of central obesity: STRIDE—a randomized controlled study. *Arch Intern Med.* 2004;164:31–39.

CHAPTER 50

Gross AJ, Paskett KT, Cheever V, et al. Periodontitis: a global disease and the primary care provider's role. *Postgrad Med J.* 2017;93(1103):560–565.

CHAPTER 51

Bonura F. Prevention, screening, and management of osteoporosis: an overview of the current strategies. *Postgrad Med.* 2009;121:5–17.

Jeremiah MP, Unwin BK, Greenawald MH, et al. Diagnosis and management of osteoporosis. *Am Fam Physician.* 2015;92(4):261–268.

CHAPTER 52

Mulheim E, Fulbright N, Duncan N. Prostate cancer screening. *Am Fam Physician.* 2015;92(8):683–688.

Nickel CJ. Prostatitis. *Can Urol Assoc J.* 2011;5(5):306–315.

Sharp VJ, Takacs EB, Powell CR. Prostatitis: diagnosis and treatment. *Am Fam Physician.* 2010;82(4):397–406.

U.S. Preventive Service Task Force (USPSTF). http://www.uspreventiveservicetaskforce.org.

CHAPTER 53

Bloomfield P. Update to CDC's sexually transmitted disease treatment guidelines, 2006: fluoroquinolones no longer recommended for treatment of gonococcal infections. *MMWR Morb Mortal Wkly Rep.* 2007;56(14):332–336.

Centers for Disease Control and Prevention. Sexually transmitted diseases treatment guidelines 2002. *MMWR Morb Mortal Wkly Rep.* 2002;51(RR-6):1–77.

Corey L, Wald A, Patel R, et al. Once-daily valacyclovir to reduce the risk of transmission of genital herpes. *N Engl J Med.* 2004;350:11–20.

Kropp R, Latham-Carmanico C, Steben M, et al. What's new in management of sexually transmitted infections? *Can Fam Physician.* 2007;53:1739–1741. Also available at https://www.cdc.gov/std/tg2015/tg-2015-print.pdf.

CHAPTER 54

Bernard P. Management of common bacterial infections of the skin. *Curr Opin Infect Dis.* 2008;21:122–128.

Stevens DL, Bisno AL, Chambers HF, et al. Practice guidelines for the diagnosis and management of skin and soft tissue infections: 2014 update by the Infectious Diseases Society of America. *Clin Infect Dis.* 2014;59:e10.

CHAPTER 55

Aveyard P, West R. Managing smoking cessation. *BMJ.* 2007;335:37–41.

Larzelere MM, Williams DE. Promoting smoking cessation. *Am Fam Physician*. 2012;85(6);591–598.

CHAPTER 56

Arnold JJ, Hehn LE, Klein DA. Common questions about recurrent urinary tract infections in women. *Am Fam Physician*. 2016;93(7):560–569.

White B. Diagnosis and treatment of urinary tract infections in children. *Am Fam Physician*. 2011;83(4):409–415.

Schaeffer AJ, Nicolle LE. Urinary tract infections in older men. *N Engl J Med*. 2016;374:562–571.

CHAPTER 57

Bernstein JA, Lang DM, Khan DA, et al. The diagnosis and management of acute and chronic urticaria: 2014 update. *J Allergy Clin Immunol*. 2014;133(5):1270–1277.

Fromer L. Treatment options for the relief of chronic idiopathic urticaria symptoms. *South Med J*. 2008;101(2):186–192.

Kaplan AP. Chronic urticaria: pathogenesis and treatment. *J Allergy Clin Immunol*. 2004;114(3):465–474.

Morgan M, Khan DA. Therapeutic alternatives for chronic urticaria: an evidence-based review, part 1. *Ann Allergy Asthma Immunol*. 2008;100:403–412.

Schaefer P. Urticaria: evaluation and Treatment. *Am Fam Physician*. 2011;83(9):1078–1084.

CHAPTER 58

American Society for Colposcopy and Cervical Pathology. www.asccp.org/asccp-guidelines.

Nayar R, Wilbur DC. The Pap test and Bethesda 2014. *Cancer Cytopathol*. 2015;59:121–132.

CHAPTER 59

Albers JR, Hull SK, Wesley RM. Abnormal uterine bleeding. *Am Fam Physician*. 2004;69(8):1915–1926.

Apgar BS, Kaufman AH, George-Nwogu U, et al. Treatment of menorrhagia. *Am Fam Physician*. 2007;75:1813–1819.

Hartmann KE, Jerome RN, Lindegren ML, et al. *Primary Care Management of Abnormal Uterine Bleeding. Comparative Effectiveness Review No. 96* (Prepared by the Vanderbilt Evidence-based Practice Center under Contract No. 290-2007-10065 I.). Rockville, MD: Agency for Healthcare Research and Quality; 2013. AHRQ Publication No. 13-EHC025-EF. www.effectivehealthcare. ahrq.gov/reports/final.cfm. Accessed February 28, 2017.

CHAPTER 60

Master-Hunter T, Heiman DL. Amenorrhea: evaluation and treatment. *Am Fam Physician*. 2006;73:1374–1382.

Schlechte JA. Clinical practice. Prolactinoma. *N Engl J Med*. 2003;349(21):2035–2041.

CHAPTER 61

Morantz C; American Cancer Society. ACS guidelines for early detection of cancer. *Am Fam Physician*. 2004;69(8):2013.

Smith RA, Cokkinides V, Eyre HJ; American Cancer Society. American Cancer Society guidelines for the early detection of cancer, 2004. *CA Cancer J Clin*. 2004;54(1):41–52.

Stein L, Chellman-Jeffers M. The radiologic workup of a palpable breast mass. *Cleve Clin J Med*. 2009;76(3):175–180.

CHAPTER 62

Amy JJ, Tripathi V. Contraception for women: an evidence based overview. *BMJ*. 2009;339:b2895.

Herndon EJ, Zieman M. New contraceptive options. *Am Fam Physician*. 2004;69(4):853–860.

CHAPTER 63

Centers for Disease Control and Prevention. Sexually transmitted diseases treatment guidelines. Diseases characterized by vaginal discharge. *MMWR Morb Mortal Wkly Rep*. 2002;51(RR-6):42–48.

Egan ME, Lipsky MS. Diagnosis of vaginitis. *Am Fam Physician*. 2000;62(5):1095–1104.

Farage MA, Miller KW, Ledger WJ. Determining the cause of vulvovaginal symptoms. *Obstet Gynecol Surv*. 2008;63(7):445–464.

Spence D, Melville C. Vaginal discharge. *BMJ*. 2007;335:1147–1151.

CHAPTER 64

American Academy of Family Physicians. Preconception care (position paper). http://www.aafp.org/about/ policies/all/preconception-care.html.

Atrash H, Jack BW, Johnson K. Preconception care: a 2008 update. *Curr Opin Obstet Gynecol*. 2008;20:581–589.

Zolotor AJ, Carlough MC. Update on prenatal care. *Am Fam Physician*. 2014;89(3):199–208. Accessed November 03, 2016.

CHAPTER 65

American College of Obstetricians and Gynecologists; Task Force on Hypertension in Pregnancy. Hypertension in pregnancy. Report of the American College of Obstetricians and Gynecologists Task Force on Hypertension in Pregnancy. *Obstet Gynecol*. 2013;122(5):1122.

Fell DB, Dodds L, Joseph KS, et al. Risk factors for hyperemesis gravidarum requiring hospital admission during pregnancy. *Obstet Gynecol*. 2006;107(2 , pt 1):277.

James AH. Venous thromboembolism in pregnancy. *Arterioscler Thromb Vasc Biol*. 2009;29:326–331.

Matthews A, Haas DM, O'Mathuna DP, et al. Interventions for nausea and vomiting in early pregnancy. *Cochrane Database Syst Rev*. 2015;(9):CD007575. doi:10.1002/14651858.CD007575.pub4.

McLaughlin SP, Carson CC. Urinary tract infections in women. *Med Clin North Am*. 2004;88(2):417–429.

Nicholson W, Bolen S, Witkop CT, et al. Benefits and risks of oral diabetes agents compared with insulin in women with gestational diabetes. *Obstet Gynecol.* 2009;113:193–205.

Stagnaro-Green A, Abalovich M, Alexander E, et al. Guidelines of the American Thyroid Association for the diagnosis and management of thyroid disease during pregnancy and postpartum. *Thyroid.* 2011;21(10):1081.

CHAPTER 66

American Academy of Pediatrics, American College of Obstetricians and Gynecologists. *Breastfeeding Handbook for Physicians.* 2nd ed. Washington, DC: American Academy of Pediatrics and American College of Obstetricians and Gynecologists; 2013.

American College of Obstetricians and Gynecologists' Committee on Obstetric Practice. Committee Opinion No. 670. Immediate postpartum long-acting reversible contraception. *Obstet Gynecol.* 2016;128(2):e32–e37.

Dildy GA III. Postpartum hemorrhage: new management options. *Clin Obstet Gynecol.* 2002;45(2):330–344.

Gray RH, Campbell OM, Zacur HA, et al. Postpartum return of ovarian activity in nonbreastfeeding women monitored by urinary assays. *J Clin Endocrinol Metab.* 1987;64(4):645.

Shaw E, Kaczorowski J. Postpartum care-what's new? *Curr Opin Obstet Gynecol.* 2007;19:561–567.

CHAPTER 67

American Academy of Pediatrics, Joint Committee on Infant Hearing. Year 2007 position statement: principles and guidelines for early hearing detection and intervention programs. *Pediatrics.* 2007;120(4):898–921.

American Board of Pediatrics. Chapter 1: Growth and development; Part E: Developmental milestones. American Academy of Pediatrics Board Content Specifications. 2010. www.abp.org. Accessed September 2012.

Bright Futures Periodicity Schedule Workgroup. 2015 Recommendations for Preventive Pediatric Health Care Committee on Practice and Ambulatory Medicine and Bright Futures Periodicity Schedule Workgroup. *Pediatrics.* 2015;136(3). doi:10.1542/peds.2015-2009.

Eissa MA, Wen E, Mihalopoulos NL, et al. Evaluation of AAP guidelines for cholesterol screening in youth: project Heart Beat! *Am J Prev Med.* 2009;37(1):S71–S77.

Food and Agriculture Organization of the United Nations (FAO), World Health Organization (WHO) and United Nations University (UNU). Human energy requirements. Chapter 3: Energy requirements of infants from birth to 12 months. www.fao.org/docrep/007/y5686e/y5686e05.htm. Accessed January 20, 2017.

Hagan JF, Shaw JS, Duncan PM, eds. *Bright Futures: Guidelines for Health Supervision of Infants, Children, and Adolescents [pocket guide].* 4th ed. Elk Grove Village, IL: American Academy of Pediatrics; 2017.

Lambert M. AAP updates recommendations for routine preventive pediatric health care. *Am Fam Physician.* 2016;94(4):324–324.

Maisels MJ, Bhutani VK, Bogen D, et al. Hyperbilirubinemia in the newborn infant ≥35 weeks' gestation: an update with clarifications. *Pediatrics.* 2009;124(4):1193–1198.

Nelson HD, Bougatsos C, Nygren P. Universal newborn hearing screening: systematic review to update the 2001 US Preventive Services Task Force Recommendation. *Pediatrics.* 2008;122(1):e266–e276.

U.S. Preventive Services Task Force. Universal screening for hearing loss in newborns: US Preventive Services Task Force recommendation statement. *Pediatrics.* 2008;122(1):143–148.

CHAPTER 68

American Cancer Society. American Cancer Society updates HPV vaccine recommendations to include males. 2016. http://m.cancer.org/cancer/news/news/american-cancer-society-updates-hpv-vaccine-recommendations-to-include-males. Accessed March 12, 2017.

Centers for Disease Control and Prevention. Advisory committee on immunization practices (ACIP). www.cdc.gov/vaccines/recs/acip. Accessed March 12, 2017.

National Diabetes Education Initiative. Diabetes management guidelines. American Diabetes Association (ADA) 2016 Guidelines. 2016. http://www.ndei.org/ADA-2013-Guidelines-Criteria-Diabetes-Diagnosis.aspx.html#children.

U.S. Preventive Services Task Force. Information for health professionals. Guide to clinical preventive services. https://www.uspreventiveservicestaskforce.org/Page/Name/tools-and-resources-for-better-preventive-care. Accessed March 12, 2017.

CHAPTER 69

Goldstein MA. Preparing adolescent patients for college. *Curr Opin Pediatr.* 2002;14(4):384–388.

Hornberger LL. Adolescent psychosocial growth and development. *J Pediatr Adolesc Gynecol.* 2006;19:243–246.

CHAPTER 70

Block RW, Krebs NF; American Academy of Pediatrics Committee on Child Abuse and Neglect; American Academy of Pediatrics Committee on Nutrition. Failure to thrive as a manifestation of child neglect. *Pediatrics.* 2005;116:1234–1237.

Guan J, Karsy M, Ducis K, et al. Surgical strategies for pediatric epilepsy. *Transl Pediatr.* 2016;5(2):55–66.

Jarrar RG, Buchhalter JR. Therapeutics in pediatric epilepsy: part 1: the new antiepileptic drugs and the ketogenic diet. *Mayo Clin Proc.* 2003;78(3):359–370.

Russell K, Wiebe N, Saenz A, et al. Glucocorticoids for croup. *Cochrane Database Syst Rev.* 2004;(1):CD001955.

Sobol SE, Zapata S. Epiglottis and croup. *Otolaryngol Clin North Am.* 2008;41:551–566.

CHAPTER 71

Banks JB. Childhood discipline: challenges for clinicians and parents. *Am Fam Physician.* 2002;66:1447–1452.

Daughton JM, Kratochvil CJ. Review of ADHD pharmacotherapies: advantages, disadvantages, and clinical pearls. *J Am Acad Child Adolesc Psychiatry.* 2009;48:240–248.

Hamilton SS, Glascoe FP. Evaluation of children with reading difficulties. *Am Fam Physician.* 2006;74:2079–2084.

CHAPTER 72

McCarthy P. Fever without apparent source on clinical examination. *Curr Opin Pediatr.* 2004;16(1):94–106.

Sur DK, Bukont EL. Evaluating fever of unidentifiable source in young children. *Am Fam Physician.* 2007;75:1805–1811.

CHAPTER 73

Lieberthal AS, Carroll AE, Chonmaitree T, et al. The diagnosis and management of acute otitis media. *Pediatrics.* 2013;131:e964–e999.

Spiro DM, Arnold DH. The concept and practice of wait-and-see approach to acute otitis media. *Curr Opin Pediatr.* 2008;20:72–78.

CHAPTER 74

Mirabelli MH, Devin MJ, Singh J, et al. The preparticipation sports evaluation. *Am Fam Physician.* 2015;92(5):371–376.

Peterson AR, Bernhardt DT. The preparticipation sports evaluation. *Pediatr Rev.* 2011;32(5):e53–e65.

Wingfield K, Matheson GO, Meeuwisse WH. Preparticipation evaluation: an evidence-based review. *Clin J Sport Med.* 2004;14:109–122.

CHAPTER 75

Centers for Disease Control and Prevention. Adult immunization schedule. http://www.cdc.gov. Accessed March 13, 2017.

Spalding MC, Sebesta SC. Geriatric screening and preventive care. *Am Fam Physician.* 2008;78(2):206–215.

U.S. Preventive Service Task Force. www.uspreventiveservicetaskforce.org.

CHAPTER 76

Amin SH, Kuhle CL, Fitzpatrick LA. Comprehensive evaluation of the older woman. *Mayo Clin Proc.* 2003;78(9):1157–1185.

Caprio TV, Williams TF. Comprehensive geriatric assessment. In: Duthie EH, Katz PR, Malone ML, eds. *Practice of Geriatrics.* 4th ed. Philadelphia, PA: Saunders Elsevier; 2007.

Devons CA. Comprehensive geriatric assessment: making the most of the aging years. *Curr Opin Clin Nutr Metab Care.* 2002;5(1):19–24.

CHAPTER 77

Bogardus ST Jr, Yueh B, Shekelle PG. Screening and management of adult hearing loss in primary care: clinical applications. *JAMA.* 2003;289(15):1986–1990.

Gohel PS, Mandava N, Olson JL, et al. Age-related macular degeneration: an update on treatment. *Am J Med.* 2008;121:279–281.

Hauser RA. Levodopa: past, present and future. *Eur Neurol.* 2009;62:1–8.

CHAPTER 78

Blennow K, de Leon MJ, Zetterberg H. Alzheimer's disease. *Lancet.* 2006;368:387–403.

Knopman DS. An overview of common non-Alzheimer dementias. *Clin Geriatr Med.* 2001;17:281–301.

CHAPTER 79

Huggins ME, Bhatia NN, Ostergard DR. Urinary incontinence: newer pharmacotherapeutic trends. *Curr Opin Obstet Gynecol.* 2003;15(5):419–427.

Martin JL, Williams KS, Abrams KR, et al. Systematic review and evaluation of methods of assessing urinary incontinence. *Health Technol Assess.* 2006;10(6):1.

CHAPTER 80

Charette SL. Hospitalization of the nursing home patient. *J Am Med Dir Assoc.* 2003;4(2):90–94.

Ferrell BA. The management of pain in long-term care. *Clin J Pain.* 2004;20(4):240–243.

King MS, Lipsky MS. Evaluation of nursing home patients. A systematic approach can improve care. *Postgrad Med.* 2000;107(2):201–204, 207–210, 215.

CHAPTER 81

Chou R, Deyo R, Devine B, et al. *The Effectiveness and Risks of Long-Term Opioid Treatment of Chronic Pain.* Evidence Report/Technology Assessment No. 218. Rockville, MD: Agency for Healthcare Research and Quality; 2014. AHRQ Publication No. 14-E005-EF.

Chou R, Fanciullo GJ, Fine PG, et al. Clinical guidelines for the use of chronic opioid therapy in chronic noncancer pain. *J Pain.* 2009;10(2):113–130.

Enthoven WT, Roelofs PD, Deyo RA, et al. Non-steroidal anti-inflammatory drugs for chronic low back pain. *Cochrane Database Syst Rev.* 2016;2:CD012087.

Pirlamarla P, Bond RM. FDA labeling of NSAIDs: review of nonsteroidal anti-inflammatory drugs in cardiovascular disease. *Trends Cardiovasc Med.* 2016;26(8):675–680.

Turk DC, Wilson HD, Cahana A. Treatment of chronic non-cancer pain. *Lancet.* 2011;377:2226–2235.

CHAPTER 82

Bush K, Bradford PA. β-lactams and β-lactamase inhibitors: an overview. *Cold Spring Harb Perspect Med.* 2016;6(6):1–22.

Deck DH, Winston LG. Tetracyclines, macrolides, clindamycin, chloramphenicol, streptogramins, & oxazolidinones. In: Katzung BG, Trevor AJ, eds. *Basic & Clinical Pharmacology*. 13th ed. New York, NY: McGraw-Hill; 2015. Accessed December 09, 2016.

Oliphant CM, Green GM. Quinolones: a comprehensive review. *Am Fam Physician*. 2002;65(3):455–465.

Petri WA Jr. Penicillins, cephalosporins, and other β-lactam antibiotics. In: Brunton LL, Chabner BA, Knollmann BC, eds. *Goodman & Gillman's: The Pharmacological Basis of Therapeutics*. 12th ed. New York, NY: McGraw-Hill; 2011.

CHAPTER 83

Antihypertensive and Lipid-Lowering Treatment to Prevent Heart Attack Trial Collaborative Research Group. Diuretic versus alpha blocker as first-step antihypertensive therapy: final results from the Antihypertensive and Lipid-Lowering Treatment to Prevent Heart Attack Trial (ALLHAT). *Hypertension*. 2003;3(42):239–246.

Braunwald E. Heart failure. *JACC Heart Fail*. 2013;1(1):1–20.

Brown NJ, Vaughan DE. Angiotensin-converting enzyme inhibitors. *Circulation*. 1998;97:1411–1420.

Buggey J, Mentz RJ, Pitt B, et al. A reappraisal of loop diuretic choice in heart failure patients. *Am Heart J*. 2015;169(3):323–333. doi:10.1016/j.ahj.2014.12.009.

Chapple CR. A comparison of varying alpha blockers and other pharmacotherapy options for lower urinary tract symptoms. *Rev Urol*. 2005;7(4):S22–S30.

Gillette M, Morneau K, Hoang V, et al. Antiplatelet management for coronary heart disease: advances and challenges. *Curr Atheroscler Rep*. 2016;18:35.

Heran BS, Galm BP, Wright JM. Blood pressure lowering efficacy of alpha blockers for primary hypertension. *Cochrane Database Syst Rev*. 2012;(8):CD004643. doi:10.1002/14651858.CD004643.pub2.

Heran BS, Wong MMY, Heran IK, et al. ACE inhibitors for the treatment of high blood pressure. *Cochrane Database Syst Rev*. 2008;(4):CD003823. doi:10.1002/14651858.CD003823.pub2

Laine M, Paganelli F, Bonello L. P2Y12-ADP receptor antagonists: days of future and past. *World J Cardiol*. 2016;8(5):327–332.

Lepor H. Alpha blockers for the treatment of benign prostatic hyperplasia. *Rev Urol*. 2007;9(4):181–190.

Medications, Lexi-Comp Online™, Lexi-Drugs Online™. Hudson, OH: Lexi-Comp, Inc. http://www.crlonline.com. Accessed November, 2016.

Michel MC, Foster C, Brunner HR, et al. A systematic comparison of the properties of clinically used angiotensin II type 1 receptor antagonists. *Pharmacol Rev*. 2013;65(2):809–848.

Miller PE, Martin SS. Approach to statin use in 2016: an update. *Curr Atheroscler Rep*. 2016;18(5):20.

Olde Engberink RH, Frenkel WJ, van den Bogaard B, et al. Effects of thiazide-type and thiazide-like diuretics on cardiovascular events and mortality: systematic review and meta-analysis. *Hypertension*. 2015;65(5):1033–1040. doi:10.1161/HYPERTENSIONAHA.114.05122.

Spence JD, Dresser GK. Overcoming challenges with statin therapy. *J Am Heart Assoc*. 2016;5(1). doi:10.1161/JAHA.115.002497.

CHAPTER 84

American Diabetes Association. Standards of medical care in diabetes. *Diabetes Care*. 2016;39(1):S1–S112.

Gallant C, Kenny P. Oral glucocorticoids and their complications: a review. *J Am Acad Dermatol*. 1986;(14):161–177.

Lipworth BJ. Airway and systemic effects of inhaled corticosteroids in asthma: dose response relationship. *Pulm Pharmacol*. 1996;(9)19–27.

Silvio EI, Lipska KJ, Mayo H, et al. Metformin in patients with type 2 diabetes and kidney disease. *JAMA*. 2014;312(24):2668–2675.

Williams HC. Atopic dermatitis. *N Engl J Med*. 2005;352(23):14–24.

CHAPTER 85

Ali T, Roberts DN, Tierney WM. Long-term safety concerns with proton pump inhibitors. *Am J Med*. 2009;122(10):896–903. doi:10.1016/j.amjmed.2009.04.014.

Sachs G, Shin JM, Howden CW. Review article: the clinical pharmacology of proton pump inhibitors. *Aliment Pharmacol Ther*. 2006;23(suppl 2):2–8.

CHAPTER 87

Cazzola M, Matera GM. Bronchodilators: current and future. *Clin Chest Med*. 2014;35:191–201.

Filleul O, Crompot E, Saussez S. Bisphosphonate-induced osteonecrosis of the jaw: a review of 2,400 patient cases. *J Cancer Res Clin Oncol*. 2010;136(8):1117–1124.

O'Connell M, Borchert JS. Chapter 73: Osteoporosis and other metabolic bone diseases. In: DiPiro JT, Talbert RL, Yee GC, et al. *Pharmacotherapy: A Pathophysiologic Approach*. 9th ed. New York, NY: McGraw-Hill; 2014. http://accesspharmacy.mhmedical.com/content.aspx?bookid=689&Sectionid=48811480. Accessed December 3, 2016.

Simons FE, Simons KJ. Clinical pharmacology of new histamine H1 receptor antagonists. *Clin Pharmacokinet*. 1999;35(5):329–352.

Wallace DV, Dykewicz MS, Bernstein DI, et al. The diagnosis and management of rhinitis: an updated practice parameter. *J Allergy Clin Immunol*. 2008;112(2 suppl):S1–S84.

Index

Index note: page references with *a b, f,* or *t* indicate a box, figure or table on the designated page; page references in bold indicate discussion of the subject in the Question and Answers sections.